SOCIETY FOR NEUROSCIENCE SYMPOSIA

Volume II

Society for Neuroscience

Officers, 1976

President   Robert W. Doty

President-Elect   Floyd E. Bloom

Secretary   David H. Cohen

Treasurer   Jennifer S. Buchwald

Program Committee

Edward V. Evarts, *Chairman*
Jesus Alanis
Claude F. Baxter
Reginald G. Bickford
William H. Calvin
Byron A. Campbell
Sven O. E. Ebbesson

Ann M. Graybiel
J. Allan Hobson
Arthur J. Hudson
Stephen R. Max
Frederick A. Miles
Robert W. Doty, *ex officio*
David H. Cohen, *ex officio*

Communication Committee

W. Maxwell Cowan, *Chairman*
Richard P. Bunge

James A. Ferrendelli
Walle J. H. Nauta

SOCIETY FOR NEUROSCIENCE SYMPOSIA
Volume II

APPROACHES TO THE CELL BIOLOGY OF NEURONS

Editors

W. Maxwell Cowan, M.D., Ph.D.
Chairman, Department of Anatomy
Washington University School of Medicine

James A. Ferrendelli, M.D.
Department of Pharmacology and Neurology
Washington University School of Medicine

Assistant Editor: Gerry Gurvitch
Society for Neuroscience

Published by the Society for Neuroscience
Bethesda, Maryland

Library of Congress Catalogue Card Number 75-27110

International Standard Book Number 0-916110-04-4

Papers presented at five symposia during the
Sixth Annual Meeting of the
Society for Neuroscience, held in Toronto, Canada, 1976.

© 1977 by the Society for Neuroscience

9650 Rockville Pike, Bethesda, Md. 20014

All rights reserved

Printed in the United States of America

PREFACE

This volume is the second in a projected series based on selected symposia presented at the Annual Meetings of the Society for Neuroscience. For the Society's first publishing venture, two of the symposia presented at the New York meeting in the fall of 1975 were published in the monograph *Neurotransmitters, Hormones and Receptors; Novel Approaches*. From the symposia presented at the Toronto meeting in November 1976, five were selected for publication by the Program and Communication Committees. Since the principal objective of the symposia organized by the Society is to provide a fairly broad coverage of modern neurobiology, the Program Committee tries to select from the vast range of potential subjects those which are both topical and likely to be of broad interest to the Society's membership. It is not always easy to identify from among these a group of symposia which, when collated, will "hang together" and form a coherent volume. However, we believe that the topics selected from the 1976 symposia do have an underlying unity, and have attempted to indicate this by the choice of the title: *Approaches to the Cell Biology of Neurons*.

It is evident that even collectively the papers included in this volume cover only a small fraction of the material that rightly comprises the cell biology of neural tissue. A volume covering all this material would be several times this size, and probably involve symposia over a decade or more. From a glance at the Table of Contents, it is also evident that the papers included in this volume vary considerably, both in length and in their breadth of coverage. Some are intentionally narrowly focused and deal with a single topic of current interest, briefly and concisely. Others survey a wider field and more nearly approximate conventional reviews. Because no restraints are placed on the authors (other than suggestions as to format), and because the organizers of the various symposia are given considerable latitude both in the selection of the subjects to be included and in the selection of participants, a greater degree of uniformity would be surprising, and not necessarily desirable. The primary objective of this series is not to compete with other published review series, but simply to make available in a permanent form and to a wider audience than those who attend the Society's annual meetings, some of the interesting material that is presented each year. And by selecting particular symposia for publication we do not mean to imply that the material presented at the other symposia is less interesting or less important. On the contrary, some of the best-attended symposia were not among those selected for publication, either because their theme did not fit comfortably into the overall plan for the forthcoming volume, or because the organizers and/or the contributors were reluctant, for various reasons, to prepare manuscripts for publication.

The first group of papers included in this volume was based on the symposium on neurogenetics organized by Dr. Verne Caviness. It had been our hope when this topic was first suggested that the symposium might bring together workers dealing with each of the several interesting experimental models currently being used in genetic studies of the nervous system. Unfortunately this was not possible, although at the meeting three different systems were considered at some length. Dr. Seymour Benzer discussed some of the exciting work from his laboratory on genetic mutants in drosophila: although he had earlier indicated that he could not submit a manuscript, his work was deemed to be of such importance and of such general interest that he was nevertheless invited to participate in the symposium. Those interested in reading about the work on drosophila are referred to the original publications from Benzer's group. Similarly, it is unfortunate that none of the important work on gene expression in neuroblastomas and other cultured neural cell lines is included. However, the papers that are presented serve to illustrate the usefulness of simple organisms for the genetic analysis of neuronal structure, and review some of the recent work on neurological mutants in the mouse. While it is still uncertain at what stage or stages in development most of these mutations exert their effects, or what the nature of the primary defect may be, these models are likely to play an increasing role in the analysis of neural development.

The second group of papers is derived from the symposium on *Extrinsic Influences on the Developing Neuron*, organized by Dr. Jack Diamond. Since they deal with a number of critical events in neural development, including the factors involved in process elongation, the capacity of isolated neurons to express certain properties associated with their differentiated state, including appropriate transmitter biosynthesis and release, and some of the trophic factors involved in initiating and maintaining normal sensory innervation, they follow fairly naturally the series on neurogenetics.

The ability to synthesize, store and release transmitter substances is, perhaps, second only to the ability to propagate impulses, the most interesting feature of most neurons. It is not inappropriate, therefore, that a sizable portion of this volume should deal with certain aspects of neurotransmitter function. This group of papers begins with a series of five from the symposium organized by Dr. Rodolfo Llinás on the pivotal role played by calcium in neural function. Once it had been shown that the influx of Ca^{2+} is an essential prelude to the exocytotic release of many secreted substances, considerable interest came to be focused on the source of the available Ca^{2+}, its mode of entry into the presynaptic axon terminal, and how rapidly it can reach the synaptic vesicles and promote their fusion with the critical foci in the presynaptic membrane. Since much of this material has never before been brought together in this way, this section is likely to remain an important reference source for some time.

The explosion in our knowledge of central neural transmitters in the past decade is one of the most exciting chapters in modern neuroscience. Of particular interest has been the discovery that a substantial array of relatively simple peptides may serve as neurotransmitters in many parts of the nervous system, in addition to the hypothalamus. The symposium organized by Dr. Jeffery Barker brought together several of those who have contributed significantly to this burgeoning field, and collectively their papers review much of the recent work on this topic. There is probably no more striking indication of the rapidity with which this subject has advanced than the paucity of references in the various bibliographies to papers published before the first meeting of the Society for Neuroscience in 1971.

The concluding group of papers addressed the fundamental issue of how synaptic activity can be modulated. That not every activation of a presynaptic process leads to the same postsynaptic response has long been known, and certain long-term changes following repeated synaptic activation, such as postsynaptic potentiation, have been of interest to neurophysiologists for almost a quarter of a century. However, it is only in the past decade that significant advances have been made in our understanding of how events in the millisecond range may lead to changes measurable in minutes or even days. The symposium organized by Dr. Floyd Bloom has provided three papers, each dealing with a different facet of this overall problem. Although much of this material has been reviewed elsewhere, it is appropriate that it be included in this volume, and since it, too, is a "fast moving" field, the reader will not be surprised to find in these papers as yet unpublished observations and new hypotheses based on older findings.

The success of the first volume in this series, despite its relatively narrow focus, encourages us to believe that the series as a whole will fulfill a significant need. The publication of this appreciably larger volume would not have been possible but for the helpfulness of many individuals. Again, our thanks must go first to the organizers and contributors of the various symposia—to the organizers for putting the symposia together and persuading the contributors to participate, and to the contributors not only for participating at the meeting, but also for preparing their manuscripts against a rather tight deadline and, by following the format guidelines, greatly easing the task of the editors. Second, we should like to thank the Executive Secretary of the Society, Mrs. Marjorie Wilson, who has shouldered the responsibility of seeing the volume through the press, with all that this entails, including having the papers copy-edited and prepared in publishable form. Her good-natured enthusiasm and commitment to the whole project has made the work of the Communication Committee more of a pleasure than a chore. And finally, we should like to thank Ms. Dorothy A. Kinscherf, Ms. Gerry Gurvitch, and Mrs. Doris Stevenson for secretarial assistance and help in the editing of the volume.

W. Maxwell Cowan
James A. Ferrendelli
St. Louis, January 1977

CONTENTS

Genetics

Use of Nematode Behavioral Mutants for Analysis of Neural Function and Development
1   *Samuel Ward*

Reeler Mutant Mouse: A Genetic Experiment in Developing Mammalian Cortex
27   *Verne S. Caviness, Jr.*

Genetic Dissection of the CNS with Mutant-Normal Mouse and Rat Chimeras
47   *Richard J. Mullen*

Extrinsic Influences on the Developing Neuron

Regulation of Neuronal Morphogenesis by Cell-Substratum Adhesion
67   *Paul C. Letourneau*

Role of Non-Neuronal Cells in the Development of Rat Sympathetic Neurons in Vitro
Linda L. Y. Chun, E. J. Furshpan, Story C. Landis, P. R. MacLeish, Colin A. Nurse, P. H. O'Lague,
82   *Paul H. Paterson, D. D. Potter, and Louis F. Reichardt*

Development of Neuronal Circuitry in the Insect Optic Lobe
92   *I. A. Meinertzhagen*

Control of Mechanosensory Nerve Sprouting in Salamander Skin
120 *Ellis Cooper, Sheryl A. Scott, and Jack Diamond*

Role of Calcium in Synaptic Transmitter Release

Calcium and Transmitter Release in Squid Synapse
139 *Rodolfo R. Llinás*

161 Considerations in Determining the Mode of Influence of Calcium on Vesicle-Membrane Interaction
V. A. Parsegian

172 Calcium Metabolism at the Mammalian Presynaptic Nerve Terminal: Lessons from the Synaptosome
M. P. Blaustein, N. C. Kendrick, R. C. Fried, and R. W. Ratzlaff

195 Calcium Electroresponsiveness and Its Relationship to Secretion in Molluscan Exocrine Gland Cells
Stanley B. Kater

215 Synaptic Vesicle Exocytosis Revealed in Quick-Frozen Frog Neuromuscular Junctions Treated with 4-Aminopyridine and Given a Single Electrical Shock
J. E. Heuser

Role of Peptides in Neuronal Function

241 Substance P and Related Peptides
J. W. Phillis

265 TRH, LHRH and Somatostatin: Distribution and Physiological Action in Neural Tissue
L. P. Renaud

291 Enkephalins, Endorphins, and Opiate Receptors
Hans W. Kosterlitz, John Hughes, John A. H. Lord, and Angela A. Waterfield

308 Angiotensin-Sensitive Sites in the Brain Ventricular System
M. Ian Phillips, D. Felix, W. E. Hoffman, and D. Ganten

340 Peptides as Neurohormones
Jeffery L. Barker and Thomas G. Smith, Jr.

Biochemical Sequelae of Synaptic Action

375 Chairman's Introduction
Floyd E. Bloom

Modulation of Receptor Sensitivity in the Pineal: The Roles of Cyclic Nucleotides
376   *John W. Kebabian, Martin Zatz, and Robert F. O'Dea*

Cyclic Nucleotides and Phosphorylated Proteins in Neuronal Function
399   *Philip Kanof, Tetsufumi Ueda, Isao Uno, and Paul Greengard*

Membrane Fluidity Implicated in the Regulation of Decay of Post-Tetanic Potentiation
435   *S. H. Barondes, W. T. Schlapfer, and P. B. J. Woodson*

PARTICIPANTS

Jeffery L. Barker
Laboratory of Neurophysiology
National Institute of Neurological
and Communicative Disorders
and Stroke, NIH
Bethesda, Maryland 20014

Samuel H. Barondes
Department of Psychiatry
University of California, San Diego,
School of Medicine
La Jolla, California 92093

Mordecai P. Blaustein
Department of Physiology and
Biophysics
Washington University School of
Medicine
St. Louis, Missouri 63110

Floyd E. Bloom
Arthur Vining Davis Center for
Behavioral Neurobiology
Salk Institute
San Diego, California 92112

Verne S. Caviness, Jr.
Eunice Kennedy Shriver Center
for Mental Retardation, Inc.
200 Trapelo Road
Waltham, Massachusetts 02154

Linda L. Y. Chun
Department of Neurobiology
Harvard Medical School
Boston, Massachusetts 02115

Ellis Cooper
Department of Neurosciences
McMaster University Medical Center
Hamilton, Ontario

Jack Diamond
Department of Neurosciences
McMaster University Medical Center
Hamilton, Ontario

D. Felix
Institute for Brain Research
University of Zürich
Zürich, Switzerland

R. C. Fried
Dept. of Physiology and Biophysics
Washington University School of
Medicine
St. Louis, Missouri 63110

E. J. Furshpan
Department of Neurobiology
Harvard Medical School
Boston, Massachusetts 02115

D. Ganten
Department of Pharmacology
University of Heidelberg
Heidelberg, West Germany

Paul Greengard
Department of Pharmacology
Yale University School of Medicine
New Haven, Connecticut 06510

John E. Heuser
Department of Physiology
University of California School of Medicine
San Francisco, California 94143

W. E. Hoffman
Neurobehavior Laboratory
Department of Physiology
University of Iowa
Iowa City, Iowa 52242

John Hughes
Unit for Research on Addictive Drugs
University of Aberdeen
Aberdeen, Scotland

Philip Kanof
Department of Pharmacology
Yale University School of Medicine
New Haven, Connecticut 06510

Stanley B. Kater
Department of Zoology
University of Iowa
Iowa City, Iowa 52242

John W. Kebabian
Experimental Therapeutics Branch
National Institute of Neurological and Communicative Disorders and Stroke
Bethesda, Maryland 20014

N. C. Kendrick
Department of Biochemistry
University of Wisconsin
Madison, Wisconsin 53704

H. W. Kosterlitz
Unit for Research on Addictive Drugs
University of Aberdeen
Aberdeen, Scotland

Story C. Landis
Department of Neurobiology
Harvard Medical School
Boston, Massachusetts 02115

Paul C. Letourneau
Department of Structural Biology
Stanford University School of Medicine
Stanford, California 94305

Rodolfo R. Llinás
Department of Physiology and Biophysics
New York University School of Medicine
New York, New York 10016

John A. H. Lord
Unit for Research on Addictive Drugs
University of Aberdeen
Aberdeen, Scotland

P. R. MacLeish
Department of Neurobiology
Harvard Medical School
Boston, Massachusetts 02115

I. A. Meinertzhagen
Department of Psychology
Dalhousie University
Halifax, Nova Scotia

Richard J. Mullen
Department of Neuropathology
Harvard Medical School
Boston, Massachusetts 02115

Colin A. Nurse
Department of Neurobiology
Harvard Medical School
Boston, Massachusetts 02115

Robert F. O'Dea
Section on Pharmacology
Laboratory of Clinical Sciences
National Institute of Mental Health
Bethesda, Maryland 20014

P. H. O'Lague
Department of Biology
University of California at Los Angeles
Los Angeles, California 90024

V. Adrian Parsegian
Physical Sciences Laboratory, DCRT
National Institutes of Health
Bethesda, Maryland 20014

Paul H. Patterson
Department of Neurobiology
Harvard Medical School
Boston, Massachusetts 02115

M. Ian Phillips
Department of Physiology
University of Iowa
Iowa City, Iowa 52242

John W. Phillis
Department of Physiology
University of Saskatchewan College of Medicine
Saskatoon, Saskatchewan

D. D. Potter
Department of Neurobiology
Harvard Medical School
Boston, Massachusetts 02115

R. W. Ratzlaff
Department of Physiology and Biophysics
Washington University School of Medicine
St. Louis, Missouri 63110

Louis F. Reichardt
Department of Neurobiology
Harvard Medical School
Boston, Massachusetts 02115

Leo P. Renaud
Division of Neurology
Montreal General Hospital
Montreal, Quebec

W. T. Schlapfer
Veterans Administration Hospital
3350 La Jolla Village Drive
La Jolla, California 92037

Sheryl A. Scott
Department of Neurosciences
McMaster University Medical Center
Hamilton, Ontario

Thomas G. Smith, Jr.
Laboratory of Neurophysiology
National Institute of Neurological and Communicative Disorders and Stroke, NIH
Bethesda, Maryland 20014

Tetsufumi Ueda
Department of Pharmacology
Yale University School of Medicine
New Haven, Connecticut 06510

Isao Uno
Department of Pharmacology
Yale University School of Medicine
New Haven, Connecticut 06510

Samuel Ward
Department of Biological Chemistry
Harvard Medical School
Boston, Massachusetts 02115

Angela A. Waterfield
Unit for Research on Addictive Drugs
University of Aberdeen
Aberdeen, Scotland

P. B. J. Woodson
Veterans Administration Hospital
3350 La Jolla Village Drive
La Jolla, California 92037

Martin Zatz
Section on Pharmacology
Laboratory of Clinical Sciences
National Institute of Mental Health
Bethesda, Maryland 20014

GENETICS

Use of Nematode Behavioral Mutants for Analysis of Neural Function and Development

Samuel Ward

Harvard Medical School, Boston, Massachusetts

The soil nematode *Caenorhabditis elegans* was selected 11 years ago by Sydney Brenner as an experimental organism suitable for the isolation of many behavioral mutants and small enough for anatomical analysis of such mutants with the electron microscope (Brenner, 1973, 1974). Two distinct goals motivated the initial studies of this organism: first, the hope that some of the mutants would have simple anatomical alterations that could be directly correlated with their behavioral defects, allowing the assignment of specific functions to specific neurons, and second, the hope that the detailed analysis of the kinds of alterations induced by individual mutations and the classes of cells affected by given mutations would reveal general features of the genetic program that specifies the development of the organism.

Over the past 11 years the number of investigators working on *C. elegans* has increased to about 75 and is still growing. Nearly 3,000 different mutants have been isolated and different investigators are pursuing their effects on different cells (see Ward, 1976; Hirsh and Vanderslice, 1976).

My own research is in the development of the nervous system. In particular, I would like to learn something about the workings of the complex black box that connects individual genes to the determination of the morphology of developing neurons. Are there gene products whose specific function is to determine the morphology of cells? If so, what are these gene products and how do they act in the developing cell? One would anticipate that mutations in such hypothetical genes would cause specific morphological alterations in cells. Because the morphology of a neuron determines its function, by selecting behavioral mutants altered in the function of the nervous system one might commonly find mutants that alter the morphology of neurons, and some of these might be in specific morphological genes. It is my hope that it will be possible to compare such mutants to the wild type in order to identify the defective gene products and thereby learn something about the role of normal gene products in determining the development of neurons (Ward, 1976).

In this paper I will first summarize the results of several years' work on one specific class of mutants in the nematode, sensory mutants, work performed both in my laboratory and that of my colleagues Jim Lewis and Jonathan Hodgkin (1977). Second, I will discuss frankly some of the difficulties and frustrations we have experienced in trying to interpret the effects of these specific mutants. Some of these difficulties illustrate problems endemic to genetic studies of development. Third, I will describe the more recent work performed in my laboratory that is being directed toward genetic analysis of the structure and function of a non-neuronal cell, the sperm.

C. elegans as an Experimental Organism

C. elegans is a filter-feeding nonparasitic nematode that normally lives on soil bacteria. In the laboratory it is grown on petri plates seeded with *Escherichia coli* in much the same way that bacteriophages are grown. It is a self-fertilizing hermaphrodite that lays about 300 eggs. These eggs hatch into small larvae that mature through a series of four moults to the adult in 3 days at 20°C. Males arise from loss of a sex chromosome at meiosis and can be maintained and mated with hermaphrodites for genetic analysis.

When the larvae hatches it has 550 somatic cells and four germ line cells. In the course of maturation the number of cells increases to 810 somatic cells and about 2,600 germ line cells in the adult (Sulston and Horvitz, 1977). In the course of the postembryonic development, 70 new neurons are added to the larval nervous system, increasing the number of neurons from 210 to 280 in the adults (Sulston, 1976). The position, structure, and connections of nearly all these neurons have been reconstructed from complete serial sections of essentially the entire animal so the location and arrangement of all the neurons is known (Ward, Thomson, White, and Brenner, 1975; Ware, Clark, Crossland, and Russell, 1975; White, Southgate, Thomson, and Brenner, 1976).

Most of the nervous system is located in the head. There is a central nerve ring with cell bodies anterior and posterior and nerve cords extending to the head and body. Fifty-eight neurons extend dendritic sensory processes to the tip of the head. The axonal processes of most of these nerves bend around into a U to enter the nerve ring synapsing there. Some sensory neurons synapse on interneurons, some of them synapse on motor neurons, and some of the sensory neurons synapse directly on muscles, making them sensory-motor neurons (Ward et al., 1975; Ware et al., 1975). The bulk of the motor nervous system is in a series of ventral ganglia and in a ventral nerve cord that extends down the length of the animal, innervating the muscles. The ventral nerve cord sends commissures to make up the dorsal nerve cord that innervates the dorsal musculature. There is also a small anal ganglion in the hermaphrodite and a larger anal ganglion in the male.

Chemotactic Behavior

To isolate mutants that would affect a limited subset of cells so that one could detect anatomical alterations easily, I chose to study the chemotaxis of the animal in order to be able to isolate sensory mutants (Ward, 1973). It was known that *C. elegans* was attracted to bacteria, so this response was used to devise several quantitative assays for chemotaxis. All these assays involve establishing a radial gradient of attractants in various media and observing the responses of worms placed in these gradients. Other assays have also been used to study chemotaxis (Dusenbery, 1973). One gradient assay is illustrated by the tracks of worms placed on a petri plate spread with agar in which a radial gradient of attractant had been established (Figure 1a). The Figure shows that the worms have moved more or less directly up the gradient to the center of the plate. Therefore, worms can orient in the gradient so their behavior is a true taxis. When they arrive at the center they remain at the peak of the gradient. In the absence of attractant the worm simply moves at random (Figure 1b). Assays such as this can be quantified by measuring the degree of orientation or by the fraction of time the worm spends in the center, because both depend on the concentration of attractant. I have identified a number of different attractants, which are summarized in Table 1. Each of these attractants has been classified by competition experiments (Ward, 1973). One class of attractants includes cyclic AMP and cyclic GMP, but not other derivatives of those molecules. Other classes included monovalent anions, monovalent

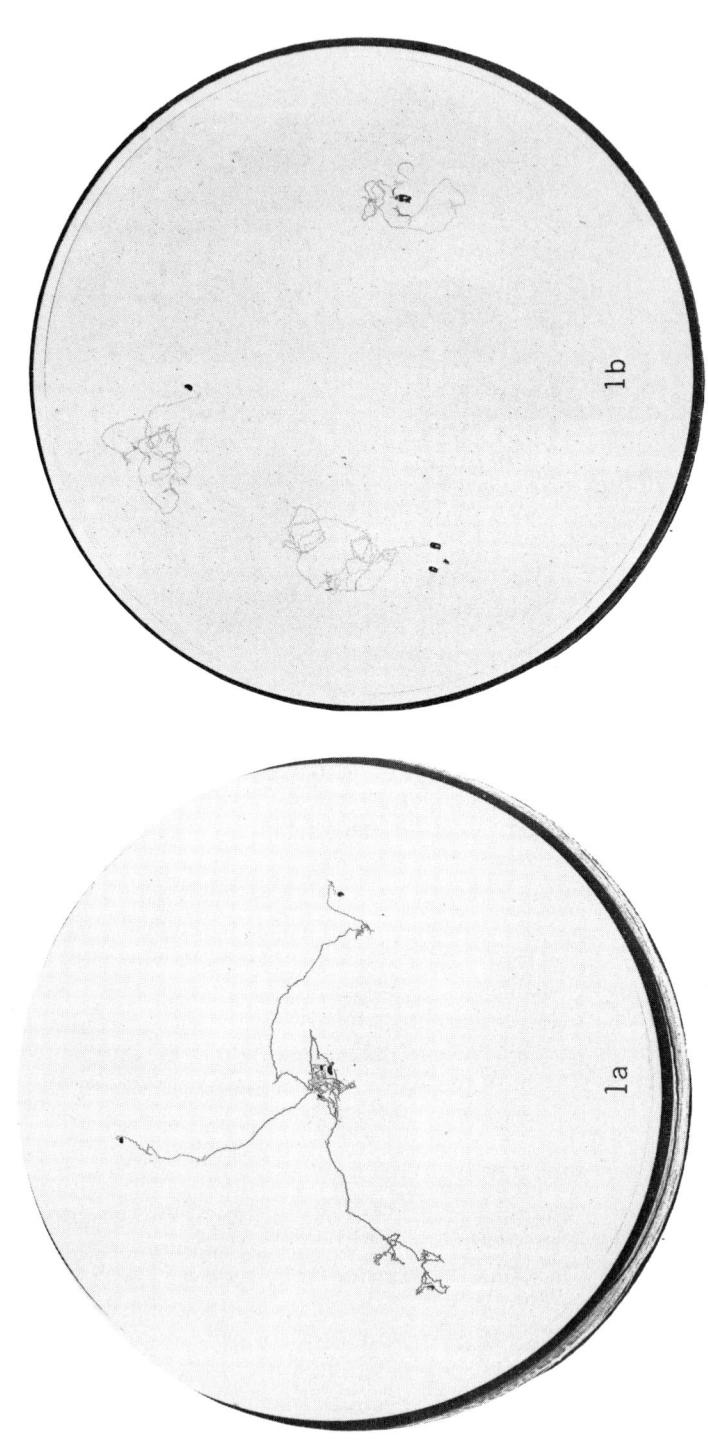

FIGURE 1. (a) Tracks of three wild-type adults responding to gradients of NH4Cl. Three worms were applied near the edge of the plate and allowed to track for 20 min. Note the orientation up the gradient and the accumulation at the center. (b) Control tracks of three animals in the absence of attractant.

TABLE 1. Attractants of C. elegans[a]

Class	Representative attractant	Accumulation threshold (mM)
Cyclic nucleotides	cAMP	0.2
Anions	Cl^-	2
Cations	Na^+	2
Basic pH	OH^-	~0.001
Bacterial filtrate	?	?

[a] The attractants that have been most studied are listed. They are grouped into classes that do not compete with one another.

cations, basic pH, and at least two unknown chemicals that are present in bacterial filtrates. In addition, there are repellents (Dusenbery, 1973). These results show that *C. elegans* has a repetoire of chemical senses and a defined behavioral response in gradients.

There must be receptors that are detecting this response. Where are those receptors located? One way to find out is to observe the behavior of the mutant shown in Figure 2, a morphological mutant that has a bent head. This bend is due to a defect in the hypodermis of the worm, causing the head to be bent either to the right or to the left at random in a population. The degree of bend varies for different individuals of this mutant genotype. If mutants of this kind are placed in a gradient of attractant, they leave tracks, such as those shown in Figure 3. The animals start from the outside and reach the center, but instead of following the direct path of the wild type, they follow a spiral path into the center. If one observes them when they are making this path, one observes that the animal orients so that its head points up the gradient. But when it does that, because its head is bent, its body is at an angle to the gradient. Therefore, when it moves, it moves at an angle to the gradient, tracing a logarithmic spiral into the center of the plate. The tracks are complicated because the bend in the head also serves as a rudder at the tip of the head, so when the poor animal tries to move forward it actually goes around in a loop. And when it goes around in a loop it then discovers that it is no longer facing up the gradient so it turns, reorients its head up the gradient, and tries again, eventually arriving in the center. This mutant demonstrates that the receptors for these attractants must be located in the head. This can be confirmed by tracking other head-defective mutants (Ward, 1973, 1976).

Sensory Anatomy

What is the structure of these receptors? An en face scanning electron micrograph is shown in Figure 4. There is a large opening in the middle,

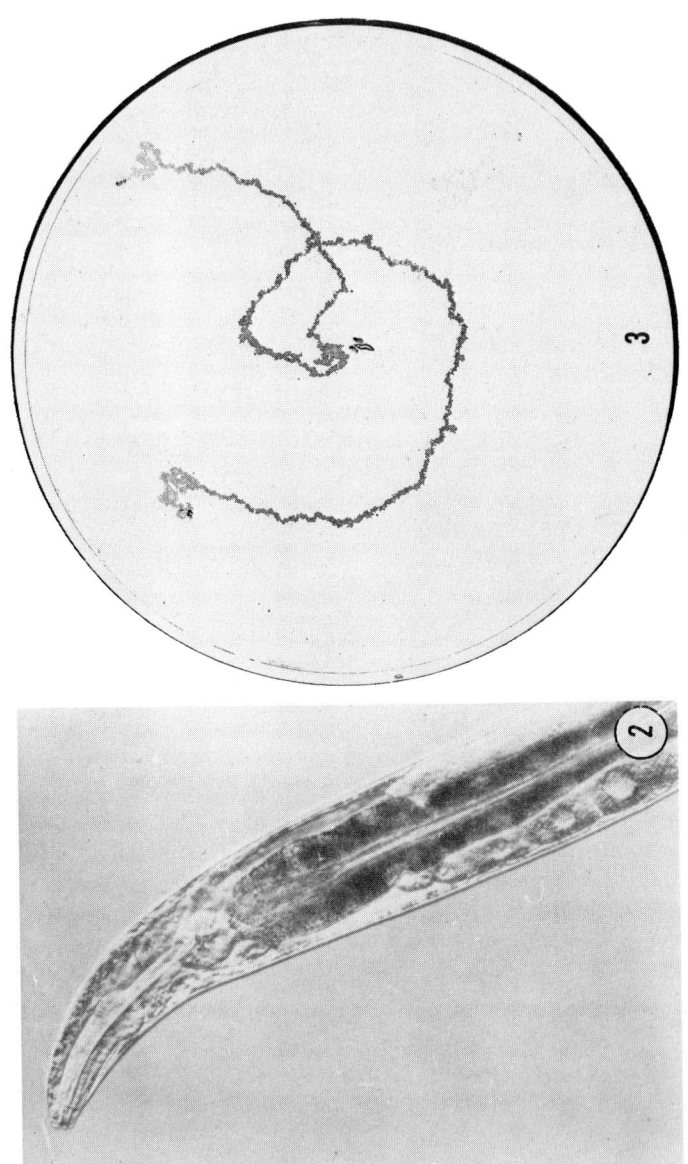

FIGURE 2. Light micrograph of an adult "bent-head" animal, mutant E611.
FIGURE 3. Tracks of two "bent-head" mutant animals responding to NH4Cl.

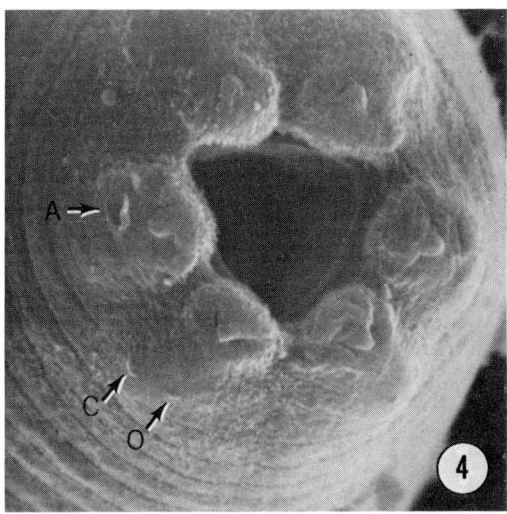

FIGURE 4. En face scanning electron micrograph. The six papillae surmounting the lips are the endings of the inner labial sensilla. Other sensilla endings are the small bumps and the inpocketing of the amphids. Abbreviations: A, amphid; C, cephalic sensilla; O, outer labial sensilla. (Figures 4 through 7 are from Ward et al., 1975.)

which is the mouth, and this is surrounded by six lips, each surmounted by a papilla. Each papilla is the ending of one particular class of sensilla. Another class of sensilla end in small bumps, two of which are visible in the cuticle. These are distributed symmetrically around these lips. A large sense organ ends laterally in an inpocketing of the cuticle and this sense organ is the chemoreceptor called the amphid. All of these sensilla have been reconstructed from serial electron micrographs (Ward et al., 1975; Ware et al., 1975). Two thin sections cut through the amphid are shown in Figure 5. The sensory neurons are modified cilia, as is common for sensory neurons throughout the animal kingdom. There are 10 ciliated processes in this region of the amphid. These arise from eight individual neurons that penetrate out through this channel, exposing themselves to the outside. There are four additional neurons in this amphid that have a more complex morphology. In addition, the amphid is comprised of two non-neuronal cells, a gland cell, called the sheath cell, and a socket cell that surrounds the whole sensillum, so that the physical structure of the sensillum is analogous to sensilla in other invertebrates. The structure of the whole amphid is shown diagrammatically in Figure 6 as a longitudinal section with

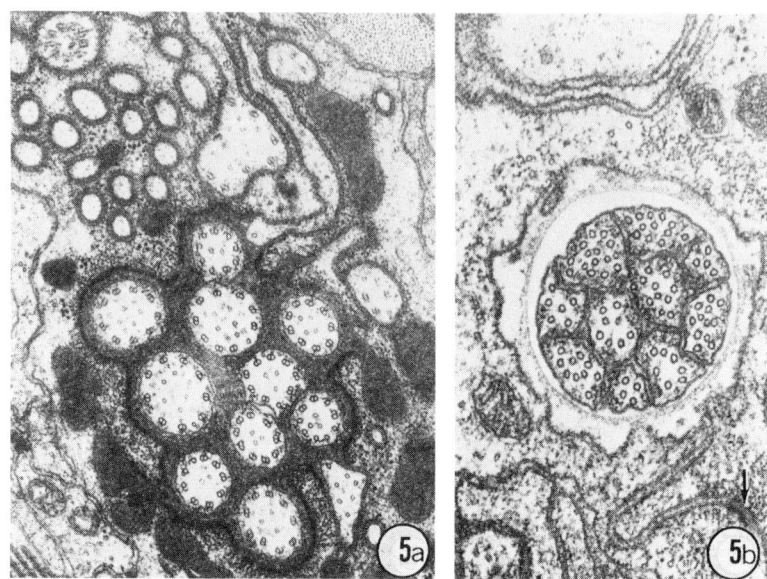

FIGURE 5. Fine structure of the amphidial neurons. High magnification electron micrographs of transverse sections of the amphidial neurons. (a) 3 μm from the amphidial opening. × 31,000. (b) 1 μm from the opening. × 45,000.

representative cross sections. The sheath cell is shown in grey and the socket cell is shaded darker. The neurons penetrate up through a cavity opening up to the outside; this was the opening that was visible in the earlier scanning electron micrograph (Figure 4). In the cross sections one sees the ciliated neurons penetrating up through this channel and four other neurons pushing their way off into the edges of the sheath cell. The morphology of the dendritic tips of those four neurons is shown in Figure 7. They have striking morphological endings for sensory neurons. One of them consists of two large sheet-like branches extending to each side, and one of them has projections looking like fingers. This cell is called the finger cell for obvious reasons. Each of these endings contains a short, modified cilium. They have a basal body in the region indicated, and short forward axonemal projections.

Sensory Mutants

The results presented so far show that this animal has a simple pattern of chemotactic behavior and that the morphology of the sense organ

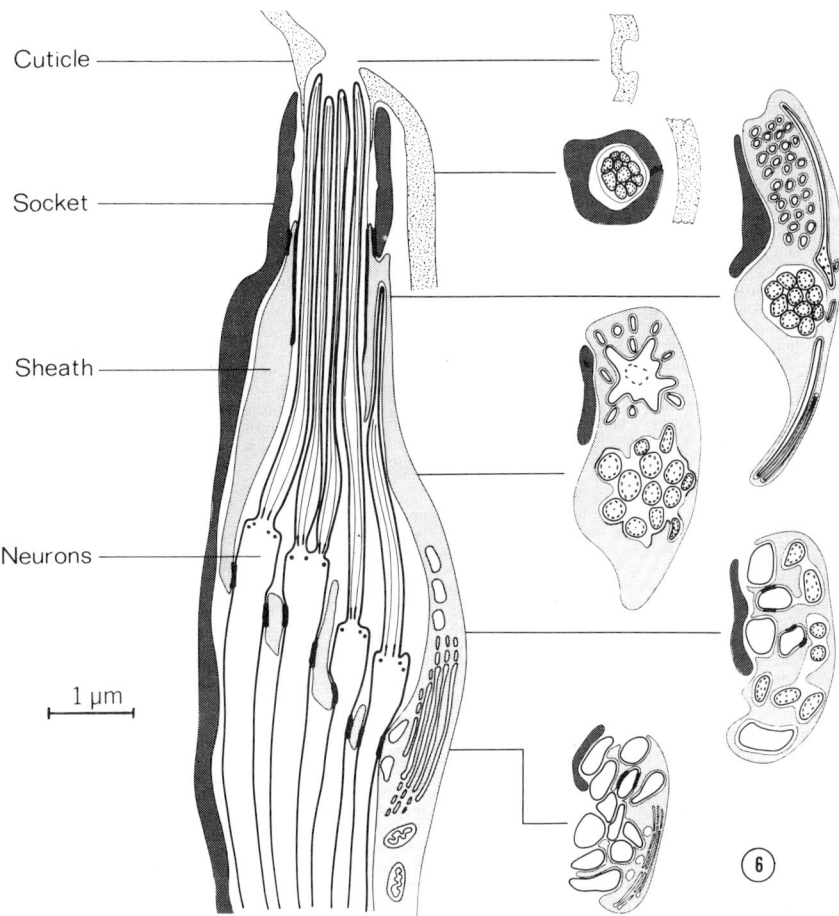

FIGURE 6. Amphid. A right amphid is shown diagrammatically in radial and transverse section. The shapes of the cells were simplified slightly for clarity. Dense vesicles are shown near the basal bodies of the neurons. A large Golgi apparatus and mitochondria are shown in the base of the sheath cell. The scale of the transverse sections is one half that shown for the longitudinal sections.

mediating this behavior is known in detail. We can now isolate nonchemotactic mutants and ask, do they affect the morphology of these individual neurons? Several schemes have been used to select these mutants. The one that has been used in my laboratory by Paul St. John and myself is simply to take the F2 progeny of a mutagenized population

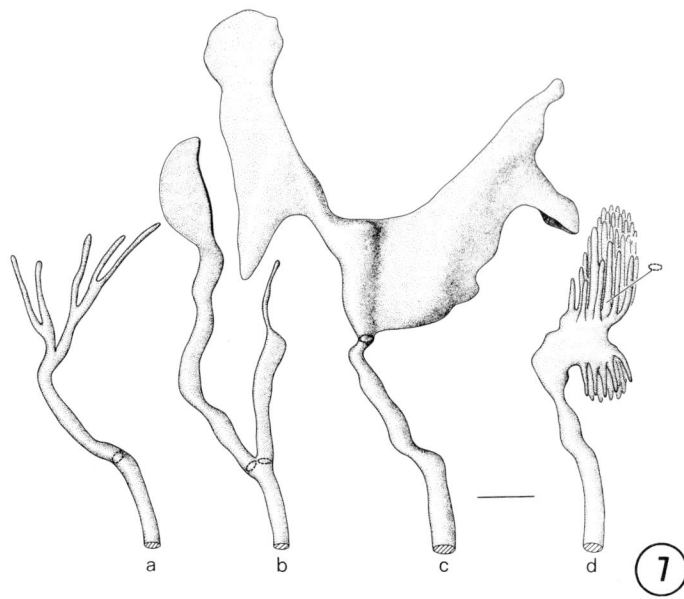

FIGURE 7. Amphidial neurons "a" through "d". The neurons are shown viewed from the side. They are based on computer reconstruction of transverse cell outlines. The rings of doublets indicate the position of the basal bodies.

of worms and to place them on the outer edge of an attractant gradient plate (Ward, 1976). All those animals that swim to the center are removed, enriching the remainder for animals that fail to respond to the attractant. After two cycles of selection, potential mutants are picked, cloned, and retested. Alternatively, Lewis and Hodgkin (1977) have mutagenized a population of worms, placed them at the peak of the gradient, and simply selected for animals that swim down the gradient. Dusenbery, Sheridan, and Russell (1975) have selected mutants by using a countercurrent apparatus. Some 40 or 50 independent mutants have been isolated by the several labs. An example of the behavioral defect in a mutant isolated in our lab is shown in Figure 8b together with a control, Figure 8a. For this Figure, three animals were put at the peak of a prepared attractant gradient. The wild-type controls remain at the peak of the gradient (Figure 8a). The sensory mutant, S1, when placed under exactly the same conditions, wanders from the center with no obvious direction. This shows clearly that the mutant has normal motility, but it doesn't respond to the attractant. The growth of the mutant is normal

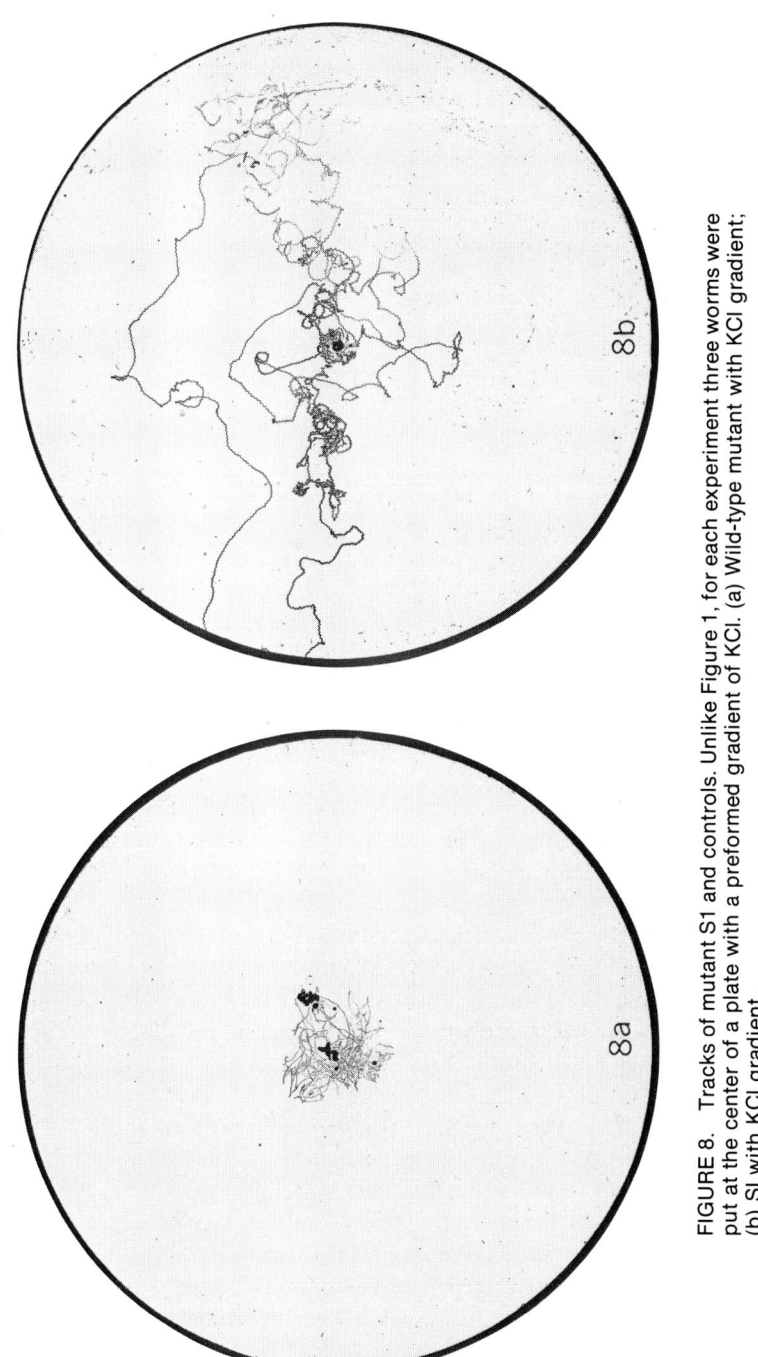

FIGURE 8. Tracks of mutant S1 and controls. Unlike Figure 1, for each experiment three worms were put at the center of a plate with a preformed gradient of KCl. (a) Wild-type mutant with KCl gradient; (b) SI with KCl gradient.

TABLE 2. Chemotaxis-defective mutants[a]

Gene	Linkage group	Mutation	Accumulation response			
			Na$^+$	Cl$^-$	cAMP	Bacteria
che-1	I	E1034 E1035 S2	0	0	0	+
che-2	X	E1033	0	0	0	0
che-3	I	E1124	0	0	0	0
che-4	V	E1066	(+)	+	+	−
—	—	S1	0	0	0	(+)

[a] Mutants are listed by gene (complementation group) when known. The mutant numbers are independently isolated strains. E1034, E1035, and E1066 were isolated by selection for worms which do not remain at the center of a gradient; E1033 and E1124 were initially isolated because their males are sterile and, subsequently, found to be chemotaxis-defective (Lewis and Hodgkin, 1977). S1 and S2 were selected for their non-response to KCl as described in the text. The accumulation behavior was assayed as described by Ward, 1973. Symbols: +, Normal response; 0, no response; (+), intermediate response; −, not determined.

and its behavior is indistinguishable from the wild-type mutant in the absence of a chemical attractant, so its only defect appears to be in its sensory response.

One can catalogue the chemotactic mutants by their behavioral defects and assign them to different genes by complementation tests and mapping. A summary of some of the mutants that we have worked with and some of those studied by Lewis and Hodgkin is shown in Table 2. The response to various attractants are shown together with the linkage data. Mutants in chemotaxis-defective gene 1 (*che-1*), for example, failed to respond to sodium, chloride, and cyclic AMP, but retained a normal response to bacteria. All these responses can be measured quantitatively and accurately by varying the concentration of attractants. Mutations in genes *che-2* and *che-3* fail to respond to any of the attractants, yet their movement is normal and they grow normally. The mutant in *che-4* has a slightly defective response to sodium and a normal response to the other attractants. The mutant S1, which was described in Figure 8, fails to respond to salts or cyclic AMP but has an intermediate response to bacteria. These results show that one can obtain mutants with a range of different behavioral phenotypes.

What sort of anatomical defects does one find in these mutants? Lewis and Hodgkin (1977) and I have sectioned a total of 21 different mutants, including the ones listed in Table 2, and found alterations in the sensory anatomy of nine of these different mutants. One example of the kinds of alterations observed is shown in Figure 9, taken from Lewis and Hodgkin (1977). Figure 9a shows a computer-aided reconstruction of the dendritic terminal of an amphidial neuron "d" in the wild type (from Figure 7) and Figure 9b shows the same neuron terminal in the mutant. In the mutant, the bulk of the cell is there, the basal body of the cilium is there, but the finger-like projections of the cell are grossly altered. One other sensory cell is slightly defective in this mutant, but the other neurons, including those in the amphid, appear normal except for minor rearrangements. This mutant appears to be in a gene which affects a specific aspect of cell morphology.

As more anatomy on the alleles of this gene was pursued, the interpretation became more complicated. The anatomical defects in the mutants are variable. If one cuts several individuals of identical genotype one finds that the finger cell is defective in some and not in others (Lewis and Hodgkin, 1977). The extent of the defect sometimes varied between the two symmetrical neurons in the same animal (Ward, unpublished observations). Such variation is not too surprising. The wild-type anatomy is extraordinarily invariant, but a mutant must perturb the normal anatomical development. This perturbation could cause an unstable situation that results in variability in the final anatomy. Alternatively, the mutant gene product itself may have variable activity.

The behavioral phenotype of *che-1* mutants is not, however, variable at all. By quantitative behavioral analysis, the mutant population is

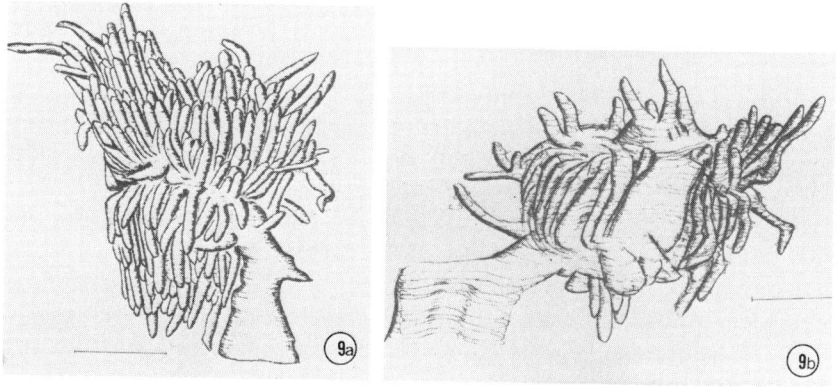

FIGURE 9. Computer-aided reconstructions of the sensory tips of amphidial neuron "d". (a) Wild type; (b) mutant E1034. From Lewis and Hodgkin (1977).

perfectly homogeneous (Ward, 1976). So here is a case of a mutant with an anatomical alteration which is variable and a behavioral phenotype which is not. In addition, if one compares strains with mutations in different alleles of this same gene one finds that the degree of the anatomical defect also varies (Lewis and Hodgkin, 1977). One of the allele strains has "fingers" that are completely missing on neuron "d", whereas in another allele, the cells are nearly normal. These strains are indistinguishable from one another by behavioral criteria.

Mutants in genes *che-2* and *che-3*, which have an overlapping behavioral phenotype with *che-1* (Table 2), have essentially all the ciliated sensory endings in the tip of the head defective, not only the amphidial sensory neurons, but the other sensory neurons as well. One exception is the finger cell, which has nearly normal morphology in these mutants. Unlike *che-1* mutants, the anatomical defects are not variable in these mutants. Although the mutants in *che-2* and *che-3* have a clearly overlapping behavioral defect with *che-1*, they have an apparently non-overlapping anatomical defect. Mutations in *che-4* have a minor anatomical defect in three amphidial neurons, but not in the fingers cell. S1 has no detectable alteration in anatomy.

Interpretation of Mutants

What these results show is that by selecting for these behavioral mutants we have obtained mutants altered in the specific morphology of cells. Yet, it is difficult to interpret these alterations. First, some of the anatomical alterations vary in the individual animals of one genotype, but the behavioral alterations do not. Second, different alleles of one gene can have identical behavioral defects, but somewhat different anatomical defects. Third, different genes have overlapping behavioral defects and non-overlapping anatomical defects. So the hope that one would find simple correlations between the anatomical defects and the behavior seems not to be the case for this class of mutants.

It is possible that the anatomical defects we have detected are not the only defects in the mutants. Only the dendritic endings of the sensory neurons have been examined in the mutants. We have not tried to reconstruct the CNS of any mutants because, although it is technically possible to do so, it is such a tedious job that we focused just on the tip of the head to see what we would find. The behavioral defects in the mutant animals may be due to defects in the CNS, and what we are seeing in the periphery may be trivial variations in morphology that do not reflect the primary defect of the mutation. It is a general problem in developmental genetics that when you first find a developmental mutant apparently affecting a single cell type it often has pleiotropic effects on other cells (Grünberg, 1973; Wright, 1970). Sometimes this is because those cells were dependent in their development on the normal presence of the first cell, or, alternatively, because animals are economical with their gene products and often use the same gene product over and over again in different cells. So it is not surprising that when one looks for mutants altered in genes controlling the development of cell morphology one finds complicated defects that are not easy to interpret.

The complications of the behavioral and developmental interpretation of mutants arose when the number of mutants available increased. The pattern was simple at first, but became more and more complicated as the number of mutations on hand increased. One might anticipate two future possibilities if one made a graph of the degree of confusion against the number of mutants. One possibility is that we are sitting at a maximum and that, if we isolated a larger number of mutants, we could resolve the complications by finding some peculiarities in the mutants already analyzed, and so identify a consistent pattern of correlation between developmental, anatomical, and behavioral defects. Alternatively, one might find that as one isolates more and more genes the confusion simply continues to increase and one continues to find a bewildering variety of defects.

I have not tried to resolve these possibilities because the problem that interests me most is what it is that the normal products genes are doing to determine the morphology of these cells. The anatomical and behavioral defects of mutants are many steps removed from the defective gene products. Are these morphological mutants actually defective in specific gene products that control cell morphology, or are they defects in the "ordinary" biochemistry of these cells? The answer is: I don't know, because I don't know what the gene products are that determine cell morphology. Finding out is a biochemical problem. It is impossible to solve such a problem in a whole organism, and difficult, at best, even if one could isolate just the nervous system, because there are so many different types of cells interacting with each other to form the normal morphology. When one has mutants that are fairly specific, affecting only a single class of cells, for example, it's hard to imagine how one would isolate the gene products that are defective from the whole worm because there would be so few of them.

Sperm- and Fertilization-Defective Mutants

In wresting with the difficulty of interpreting behavioral mutants, I discovered that two of the mutant alleles of *che-1* have a third phenotype. In addition to being defective in their response to several attractants and having a specific anatomical defect, they are sterile when grown at elevated temperatures. This defect is readily detected in the hermaphrodite because when grown at 25°C these mutants lay nothing but unfertilized oocytes instead of normal fertile zygotes. One can quantify this phenotype by simply counting the production of these unfertilized oocytes in the mutant and comparing it to the wild type as shown in Table 3. This Table shows that the wild-type hermaphrodite normally lays about 280 progeny and then produces about 50 excess oocytes. The mutant E1034 is similar to the wild type at 16°C. At 25°C, wild-type progeny are slightly reduced, but the mutant produces less than 0.1 progeny per animal. Instead, at 25°C, it lays unfertilized oocytes in numbers comparable to the number of progeny that the wild type would have laid. So there is a temperature-sensitive mutation in the nonchemotactic E1034 strain that causes the animal to be sterile and produce infertilized eggs. Is this due to a defect in the mutant's oocytes or a defect in its sperm? One can easily distinguish these possibilities by taking the hermaphrodites grown at 25°C and mating them with wild-type males. As shown in Table 2, outcross progeny are produced from this mating, demonstrating that the oocytes are capable of being fertilized if wild-type sperm are provided. Therefore, the sterility must be due to a defect in the sperm.

I was excited when this phenotype was first found because there is a precedent for mutations affecting the sperm and the nervous system in mice. Several neurological mouse mutants are sterile as males, and the

TABLE 3. *The sterile phenotype of E1034[a]*

Strain	Temp (°C)	Progeny/Worm	Oocytes/Worm
Wild	16	284 ± 37	45
E1034	16	225 ± 34	43
tsH1	16	302 ± 21	17
Wild	25	253 ± 14	14
E1034	25	0.1	242 ± 36
tsH1	25	<0.06	205 ± 49
E1034 + Wild ♂	25	240	

[a] tsH1 is the reisolated sterile mutant strain that has normal chemotactic behavior. Each number is the average of eight individuals that were counted, and the uncertainty is the standard deviation of the mean.

defect is due to a defect in their sperm (Bennett, Gall, Southard, and Sidman, 1971). Before we could establish that mutations affecting nervous systems and sperm were common, it was important to rule out an alternative hypothesis to explain these multiple phenotypes: the stocks might contain more than one mutation, each causing a different phenotype. We have recently shown that the sterility in the E1034 strain is indeed due to a different mutation from that causing the chemotaxis defect, and we have separated these two mutations by recombination. The reisolated sterile mutant strain is designated *tsH1*, and its phenotype is shown in Table 3 and discussed in detail elsewhere (Ward and Miwa, 1977).

Although we were disappointed to have separated these phenotypes, the original double mutation led us to study the morphology and properties of the nematode's sperm, thinking that we might learn about the nervous system. In the course of our study, we discovered that sperm are interesting cells in their own right and that they have an attractive property for someone who is interested in biochemistry: they are isolatable as homogeneous cells, so that one can compare mutant to wild-type sperm biochemically much more easily than one can with mutant neurons.

In the remainder of this paper I will describe our preliminary studies of the morphology of sperm and our studies of the behavior of wild-type and mutant *C. elegans* sperm at fertilization. I will show that sperm face some of the same problems in finding oocytes that neurons must face in developing their own morphology and finding targets, so that the study of sperm is not entirely irrelevant to neurobiology.

The mutants E1034 or *tsH1* do make sperm when grown at 25°C. The process of meiosis in the sterile mutant (either E1034 or *tsH1*) is indistinguishable by light microscopy from the wild type in both hermaphrodites and males when grown at 25°C. The mutant accumulates as many sperm as the wild type, about 200 in the hermaphrodite and as many as 4,000 in the male, yet both mutant hermaphrodites and males are sterile at 25°C.

Nematode sperm are unlike mammalian sperm. They are not flagellated but, instead, are ameboid (Chitwood and Chitwood, 1974). In addition, *C. elegans* sperm can have long filamentous processes. When wild-type *C elegans* sperm are squashed out of a male into an appropriate buffer they first appear as roughly spherical cells about 6 μm in diameter, sometimes with pseudopod-like extensions. After they have been in buffer for a few minutes, they begin to extend filamentous processes that

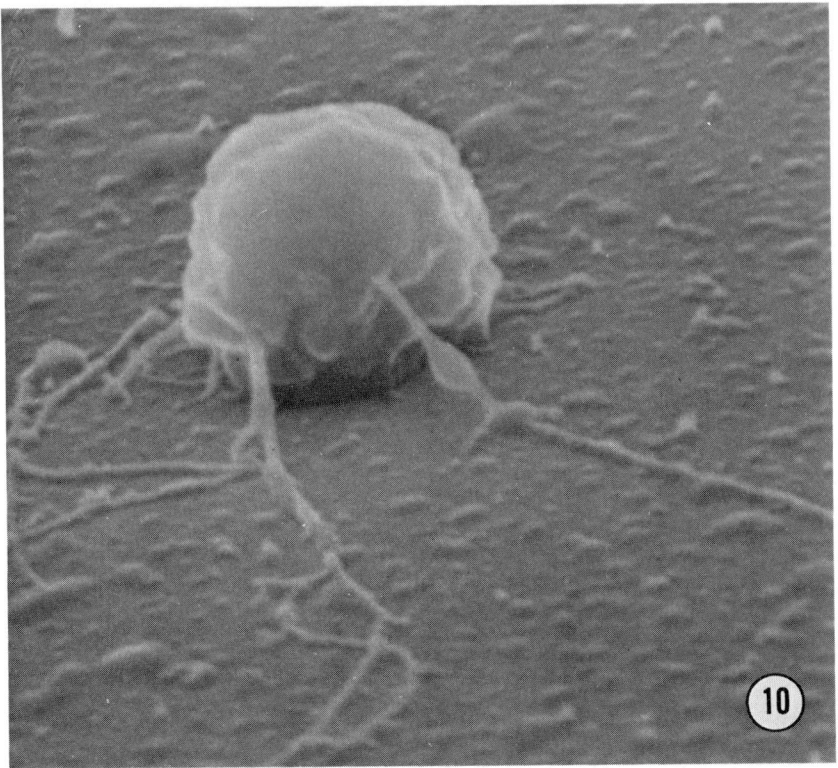

FIGURE 10. Scanning electron micrograph of a male sperm 30 min after squashing. The sperm was fixed with glutaraldehyde to a polylysine-coated cover slip, dehydrated, and critical point dried before shadowing.

can grow in length to as long as 40 μm. These are seen in the scanning electron micrograph (Figure 10). When viewed unfixed with dark field illumination, these filaments can be observed to wiggle rapidly. This motion is apparently passive because formaldehyde-fixed sperm can have filaments wiggling as actively as do unfixed sperm. The filamentous processes from a single sperm vary in length and number, but a sperm

FIGURE 11. Transmission electron micrograph of a section of hermaphrodite sperm in spermatheca. Abbreviations: N, nucleus; V, special membrane vesicles; P, pseudopodial region.

FIGURE 12. Transmission electron micrograph of hermaphrodite sperm in spermatheca showing the fusion of the special membrane vesicles (V) with the plasma membrane.

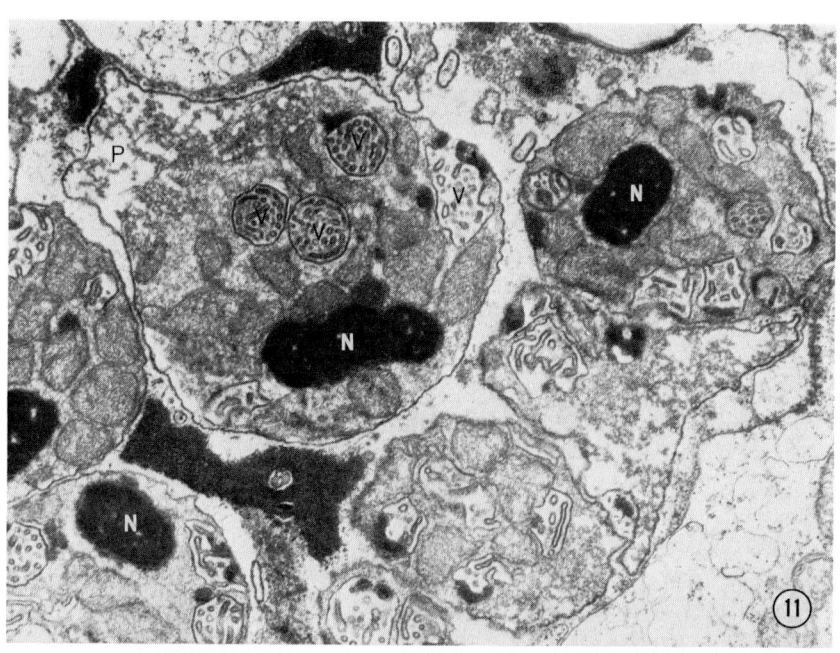

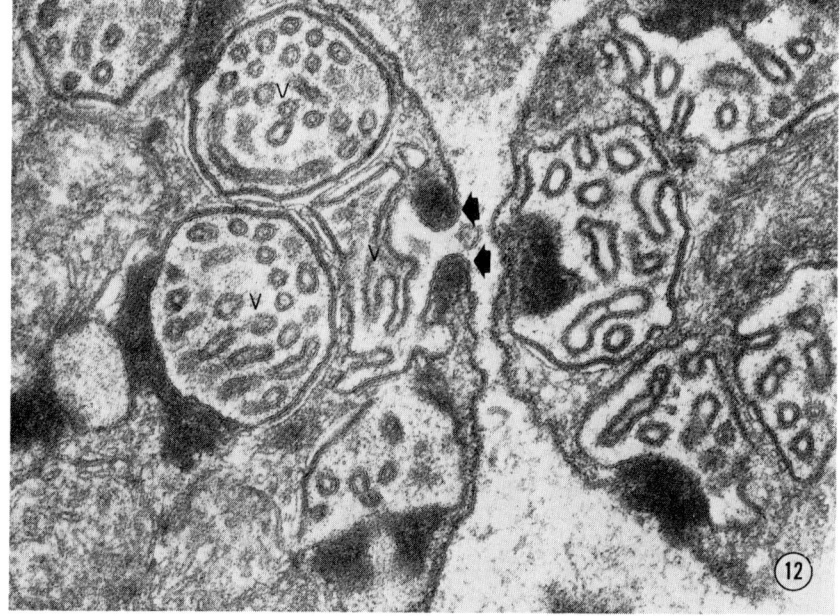

can have as many as 15 processes. When the sperm are examined inside the hermaphrodite by scanning electron microscopy of broken animals, they do not have filaments visible, so we do not yet know whether or not they have a normal function.

Where are the filaments when the sperm are inside the hermaphrodite or immediately after release, and what is their structure? By fixing hermaphrodites or males and sectioning them for examination with the transmission electron microscope, one can see that the sperm resemble those of some other nematodes (Beams and Sekhon, 1972; Foor, 1970). They have a pseudopodial region and a region containing organelles, including the highly condensed nucleus and mitochondria (Figure 11). The sperm also contain peculiar organelles containing membrane bound filamentous processes. These unusual organelles have been called special membrane vesicles in other nematode sperm.

These special membrane vesicles fuse with the plasma membrane of the sperm in some of the sperm in the spermatheca, as shown in Figure 12. Parts of two adjacent sperm are visible in this Figure, and the fusion of a special membrane vesicle with the plasma membrane is visible in one of them. It is also apparent in other special membrane vesicles that the tubular membranes visible inside these vesicles are invaginations of the vesicle membrane. These invaginated tubular membranes may become the filaments extending from the cell when the special membrane vesicle fuses with the plasma membrane.

We have only just begun to examine sperm in *tsH1* grown at 25°C. So far they appear indistinguishable from the wild type. They do contain special membrane vesicles and they extend filaments visible with the light or scanning electron microscope when the sperm are squashed out of 25°C grown males or hermaphrodites.

Why does fertilization fail to take place in this mutant? To answer this question we have begun to study the normal process of fertilization with the light and electron microscopes (Ward and Carrel, 1977). The live animal can be examined with the light microscope by using Nomarski optics with the specimen mounted in an agar chamber (Sulston, 1976). One view of the gonad immediately prior to fertilization is shown in Figure 13. Sperm are visible as round cells with a prominent nucleus. Several can be seen contacting the oocyte and more can be seen clustered in the spermatheca. Twenty or so sperm contact the oocyte as it reaches maturity at the end of the oviduct and presses against the spermatheca. The oocyte then is squeezed into the spermatheca carrying this cap of sperm. It then passes into the uterus through a narrow constriction. It continues to be contacted by its cap of sperm and

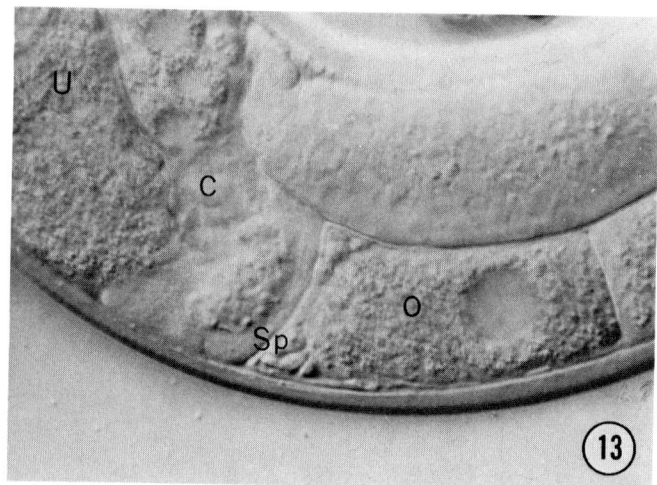

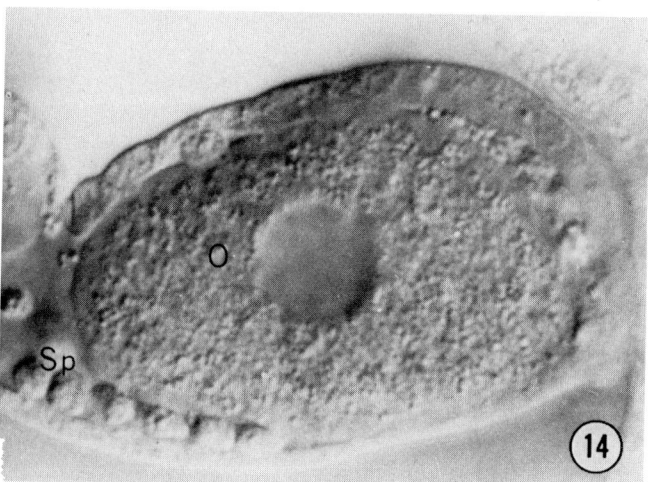

FIGURE 13. Light micrograph of a hermaphrodite gonad in the region of the spermatheca. Abbreviations: Sp, sperm; O, oocyte; C, constriction; U, uterus.

FIGURE 14. Light micrograph of a 25°C grown E1034 hermaphrodite oocyte dissected out of the gonad. Note sperm contacting the oocyte.

carries these into the uterus. Fertilization takes place somewhere along the oocyte's passage. The sperm carried into the uterus that do not fertilize the oocyte abruptly migrate back to the spermatheca to be able to fertilize other oocytes. Every sperm in the hermaphrodite fertilizes an oocyte because the number of zygotes produced by the hermaphrodite corresponds exactly to the number of sperm (Ward and Carrel, 1977).

As shown in Figure 14, which is a light micrograph of an oocyte dissected out of a E1034 mutant hermaphrodite grown at 25°C, sperm contact the oocyte normally. In the intact mutant hermaphrodite grown at 25°C, the oocytes pass through the spermatheca normally with their cap of sperm, but fertilization fails to take place. In addition, the supernumerary sperm carried into the uterus fail to migrate back to the spermatheca. After twenty or so oocytes have passed into the uterus, about half of the sperm are swept out of the spermatheca, many of these getting expelled when the unfertilized oocytes are laid (Ward and Miwa, 1977).

We have also examined the process of fertilization by male sperm (Ward and Carrel, 1977). Males mate with the hermaphrodite and deposit their sperm in the uterus in the region of the vulva. These sperm then move, apparently by active amoeboid motion, around the eggs or oocytes in the uterus up to the region of the spermatheca and through the hermaphrodite sperm that are accumulated there.

One can ask how the male sperm compete with the hermaphrodite's own sperm for the oocytes by using genetic markers to distinguish outcross progeny (male sperm fertilized) from self-cross progeny (hermaphrodite sperm fertilized). Results of mating two individual hermaphrodites with males for 3 h are shown in Figure 15; also shown in this Figure is the production of outcross progeny with time after mating. In Figure 15a we see that outcross progeny begin to appear within 5 h of mating and shortly after that *only* outcross progeny are produced. The hermaphrodite shown in Figure 15a was not mated by many males and, after producing some outcross progeny, it returned to producing self-cross progeny. The hermaphrodite shown in Figure 15b was heavily mated and only produced outcross progeny after mating. This shows that, in spite of the hermaphrodite sperm already present in the spermatheca, male sperm have a selective advantage at fertilization and successfully compete with the hermaphrodite's own sperm for the oocytes.

The reisolated sterile mutant *tsH1* males grown at 25°C transfer sperm to the hermaphrodite. At least some of these reach the spermatheca, although most transferred sperm are found in the region of the vulva. These transferred sperm fail to fertilize the oocytes.

What does this study of sperm and fertilization have to do with the nervous system? Perhaps nothing, but I think that fertilization in this

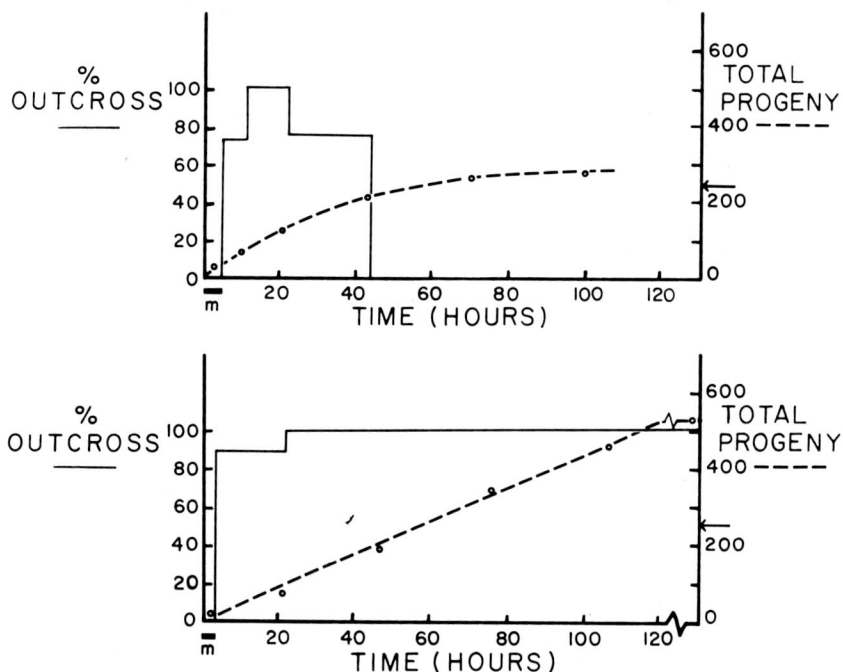

FIGURE 15. Distribution of outcross progeny after mating by wild-type males. Upper figure is a *dpy-11*^{e224} hermaphrodite; lower figure is a *dpy-1*^{e1} hermaphrodite. Outcross progeny were distinguished from self-cross progeny by their nondumpy appearance. M is the time of mating. The arrow marks the progeny yield from unmated controls.

nematode has features in common with neuron development that may reflect common biochemical mechanisms. (1) The sperm are motile cells moving by amoeboid motion as do developing neurons; (2) sperm must locate a specific target cell, the oocyte, and recognize its membrane to adhere as do developing neurons; (3) sperm contain internal vesicles that fuse with the plasma membrane as do neurons; (4) male and hermaphrodite sperm compete with one another for the oocyte targets, the male sperm winning. Competition between neurons for their targets may be an important mechanism of proper synapse formation in vertebrate nervous systems (e.g., Clarke and Cowan, 1975).

More important from a practical biochemist's point of view is the fact that sperm cells can be isolated in homogeneous form from males so that it is possible to characterize them biochemically.

One way that we are doing this is to raise antisera to the sperm and try to use these antisera to identify alterations in mutants by cross-absorption of antisera raised against mutant and wild-type sperm. One attractive biochemical hypothesis to explain the fertilization defect in strain *tsH1* grown at 25°C is that the mutant sperm are defective in a cell surface component that is necessary for proper interaction with the surface of the oocyte. If this were so, the difference might be detectable as a change in a cell surface antigen on the sperm.

CONCLUSIONS

The sensory mutants described in the first part of this talk do not provide a set of simple interpretable alterations in the sensory nervous system. In two of the genes characterized by Lewis and Hodgkin, anatomical alterations were reproducible and uniform, but nearly all the sensory neurons in the worm were defective, so these mutants did not help to establish the functions of individual neurons. In the gene most thoroughly examined, *che-1*, a specific anatomical alteration was found, but this was variable between individuals of the same mutant allele and varied between alleles of the same mutant gene. Yet the behavioral phenotypes did not vary. It may have been bad fortune to have hit first upon mutants that gave results difficult to interpret, and if more mutants were isolated and sectioned it would be possible to find more straightforward mutant defects. But it might also be that in an organism like *C. elegans* with a small genome, gene products are used with great economy in development by being used again and again in many cells so that most mutants have pleiotropic effects, making correlation of behavioral and anatomical defects difficult.

The process of development of the sensory neurons has not been described. We do not know the sequence of events by which the sensory neurons take up their final positions; we do not know the lineage relationships among the different sensory neurons. Such information is essential for interpretation of developmental mutants. It is clear now that the sensory nervous system is a poor part of the nervous system for studying development of mutants because it develops entirely in the embryo, where it is hard to observe (Ward et al., 1975). The motor nervous system is a much better place for developmental analysis because some of it develops postembryonically and the entire lineage of every postembryonic cell has been described (Sulston, 1976; Sulston and Horvitz, 1977). Therefore, in this part of the nervous system the classes of cells affected by developmental mutations can be interpreted in terms of their lineage relationships and developmental histories and some of the difficulties in interpreting sensory mutants can be avoided.

But even in the postembryonic nervous system, if one is interested in biochemistry, one must always face the difficult problem of how to identify the defective gene products. For biochemical analysis of mutants, the inability to isolate a homogeneous population of cells from the nervous system has led me to turn my interest to the study of sperm by using fertilization-defective mutants. It is my hope that some of the basic biochemistry of development will be the same, so that what is learned about sperm can be applied to the difficult task of finding out more about the biochemical basis of the genetic control of neural development.

ACKNOWLEDGMENTS

I thank Jim Lewis and Jonathan Hodgkin for communicating their results prior to publication and for permission to reproduce figures. I thank Gail Korman and Greg Nelson for preparation of electron micrographs, and John Carrel for capable technical assistance. Support from the National Science Foundation and the National Institute of General Medical Sciences is gratefully acknowledged.

REFERENCES

Beams, H. W. and S. S. Sekhon (1972). Cytodifferentiation during spermogenesis in *Rabditis pellio*, *J. Ultrastruct. Res.* **38**:511–527.

Bennett, W. I., A. M. Gall, J. L. Southard, and R. L. Sidman (1971). Abnormal spermogenesis in quaking, a myelin-deficient mutant mouse, *Biol. Reprod.* **5**: 30–58.

Brenner, S. (1973). The genetics of behavior, *Br. Med. Bull.* **29**:269–271.

Brenner, S. (1974). The Genetics of *Caenorhabditis elegans*, *Genetics* **77**:71–94.

Chitwood, B. G. and M. B. Chitwood (1974). *An Introduction to Nematology*. University Park Press, Baltimore.

Clarke, P. G. H. and W. M. Cowan (1975). Ectopic neurons and aberrant connection during neural development, *Proc. Natl. Acad. Sci. U.S.A.* **72**:4455–4458.

Dusenbery, D. B. (1973). Countercurrent separation: a new method for studying behavior of small aquatic organisms, *Proc. Natl. Acad. Sci. U.S.A.* **70**:1349–1352.

Dusenbery, D. B., R. E. Sheridan, and R. L. Russell (1975). Chemotaxis-defective mutants of the nematode *Caenorhabditis elegans*, *Genetics* **80**: 297–309.

Foor, W. E. (1970). Spermatozoan morphology and zygote formation in nematodes, *Biol. Reprod. (Suppl.)* **2:**177–202.

Grüneberg, H. (1973). *The Pathology of Development, A Study of Inherited Skeletal Disorders in Animals*. John Wiley and Sons, New York.

Hirsh, D. and R. Vanderslice (1976). Temperature-sensitive developmental mutants of *Caenorhabditis elegans, Dev. Biol.* **49:**220–235.

Lewis, J. A. and J. A. Hodgkin (1977). Specific neuroanatomical changes in chemosensory mutants of the nematode *Caenorhabditis elegans, J. Comp. Neurol.*, in press.

Sulston, J. E. (1976). Post-embryonic development in the ventral cord of *Caenorhabditis elegans, Philos. Trans. R. Soc. London Ser. B* **275:**287–297.

Sulston, J. E. and H. R. Horvitz (1977). Post-embryonic cell lineages of the nematode *Caenorhabditis elegans, Dev. Biol.*, in press.

Ward, S. (1973). Chemotaxis by the nematode *Caenorhabditis elegans:* identification of attractants and analysis of the response by use of mutants, *Proc. Natl. Acad. Sci. U.S.A.* **70:**817–821.

Ward, S. (1976). The use of mutants to analyze the sensory nervous system of *Caenorhabditis elegans*, pp. 365–382 in *The Organization of Nematodes*, Croll, N., ed. Academic Press, New York.

Ward, S. and J. Carrel (1977). The process of fertilization in the nematode *Caenorhabditis elegans*, manuscript in preparation.

Ward, S. and J. Miwa (1977). A temperature-sensitive fertilization defective mutant in the nematode *Caenorhabditis elegans*, manuscript in preparation.

Ward, S., N. Thomson, J. White, and S. Brenner (1975). Electron microscopical reconstruction of the anterior sensory anatomy of the nematode *Caenorhabditis elegans, J. Comp. Neurol.* **160:**313–338.

Ware, R. W., D. Clark, K. Crossland, and R. L. Russell (1975). The nerve ring of the nematode *Caenorhabditis elegans*: sensory input and motor output, *J. Comp. Neurol.* **162:**71–110.

White, J. G., E. Southgate, J. N. Thomson, and S. Brenner (1976). The structure of the ventral nerve cord of *Caenorhabditis elegans, Philos. Trans. R. Soc. London Series B* **275:**327–348.

Wright, T. R. F. (1970). The genetics of embryogenesis in *Drosphila, Adv. Genet.* **15:**261–395.

Reeler Mutant Mouse: A Genetic Experiment in Developing Mammalian Cortex

Verne S. Caviness, Jr.

Eunice Kennedy Shriver Center for Mental Retardation, Inc., Waltham, Massachusetts

Reeler is an autosomal recessive mutation occurring in mice (Falconer, 1951; Committee on Standard Nomenclature for Mice, 1972). Animals homozygous for the mutated allele at the reeler locus have generalized high amplitude action tremor, dystonic postures, and a reeling ataxia of gait. There are abnormalities in the pattern of neuron position throughout all the cortical structures of the brain, with the exception of the olfactory bulb, which is cytoarchitectonically normal (Hamburgh, 1960, 1963; Meier and Hoag, 1962; Caviness and Sidman, 1972, 1973a; Caviness, 1976). The characters of the abnormal cell patterns appear not to be altered by variations in genetic background in that they are identical in reelers of the C3H strain, the C57 strain, and in hybrid mutants resulting from cross-breeding between those two strains (Caviness, So, and Sidman, 1972). The abnormal cell patterns do not occur in animals that are heterozygous for the mutated allele.

The abnormalities in cortical cell pattern associated with the reeler mutation pose two broad questions of interest in developmental neurobiology: (1) To what extent are the morphogenetic mechanisms that govern connections between cells and those that govern the morphology of cells dependent upon the relative positions of neurons? (2) What are the morphogenetic events, their molecular mechanisms, and genetic control that govern the position of neurons within cortical structures? In the present report, partial answers to these questions are considered in terms of the comparative structure and development of neocortex and piriform cortex of the forebrain in normal and reeler mice.

MATERIALS AND METHODS

Mice of the C57BL/6J or C3H/HEJ strains or hybrid animals resulting from cross-breeding between these strains were used in all comparative studies of normal and reeler animals (Caviness et al., 1972). Studies of connectivity of major afferent systems were based upon orthograde degeneration of axons and terminals (Fink and Heimer, 1967; Devor, Caviness, and Derer, 1975; Caviness, Korde, and Williams, 1977); retrograde transport of horseradish peroxidase (LaVail, Winston, and Tisch, 1973; Yorke and Caviness, 1975); and Timm's histochemical method (Haug, 1974; Caviness, Frost, and Hayes, 1976). The corpus callosum (Yorke and Caviness, 1975; Caviness and Yorke, 1976) and the olfactory bulb (Devor et al., 1975; Caviness et al., 1977) were destroyed by suction through a craniectomy, under direct visualization. Electrolytic lesions were delivered to the thalamus by a transcerebellar approach (Caviness et al., 1976). Normal fiber impregnations were based upon the silver-pyridine method of Schneider (1969), Golgi impregnations were based upon the method of Lund (1970), and labeling of cohorts of dividing neurons with tritiated thymidine were based upon the method of Sidman (1970). Animals whose brains were studied by electron microscopy were perfused transcardially with Karnovsky's fixative, and the tissue was processed by standard methods (Karnovsky, 1965; Caviness et al., 1977).

RESULTS

The principal neuronal classes that may be recognized in the neocortex and the piriform cortex of the normal animal are also present in reeler (Caviness and Sidman, 1972; Caviness, 1976). As in the normal animal, neurons are to some extent segregated by class into tangential laminae. However, the relative positions of the different neuronal classes are abnormal in the mutant (Figure 1A and C). In both the neocortex and the piriform cortex, for example, the relative positions of polymorphic cells and pyramidal cells are inverted. The polymorphic cells, those varying widely in size and shape, occupy the deepest stratum of normal neocortex. In the mutant, these cells occupy the most superficial plane, which is normally given to the molecular layer. Pyramidal cells occupy a wide field in both normal and reeler cortex. In the normal animal, the pyramidal field lies above the polymorphic cell zone and extends to the molecular layer. In the mutant, the field of pyramidal cells lies subjacent to the zone of polymorphic cells and

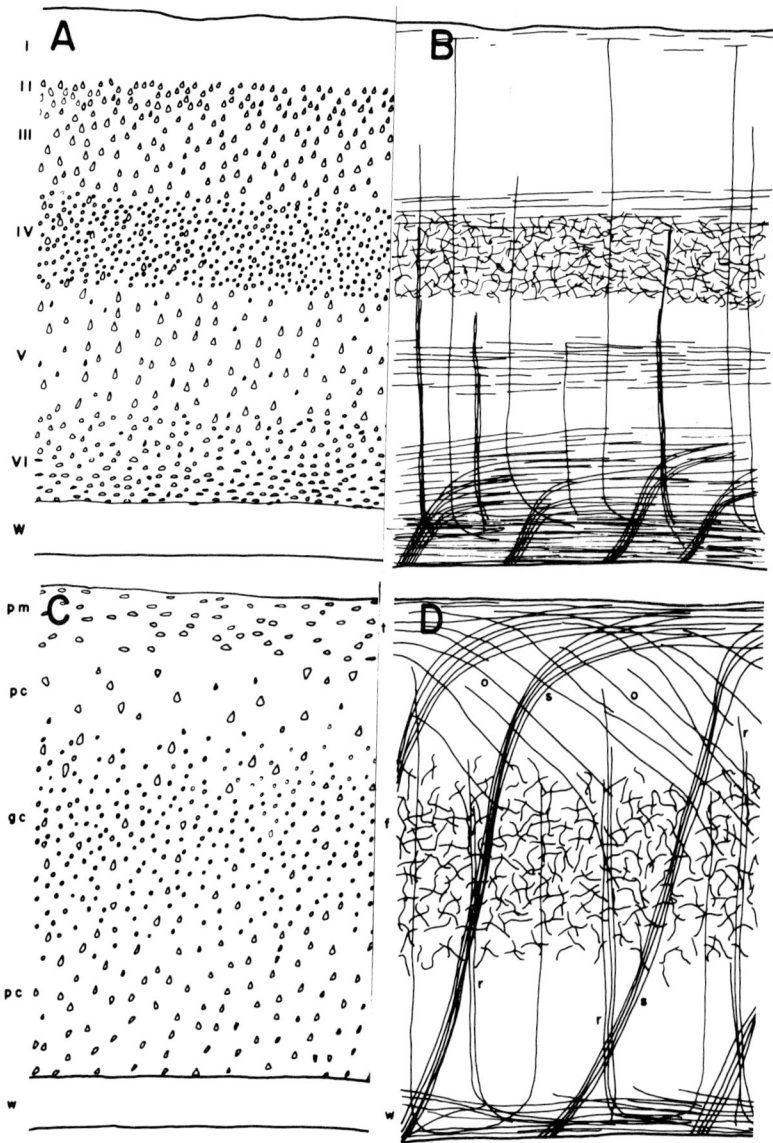

FIGURE 1. Schematic representation of cell and fiber patterns in the neocortex of normal (A and B) and reeler (C and D) mice (Caviness, 1976). Roman numerals refer to the cortical laminae in the normal animal. The polymorphic cell zone (pm) lies superficially in the mutant cortex. Granule cells (gc) are concentrated at an intermediate level within the pyramidal cell zone (pc).

extends to the central white matter. In the normal animal, the largest of the pyramidal cells are concentrated in the depths of the cortex, whereas medium-sized and small pyramids lie at successively more superficial levels. In the mutant, by contrast, the largest pyramidal cells are found superficially, immediately below the polymorphic cell zone. Medium-sized and small pyramidal cells are most densely concentrated in the depths of the cortex of the mutant cortex. In mutant and normal animals alike, the granule cells of the neocortex lie at an intermediate cortical depth, intercallated between large and medium-sized pyramidal cells. To a greater extent than in normal animals, there is intermixing of the granule cells and adjacent pyramidal cell classes.

Patterns of Distribution of Principal Afferent Systems
Corpus callosum

The tangential pattern of distribution of terminals of axons of the corpus callosum is identical in the neocortex of normal and reeler mice (Figure 2A) (Yorke and Caviness, 1975; Caviness and Yorke, 1976). There is a generalized high density distribution of terminals in frontal fields 6, 10, and 11. High density peaks follow the boundaries of field 17 with 18a laterally, and 18b medially. A similar high density peak lies laterally at the border of parietal field 3 with 40, and at the border of the medial limb of field 3 with field 1. Within the cortex of both reeler and normal animals, axon terminals are concentrated in laminar fashion among the somata of small and medium-sized pyramidal neurons (Figure 2B and C). In the normal animal, these cells are located superficially, whereas in the mutant they are concentrated in the depths of the cortex. In both mutant and normal neocortex, terminals of the corpus callosum are also distributed sparsely among the large pyramids and polymorphic cells. In the normal animal, these lie in the depths of the cortex, whereas they occupy the most superficial level of the reeler cortex.

Thalamo-Cortical Connections

The patterns of projection of thalamic nuclei upon cytoarchitectonic fields of the neocortex are also identical in normal and reeler mice. For example, the ventrobasal nucleus in both normal and reeler mice projects a tangetial mosaic of columns that is coextensive with a cellular barrel (Figure 3) (Caviness et al., 1976) in cytoarchitectonic field 3, the barrel field (Woolsey and Van der Loos, 1970; Caviness, 1975, 1976). The thalamo-cortical axons ascend to a subcortical level grouped in large fascicles in both mutant and normal animals. In the normal animal, these fascicles enter a fiber stratum coursing in the polymorphic cell

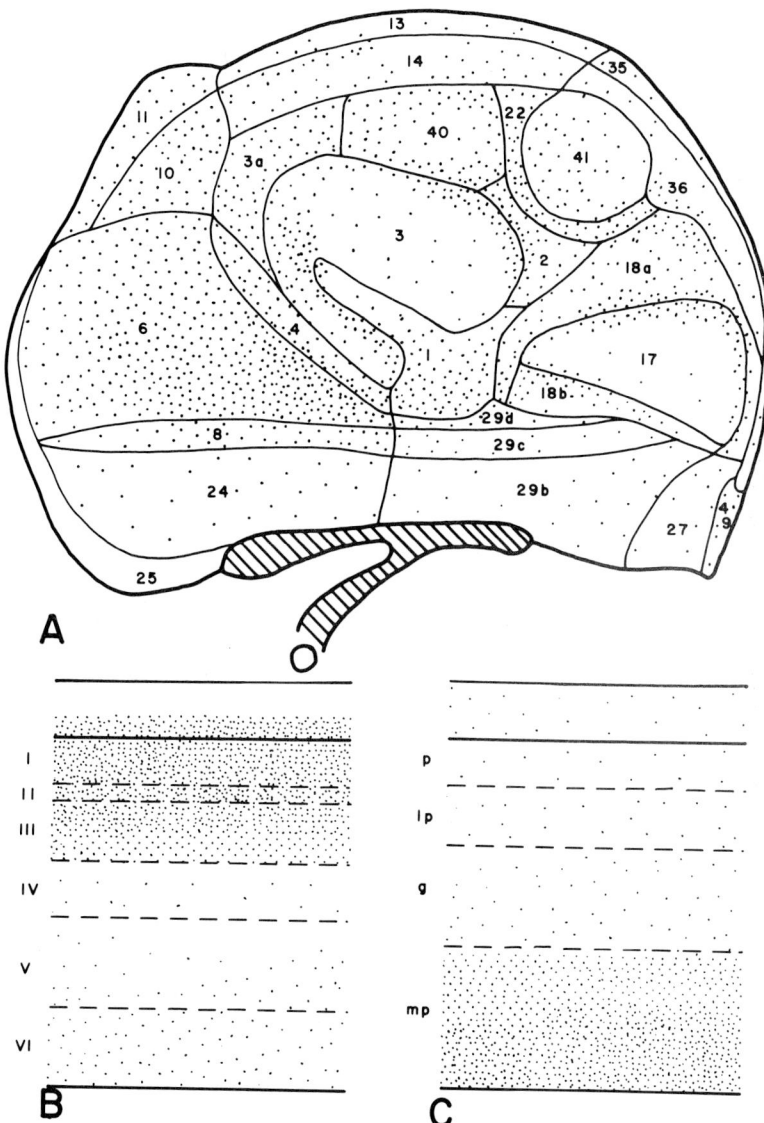

FIGURE 2. The distribution of terminals of callosal axons (stippling) is projected upon the cytoarchitectonic map of the neocortex of normal and reeler mice (A) (Yorke and Caviness, 1975; Caviness and Yorke, 1976). In most cytoarchitectonic fields of the normal cortex, terminals are most densely concentrated at the level of the somata of small and medium-sized pyramidal cells of layers II and III (Yorke and Caviness, 1975). In the reeler, also, they are most densely concentrated at the level of small and medium-sized pyramidal cells (m), but these lie in the depths of the mutant cortex (Caviness and Yorke, 1976).

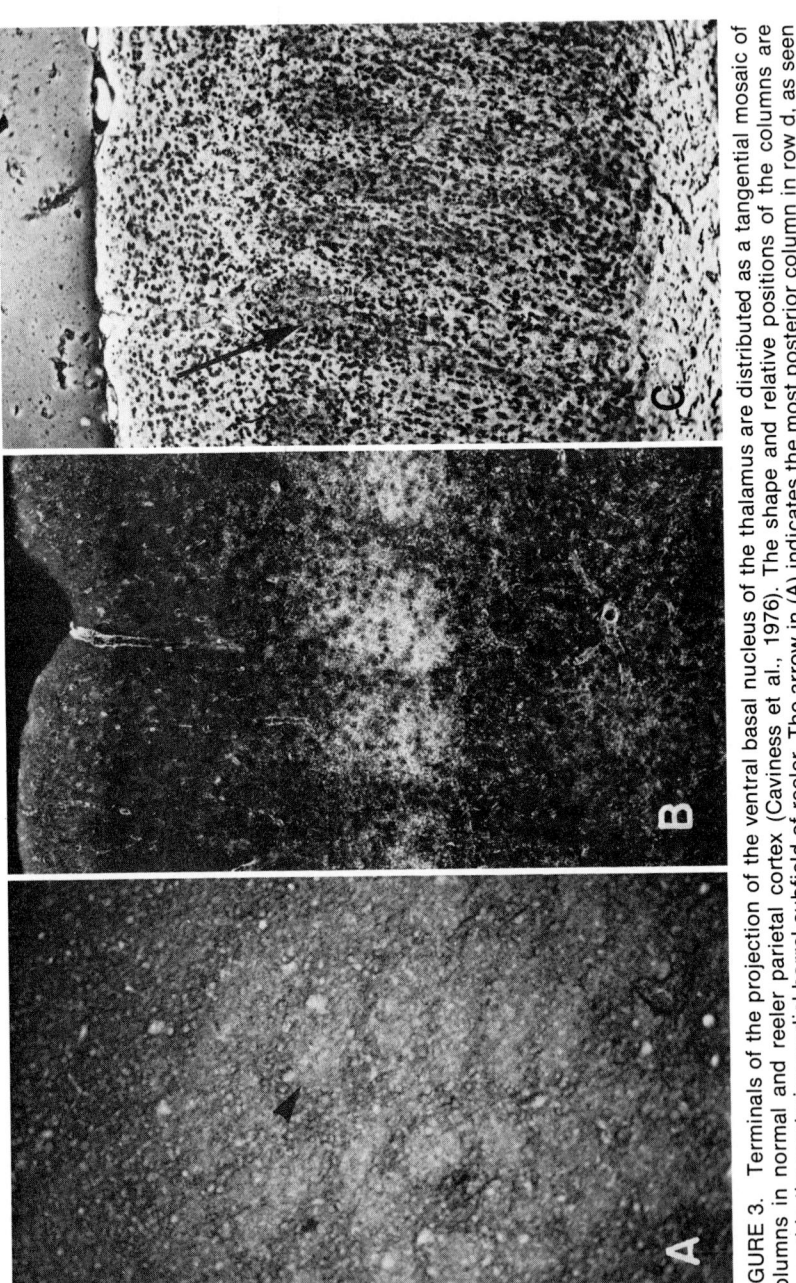

FIGURE 3. Terminals of the projection of the ventral basal nucleus of the thalamus are distributed as a tangential mosaic of columns in normal and reeler parietal cortex (Caviness et al., 1976). The shape and relative positions of the columns are normal in the posterior medial barrel subfield of reeler. The arrow in (A) indicates the most posterior column in row d, as seen in a tangential section impregnated by Timm's histochemical method (Caviness et al., 1976; Haug, 1974). ×53. The terminals are concentrated at the level of the granule cells, where they are coextensive with cellular barrels in both normal (B) and reeler (C) (arrow) animals. They continue among medium-sized pyramids above the barrels in the normal cortex (B) and below the barrels in the reeler cortex (C). (B) and (C), coronal sections, Fink-Heimer impregnations; (B) dark field illumination, ×150; (C) bright field illumination, ×100.

zone in the depths of the cortex (Figure 1B). In the mutant, the fascicles of thalamo-cortical axons also enter a fiber stratum in the polymorphic cell zone, but must traverse the full width of the cortex to do so (Figure 1D). In mutant and normal neocortex, the fibers pass through the polymorphic cell zone until they reach their target cytoarchitectonic field. They then penetrate more deeply into the cortex, ascending from below in the normal animal, but descending from above in reeler. In both normal and reeler animals, the afferents from the ventrobasal nucleus terminate densely as a mosaic of columnar aggregates within the barrels formed by granule cells at the mid-cortical level and among adjacent medium-sized pyramids (Figure 3B and C). The latter are supragranular in the normal animal, but lie at an infragranular level in the mutant.

Lateral Olfactory Tract

Axons from the olfactory bulb of normal and reeler mice course in the lateral olfactory tract (Devor et al., 1975). Terminals of this afferent system are distributed densely to a superficial laminar zone (Figure 4A and B) where they contact the distal segments of the apical shafts of pyramidal cells whose somata lie in the subjacent cortex. In the normal animal, somata of these pyramidal cells are most densely concentrated superficially in the cellular zone of the cortex. Golgi impregnations establish that in reeler, a small number of the pyramidal cells are aligned tangentially (Devor et al., 1975). Their apical dendrites do not extend into the zone of terminals from the lateral olfactory tract. Axons of the lateral olfactory tract appear not to penetrate the cortex to engage these aberrantly aligned pyramidal cells.

Cells of Origin of Major Neocortical Efferent Systems

The laminar pattern of neuronal position in the neocortex of the normal animal corresponds to a laminar segregation of the cell bodies of origin of the principal cortical efferent systems (e.g., Wise, 1975). Horseradish peroxidase (HRP) injected into the superior colliculus becomes concentrated, by retrograde axonal transport, in the somata of pyramidal cells, which are located exclusively in layer V of occipital cortex. HRP injected into the lateral geniculate nucleus becomes concentrated in the somata of neurons lying in layer VI (Figure 5A). When the tracer is injected into the neocortex itself, it becomes concentrated most densely within the somata of the medium-sized

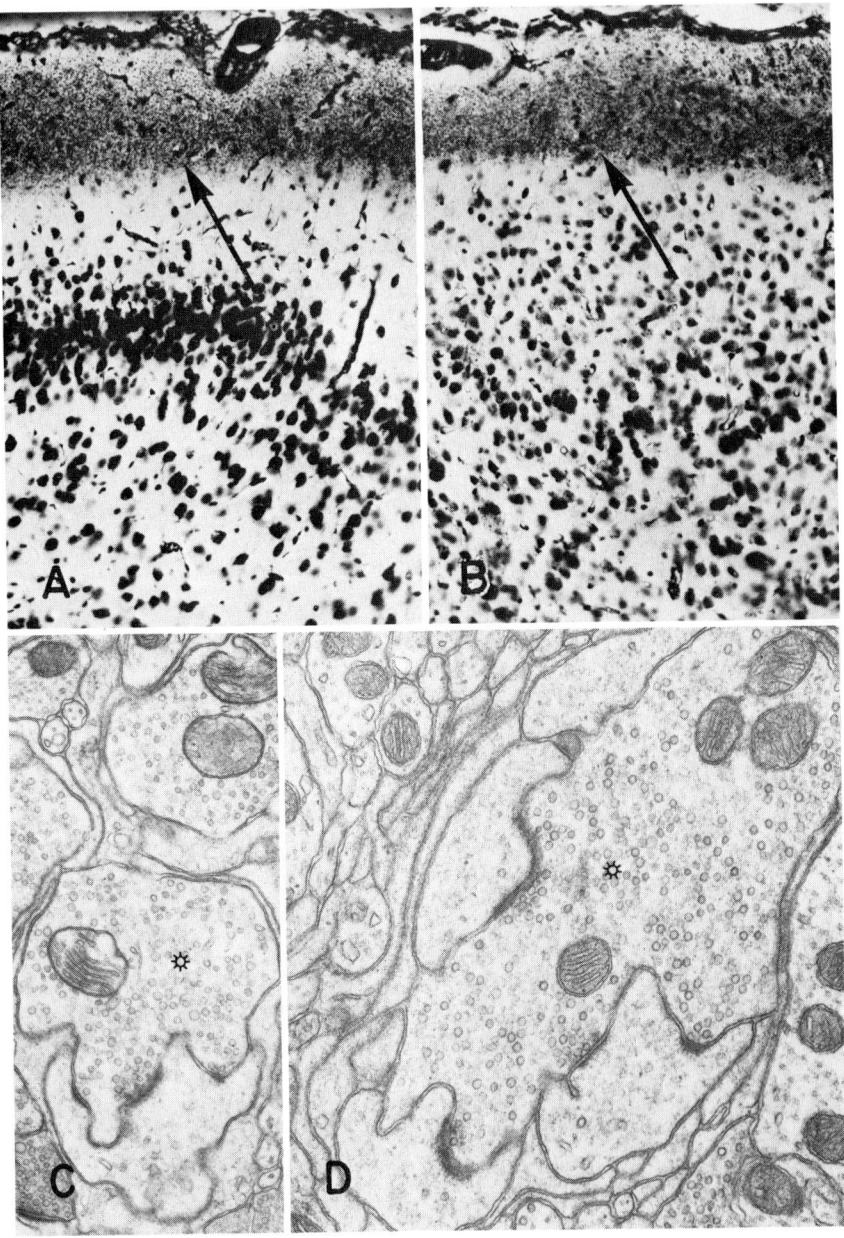

FIGURE 4. Degenerating terminals of axons of the lateral olfactory tract in superficial lamina zone (arrows) of normal (A) and reeler (B) piriform cortex. (A) and (B), coronal plane, Fink-Heimer impregnations, ×125. Electron micrographs of terminals of axons of the lateral olfactory tract (asterisks) in normal (C) and reeler (D) piriform cortex. (C) ×25,000; (D) ×31,000.

pyramids at the superficial level of contralateral cortex (Figure 5C). A few cells of layers V and VI will also concentrate the label.

Relatively large injections of HRP into the tectum of reeler, with diffusion through the posterior region of the thalamus as well, label numerous somata that lie within and above the granule cell zone in the outer half of the neocortex of the mutant (Figure 5B). Only infrequently, a labeled cell may also be identified below the granule cells in the depths of the cortex. When HRP is injected into the neocortex of reeler, it is concentrated, principally, within the somata of medium-sized pyramids lying in the depths of the contralateral cortex (Figure 5D). Only infrequently a labeled cell is identified in a supragranular position among the contralateral large pyramidal and polymorphic cells.

Intrinsic Organization of the Neocortex

A similar range of pyramidal and stellate neuronal classes may be identified in rapid-Golgi impregnations of the neocortex of reeler and normal mice (Figure 6) (Caviness, 1977). In the visual cortex, for example, spiny stellate cells (cell a in Figure 6A and B) are most densely concentrated at the intermediate cortical level corresponding to the granule cell zone. These cells, presumably a major target of thalamo-cortical afferents in normal and reeler alike, deploy their dendrites and axons in the region of the cell body. Their axons, either ascending or descending, extend for short distances among adjacent pyramidal cells.

The pyramidal cells of the normal cortex are, with rare exception, radially aligned with ascending orientation of the dominant apical dendrite (Figure 6A, cells c through d). Those pyramidal neurons whose somata are located well within the cortex in reeler likewise tend to be radially aligned, but the orientation of the cell may be either ascending (Figure 6B, cells b and d) or descending (Figure 6B, cells c and e). Those lying at the superficial or deep extremes of the cortex, by contrast, tend to be more tangential in their alignment. The axons of the largest pyramidal cells, located in the depths of the normal cortex, descend to the central white matter or to the tangential fiber stratum in the polymorphic cell zone (Figure 6A, cell b). They give off relatively few ascending collaterals. The homologous cells, lying superficially in the reeler cortex, may direct their principal axonal trunks superiorly into the fiber stratum of the polymorphic cell zone. Alternatively, the axons of such cells may descend radially to the central white matter. Just as

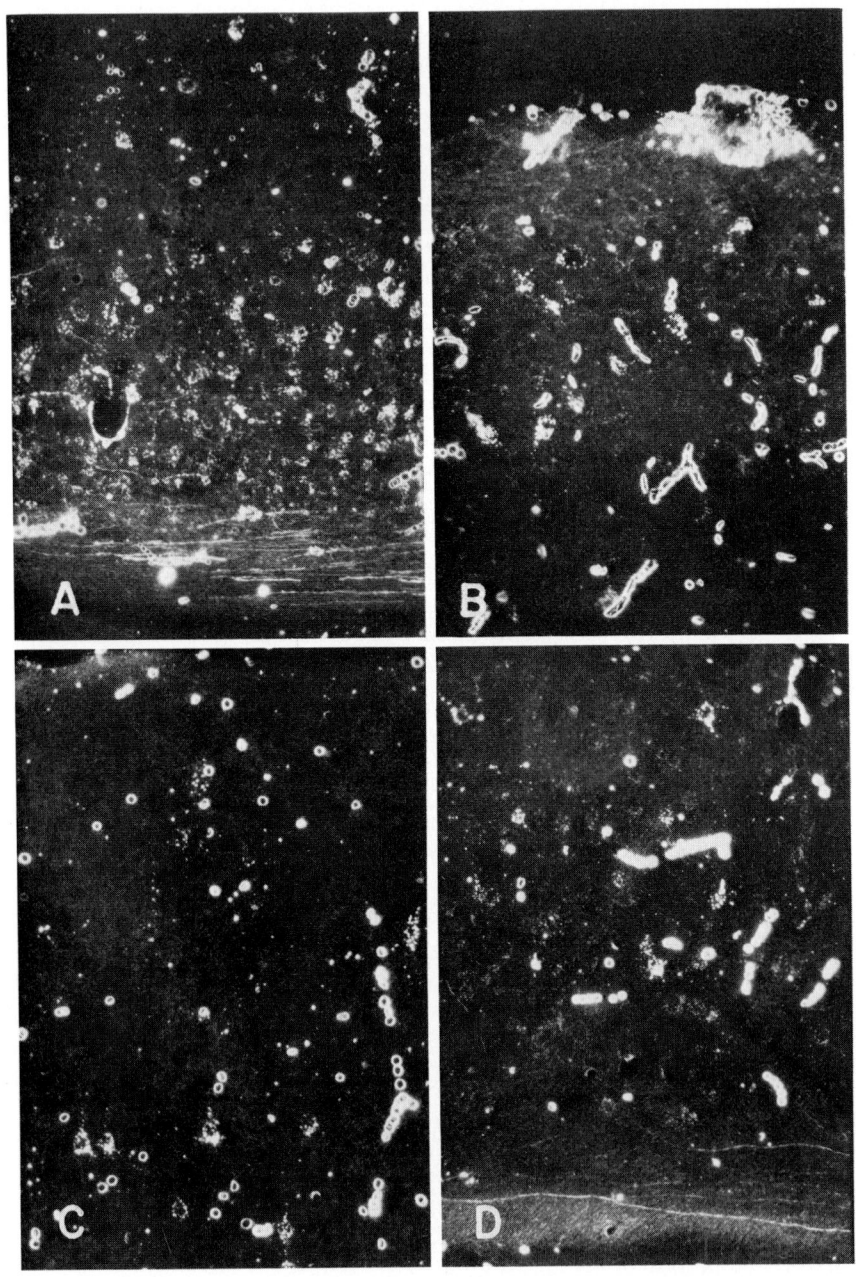

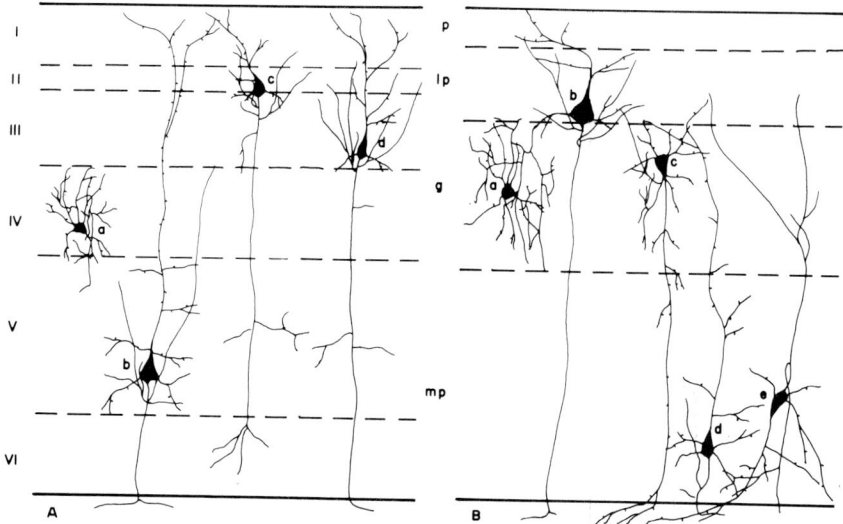

FIGURE 6. Drawings of neurons of normal (A) and reeler (B) visual cortex impregnated by the rapid-Golgi method. See text for details.

with the axons of their homologues in the normal animal, however, they give off few or no collaterals to other cellular zones as they traverse the cortex (Figure 6B, cell b). The axons of medium-sized and small pyramids, lying superficially in the cortex of the normal animal, descend radially and, in general, reach the central white matter. In their descent they give off a rich collateral arbor, particularly within the granule cell zone and among the large pyramids of layer V (Figure 6A, cells c and d). The homologous cells lying in the depths of the cortex of the mutant likewise direct their principal axonal trunks into the subjacent central white matter. Like their homologues in the normal animal, they may direct a rich collateral system among the granule and large pyramidal cell groups that lie more superficially in the mutant cortex. Often this is achieved by a dramatically ascending and descending hairpin arc of the axon, with the collateral system springing from the apex of the hairpin turn (Figure 6B, cell c).

FIGURE 5. HRP-labeled neuron somata of origin of cortical projections to lateral geniculate and tectum of normal (A) and reeler (B) mice. In the normal animal, these lie in an infragranular position, whereas in reeler, they lie in a supragranular position. HRP-labeled neuron somata of origin of callosal axons, by contrast, lie principally at a supragranular level of normal cortex (C), but at an infragranular level of reeler cortex (D). (A) through (D), dark field illumination, ×200.

Synaptology of the Lateral Olfactory Tract

In both normal and reeler animals, the terminals of axons of the lateral olfactory tract, identified by degenerative changes after olfactory bulb ablation (Caviness et al., 1977; Caviness and Korde, unpublished observations), contain spherical vesicles 400 to 500 Å in diameter and form only asymmetric synapses with dendritic spines or small dendritic branches (Figure 4C and D). The density, and presumably the total number, of these terminals is substantially less in reeler than in the normal animal. In the normal animal, this type of terminal usually engages only a single spine, with which it is generally deeply interdigitated. In reeler, by contrast, such terminals may be larger than in the normal animal. They may contact as many as three or four spines, and the reciprocal interdigitations of spine and terminal are relatively shallow. In reeler, but not in the normal animal, these terminals are invariably surrounded by a conspicuous multilaminate glial envelope.

Developmental Events Leading to Cell Malposition in the Reeler Cortical Malformation

Homologous cells are generated simultaneously in reeler and normal litter mates (Caviness and Sidman, 1973b; Caviness, 1973; Devor et al., 1975). In the normal animal, statistically speaking, the earliest generated cells will come to occupy the deepest layers, whereas the latest generated cells will be found in the most superficial layers of the cortex (Figure 7). However, on E12 and E13, when cell generation is proceeding maximally in the piriform cortex (Figure 7), or between E13 and E15 in the neocortex, cells of all classes are generated simultaneously. Among these are cells destined for positions at all depths in the cortex.

In reeler, the normal vectorial relationship between sequence of cell generation and cell position in the cortex is reversed. The earliest generated cells tend to occupy the more superficial positions, whereas the latest generated cells come to lie at deeper levels. As in the normal animal, neurons of all cell classes are formed during the period of maximal cell generation in the mutant. As in the normal animal, neurons formed at this time will come to lie at all radial levels of the cortex (Figure 7).

Radial glial fibers, which serve as guides to migrating neurons in the normal animal (Rakic, 1972), appear in Golgi impregnations to be of

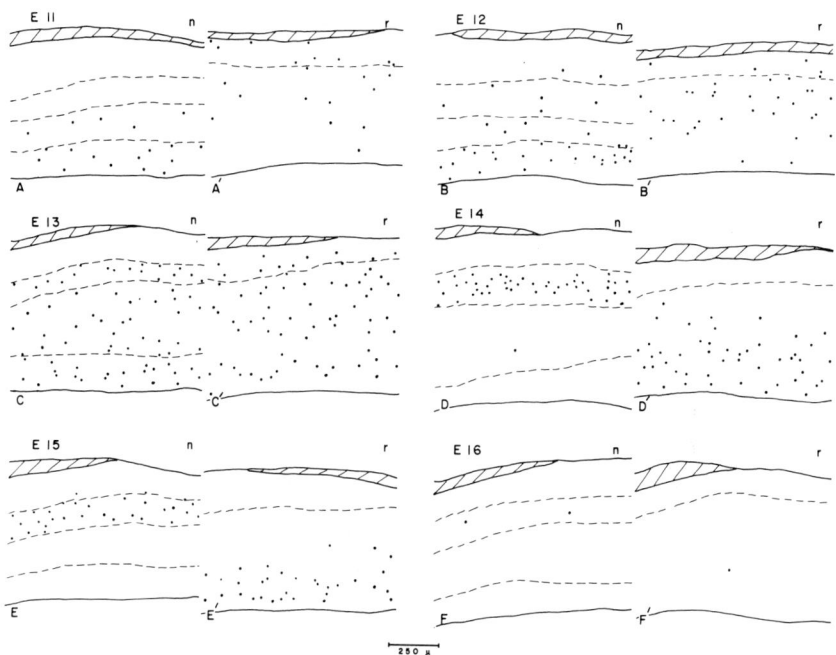

FIGURE 7. Autoradiographic plots of piriform cortex from adult normal (A through F) and reeler mutant mice (A' through F') (Devor et al., 1975). Each dot represents the position of a heavily labeled neuron, marked at the time of its last division by ^{3}H-labeled thymidine injected into the pregnant dam on embryonic days E11-E16. The lateral olfactory tract is cross-hatched. Horizontal plane.

normal morphology and to be deployed in a normal pattern in reeler (Figure 8) (Pinto and Caviness, unpublished observations). Cell migration appears to proceed according to the normal schedule in reeler. In the mutant, as in the normal animal, the earliest neocortical neurons to be formed complete their migrations by embryonic day 13. These early formed neurons are stellate in configuration. They are diffusely distributed through the postmigratory zone on E13 in a fashion that is indistinguishable in reeler and normal embryos. Over the next 24 to 48 h, a cortical plate, bracketed above and below by cell-sparse plexiform and subplate zones, respectively, emerges in the normal embryo (Figure 9A). As this occurs, the neurons generated on E11 become subdivided into two populations in the normal animal (Derer, Caviness, and Sidman, 1977). A small number remain superficially in the external plexiform layer. A somewhat larger contingent is displaced deeply to the subplate

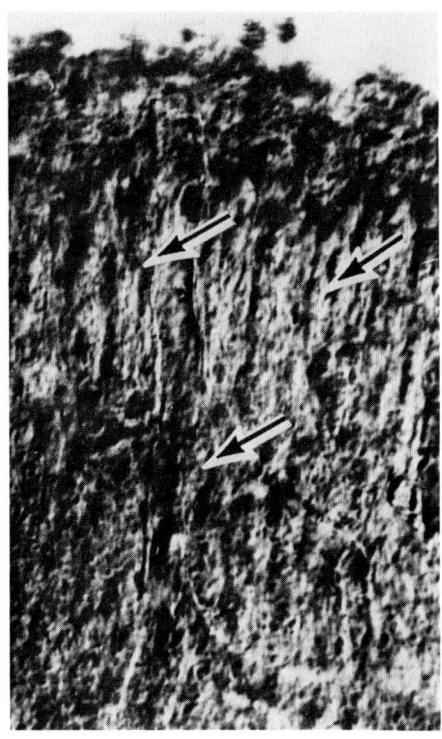

FIGURE 8. Regularly spaced, radially ascending glial fibers in the neocortex of an E16 reeler embryo (3 are marked with arrows) appear "elevated," with highlights to the left. Cell bodies appear "depressed." The black-white photograph was printed from a color transparency. The latter, in turn, was photographed with Nomarski optics, substage diaphragm at minimum aperture, from a "nonimpregnated" sector of cortex in a rapid-Golgi impregnation. Optical conditions were such that fibers were a brillant scarlet and cortical neurons were blue. ×450.

region as cells that arrive subsequently enter the cortical plate (Figure 9C).

The early events of cortical histogenesis are dramatically different in reeler. Between E13 and E15, a cell-sparse plexiform zone appears at an intermediate cortical depth (Figure 9B). The superficial and subplate zone is more cellular than in the normal animal. The behavior of the earliest formed postmigratory cells is distinctly anomalous in the mutant. Rather than becoming subdivided into separate, superficially, and deeply directed subpopulations, all of the early formed cells remain together as a single population at the most superficial level of the mutant cortex (Figure 9D).

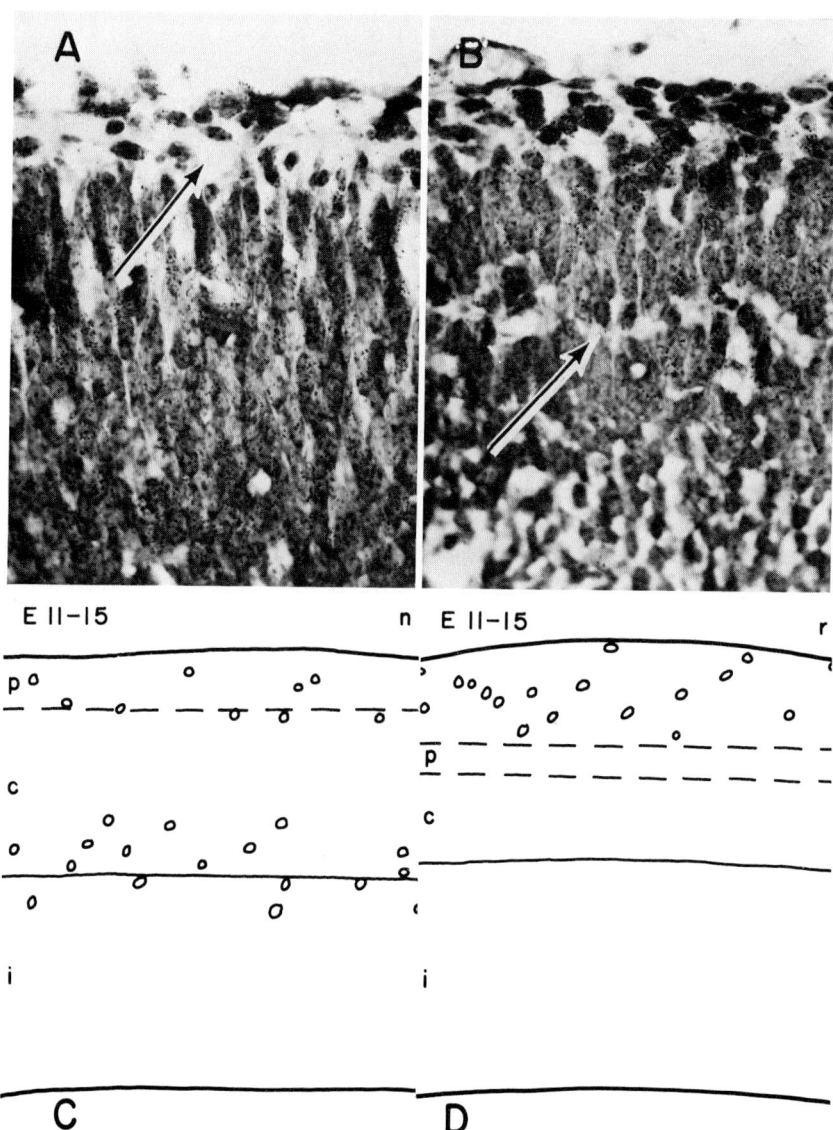

FIGURE 9. Neocortex of normal (A) and reeler (B) E15 embryos. Arrows indicate external plexiform and intermediate plexiform zones of normal and reeler cortex, respectively. (A) and (B), cresyl violet, ×540. Autoradiographic plots of the positions within the neocortex of heavily labeled neurons (circles) in normal (C) and reeler (D) E15 embryos. Neurons were marked at the time of their last division by ^{3}H-labeled thymidine injected into the pregnant dam on embryonic day E11. External and intermediate plexiform zones in normal and reeler cortex, respectively, are marked by p. The cortical plate and intermediate zones of both normal and reeler specimens are marked by c and i, respectively.

DISCUSSION

The cells of a class of neurons have in common a characteristic somatic and dendritic morphology and a characteristic pattern of axon deployment. These cytologic characteristics serve, generally, as the defining attributes of a cell class. The neurons of a class also have in common a characteristic pattern of afferent and efferent connections vis-a-vis neurons of the same or other classes. Further, the neurons of a class have in common a characteristic position relative to neurons of the same or other classes. These latter two characteristic patterns of connectivity and relative position, might, therefore, also be regarded as defining attributes of cell class.

Cells of each neuronal class in the neocortex and the piriform cortex of the reeler share the principal cytologic features of homologous cells in normal littermates: somatic size and shape, overall size, branching patterns, and character of spine investment of the dendritic arbor and general patterns of axon deployment. Evidently, these aspects of neuronal form are expressed normally despite mutation at the reeler locus. Orientation and alignment of somata and dendrites, and, to some extent, of axons are, in some instances, atypical and presumably reflect the capacity of neurons to adapt to abnormal positions rather than the direct consequences of the reeler mutation itself.

The patterns of intercellular connections, like principal cytologic features, also appear to be little modified in the reeler cortical malformation, at least in their qualitative aspects. Just as in the normal animal, the medium-sized pyramids of the neocortex are the principal cells of origin of the callosal axons, and large pyramids and polymorphic neurons are the cells of origin of diencephalic and other subcortical projections. The distribution of principal afferent systems to the neocortex and piriform cortex is normal in the tangential sense in the mutant. Terminals of extrinsic afferents to the neocortex and piriform cortex, as well as intrinsic neocortical intercellular connections, appear to be directed to the same neuronal classes in reeler as in the normal animal. As in the normal animal, terminals of axons of the lateral olfactory tract in reeler form only Type 1, asymmetric synapses with dendritic spines and branches. These are concentrated in a laminar zone, immediately subjacent to the tract. The observations of Dräger (1975) and Mangini and Pearlman (personal communication), in harmony with the findings of structural studies, establish by single cell recordings that many of the neurons of the visual cortex of reeler have normal receptive field properties with respect to size, shape, binocularity, and stimulus orientation requirements.

Collectively, these anatomic and physiologic observations imply that intercellular connections are formed according to an identical set of developmental rules in normal and reeler animals. These rules are, evidently, unaltered by the mutation of the reeler locus. To the extent that axons locate their target cells in reeler, they must do so according to rules that do not depend upon the positions of neurons.

The dystonic postures, the tremor, and the gait disturbance that are such conspicuous behavioral abnormalities in reeler may be only the most readily observable manifestations of CNS malfunction in the mutant. Functional abnormalities, obviously, may have their basis in quantitative rather than qualitative anomalies of connectivity. The number of terminals of the olfactory bulb projection upon the piriform cortex appears to be much reduced in the mutant. This may reflect a decreased efficiency of innervation posed by obstacles attendant upon neuronal malposition. The innervation ratio of spine to axon terminal in this system is much increased, and the terminals and the spines they engage are invested by dense glial envelopes. Similar abnormalities of innervation ratio and glial investment are characteristics of this neuropil during the period of restitution of connections after incomplete ablation of the olfactory bulb in the normal animal (Caviness et al., 1977). Conceivably, these cytologic features could reflect the incompleteness of innervation or even a continuous process of dennervation and reinnervation in the mutant neuropil.

The relative positions of neurons in the cortex are correlated with neuronal class in both normal and reeler cortex. The relative positions of neurons in the rodent cortex are less well correlated and may be only incidentally related to the sequence of cell formation. For example, large pyramids are segregated together in laminar fashion in both reeler and normal cortex, independent of whether they are formed on E11 or E14 (Caviness and Sidman, 1973b). This implies that the developmental mechanisms that govern neuronal position in the cortex of both normal and reeler animals are keyed to, and, in some way are, an expression of neuronal class. The systematic inversion of the normal relative positions of different classes of neurons in reeler suggests that the morphogenetic mechanism that governs cell position derives from the action of the gene at the reeler locus. The normal allele at this locus is dominant: the abnormal cortical pattern is not expressed in animals heterozygous for both normal and reeler alleles. The neuronal pattern created by the homozygous state of the reeler mutant allele is independent of substantial variations in genetic background in that it is indistinguishable in the C57 strain, in the C3H strain, or in animals resulting from cross-breeding between these two strains (Caviness et al., 1972).

The property conferred upon the cell by the gene at the reeler locus may be the first specific attribute of neuronal class to differentiate. The cell apparently becomes committed to its relative position in the cortex before its distinctive somatic and dendritic forms become established, and before its pattern of afferent and efferent connections is achieved (e.g., see Caviness et al., 1976). Evidently, that portion of the genetic code that controls cell position, that is, the gene at the reeler locus, is different and acts independently of those portions of the genetic code subserving other specific attributes of neuronal class, which appear to be normal in the mutant.

The events through which differential grouping of neurons by class occurs in the developing cortex, and the role played by the action of the gene at the reeler locus in these events are at present not understood. It is provocative, however, that the pattern of segregation of the earliest formed postmigratory neurons in the emerging cortical plate of the rostral forebrain is radically different in normal and reeler embryos. In the normal embryo, the earliest neurons to complete their migrations segregate into two subpopulations: one that remains superficially in the emerging external plexiform layer, and a second that comes to lie deeply in the subplate region. In reeler embryos, this primary segregation does not occur. The entire contingent of early postmigratory neurons remains at a superficial level, and a normally cell-sparse external plexiform zone does not develop. A variety of mechanisms might cause this early systematic error in the positional behavior of postmigratory neurons in reeler. For example, there might be a greater than normal affinity of the entire contingent for each other or for other non-neural structures, perhaps, at the superficial margin of the cortex. Alternatively, one might consider these cells to have a reduced affinity for, and hence fail to engage, structures at basal cortical levels. Such hypothetical mechanisms are based upon the premise that differential affinities between like and unlike cellular elements, deriving from the action of the gene at the reeler locus, govern the relative positions of neurons in the developing cortex (DeLong and Sidman, 1970).

ACKNOWLEDGMENTS

This study was supported in part by Public Health Service Grant H D 04147 and 1 R01 NS12005-02 from the National Institutes of Health, and by the Joseph P. Kennedy, Jr., Memorial Foundation.

REFERENCES

Caviness, V. S., Jr. (1973). Time of neuron origin in the hippocampus and dentate gyrus of normal and reeler mutant mice: an autoradiographic analysis, *J. Comp. Neurol.* **151**:113–120.

Caviness, V. S., Jr. (1975). Architectonic map of neocortex of the normal mouse, *J. Comp. Neurol.* **164**:247–264.

Caviness, V. S., Jr. (1976). Cellular and fiber patterns of the neocortex of the reeler mutant mouse, *J. Comp. Neurol.* **170**:435–448.

Caviness, V. S., Jr. (1977). Reeler mutant mice and laminar distribution of afferents, *Exp. Brain Res.,* in press.

Caviness, V. S., Jr., D. O. Frost, and N. L. Hayes (1976). Barrels in somatosensory cortex of normal and reeler mutant mice, *Neurosci. Lett.* **3**:7–14.

Caviness, V. S., Jr., M. G. Korde, and R. S. Williams (1977). Cellular events induced by ablation of the olfactory bulb in the molecular layer of the piriform cortex of the mouse, *Brain Res.,* in press.

Caviness, V. S., Jr., and R. L. Sidman (1972). Olfactory structures of the forebrain in the reeler mutant mouse, *J. Comp. Neurol.* **145**:85–104.

Caviness, V. S., Jr., and R. L. Sidman (1973a). Retrohippocampal, hippocampal, and related structures of the forebrain in the reeler mutant mouse, *J. Comp. Neurol.* **147**:235–253.

Caviness, V. S., Jr., and R. L. Sidman (1973b). Time of origin of corresponding cell classes in the cerebral cortex of normal and reeler mutant mice: an autoradiographic analysis, *J. Comp. Neurol.* **148**:141–152.

Caviness, V. S., Jr., D. K. So, and R. L. Sidman (1972). The hybrid reeler mouse, *J. Hered.* **63**:241–246.

Caviness, V. S., Jr., and C. H. Yorke, Jr. (1976). Interhemispheric neocortical connections of the corpus callosum in the reeler mutant mouse: a study based on anterograde and retrograde methods, *J. Comp. Neurol.* **170**:449–460.

Committee on Standard Genetic Nomenclature for Mice (1972). Standard karyotype of the mouse, Mus musculus, *J. Hered.* **63**:69–72.

DeLong, G. R. and R. L. Sidman (1970). Alignment defect of reaggregating cells in cultures of developing brains of reeler mutant mice, *Dev. Biol.* **22**:584–600.

Derer, P., V. S. Caviness, Jr., and R. L. Sidman (1977). Early cortical histogenesis in the primary olfactory cortex of the mouse, *Brain Res.,* in press.

Devor, M., V. S. Caviness, Jr., and P. Derer (1975). A normally laminated afferent projection to an abnormally laminated cortex: some olfactory connections in the reeler mouse, *J. Comp. Neurol.* **164**:471–482.

Dräger, U. C. (1975). Physiologic properties of cells in the primary visual cortex of the reeler mutant mouse, *Abstr. Annu. Meet. Soc. Neurosci.,* 5th, New York, p. 102.

Falconer, D. S. (1951). Two new mutants, "trembler" and "reeler," with neurological actions in the house mouse (Mus musculus L.), *J. Genet.* **50**:192–201.

Fink, R. P. and L. Heimer (1967). Two methods for selective silver impregnation of degenerating axons and their synaptic endings in the central nervous system, *Brain Res.* **4**:369–374.

Hamburgh, M. (1960). Observations on the neuropathology of "reeler," a neurobiological mutation in mice, *Experientia* **16**:460–461.

Hamburgh, M. (1963). Analysis of the postnatal developmental effects of "reeler," a neurological mutation in mice. A study in developmental genetics, *Dev. Biol.* **8**:165–185.

Haug, F.-M. Š. (1974). Light microscopical mapping of the hippocampal region, the pyriform cortex and the corticomedial amygdaloid nuclei of the rat with Timm's sulphide silver method. I. Area dentata, hippocampus and subiculum, *Z. Anat. Entwicklungsgesch.* **145**:1–27.

Karnovsky, M. J. (1965). A formaldehyde-gluteraldehyde fixative of high osmolarity for use in electron microscopy, *J. Cell Biol.* **27**:137A–138A.

LaVail, J. H., K. R. Winston, and A. Tish (1973). A method based on retrograde intraaxonal transport of protein for identification of cell bodies of origin of axons terminating within the central nervous system, *Brain Res.* **58**:470–477.

Lund, J. S. (1970). Organization of neurons in the visual cortex, area 17, of the monkey (Macaca mulatta), *J. Comp. Neurol.* **147**:455–496.

Meier, H. and W. G. Hoag (1962). The neuropathology of "reeler," a neuromuscular mutation in mice, *J. Neuropathol. Exp. Neurol.* **21**: 649–654.

Rakic, P. (1972). Mode of cell migration to the superficial layers of fetal monkey neocortex, *J. Comp. Neurol.* **145**:61–84.

Schneider, G. E. (1969). Two visual systems, *Science* **163**:895–902.

Sidman, R. L. (1970). Autoradiographic methods and principles for study of the nervous system with thymidine-H^3, pp. 252–274 in *Contemporary Research Methods in Neuroanatomy*, Nauta, W. J. H. and S. O. E. Ebbesson, eds. Springer-Verlag, New York.

Wise, S. P. (1975). The laminar organization of certain afferent and efferent fiber systems in the rat somatosensory cortex, *Brain Res.* **90**:139–142.

Woolsey, T. A. and H. Van der Loos (1970). The structural organization of layer IV in the somatosensory region (SI) of mouse cerebral cortex, *Brain Res.* **17**:205–242.

Yorke, C. H., Jr., and V. S. Caviness, Jr. (1975). Interhemispheric neocortical connections of the corpus callosum in the normal mouse: a study based on anterograde and retrograde methods, *J. Comp. Neurol.* **164**:233–246.

Genetic Dissection of the CNS With Mutant-Normal Mouse and Rat Chimeras

Richard J. Mullen

Harvard Medical School and Children's Hospital Medical Center, Boston, Massachusetts

One of the central problems in the genetic approach to the study of the central nervous system is to determine in which cell population the various mutant genes are acting most directly. Histologically, one might observe the most obvious effect of a mutation, but that effect could be the final consequence of one or several events secondary to the primary lesion. For example, degeneration of cell type "A" might be the result of the mutant gene acting in cell type "B" with which "A" must interact to survive. A mosaic system is needed that will allow genetically mutant cells access to genetically normal cells and/or a normal environment and vice versa so that we can determine in which cell type the mutant gene is acting. In mammals, such a mosaic system can be achieved by producing experimental chimeras (also known as allophenics or tetraparentals) containing mixtures of mutant and normal cells. In addition, the mosaic distribution of cells in chimeras provides the opportunity to study cell lineages and to determine whether any cell types or regions of the CNS are clonally derived.

After techniques for culturing preimplantation mouse embryos were worked out by Whitten (1956), techniques for producing mouse chimeras were developed by Tarkowski (1961) and Mintz (1962, 1965). The use of chimeric mice in a great variety of disciplines has been reviewed by Mintz (1974). More detailed descriptions of cell interactions in the developing nervous system may be found in the reviews by Sidman (1972, 1974) and Rakic (1974).

Production of Chimeras

The technique for producing mouse chimeras begins with the flushing of eight-cell embryos from the oviducts of pregnant mice on embryonic day 2 (vaginal plug = day 0). After removing the zona pellucida with the enzyme pronase, two embryos are placed in contact at 37°C in a small drop of culture medium and cultured overnight. In most of the studies described here, each pair consists of one embryo from a normal strain and one from a neurological mutant strain. The symbol "↔" indicates aggregation of two embryos (e. g., $rd/rd \leftrightarrow +/+$). By the following day, the embryos have grown together to form single blastocysts that are twice the normal size. It should be emphasized that the cells have mixed together; they have not fused. The blastocysts are surgically transplanted to the uteri of host females that have been made pseudopregnant by mating with vasectomized males. The original parental strains are usually chosen to differ in pigmentation genes so that the resulting chimeras can be overtly identified by coat color (Figure 1). The success rate varies, especially when working with the neurological mutants, but in general, 25 to 40% of the chimeric embryos transplanted will be born. Of those born, about 60 to 70% will be overt (i.e., multicolored) chimeras, and others will have cellular mosaicism internally, so that perhaps a total of 80 to 90% will actually be chimeric. There does not appear to be any developmental selection against chimerism, for the embryos are as viable as similarly treated nonchimeric embryos (Bowman and McLaren, 1970; Mullen and Carter, 1973), and adult chimeras are normal in size and healthy. Details of the techniques we use have been presented elsewhere (Mullen and Whitten, 1971; Mullen and Carter, 1973).

The chimeric rats were produced by similar techniques, except that the eight-cell embryos were collected on embryonic day 3, and host females were pregnant rather than pseudopregnant (Mullen and LaVail, 1976).

Retinal Degeneration

One of the first areas of the central nervous system to be studied with chimeric mice was the retina (Mintz and Sanyal, 1970; Wegmann, LaVail, and Sidman, 1971). In retinal degeneration (rd) chimeras, $rd/rd \leftrightarrow +/+$ (i.e., chimeras derived from aggregation of embryos homozygous for rd with genetically normal embryos), patches of normal retina, completely degenerated retina, and patches with an intermediate

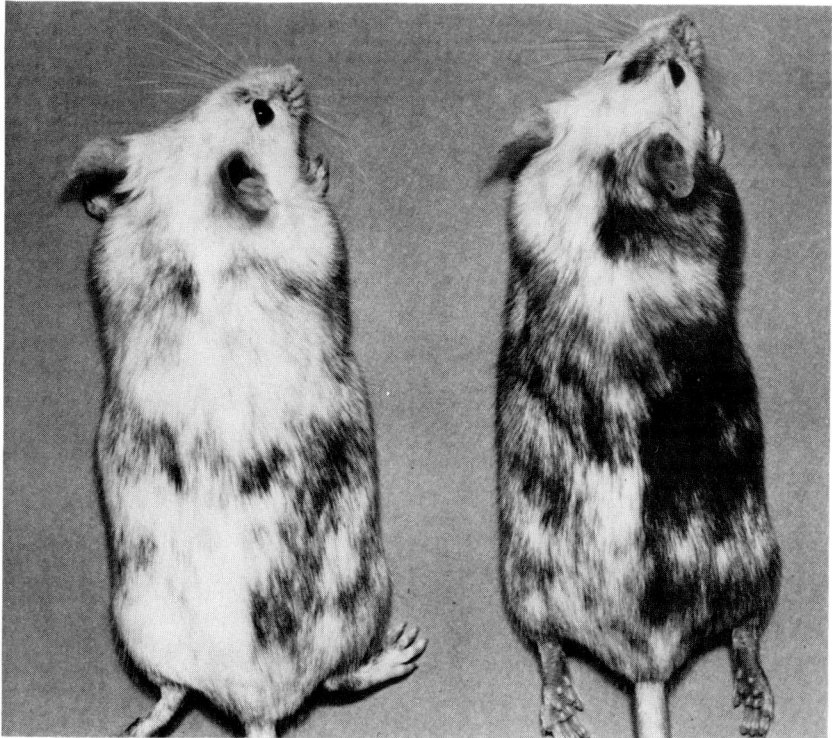

FIGURE 1. Two chimeras derived from aggregation of embryos from an albino strain with ones from a pigmented strain.

amount of photoreceptor degeneration were observed. In chimeras that had both pigmentation and retinal degeneration mosaicism, Mintz and Sanyal (1970) reported that there was no correlation between the genotype of the pigment epithelial cells (i.e., either pigmented or albino) and the underlying photoreceptors (i.e., normal or degenerated), suggesting that the two cell types have independent cell lineages.

The pigment epithelium interacts with photoreceptor cells in several ways, so that a defect in pigment epithelial cells could secondarily affect photoreceptor cells. To determine whether the pigment epithelium was involved in any way in the photoreceptor degeneration, Dr. Matthew LaVail and I examined retinal degeneration chimeras that had the pigmentation marker for pigment epithelial cells. Both of the possible combinations of genotypes, $rd/rd\ +/+ \leftrightarrow +/+\ c/c$ (rd/rd epithelial cells pigmented) and *rd/rd c/c* ↔ +/+ +/+ (*rd/rd* epithelial cells albino, *c/c*), were studied. Photoreceptor cell degeneration was found under both normal and mutant pigment epithelium and, likewise, normal photoreceptor cells were found under both types of pigment epithelium. Autoradiographic analysis indicated that rod outer segment renewal in photoreceptor cells that were under mutant pigment epithelium was proceeding at the normal rate. In addition, electron micrographs showed that genetically mutant pigment epithelial cells were functioning normally in phagocytizing shed outer segment discs. Thus, the pigment epithelial cell does not appear to be a primary site of *rd* gene action. The *rd* gene is acting in the neural retina, probably in the photoreceptor cell, although an independent cell marker is needed to prove this. These results have recently been described in detail (LaVail and Mullen, 1976*a*, *b*).

Retinal Dystrophy in Rats

The inherited retinal dystrophy (*rdy*) disease in rats is quite distinct from the mouse *rd* disease. In dystrophic rats, relatively normal rod outer segments are formed, but then the photoreceptor cells degenerate between 20 to 60 days (Dowling and Sidman, 1962). It has been postulated, however, that the disease may be primarily a pigment epithelial cell disorder because several laboratories have shown that in dystrophic rats, these cells fail to phagocytize shed rod outer segment discs (Herron, Riegel, Myers, and Rubin, 1969; Bok and Hall, 1971; LaVail, Sidman, and O'Neil, 1972) as they do in normal animals (Young and Bok, 1969). This failure leads to an accumulation of debris between the outer segments and the pigment epithelium.

Where is the primary site of *rdy* gene action? Is the gene acting in the pigment epithelial cell? Or is it acting in the photoreceptor cell, perhaps resulting in an altered outer segment that the pigment epithelial cell does not recognize? Or is there some factor extrinsic to the eye that alters either the pigment epithelial or photoreceptor cell? Although when we started this project chimeric rats had never been made (Mayer and Fritz [1974] have subsequently reported producing chimeric rats), we felt that a few chimeras might answer the question because of the high degree of mosaicism seen in the retinas of mouse chimeras. As with the mouse chimeras, pigmentation was used as a cell marker for the pigment epithelial cells; the *rdy/rdy* pigment epithelial cells, which were homozygous for the pink-eye dilution (p) gene, were nonpigmented, while the genetically normal pigment epithelial cells were pigmented. When we examined the retinas from the two chimeras we produced, accumulation of debris and/or photoreceptor degeneration was found underlying all of the 200 patches of mutant pigment epithelium examined (Figure 2), and only normal-appearing photoreceptors were found underlying genetically normal pigment epithelium (Mullen and LaVail, 1976). Thus, in rats with inherited retinal dystrophy, although it is the photoreceptor cell that degenerates, the *rdy* gene is actually acting in the pigment epithelial cell.

Although it has not affected our interpretation of the pigment epithelial cell as being the site of gene action, it is significant to note that there was some amelioration of the rate and severity of the disease, especially in regions near normal pigment epithelium and where outer segments leaned toward or into a patch of normal pigment epithelium (described by Mullen and LaVail, 1976).

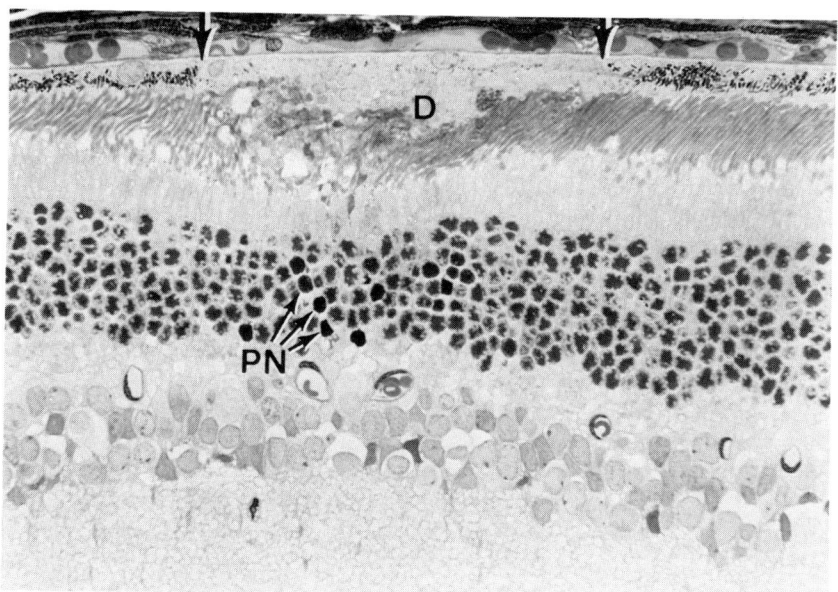

FIGURE 2. Section of retina from a rat retinal dystrophy chimera (*rdy/rdy p/p* ↔ +/+ +/+). Outer segment debris (D) and photoreceptor cell degeneration (pyknotic nuclei, PN) are present only under mutant *rdy/rdy* pigment epithelium (i.e., nonpigmented, *p/p*, pigment epithelium, between vertical arrows). A 1- to 1.5-μm plastic section was stained with toluidine blue. From Mullen and LaVail (1976).

β-Glucuronidase as a Purkinje Cell Marker

When we turn our attention to the brains of chimeras we, of course, lose pigmentation as an independent cell marker. What is needed, therefore, is some way to make cells from one parental component appear "pigmented," while cells from the other component remain "nonpigmented." Strains of mice (e.g., C57BL/6) that are homozygous for the Gus^b allele at the glucuronidase locus have normal or high β-glucuronidase enzyme activity, whereas other strains (e.g., C3H/HeJ) that are homozygous for the Gus^h allele have low enzyme activity. Histochemistry for β-glucuronidase has been used previously as a cell marker for chimeric livers (Condamine, Custer, and Mintz, 1971); Gus^b cells showed intense red staining, whereas Gus^h cells showed little or no staining. The standard histochemical techniques, however, are too insensitive for use on the central nervous system. Feder (1976) has developed a more sensitive histochemical technique, and we have found that with this technique, β-glucuronidase can be used as a cell marker for cerebellar Purkinje cells and perhaps other cell types in the CNS (Mullen and Sidman, unpublished observations). The brains were processed according to methods described by Feder, except that the mice were perfused with cold 4°C fixative. Sections were cut at 7 μm and histochemically stained in a reaction solution containing hexazotized pararosanilin and naphthol-AS-BI-β-D-glucuronide (Sigma Chemical Co.) (Hayashi, Nakajima, and Fishman, 1964) with 5% gelatin added. The enzyme reaction resulted in a red precipitate. Methyl green was used as a counterstain. In Gus^b/Gus^b (i.e., normal or high activity) mice, virtually every Purkinje cell showed enzyme activity, whereas Gus^h/Gus^h (low activity) mice exhibited no enzyme activity in Purkinje cells (Figure 3A and B). In these studies, the sections were stained for 2 or 3 days (i.e., 48 to 72 h) with the reaction solution changed daily (because the reaction solution deteriorates with time, the 2 to 3 days probably equals approximately 15 to 25 h actual staining time if the solution were changed more often). In $Gus^b/Gus^b \leftrightarrow Gus^h/Gus^h$ chimeras, Purkinje cell mosaicism is obvious; some cells are stained and are therefore from the Gus^b component, whereas other cells are not stained and are therefore Gus^h (Figure 3C).

It should be emphasized that both Gus^b/Gus^b and Gus^h/Gus^h mice are normal and healthy and that, as far as we know, β-glucuronidase has nothing to do with any of the cerebellar mutants to be discussed. Also, because β-glucuronidase is an independent locus, it is possible to make either chimeras in which the genetically mutant cells have high glucuronidase activity, or ones in which the mutant cells have low

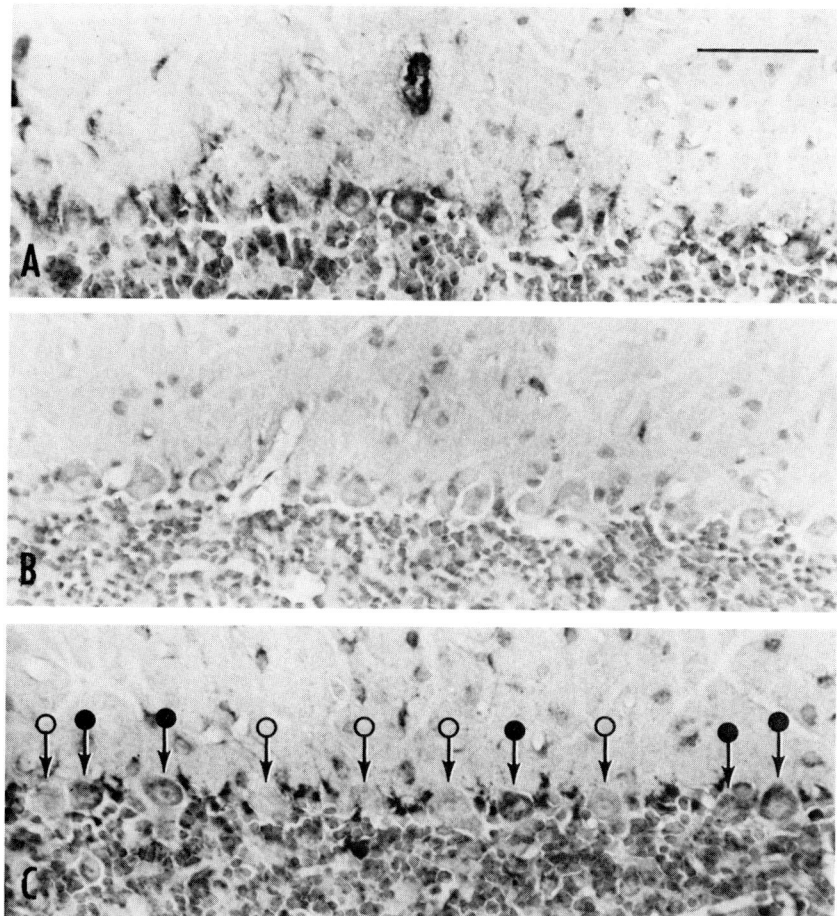

FIGURE 3. Histochemistry of β-glucuronidase activity in mouse cerebellar Purkinje cells. The red precipitate deposited at sites of enzyme activity appears dark gray or black in these photographs. (A) Cerebellum of a Gus^b/Gus^b control. Every Purkinje cell has enzyme activity. (B) Cerebellum of Gus^h/Gus^h control. None of the Purkinje cells show enzyme activity. (C) Cerebellum of a $Gus^b/Gus^b \leftrightarrow Gus^h/Gus^h$ chimera. Some of the Purkinje cells are stained and are, therefore, Gus^b/Gus^b (arrows with filled circles); other cells are not stained and are, therefore, Gus^h/Gus^h (arrows with open circles). Bar in A represents 50 μm.

glucuronidase activity. In all of the following studies, however, the genetically mutant cells are Gus^b/Gus^b and therefore have high glucuronidase activity, whereas the genetically normal cells have low activity (i.e., are not stained).

Purkinje Cell Degeneration

The first cerebellar mutant I would like to discuss is a new mutant, Purkinje cell degeneration (*pcd*), which we have recently described (Mullen, Eicher, and Sidman, 1976). Adult *pcd/pcd* mutants have virtually no Purkinje cells; this must be the result of postnatal degeneration, since they have a normal number of Purkinje cells up to about 3 weeks after birth. The subsequent degeneration is rapid, occurring in 2 to 3 weeks.

In three adult *pcd/pcd* ↔ +/+ chimeras, we found that in this mosaic environment some Purkinje cells degenerate, but others survive. What is the genotype of these surviving cells? Are these the +/+ cells, or is the gene acting extrinsically, in which case the surviving population should contain both +/+ and *pcd/pcd* cells? One of our *pcd* chimeras was also mosaic for β-glucuronidase. The *pcd/pcd* component had high glucuronidase, whereas the +/+ component had low glucuronidase (i.e., *pcd/pcd* Gus^b/Gus^b ↔ +/+ Gus^h/Gus^h). When we stained the sections for enzyme activity, none of the surviving Purkinje cells stained (Figure 4); therefore, these were the +/+ cells; the *pcd/pcd* Purkinje cells had all degenerated (Mullen, 1975, 1977). This indicates that the *pcd* gene acts intrinsically within the Purkinje cells. Although there is

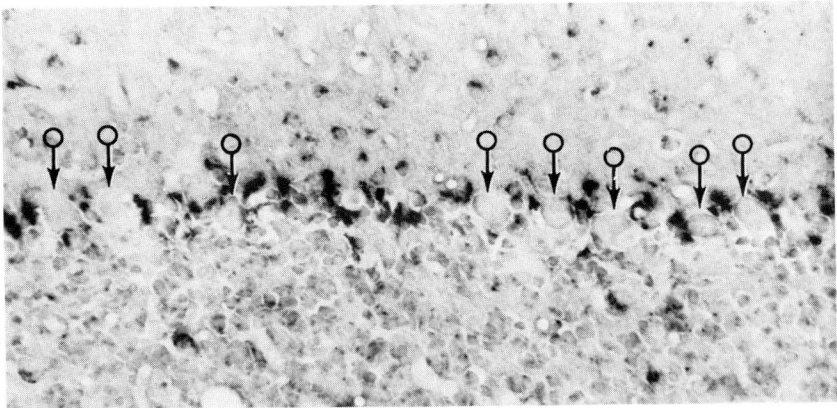

FIGURE 4. Purkinje cell lamina of a Purkinje cell degeneration, *pcd/pcd* Gus^b/Gus^b ↔ +/+ Gus^h/Gus^h, chimera. There are gaps where Purkinje cells have degenerated. None of the surviving Purkinje cells (arrows with open circles) exhibit enzyme activity (i.e., they are Gus^h/Gus^h) and are, therefore, genetically normal, +/+ cells. The intense staining in the Purkinje cell layer is probably in glia. Same magnification and exposure as in Figure 3.

the possibility that the gene acts in another cell type that has a mosaic distribution identical to the Purkinje cells, this seems to be highly improbable, especially when we consider the extremely fine mosaic pattern of Purkinje cells as described below.

This study also does not rule out the possibility that the gene acts in other cell types and, in fact, we know that the *pcd* gene does act elsewhere. Mutants also exhibit a slow loss of photoreceptor cells (Mullen and LaVail, 1975) and a loss of mitral cells in the olfactory bulb (Mullen et al., 1976). Speculations about what these three neuronal cell types have in common were somewhat dampened when we found that *pcd/pcd* males also have abnormal sperm. These pleiotropic effects of the *pcd* locus were also expressed in the chimeras, but at present we have no evidence whether the gene is also acting intrinsically within these other cell types.

Reeler

The problem in the cerebellum of the reeler (*rl*) mutant is basically the same as in the cerebral cortex that Dr. Caviness described in the preceding paper (see references cited by Caviness, 1977). In the cerebellum of reeler mutants, the Purkinje cells are in the wrong position, most of them lying below the granule cells. In addition, foliation is so drastically affected that there are practically no folia (compare near normal foliation in Figure 5A with that of reeler in Figure 6A). Are the Purkinje cells in abnormal positions because the reeler gene is acting within them, causing them to take up abnormal positions, or are factors extrinsic to the Purkinje cell responsible for aberrant positioning? Figure 5A shows a section of the cerebellum from a *rl/rl* ↔ +/+ chimera. The foliation is normal and the Purkinje cells are in normal position except for a small patch of aberrantly positioned cells in the declive-tuber vermis. The genetically reeler cells were of the high β-glucuronidase genotype (Gus^b), and the genetically normal cells were of the low genotype. Histochemistry of nearby sections revealed that some of the aberrantly positioned cells in this small patch were stained and were, therefore, *rl/rl*, but others were not stained and were, therefore, genetically normal, +/+ cells. Thus, there were genetically normal cells in abnormal position.

There were also genetically reeler cells in the normal Purkinje cell layer. In fact, in the section shown in Figure 5A, approximately 50% of the normally positioned Purkinje cells were genetically reeler. This,

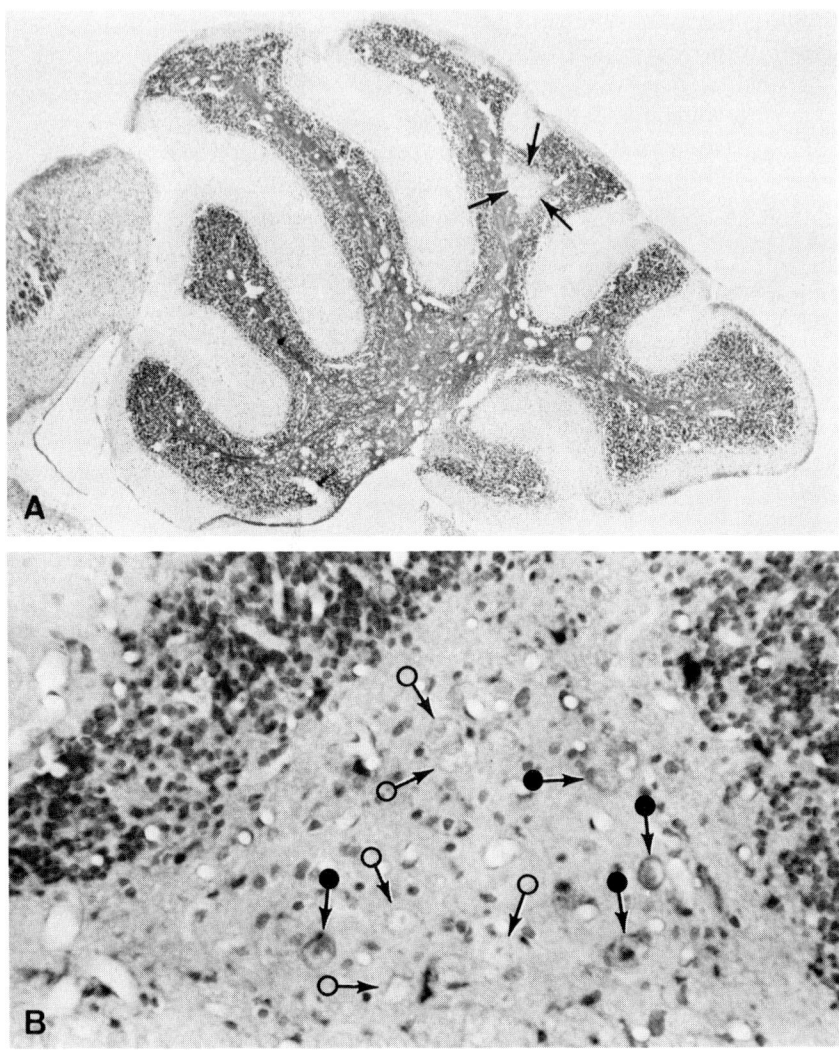

FIGURE 5. Cerebellum of a reeler chimera (rl/rl Gus^b/Gus^b ↔ +/+ Gus^h/Gus^h). (A) Sagittal section of whole cerebellum stained with cresyl violet and luxol fast blue. Except for a small patch (arrows) of aberrantly positioned Purkinje cells, the cortex appears normal. (B) Adjacent section through the same patch as shown in A, stained for β-glucuronidase. The Purkinje cells that are stained (i.e., Gus^b/Gus^b, arrows with filled circles) are genetically reeler; those cells that are not stained (i.e., Gus^h/Gus^h, arrows with open circles) are genetically normal, +/+ cells.

however, is somewhat less significant than the aberrantly positioned normal cells, for in homozygous reeler mutants some Purkinje cells do attain normal positions. Quantitatively, however, there were many more cells in normal position in the chimera.

Figure 6B shows the cerebellum of another reeler chimera, one that exhibited reeler behavior. β-Glucuronidase histochemistry showed that approximately 99% of the Purkinje cells (in both normal and abnormal positions) were genetically reeler, and yet the cerebellum as a whole was more normal appearing than a reeler cerebellum with more Purkinje cells in proper position, and, perhaps as a consequence, better developed folia. In this chimera also, there were genetically normal Purkinje cells in abnormal positions (Figure 6C).

The above data, in particular the presence of the genetically normal cells in an abnormal position, suggest that the Purkinje cells are not being positioned according to their own genetic information, but rather by factors extrinsic to the Purkinje cells (Mullen, 1975; Mullen and Sidman, manuscript in preparation).

Staggerer

The last mutant I would like to describe is the staggerer (sg) mutant (Sidman, Lane, and Dickie, 1962). In this mutant, the cerebellar granule cells degenerate after they have migrated to the internal granule cell layer (Sidman, 1968). However, several reports, including those by Landis (1971), Sidman (1972), and Hirano and Dembitzer (1975), have shown that there are also abnormalities in the Purkinje cell, the most intriguing being the absence of tertiary branchlet spines—the site of synapse between granule cell parallel fibers and the Purkinje cell dendrite. Again, the question of cellular site of gene action arises. Does the staggerer gene act in the granule cell, Purkinje cell, both, or neither (e.g., defect in a circulating metabolite)? Dr. Karl Herrup and I have begun to study staggerer chimeras, and the first one we examined was remarkably informative and was described in detail elsewhere at the Annual Meeting of the Society for Neuroscience (Herrup and Mullen, 1976). A section from the lateral hemisphere of this chimera is shown in Figure 7. Using β-glucuronidase as a marker, we found that the Purkinje cells that were normal in appearance and in position were genetically normal. However, in the granule cell layer, there were unusually large numbers of medium-sized cells (too numerous to be Golgi type II cells) that resembled staggerer Purkinje cells. The glucuronidase cell marker

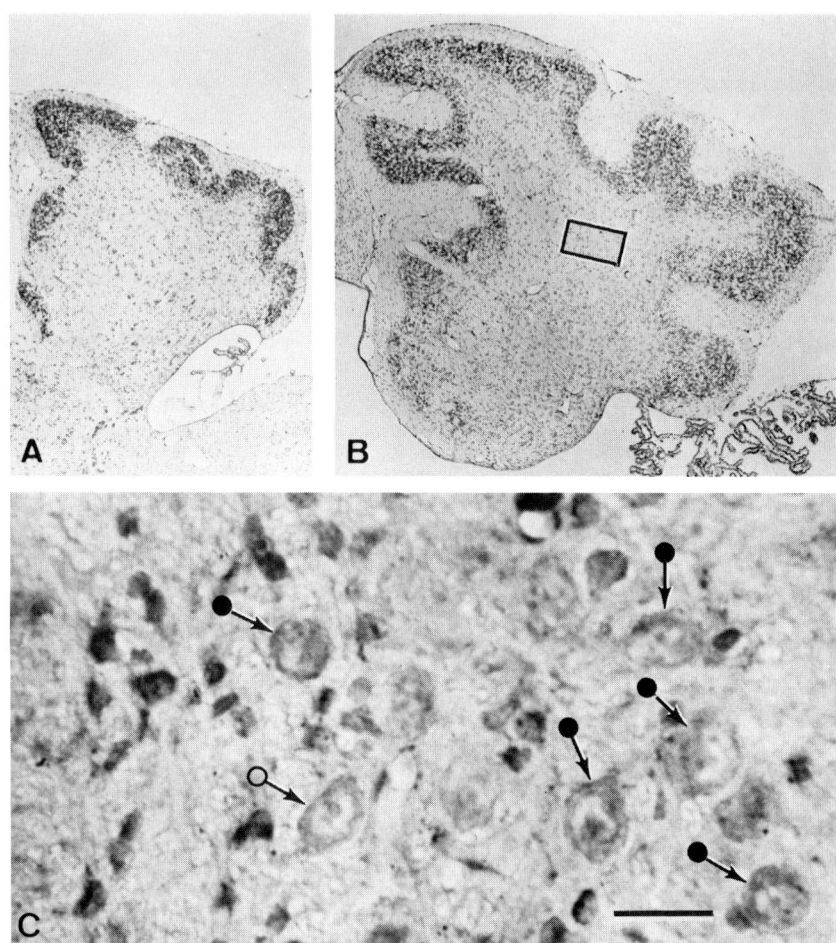

FIGURE 6. Cerebella of reeler and reeler chimera. (A) Cerebellum of adult homozygous reeler mutant showing almost complete absence of folia. (B) Cerebellum of a reeler chimera (same magnification as A) showing better developed folia but not normal (see Figure 5A). (C) Higher magnification of box in B showing Purkinje cells that lie deep to the granule cells. β-Glucuronidase histochemistry indicates that one of the Purkinje cells (arrow with open circle) is genetically normal; the other cells are genetically reeler (arrows with filled circles). Bar in C represents 20 μm.

indicated that these abnormal cells were genetically sg/sg. We interpret this to mean that the sg gene does act intrinsically within the Purkinje cell. Unfortunately, our cell marker does not work on granule cells (i.e., we could not determine the genotype of the granule cells in the chimera),

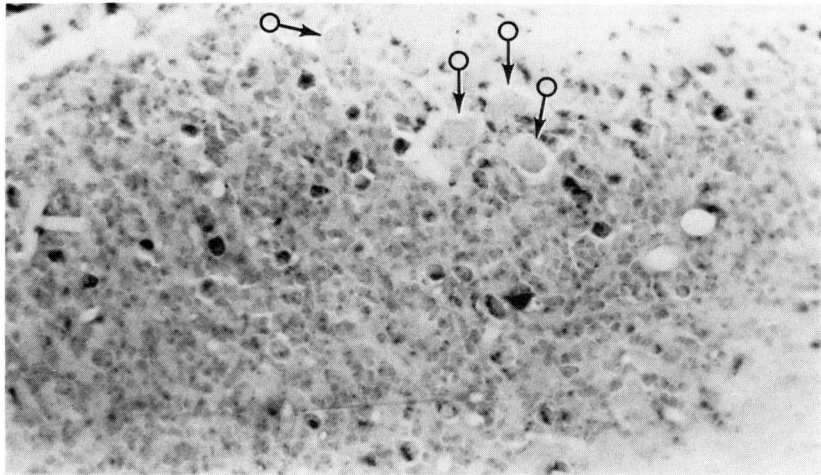

FIGURE 7. Lateral hemisphere of the cerebellum of a staggerer chimera (sg/sg Gus^b/Gus^b ↔ +/+ Gus^h/Gus^h) stained for β-glucuronidase. Purkinje cells that are normal in size and position (arrows with open circles) are genetically normal. Numerous medium-sized neurons in granule cell layer resemble staggerer Purkinje cells; they are intensely stained for β-glucuronidase and are, therefore, sg/sg in genotype.

so we cannot yet rule out the possibility that the gene also acts in granule cells. This staggerer chimera also led us to reexamine the staggerer mutant, for it revealed effects on Purkinje cells that were previously not fully appreciated. In particular, the effect of the sg gene on Purkinje cells appears to vary in different regions of the cerebellum (Herrup and Mullen, 1976).

Site of Gene Action: A Summary

The results of our studies are summarized in Table 1. It is interesting to note how frequently the most obviously affected cell type does not appear to be the primary site of gene action (rdy, rl, and sg if future studies rule out sg granule cells). To this list we should also add the studies on muscular dystrophy chimeras by Dr. Alan Peterson, who has shown that the dy gene also acts extrinsically (Peterson, 1974, 1976). With dystrophic chimeras, Peterson has shown that muscles that are entirely dystrophic in genotype (determined by isozyme analysis) can be completely normal in appearance.

I would like to emphasize that when we say that a gene acts in a particular cell type we do not rule out the possibility that it might also act elsewhere. Conversely, when we say that a gene acts extrinsically or that

TABLE 1. *Sites of mutant gene action revealed by rodent chimeras*

Mutant gene	Degenerating cell	Site of gene action
Retinal degeneration (rd)	Photoreceptor	Probably photoreceptor, not pigment epithelium
Rat retinal dystrophy (rdy)	Photoreceptor	Pigment epithelium
Purkinje cell degeneration (pcd)	Purkinje cell	Purkinje cell
Staggerer (sg)	Granule cell	Purkinje cell (granule cell?)
Reeler (rl)	No degeneration, aberrantly positioned Purkinje cells[a]	Factors extrinsic to aberrantly positioned cells

[a] An example of a cortical neuron affected by rl mutation.

it does not act in a particular cell type, we mean that if it is acting there, its action alone is not sufficient to elicit the mutant phenotype. Differences between the multitude of cell types in the nervous system may result from quantitative differences in gene expression, as well as from qualitative differences and the local milieu.

Mosaic Pattern

In addition to being useful in determining sites of gene action, chimeras provide material for studying mosaic patterns in the central nervous system. Most cortical neuronal cell types, including Purkinje cells, are born in germinal centers, such as embryonic ventricular zones, and then migrate to the position they will occupy in the adult cortex (reviewed by Sidman and Rakic, 1973). From the earliest stages, when the nervous system is a columnar epithelium, the orientation and migration of cells appears radial. One might expect that daughter cells would tend to remain in proximity to one another, giving rise to the appearance of patches or clones in adults, such as those seen in the coats of chimeras (e.g., Figure 1).

In studying Purkinje cell degeneration chimeras, I have done a serial reconstruction of part of one folium, the lobulus centralis, to determine the distribution of surviving Purkinje cells. The positions of surviving Purkinje cells along the Purkinje cell lamina in 18 20-μm sections were marked on tracing paper. The tracings were aligned by superimposing them, and then, after marking a fixed point, a map reader was used to determine the position of Purkinje cells in linear distance along the lamina. The data points were then plotted in a straight line on graph paper, with the distance between adjacent lines being scaled to the thickness of the section. In the folium studied, 75% of the Purkinje cells had degenerated. The distribution of the 25% that survived is shown in Figure 8. The mosaicism is extremely fine and appears indistinguishable from a random distribution of cells and spaces. There is no obvious pattern, nor are there any obvious clones. It seems unlikely that this distribution is the result of rearrangement of Purkinje cells after degeneration of the mutant cells, since in β-glucuronidase chimeras (i.e., $Gus^b/Gus^b \leftrightarrow Gus^h/Gus^h$), in which there was no cell loss, the mosaicism in single sections is equally fine. This fine mosaicism of Purkinje cells in single sections has also been observed recently by Dewey, Gervais, and Mintz (1976) by using a different cell-marking technique. These results suggest that in mammals there may be considerable cell mixing, either during cell migration to the cortical plate or during subsequent growth of the cortex, and that additional studies are obviously warranted. When improved cell markers become available, it will be particularly interesting to examine other regions of the CNS, because Purkinje cells may be the exception, rather than the rule, since they are subjected to thinning out into a single cell lamina during the massive foliation of the cerebellum that is unique in the development of the mouse CNS.

SUMMARY

In the past, the use of genetic mutations to dissect the intricacies of the developing and mature CNS of mammals has proven to be a powerful approach. It has been so useful in elucidating cell interactions that we are now keenly aware that the most obvious effect of a mutation may not be the primary action of the gene. The studies presented here have demonstrated that by using mutant $\leftrightarrow$ normal chimeras to aid in this genetic dissection, we can begin to unravel the problem of where these mutant genes are acting and expose new facets of gene expression and cell interactions. Our studies indicate that in mice, the retinal degeneration (rd) gene probably acts in the photoreceptor cell, whereas in rats the retinal dystrophy (rdy) gene acts in the pigment epithelial cell. In the mouse cerebellum, the Purkinje cell degeneration (pcd) and staggerer (sg) genes act in the Purkinje cell, whereas the reeler (rl) gene appears to act extrinsically to the aberrantly positioned Purkinje cells. In

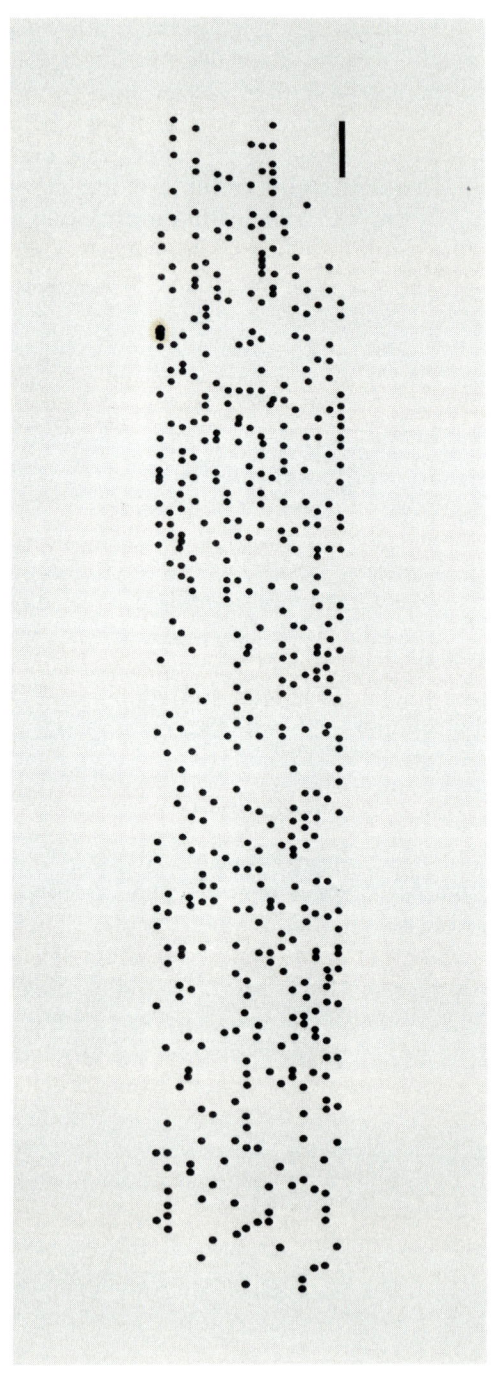

addition, the study of the mosaic distribution of cells in chimeras has the potential of adding a new dimension to the study of cell migrations and movements within the developing nervous system. The very fine, perhaps random, distribution of Purkinje cells in chimeras suggests there may be more cell mixing in the developing nervous system than we had previously thought.

ACKNOWLEDGMENTS

In many of the above studies I was fortunate to have the unique opportunity to collaborate with Drs. Matthew M. LaVail, Karl Herrup, and Richard L. Sidman. This research was supported by a Basil O'Connor Starter Research Grant from The National Foundation-March of Dimes (R.J.M.) and by grants EY01202 (M. M. LaVail) and NS11237 (R. L. Sidman) from the National Institutes of Health.

REFERENCES

Bok, D. and M. O. Hall (1971). The role of the pigment epithelium in the etiology of inherited retinal dystrophy in the rat, *J. Cell Biol.* **49**:664–682.

Bowman, P. and A. McLaren (1970). Viability and growth of mouse embryos after in vitro culture and fusion, *J. Embryol. Exp. Morphol.* **23**:693–704.

Caviness, V. S., Jr. (1977). Reeler mutant mouse: a genetic experiment in developing mammalian cortex, pp. 27–46 in *Society for Neuroscience Symposia*, Vol. 2, Cowan, W. M. and J. A. Ferrendelli, eds. Society for Neuroscience, Bethesda, Md.

Condamine, H., R. P. Custer, and B. Mintz (1971). Pure-strain and genetically mosaic liver tumors histochemically identified with the β-glucuronidase marker in allophenic mice, *Proc. Natl. Acad. Sci. U.S.A.* **68**:2032–2036.

Dewey, M. J., A. G. Gervais, and B. Mintz (1976). Brain and ganglion development from two genotype classes of cells in allophenic mice, *Dev. Biol.* **50**:68–81.

Dowling, J. and R. L. Sidman (1962). Inherited retinal dystrophy in the rat, *J. Cell Biol.* **14**:73–109.

Feder, N. (1976). Solitary cells and enzyme exchange in tetraparental mice, *Nature (London)* **263**:67–69.

Hayashi, M., Y. Nakajima, and W. H. Fishman (1964). The cytologic demonstration of β-glucuronidase employing naphthol-AS-BI-β-D-glucuronide and hexazonium pararosanilin; a preliminary report, *J. Histochem. Cytochem.* **12**:293–297.

FIGURE 8. Serial reconstruction of part of a folium of a Purkinje cell degeneration, *pcd/pcd* ↔ +/+ , chimera showing the distribution of surviving +/+ Purkinje cells after 75% of the Purkinje cells (presumably all *pcd/pcd*) had degenerated. The Figure represents the location of cells as they would appear if the folia were flattened out and viewed from above. The bar represents 100 μm. The dots are approximately to scale (i.e., the size of an average Purkinje cell).

Herron, W. L., Jr., B. W. Riegel, O. E. Myers, and M. L. Rubin (1969). Retinal dystrophy in the rat—a pigment epithelial disease, *Invest. Ophthalmol.* **8:**595–604.

Herrup, K. and R. J. Mullen (1976). Intrinsic Purkinje cell abnormalities in staggerer mutant mice revealed by analysis of a staggerer ↔ normal chimera, *Abstr. Annu. Meet. Soc. Neurosci.,* 6th, Toronto, p. 101.

Hirano, A. and H. M. Dembitzer (1975). The fine structure of staggerer cerebellum, *J. Neuropathol. Exp. Neurol.* **34:**1–11.

Landis, D. (1971). Cerebellar cortical development in the staggerer mutant mouse, *J. Cell Biol.* **51:**159 (Abstr.).

LaVail, M. M. and R. J. Mullen (1976*a*). Role of the pigment epithelium in inherited retinal degeneration analyzed with experimental mouse chimeras, *Exp. Eye Res.* **23:**227–245.

LaVail, M. M. and R. J. Mullen (1976*b*). Experimental chimeras: a new approach to the study of inherited retinal degeneration in laboratory animals, pp. 153–173 in *Retinitis Pigmentosa: Clinical Implications of Current Research*, Landers, M. B., M. L. Wolbarsht, J. E. Dowling, and A. M. Laties, eds. Plenum Press, New York.

LaVail, M. M., R. L. Sidman, and D. O'Neil (1972). Photoreceptor-pigment epithelial cell relationships in rats with inherited retinal degeneration, *J. Cell Biol.* **53:**185–209.

Mayer, J. F., Jr., and H. I. Fritz (1974). The culture of preimplantation rat embryos and the production of allophenic rats, *J. Reprod. Fertil.* **39:**1–10.

Mintz, B. (1962). Formation of genotypically mosaic mouse embryos, *Am. Zool.* **2:**432 (Abstr.).

Mintz, B. (1965). Genetic mosaicism in adult mice of quadriparental lineage, *Science* **148:**1232–1233.

Mintz, B. (1974). Gene control of mammalian differentiation, *Annu. Rev. Genet.* **8:**411–470.

Mintz, B. and S. Sanyal (1970). Clonal origin of the mouse visual retina mapped from genetically mosaic eyes, *Genetics (Suppl.)* **64:**43–44.

Mullen, R. J. (1975). Neurological mutants: use of chimeras to determine site of gene action, *Genetics (Suppl.)* **80:**56.

Mullen, R. J. (1977). Site of gene action and Purkinje cell mosaicism in *pcd* ↔ + chimeric mice, submitted for publication.

Mullen, R. J. and S. C. Carter (1973). Efficiency of transplanting normal, zona-free, and chimeric embryos to one and both uterine horns of inbred and hybrid mice, *Biol. Reprod.* **9:**111–115.

Mullen, R. J., E. M. Eicher, and R. L. Sidman (1976). Purkinje cell degeneration, a new neurological mutation in the mouse, *Proc. Natl. Acad. Sci. U.S.A.* **73:**208–212.

Mullen, R. J. and M. M. LaVail (1975). Two new types of retinal degeneration in cerebellar mutant mice, *Nature (London)* **258:**528–530.

Mullen, R. J. and M. M. LaVail (1976). Inherited retinal dystrophy: primary defect in pigment epithelium determined with experimental rat chimeras, *Science* **192:**799–801.

Mullen, R. J. and W. K. Whitten (1971). Relationship of genotype and degree of chimerism in coat color to sex ratios and gametogenesis in chimeric mice, *J. Exp. Zool.* **178:**165–176.

Peterson, A. C. (1974). Chimaera mouse study shows absence of disease in genotypically dystrophic muscle, *Nature (London)* **248:**561–564.

Peterson, A. C. (1976). Developmental interaction of dystrophic and normal cells in the neuromuscular system of mouse chimeras, *Abstr. Annu. Meet. Soc. Neurosci.*, 6th, Toronto, p. 1045.

Rakic, P. (1974). Intrinsic and extrinsic factors influencing the shape of neurons and their assembly into neuronal circuits, pp. 112–132 in *Frontiers in Neurology and Neuroscience Research*, Seeman, P. and G. M. Brown, eds. Toronto Univ. Press, Toronto.

Sidman, R. L. (1968). Development of interneuronal connections in brains of mutant mice, pp. 163–193 in *Physiological and Biochemical Aspects of Nervous Integration*, Carlson, F. D., ed. Prentice-Hall, Englewood Cliffs, N.J.

Sidman, R. L. (1972). Cell interactions in developing mammalian central nervous system, pp. 1–13 in *Cell Interactions: Proceedings of the Third Lepetit Colloquium*, Silvestri, L. G., ed. North-Holland Publishing Co., Amsterdam.

Sidman, R. L. (1974). Contact interaction among developing brain cells, pp. 221–253 in *The Cell Surface in Development*, Moscona, A. A., ed. John Wiley and Sons, New York.

Sidman, R. L., P. Lane, and M. Dickie (1962). Staggerer, a new mutation in the mouse affecting the cerebellum, *Science* **137:**610–612.

Sidman, R. L. and P. Rakic (1973). Neuronal migration, with special reference to developing human brain: a review, *Brain Res.* **62:**1–35.

Tarkowski, A. K. (1961). Mouse chimaeras developed from fused eggs, *Nature (London)* **190:**857–860.

Wegmann, T. G., M. M. LaVail, and R. L. Sidman (1971). Patchy retinal degeneration in tetraparental mice, *Nature (London)* **230:**333–334.

Whitten, W. K. (1956). Culture of tubal mouse ova, *Nature (London)* **177:**96.

Young, R. W. and D. Bok (1969). Participation of the retinal pigment epithelium in the rod outer segment renewal process, *J. Cell Biol.* **42:**392–403.

Extrinsic Influences on the Developing Neuron

REGULATION OF NEURONAL MORPHOGENESIS BY CELL-SUBSTRATUM ADHESION

Paul C. Letourneau

Stanford University School of Medicine, Stanford, California

Regulation of Neuronal Morphogenesis

In describing the anatomy of the nervous system, the term "neuronal specificity" has been applied to two morphological characteristics of neurons (Jacobson, 1970). First, neuronal specificity describes the fact that a number of nerve cell types display a similar morphology, orientation, and location from one animal to the next. Such regularity within a tissue cell type appears in the tissues of many organs. The second type of specificity occurs in the organization of synapses between two groups of neurons, such as the retina and the tectum. This spatial organization of retinal synapses with tectal cells may reflect intrinsic properties of the interacting neurons, for if the optic nerve is cut and the eye is rotated, the original arrangement of synapses will reform in spite of the rotation of the eye and the cut nerve.

Specificity of this type implies a cellular identity much more individual than is expressed in other organs. It is a challenge to developmental biologists to elucidate the mechanisms that determine how such precise morphology arises.

Studies of embryonic nervous systems indicate that the movements of neuroblasts and the elongation of nerve processes are often orderly and predictable (Lopresti, Macagno, and Levinthal, 1973; Rakic, 1971). One might immediately ask whether these movements are intrinsic to the motile cells involved or whether they arise from conditions within the local environment. Growing fibers that have been experimentally or naturally displaced from their normal pathways can adjust and reacquire the proper direction (Hibbard, 1965; Sperry and Hibbard, 1968; Van der Loos, 1965). This result would not be expected if axonal growth were simply a readout of internal programs. Consequently, consideration should be given to the view that interactions of growing fibers with their environment may be crucial to neuronal growth.

It is not surprising that cellular interactions may be important to this aspect of neuronal development (Wessells, 1973). What is most interesting is this: whereas developmental interactions are generally considered to occur at the level of tissues or large groups of cells, in the nervous system the interactions may be at the level of individual cells and may be unique in each case. It is my view that examination of the interactions that occur between neurons and their microenvironment within the embryo may clarify the basis for neuronal specificity and how it is expressed.

It is becoming clear that components of the cell surface play active roles in the exchange between a cell and its environment. In my own work, I have focused on one cell surface function, namely cell adhesion, and have asked what role this may have in the development of nerve cell shape. To directly measure cell adhesion and determine its influence on developing neurons, an in vitro system has been used.

Sensory Neurons In Vitro

The neurons used in these studies were sensory neurons from dorsal root ganglia of 4- to 8-day-old chick embryos. The ganglia were dissociated with trypsin and suspensions of single cells were plated in F_{12} medium containing 10% fetal calf serum and nerve growth factor (Letourneau, 1975a). Two cell types are cultured from sensory ganglia: sensory neurons and a non-neuronal population of glia and fibroblasts. The identifiable morphology of cultured neurons includes the cell body, fibers, or axons formed from the cell body in vitro, and growth cones, the enlarged distal ends of fibers (Figure 1). The growth cone is important for two reasons. First, it is believed to be the site where material is assembled into axonal structures after transport from the cell body, and second, it is the locomotory organelle responsible for elongation of the axon (Bray, 1970; Yamada, Spooner, and Wessells, 1971). Growth cone activity is characterized by the extension and movement of cellular processes, such as microspikes, which move about in the medium, make contact with the substratum and other objects, and regress back into the

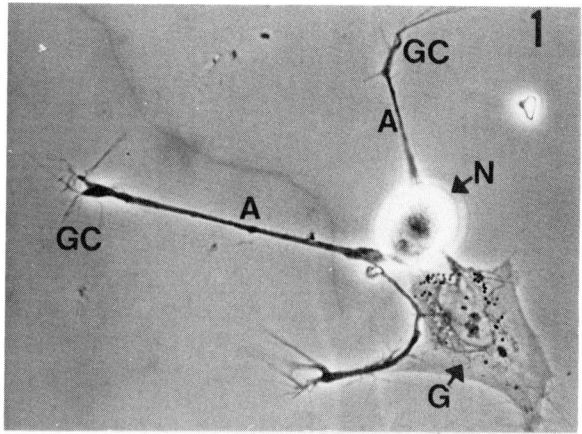

FIGURE 1. A single neuron and a non-neuronal glia or fibroblast cultured from dissociated dorsal root ganglia. Note the nerve cell body (N); axons (A); growth cones (GC); non-neuronal cell (G). ×550.

growth cone. This locomotory function, plus the microfilamentous ultrastructure of growth cones, is similar to that of the leading edge of motile fibroblasts (Ludueña and Wessells, 1973). Another similarity between these two locomotory structures is that the extension and advance of cellular processes involves formation of cell-substratum adhesions that may be basic to the mechanism of cell movements (Abercrombie, Heaysman, and Pegrum, 1971; Harris, 1973b; Ludueña, 1973). In these studies embryonic neurons were cultured on in vitro substrata to which growth cones adhered with varying strength, and correlations were made between cell-substratum adhesion and the formation and growth of nerve fibers.

Measurement of Cell-Substratum Adhesion

The adhesion of growth cones to in vitro substrata was measured with the air blaster, a device that produces shearing forces in the liquid medium that detach growth cones from the substratum (Gail and Boone, 1972; Letourneau and Wessells, 1974). These forces are reproducible, and data were obtained by counting the number of growth cones adherent to a small area of substratum immediately before and after an individual airblast. Table 1 presents the results of a number of comparisons of growth cone-substratum adhesion. From these data a

TABLE 1. *Adhesion of growth cones to substrata*[a]

Expt	Substratum	% Detached
1	TC dish 10 mM Ca	15 (n = 33)
	TC dish 0.3 mM Ca	44 (n = 25)
2	Polyornithine, polylysine coated	5 (n = 311)
	Polyglutamate coated	73 (n = 22)
	TC dish	56 (n = 25)
3	Upper surface of glia	17 (n = 138)
	TC dish	60 (n = 160)
4	Pd	48 (n = 54)
	TC dish	53 (n = 95)
5	Collagen	71 (n = 49)
	TC dish	88 (n = 25)

[a] Adhesion was assayed at a blasting distance of 2.4 cm, except for experiment 5, which was done at 2.2 cm and an air-flow rate of 3.0 liters/min. Duration of blast in all cases was 0.085 sec. Abbreviations: TC, tissue culture; n, number of neurons counted. Adapted from Letourneau (1975a,b).

hierarchy of substrata can be postulated with respect to growth cone adhesion:

polylysine-, polyornithine-coated surface ≈ glial surface > collagen > tissue culture plastic ≈ Pd.

The hydrophobic, nonwettable plastic of bacteriological petri dishes should be added at the low end of this spectrum. Many cells do not adhere to petri plastic, and because such a small number of neurons form axons when cultured in petri dishes, quantitative measurements of growth cone-substratum adhesion were not made (Martin and Rubin, 1974).

Effect of Adhesion on Neuronal Growth

Two of these substrata, tissue culture plastic and the more adhesive substratum, polyornithine-coated tissue culture plastic, were used as test substrata for assessing the roles of cell adhesion in axonal growth. Figure 2 is a graph of the initiation of axons as a function of time in culture. Neurons began to form axons earlier on polyornithine and, as seen in Table 2, a greater percentage of neurons eventually formed axons on the more adhesive substratum. As seen in Table 3, the average length of axon per neuron and the average length of individual axons were

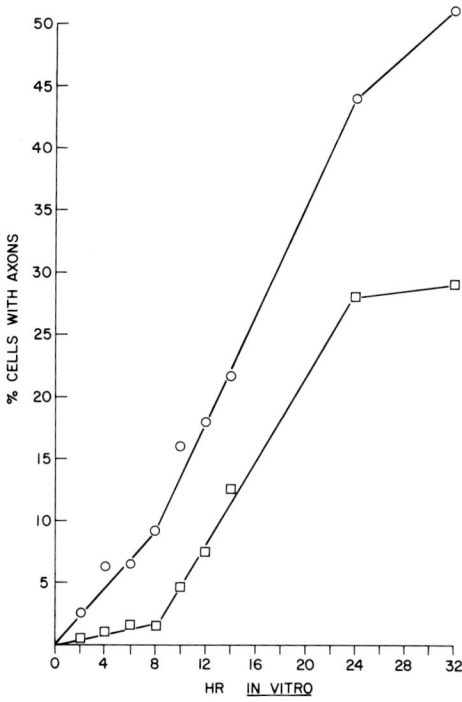

FIGURE 2. The time course of axon initiation in tissue culture dishes and in polyornithine-coated dishes. At the indicated time points, six to nine microscope fields of a dish were counted to determine the percentage of neurons with axons. Neurons were identified as spherical, refractile cell bodies with a diameter of about 15 μm. A new dish was counted for each time point. Symbols: ○, data from polyornithine dishes; □, data from tissue culture dishes. From Letourneau (1975a).

markedly higher on polylysine. This difference appeared to be due to the increased rate of axon elongation on polylysine as shown in Figure 3, which presents the average length of axon/neuron as a function of time in culture. The number of processes per neuron and the number of growth cones per neuron were also greater for neurons cultured on the more adhesive polylysine substratum (Figures 4 and 5, and Table 4).

These experimental results indicate that axonal formation, growth, and branching are all increased when neurons are cultured on substrata to which growth cones adhere tightly. This suggests that adhesive interactions of embryonic neurons with their microenvironment could determine the time, place, and initial orientation of nerve fiber

TABLE 2. *Percentage of neurons with axon(s) at 24 h in vitro*[a]

Age of embryo	Substratum	% ± SD neurons with axon(s)	
8 Days	PORN or PLYS	54 ± 8.7	(n = 739)
8 Days	Tissue culture	25 ± 2.6	(n = 642)
6 Days	PORN or PLYS	31	(n = 165)
6 Days	Tissue culture	7	(n = 123)
4 Days	PORN or PLYS	22 ± 3.9	(n = 439)
4 Days	Tissue culture	11 ± 1.6	(n = 626)

[a] Data for 8-day-old embryonic neurons are the combined results from five experiments; 6-day-old neurons are from one experiment; and 4-day-old neurons are from three experiments. Neurons were identified as spherical, refractile cells with an approximate diameter of 15 μm. Axons were identified as thin processes with a terminal growth cone, which had visible microspikes. Abbreviation: n, number of neurons counted. From Letourneau (1975a).

formation. In addition, adhesion may be important in the branching of processes, possibly by promoting the splitting of a growth cone into two individual growth cones.

Regulation of Direction of Axonal Growth

The following results indicate that adhesive interactions might also regulate the directions or pathways of axonal elongation. The hierarchy of adhesion for in vitro substrata presented earlier was used to confront

TABLE 3. *Average axon lengths after 24 h in vitro*[a]

Expt	Substratum	Avg μm/axon	Avg μm of axon/neuron
1	PORN	291	626
	Tissue culture	68	106
2	PORN	245	524
	Tissue culture	115	189
3	PORN	285	651
	Tissue culture	105	168
Combined results	PORN	275	600
	Tissue culture	96	154

[a] The lengths of the axons of 20 randomly selected neurons were measured on each experimental substratum. In each of the three experiments, the statistical significance on tissue culture plastic is $P < 0.0002$, as determined by the Mann-Whitney U test. From Letourneau (1975a).

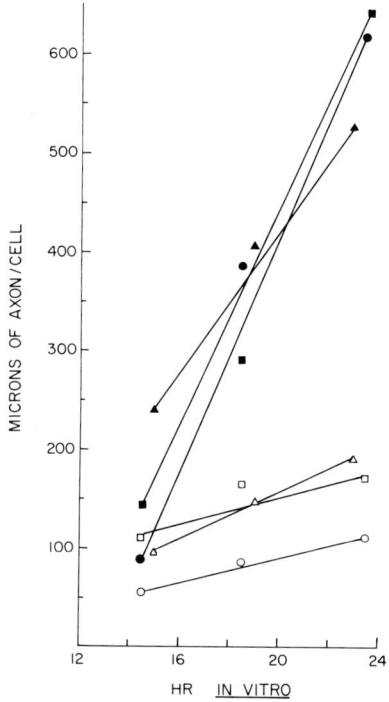

FIGURE 3. The average rates of axonal elongation per neuron for three experiments in tissue culture dishes and in polyornithine-coated dishes. Symbols: ●, ▲, ■, data from polyornithine dishes; ○, △, □, data from tissue culture dishes. At each time point the total axon lengths of 20 neurons were measured. A new dish was used for each time point. The circles, squares, and triangles denote separate experiments on both substrata. From Letourneau (1975a).

neurons with substrata made of patterned variations in adhesivity for growth cones. Patterned substrata were prepared by shadowing Pd wire onto dishes containing electron microscope grids (Harris, 1973a; Letourneau, 1975b). When the grids were removed, clear patterns of 80-μm squares of Pd deposition surrounded by 27-μm wide lanes of unshadowed dish substratum were seen. Therefore, according to the adhesion hierarchy, neurons could be confronted with Pd squares surrounded by (1) a substratum to which growth cones adhere less, i.e., petri plastic, (2) a substratum to which growth cones adhere equally well as to Pd, i.e., tissue culture plastic, or (3) a substratum to which they adhere more tightly than to Pd, such as collagen or polyornithine-coated

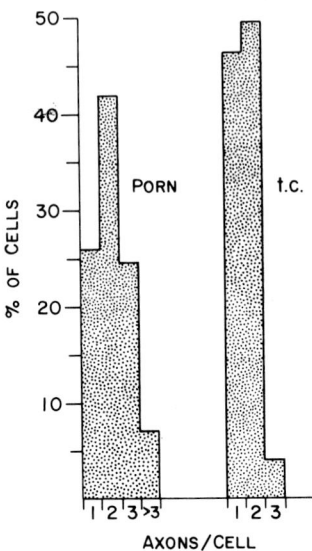

FIGURE 4. The distribution of the number of axons per neuron in polyornithine dishes and in tissue culture dishes after 24 h in vitro. The data are the combined results of three experiments. From Letourneau (1975a).

tissue culture plastic. As seen in Figures 6 through 12, the patterns of axonal growth are different under these different conditions. In petri dish cultures, neurons on the Pd squares sent out axons that grew across the Pd to the boundary with the petri plastic (Figures 6 through 8). At this point, microspike activity would continue; however, the growth cone usually did not cross onto the petri plastic. In contrast, the growth cones of neurons cultured in tissue culture dishes grew well on both substrata and often crossed from plastic to Pd and vice versa (Figures 9 and 10). In polyornithine-coated or collagen-coated dishes with Pd squares, axons extended for great distances, up to 1,000 μm or more, staying on the unshadowed substratum between the Pd squares. Axons turned corners at the intersection of two unshadowed lanes, and axons were seen with branches extending in several directions at an intersection of polyornithine-coated lanes (Figures 11 and 12). Table 5 provides numerical evidence that growth cones tend to remain on substrata to which they adhere more strongly. It should be emphasized that the strength of growth cone adhesion to Pd is the same in all cases; these differences in the patterns of nerve fiber growth depend on the relative adhesion of growth cones to the unshadowed substratum compared to

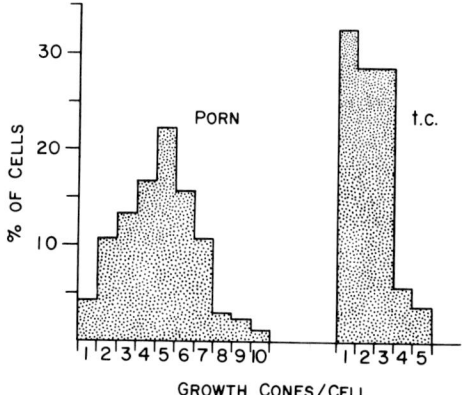

FIGURE 5. The distribution of the number of growth cones per neuron in polyornithine dishes and in tissue culture dishes after 24 h in vitro. The data are the combined results of three experiments. From Letourneau (1975a).

the Pd. This suggests that growth cone function includes comparative interactions with alternative areas of substratum. Observation of time-lapse movies of neurons cultured in collagen- or polyornithine-coated dishes with Pd squares revealed that even though growth cones remained on the more adhesive unshadowed substratum, they did not merely advance straight down the middle of the unshadowed lane, but moved back and forth between the Pd-coated surface on both sides

TABLE 4. Average number of axons and growth cones per neuron at 24 h in vitro

Expt[a]	Substratum	Axons/ neuron	Growth cones/ axon	Growth cones/ neuron
1	PORN	2.35	2.25	5.3 (n = 52)
	Tissue culture	1.59	1.42	2.25 (n = 54)
2	PORN	2.10	2.22	4.65 (n = 52)
	Tissue culture	1.59	1.40	2.21 (n = 58)
3	PORN	1.97	2.16	4.25 (n = 63)
	Tissue culture	1.59	1.33	2.11 (n = 44)
Combined results	PORN	2.13 ± 0.05	2.20 ± 0.05	4.8 ± 0.05 (n = 167)
	Tissue culture	1.59	1.39 ± 0.05	2.20 ± 0.07 (n = 156)

[a] The numbers of axons and growth cones per neuron of a random sample of cells were counted for each experimental substratum. Only neurons whose cell body and axons were not touching those of another neuron were counted. Abbreviation: n, number of neurons counted. From Letourneau (1975a).

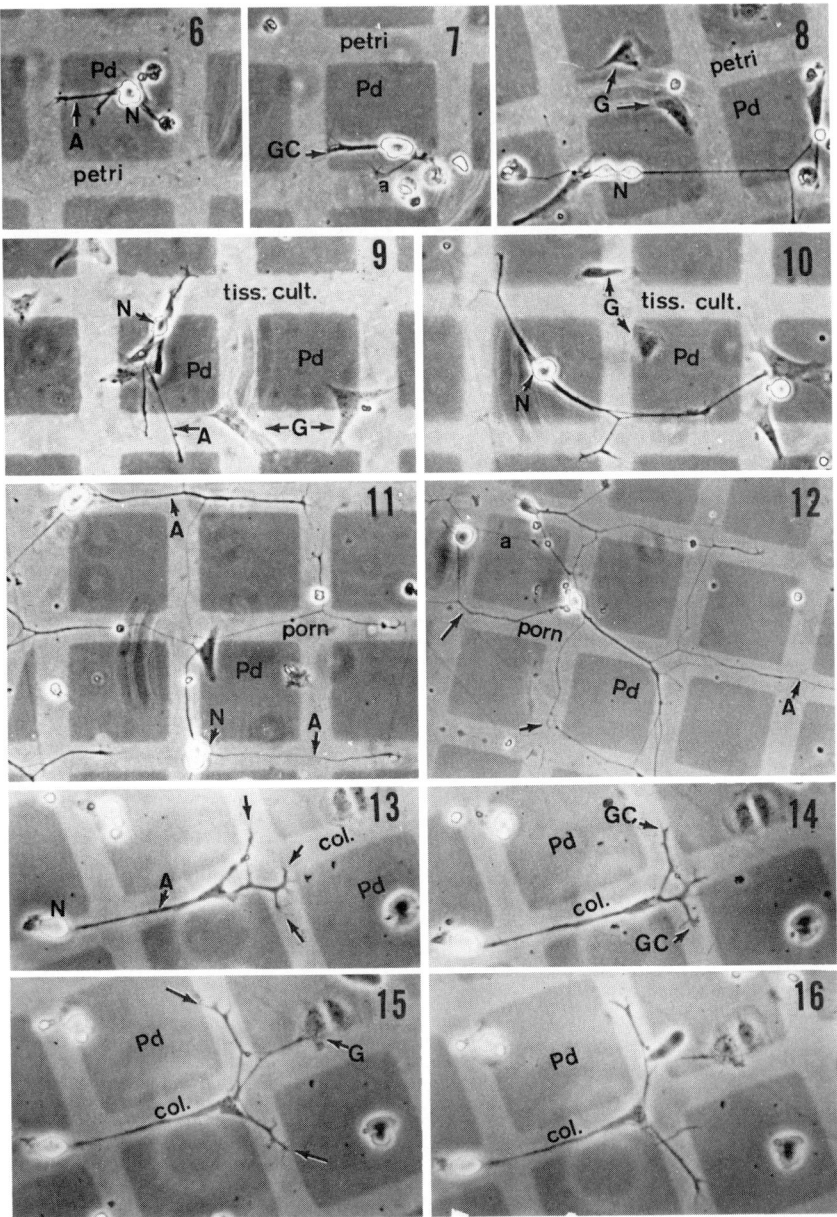

FIGURE 6. A neuron cultured in a Pd-shadowed plastic petri dish. The nerve cell body (N) and the axons (A) are on a Pd square (Pd) surrounded by unshadowed petri plastic. One axon extends to the edge of the Pd surface. All of these photographs were taken after 16 to 24 h of culture. ×180.

ADHESION AND NEURONAL MORPHOGENESIS

(Figures 13 through 16). It appeared that in these instances some of the microspikes of a growth cone would adhere to the Pd and others to the unshadowed substratum (Figures 17 through 22).

A Model for Growth Cone Function

A model for growth cone function can be presented to explain how strong growth cone-substratum adhesion enhances axonal growth and may determine the pathways of axonal growth. The motile activity of growth cones is dominated by microspikes and similar cellular extensions whose formation is asssociated with adhesive contacts with the substratum. Suppose that the adhesion of a microspike to the substratum stabilizes its structure. This stabilization might then allow or

---

FIGURE 7. Neurons cultured in a Pd-shadowed petri dish. One axon tip (GC) is at the edge of the Pd, and another (a) is on the unshadowed side of the boundary. ×180.

FIGURE 8. These growth cones have crossed the unshadowed petri plastic from one Pd square to another. Note that the glial cells (G) tend to be on the Pd squares. Axon (A); nerve cell body (N). ×180.

FIGURE 9. A neuron cultured in a Pd-shadowed tissue culture dish. The axons (A) have elongated from the Pd surface (Pd) across the unshadowed lanes. Nerve cell body (N); glial cell (G). ×170.

FIGURE 10. Neurons cultured in a Pd-shadowed tissue culture dish. Nerve cell bodies (N); glial cells (G). ×180.

FIGURE 11. Neurons cultured in a Pd-shadowed, polyornithine-coated tissue culture dish. Note how the axons extend only along the unshadowed lanes of the dish. Nerve cell body (N). Polyornithine surface (porn). ×170.

FIGURE 12. Neurons cultured in a Pd-shadowed, polyornithine-coated tissue culture dish. One axon (a) has elongated on the Pd surface, but most axons (A) stay on the unshadowed lanes. Several axons appear to have made 90° turns (arrows). Polyornithine surface (porn). ×145.

FIGURES 13–16. Four frames from a time-lapse movie of a neuron cultured on Pd-shadowed collagen.

FIGURE 13. The axon (A) has several terminal growth cones (arrows). Nerve cell body (N); collagen (col.). ×215.

FIGURE 14. Taken 36 min after Figure 13. Two growth cones (GC) have elongated along the unshadowed lane. Collagen (col.). ×215.

FIGURE 15. Taken 53 min after Figure 14. Note how the growth cones do not stay in the middle of the unshadowed lane (arrows), but wander from one side of the lane to the other (compare with Figure 14). One growth cone has contacted a glial cell (G). Collagen (col.). ×215.

FIGURE 16. Taken 35 min after Figure 15. The axons have elongated further along the unshadowed lane. Collagen (col.). ×215.

TABLE 5. *Percentage of growth cones on a substratum*[a]

| | Substratum | | |
Dish	Pd	Unshadowed lane	Glia
Petri plastic	35	18	47 (n = 98)
Tissue culture plastic	32	31	36 (n = 207)
Polyornithine coated	4	74	22 (n = 274)

Percentage of growth cones on Pd or unshadowed lane

| | Substratum | |
Dish	Pd	Unshadowed lane
Petri plastic	65	35 (n = 52)
Tissue culture plastic	51	49 (n = 132)
Polyornithine coated	5	95 (n = 214)

[a] The distribution of growth cones on Pd, unshadowed lanes, and glia, respectively, was determined by counting the number of growth cones on these substrata in several randomly selected microscopic fields. The data for growth cones on glial cells were omitted in calculating the percentages shown in the lower panels. Abbreviation: n, number of neurons counted. From Letourneau (1975b).

favor the addition of new material to the microspike. If the microspike does not adhere, then it may move about, but will eventually regress into the growth cone mass. However, if the microspike remains adherent and forms new adhesions as it expands, the net effect will be advancement of the growth cone and net axonal elongation. So on a very adhesive substratum, such as polyornithine, microspike contacts will be stronger, more frequent, or of longer duration, leading to a more efficient, and, hence, more rapid rate of axonal elongation. Similarly, increased adhesion of microspikes formed from a nerve cell body would favor establishment of a growth cone and eventually an axon, explaining the increased initiation of axons on polyornithine. Finally, if microspike-substratum adhesions were more frequent or stronger in one area adjacent to a growth cone, then axonal elongation would tend to occur in that direction, as new material is preferentially added at the more adhesive side.

CONCLUSION

These results demonstrate how genetic regulation of neuronal morphogenesis could be expressed via the adhesive interactions of embryonic neurons and their growth cones with the embryonic microenvironment. Cell-specific patterns of axonal growth could arise from cell-specific differences in adhesive interactions. These differences

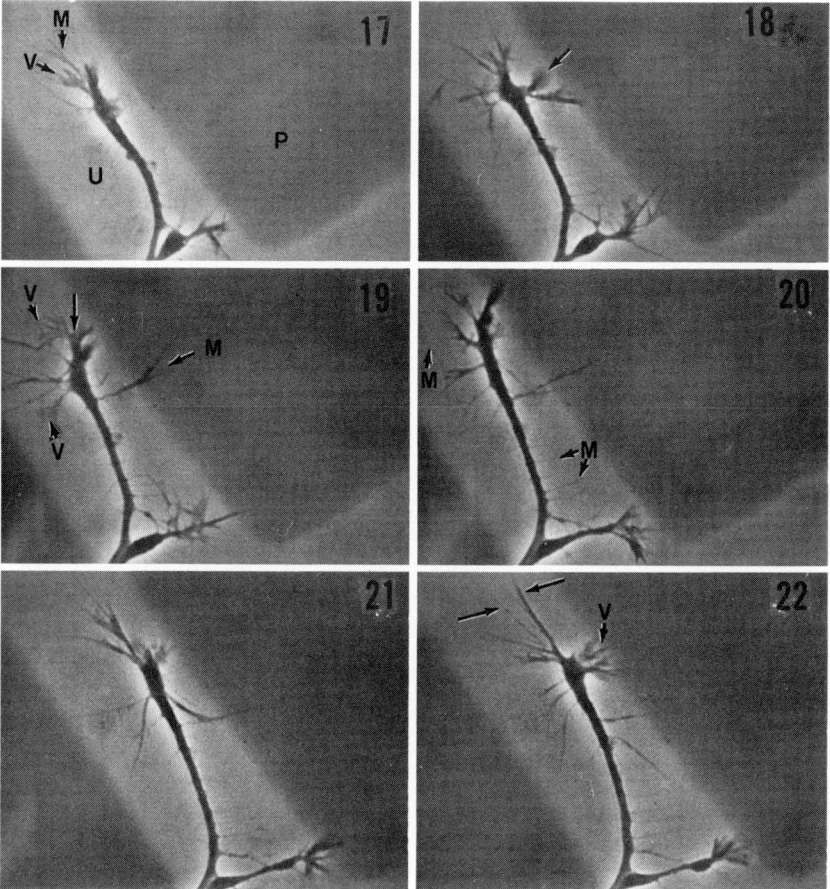

FIGURES 17–22. Frames from a time-lapse movie of a growth cone elongating along the unshadowed lane between 2 Pd-shadowed squares in a polyornithine-coated tissue culture dish.

FIGURE 17. Note the microspikes (M) and veil-like expansions of cell surface. The microspikes are distributed over the substratum adjacent to the growth cone. Pd surface (P); unshadowed lane (U). ×880.

FIGURE 18. Taken 200 sec after Figure 17. Note how the morphology of the growth cone has changed due to microspike formation and movement. Some microspikes (arrow) are out of the plane of focus, meaning they are moving in the fluid medium. ×880.

FIGURE 19. Taken 200 sec after Figure 18. The growth cone has elongated in the area indicated by the arrow. A microspike has extended onto the Pd surface. Veil (V). ×880.

FIGURE 20. Taken 200 sec after Figure 19. Note the microspikes (M) that extend from the growth cone and the sides of the axon. ×880.

FIGURE 21. Taken 200 sec after Figure 20. ×880.

FIGURE 22. Taken 200 sec after Figure 21. Note the forward extending microspikes (arrows), and the veil-like expansion (V) that is close to the Pd surface. ×880. Figures 6 through 22 are from Letourneau (1975b).

could be a function of the cell, its possible substrata, or both. For example, there are regional differences in the adhesive properties of embryonic retinal and tectal cells that could be the basis for the distribution of growing retinal fibers over the tectum (Barbera, 1975; Gottlieb, Rock, and Glaser, 1976). A more basic understanding of these problems will come from an elucidation of the cell surface components involved in cell adhesion, from the analysis of how they are distributed spatially and temporally on cells, and from the clarification of what regulates the distribution of adhesion-mediating molecules.

In summary, these experiments demonstrate the utility of in vitro studies for analysis of developmental mechanisms within the nervous system. With the in vitro approach, a simple, yet crucial, correlation has been made between strength of adhesion and several parameters of neuronal morphogenesis. Similar systems are proving useful for the examination of important aspects of neural development, such as synaptogenesis, transmitter functions, and the determinative interactions of neural crest cell populations (Fischbach, Berg, Cohen, and Frank, 1975; Norr, 1973; Patterson and Chun, 1974).

ACKNOWLEDGMENTS

I thank Professor Norman Wessells for advice, support, and encouragement in conducting these experiments. This work was supported by a National Institutes of Health predoctoral traineeship award to the author, and by National Institute of Child Health and Human Development grant HD-04708 to Dr. Wessells.

REFERENCES

Abercrombie, M., J. E. M. Heaysman, and S. M. Pegrum (1971). The locomotion of fibroblasts in culture. IV. Electron microscopy of the leading lamella, *Exp. Cell Res.* **67**:359–367.

Barbera, A. (1975). Adhesive recognition between developing retinal cells and the optic tecta of the chick embryo, *Dev. Biol.* **46**:167–191.

Bray, D. (1970). Surface movements during the growth of single explanted neurons, *Proc. Natl. Acad. Sci. U.S.A.* **65**:905–910.

Fischbach, G. D., D. K. Berg, S. A. Cohen, and E. Frank (1975). Enrichment of nerve-muscle synapses in spinal cord-muscle cultures and identification of relative peaks of ACh sensitivity at sites of transmitter release, *Cold Spring Harbor Symp. Quant. Biol.* **40**:347–358.

Gail, M. H. and C. W. Boone (1972). Cell-substrate adhesivity, *Exp. Cell Res.* **70**:33–40.

Gottlieb, D. I., K. Rock, and L. Glaser (1976). A gradient of adhesive specificity in developing avian retina, *Proc. Natl. Acad. Sci. U.S.A.* **73**:410–414.

Harris, A. (1973a). Behavior of cultured cells on substrata of variable adhesiveness, *Exp. Cell Res.* **77**:285–297.

Harris, A. (1973b). Location of cellular adhesions to solid substrata, *Dev. Biol.* **35**:83–96.

Hibbard, E. (1965). Orientation and directed growth of Mauthner's cell axons from duplicate vestibular nerve roots, *Exp. Neurol.* **13**:289–301.

Jacobson, M. (1970). *Developmental Neurobiology*. Holt, Rinehart, and Winston, Inc., San Francisco.

Letourneau, P. C. (1975a). Possible roles for cell-to-substratum adhesion in neuronal morphogenesis, *Dev. Biol.* **44**:77–91.

Letourneau, P. C. (1975b). Cell-to-substratum adhesion and guidance of axonal elongation, *Dev. Biol.* **44**:92–101.

Letourneau, P. C. and N. K. Wessells (1974). Migratory cell locomotion versus nerve axon elongation. Differences based on the effects of Lanthanum ion, *J. Cell Biol.* **61**:56–69.

Lopresti, V., E. R. Macagno, and C. Levinthal (1973). Structure and development of neuronal connections in isogenic organisms: cellular interactions in the development of the optic lamina of *Daphnia*, *Proc. Natl. Acad. Sci. U.S.A.* **70**:433–437.

Ludueña, M. A. (1973). The growth of spinal ganglion neurons in serum-free medium, *Dev. Biol.* **33**:470–476.

Ludueña, M. A. and N. K. Wessells (1973). Cell locomotion, nerve elongation, and microfilaments, *Dev. Biol.* **30**:427–440.

Martin, G. R. and H. Rubin (1974). Effects of cell adhesion to the substratum on the growth of chick embryo fibroblasts, *Exp. Cell Res.* **85**:319–333.

Norr, S. C. (1973). *In vitro* analysis of sympathetic neuron differentiation from chick neural crest cells, *Dev. Biol.* **34**:16–38.

Patterson, P. H. and L. L. Y. Chun (1974). The influence of non-neuronal cells on catecholamine and acetylcholine synthesis and accumulation in cultures of dissociated sympathetic neurons, *Proc. Natl. Acad. Sci. U.S.A.* **71**:3607–3610.

Rakic, P. (1971). Neuron-glia relationship during granule cell migration in developing cerebellar cortex. A golgi and EM study in *Macacus rhesus*, *J. Comp. Neurol.* **141**:283–312.

Sperry, R. W. and E. Hibbard (1968). Regulative factors in the orderly growth of retino-tectal connexions, pp. 41–52 in *Growth of the Nervous System (Ciba Symposium)*, Wolstenholme, G. E. and M. O'Connor, eds. J. and A. Churchill, London.

Van der Loos, H. (1965). The "improperly" oriented pyramidal cell in the cerebral cortex and its possible bearing on problems of growth and cell orientation, *Bull. Johns Hopkins Hosp.* **117**:228–250.

Wessells, N. K. (1973). *Tissue Interactions in Development*. Addison-Wesley Publishing Co., Reading, Mass.

Yamada, K. M., B. S. Spooner, and N. K. Wessells (1971). Ultrastructure and function of growth cones and axons of cultured nerve cells, *J. Cell Biol.* **49**:614–635.

THE ROLE OF NON-NEURONAL CELLS IN THE DEVELOPMENT OF RAT SYMPATHETIC NEURONS IN VITRO

Linda L. Y. Chun, E. J. Furshpan, Story C. Landis, P. R. MacLeish, Colin A. Nurse, P. H. O'Lague, Paul H. Patterson, D. D. Potter, and Louis F. Reichardt

Harvard Medical School, Boston, Massachusetts

During development, neurons are influenced by a variety of hormonal signals and cellular interactions. In the sympathetic nervous system, maturation of postganglionic neurons is influenced by the protein nerve growth factor (NGF), by neuronal input from the spinal cord, and by the target organs that the neurons innervate. Levi-Montalcini and her colleagues have shown that NGF is essential for the development of sympathetic neurons both in vivo and in vitro. Injection of a NGF antiserum into newborn mice (Levi-Montalcini and Booker, 1960) or exclusion of NGF from cultures of dissociated sympathetic neurons (Levi-Montalcini and Angeletti, 1963), results in neuronal death. Intact preganglionic input to the mouse superior cervical ganglion (SCG) at birth is also important for sympathetic neuronal maturation. Removal of this inhibits development of tyrosine hydroxylase activity in both the soma and the terminals of the SCG cells (Black, Hendry, and Iversen, 1971; Black and Mytilineou, 1976). That the state of innervation of target organs can regulate growth of sympathetic neurites was demonstrated by Olson and Malmfors (1970). When an iris is transplanted to the anterior chamber of the eye, it causes sprouting of, and becomes innervated by, the adrenergic plexus of the host iris. Furthermore, a SCG transplanted into the anterior chamber becomes vascularized but does not sprout into the host iris if the normal innervation is present. However, if the host iris is denervated, then fibers from the transplanted ganglion innervate it. Thus, the target organ seems to regulate its own innervation.

One way to investigate cellular and hormonal influences and their mechanisms of action is to study the development of dissociated rat sympathetic neurons in cultures virtually free of other cell types. A major advantage of this approach is that it facilitates control of the cellular and fluid environments and the substratum on which the cells grow. In particular, it is possible to investigate the role of non-neuronal cells in the development of the sympathetic nervous system by comparing the development of these neurons in the presence and absence of non-neuronal cells.

Sympathetic neurons are mechanically dissociated from SCG of neonatal rats (Bray, 1970). The cells are plated on a collagen substratum and cultured in a modified Leibowitz medium containing adult rat serum, NGF, and vitamins (Mains and Patterson, 1973a). If bicarbonate is included in this medium, mixed cultures of neurons and ganglionic non-neuronal cells can be obtained (Figure 1a). On the other hand, neurons grown in medium lacking bicarbonate, or in the presence of mitotic poisons, develop in the virtual absence of ganglionic non-neuronal cells (Figure 1b). Considerable information on the development of these sympathetic neurons cultured in the virtual absence of other cell types has been obtained (Table 1). Under these conditions, the neurons develop many of the properties expected for mature sympathetic neurons. They synthesize and accumulate the adrenergic transmitters dopamine (DA) and norepinephrine (NE) from tyrosine (Mains and Patterson, 1973a), and develop this ability along a time course that qualitatively parallels that seen in vivo. Because it differs in magnitude and time course from overall growth, measured by the synthesis and accumulation of protein, lipid, and RNA from radioactive precursors (Mains and Patterson, 1973b), this development of catecholamine (CA) metabolism represents neuronal differentiation. As expected, these cultures do not synthesize and accumulate detectable amounts of the transmitters γ-aminobutyric acid (GABA), serotonin (5-HT), or histamine from their respective labeled precursors. However, in older cultures small amounts of acetylcholine (ACh) made from radioactive choline (Ch) could sometimes be detected (Mains and Patterson, 1973a). The significance of this finding will be considered below. Evidence for the storage of NE in vesicles comes from pharmacological, biochemical, and morphological studies (Patterson, Reichardt, and Chun, 1975). First, reserpine almost completely inhibits the ability of neurons to store NE. Second, [^{3}H]NE can be found in osmotically labile subcellular particles. Finally, EM autoradiographic

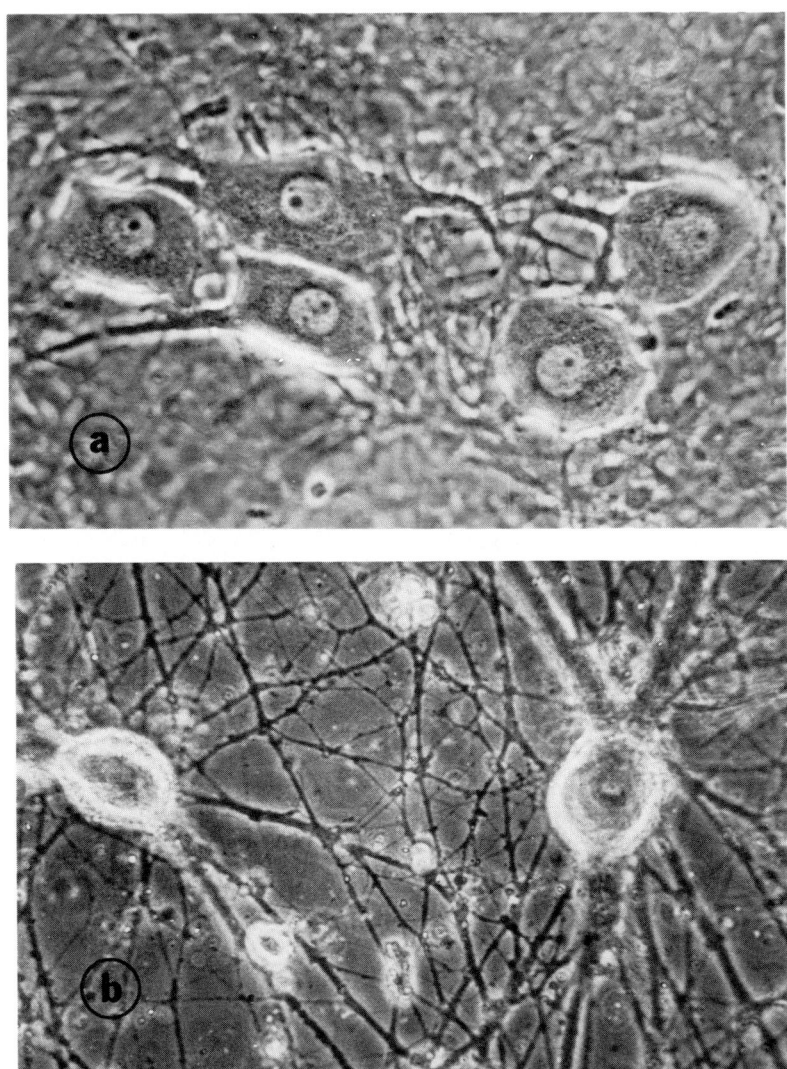

FIGURE 1. Morphology of neurons grown with or without non-neuronal cells. (a) Culture of neurons and ganglionic non-neuronal cells grown in the presence of bicarbonate. (b) Culture of neurons virtually free of non-neuronal cells grown in the absence of bicarbonate.

studies by Rowe and Claude (unpublished observations) indicate that most of the [^{3}H]NE is stored in vesicles. This stored NE can be released by depolarization with high K$^+$ or veratridine. The release of [^{3}H]NE is Ca^{2+} dependent and can be blocked by the Ca^{2+} antagonists Mn^{2+}, Mg^{2+},

> **TABLE 1.** *Properties of sympathetic neurons grown in the absence of other cell types*
>
> Synthesis and accumulation of DA and NE.
>
> Development of this ability parallels in vivo time course and is different in magnitude and time course from overall neuronal growth.
>
> No detectable synthesis and accumulation of GABA, 5-HT, or histamine, and little or no detectable synthesis and accumulation of acetylcholine.
>
> Storage of NE in vesicles.
>
> Release of NE by depolarization that is Ca^{2+}-dependent and blocked by Mn^{2+}, Mg^{2+}, or Co^{2+}.
>
> NE uptake system that is saturable, has high affinity, and is blocked by the appropriate drugs.
>
> Generation and conduction of action potentials and sensitivity to acetylcholine.
>
> EM evidence of adrenergic synapses between the neurons.

or Co^{2+} (Patterson et al., 1975; Burton and Bunge, 1975). The neurons can also take up [^{3}H]NE. The uptake process is saturable, has an apparent K_m of 1 μM, and is blocked by cocaine and desmethylimipramine (Patterson et al., 1975). Electrophysiological studies by O'Lague, MacLeish, Nurse, Claude, Furshpan, and Potter (1975) indicate that these cells can generate and conduct action potentials and are sensitive to iontophoresed ACh. Finally, Rees and Bunge (1974) have shown that these cells form morphological synapses with each other that have the ultrastructure characteristic of adrenergic neurons. They have both pre- and postsynaptic membrane specializations, numerous small granular vesicles (SGV), and occasional large granular vesicles. In summary, these neurons grown in the virtual absence of other cell types develop many of the properties expected of adrenergic neurons.

On the other hand, when these neurons were cocultured with ganglionic non-neuronal cells, the mixed cultures produced 100- to 1,000-fold more [^{3}H]ACh than neuron-alone cultures (Patterson and Chun, 1974). Furthermore, the ACh was secreted at functional cholinergic synapses between the neurons themselves (O'Lague, Obata, Claude, Furshpan, and Potter, 1974; O'Lague et al., 1975; see also Johnson, Ross, Meyers, Rees, Bunge, Wakshull, and Burton, 1976) and between neurons and skeletal myotubes (Nurse and O'Lague, 1975). Because substantial ACh production was found only in mixed cultures, it was not clear whether the neurons were being stimulated to produce ACh by the non-neuronal cells or vice versa. However, because neurons in these mixed cultures formed functional cholinergic synapses, it was likely that at least some of the ACh was produced by the neurons. To demonstrate this, neuron-alone cultures were grown in medium that had been conditioned by certain non-neuronal cells. Under these conditions, neuronal ACh production induced by the conditioned medium (CM) increased 300- to 1,000-fold over controls (Patterson et al., 1975). These experiments also showed that the non-neuronal cells could exert their effect via the bulk medium without cell-cell contact with the neurons.

Because CM induces such a large change in neuronal ACh production, it was of interest to determine what other effects it has on these neurons. We previously reported that the induction of ACh production by certain non-neuronal cells did not appreciably affect the ability of the cultures to produce CA (Patterson and Chun, 1974; Patterson et al., 1975). More recently, we have found that as the intensity of the non-neuronal influence is increased, CA production decreases significantly (Patterson and Chun, 1977). CM dose-response curves for neuronal survival and transmitter production are shown in Figure 2. ACh production rose 40-fold over this concentration range, whereas CA production decreased 25-fold. Therefore, the ratio of ACh to CA produced by neurons cultured in high CM was 1,000-fold higher than that of controls. In addition, neuronal survival does not change over this concentration range. This difference in ACh/CA with no change in neuronal number is consistent with the hypothesis that single sympathetic neurons express adrenergic or cholinergic properties depending on the environment in which they develop. It was also found that CM does not affect overall neuronal growth as measured by total neuronal protein or total neuronal lipid phosphate (Patterson and Chun, 1977). Therefore, CM seems to be a specific differentiation signal that influences transmitter functions but not neuronal survival or growth.

Electrophysiological and morphological studies of the effect of CM were carried out (Landis, MacLeish, Potter, Furshpan, and Patterson, 1976). It was found that CM not only increased production of ACh, but also induced formation of cholinergic synapses. Nicotinic synapses were very frequent in cultures grown with high CM, less so with intermediate CM, and very infrequent in unconditioned medium. There was also a concomitant decrease in the proportion of synaptic endings and varicosities that contained small granular vesicles as the CM concentration was increased. Therefore, CM not only gives rise to the

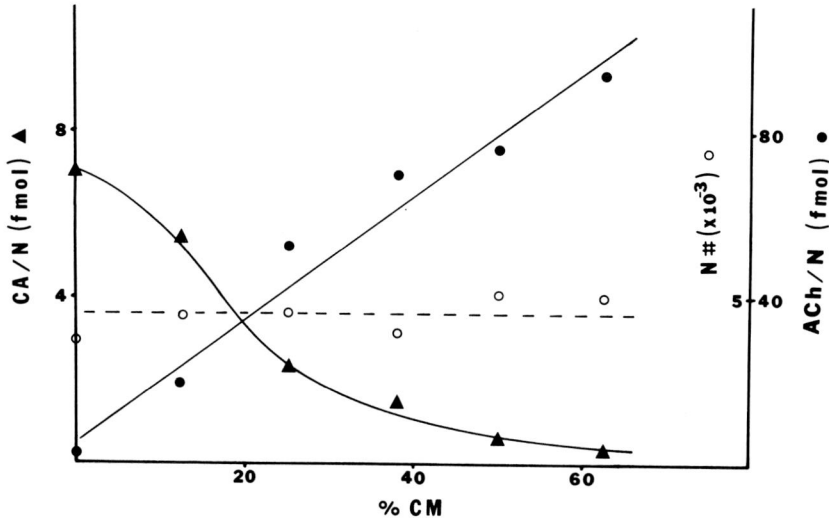

FIGURE 2. The dependence of ACh and CA production and neuronal survival on CM concentration was determined on 20-day-old L15-CO_2 cultures that had been treated with 10^{-5}M cytosine arabinoside on days 2 and 8 to virtually eliminate all non-neuronal cells. CM from confluent rat heart flasks was mixed with fresh medium at the concentrations shown and added every 2 days, beginning at day 2. On day 20, neuronal somas were counted (O) and the cultures were incubated with [^{3}H]choline and [^{3}H]tyrosine. Radioactive ACh (●) and CA (▲) were determined by high-voltage electrophoresis and the values are expressed on a per neuron basis. From Patterson and Chun (1977).

synthesis and accumulation of substantial amounts of ACh, but can induce the formation of large numbers of functional cholinergic synapses with typical cholinergic fine structure.

In intermediate CM concentrations, the cultures are capable of producing substantial amounts of both transmitters. This raises the question whether individual neurons are exclusively adrenergic or cholinergic, or whether they can display both characteristics simultaneously. To investigate this, single neurons were grown in unconditioned medium, in various CM concentrations, or on heart monolayers. A microculture containing a single neuron on an island of heart cells is shown in Figure 3. The neurites form a network confined to the island. The heart myocytes, as in vivo, beat spontaneously and are sensitive to both NE, which increases their beating frequency, and ACh, which decreases it. Single cell cultures (aged 30 to 40 days) have been analyzed for their ability to synthesize and accumulate ACh and CA, and the

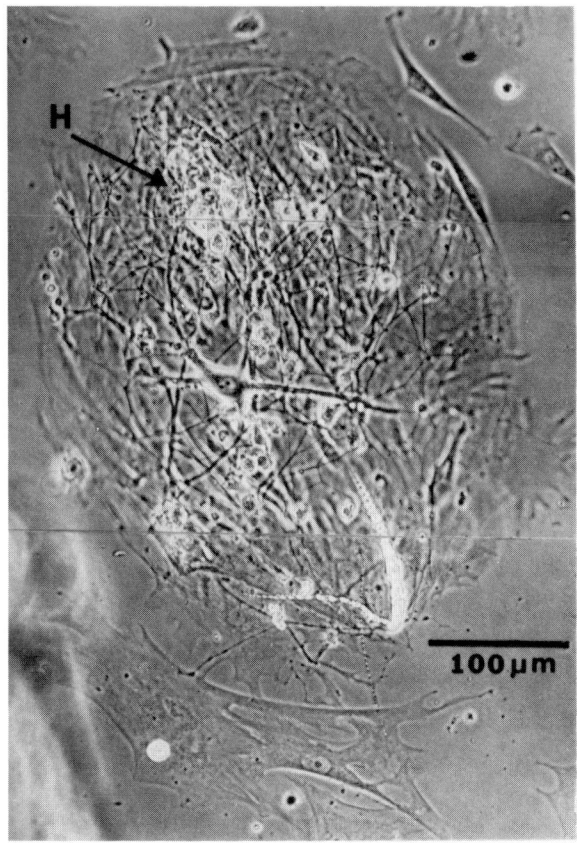

FIGURE 3. A microculture containing a solitary neuron; arrow at H indicates a cluster of myocytes. Neuron was 13 days in culture. From Furshpan et al. (1976).

majority of the neurons have thus far been found to produce predominantly one transmitter; that is, a particular neuron produced 5 to 50 fmol of one transmitter and less than 1 fmol of the other (Reichardt, Patterson, and Chun, 1976).

Furshpan, MacLeish, O'Lague, and Potter (1976) studied similar microcultures (aged 13 to 17 days) and observed single neurons with the following types of synaptic activity. (1) Many single neurons made excitatory cholinergic synapses on themselves (called autapses). These excitatory postsynaptic potentials (EPSP) had short latencies and were blocked by the nicotinic antagonists hexamethonium or D-tubocurarine. (2) The single neurons that made cholinergic autapses usually also hyperpolarized cardiac myocytes and inhibited the beating. The hyperpolarization had a longer latency and slower time course than the autaptic EPSPs, was mimicked by ACh, and was blocked by the muscarinic antagonist atropine. (3) Many single neurons depolarized the cardiac myocytes and accelerated the beating. The depolarization had a slow onset and time course, was mimicked by NE, and was blocked by the β-adrenergic antagonist propranolol. (4) Some single neurons first inhibited and then accelerated the beating of the myocytes. The inhibition was blocked by atropine as in (2), and the acceleration was blocked by propranolol as in (3). This suggests that the dual-function single neurons secreted both ACh and CA. The physiological functions were correlated with synaptic fine structure. Landis (1976) found that varicosities of neurons that secreted CA contained many SGV, whereas varicosities of cholinergic cells contained none. The dual-function neurons contained only occasional SGV. It remains to be seen how frequent the occurrence of such dual-function cells are and whether they can be detected with biochemical methods. It will also be of interest to determine if dual function is stable or a developmental phase on the way to producing one or the other transmitter.

The finding that these sympathetically derived neurons can be induced to produce ACh and to form functional cholinergic synapses requires comment. At least two hypotheses can be offered to explain these observations. (1) The neurons are behaving as they would in vivo, or (2) they are reacting to developmental signals that they normally do not receive in vivo. In support of the first hypothesis is the finding by Yamauchi, Lever, and Kemp (1973) that approximately 5% of the principal neurons in the adult rat SCG may be cholinergic. The culture conditions may select neurons that express cholinergic characteristics in the presence of non-neuronal cells or in medium conditioned by them. Several observations are relevant to this possibility. First, the neurons that form cholinergic synapses are not a small minority, but can make up more than half the neuronal population (O'Lague et al., 1975). Second, treatment with high concentrations of CM does not cause an increase in neuronal number. This suggests that the neurons that are capable of making cholinergic synapses are also present in the cultures grown without CM, but do not express this property. These observations argue against the selection of a population of predetermined cholinergic neurons, but support the second hypothesis that neurons are capable of expressing cholinergic and/or adrenergic properties depending on their developmental environment.

The importance of environment in controlling development of

transmitter metabolism in vivo has been demonstrated by LeDouarin, Renaud, Teillet, and LeDouarin (1975) in experiments in which they transplanted neural crest cells to abnormal sites. Cells from a region of presumptive adrenergic crest, which normally gives rise to sympathetic neurons and adrenal medullary cells, differentiate into parasympathetic cholinergic neurons when transplanted to the presumptive cholinergic region of the crest. Thus, the environment in which neurons develop controls their development both in vivo and in vitro. The decision to become adrenergic or cholinergic has crucial functional consequences because NE and ACh have antagonistic effects on many autonomic target tissues such as the heart, iris, and blood vessels. Studying sympathetic neuronal development in culture offers the opportunity for identifying normal developmental signals by facilitating control of the culture environment.

ACKNOWLEDGMENTS

It is a pleasure to acknowledge the assistance of William Dragun, Karen Fischer, Joseph Gagliardi, James La Fratta, Michael La Fratta, Doreen McDowell, and Shirley Wilson in various aspects of this work.

REFERENCES

Black, I. B., I. A. Hendry, and L. L. Iversen (1971). Trans-synaptic regulation of growth and development of adrenergic neurones in a mouse sympathetic ganglion, *Brain Res.* **34:**229–240.

Black, I. B. and C. Mytilineou (1976). Trans-synaptic regulation of the development of end organ innervation by sympathetic neurons, *Brain Res.* **101:**503–521.

Bray, D. (1970). Surface movements during the growth of single explanted neurons, *Proc. Natl. Acad. Sci. U.S.A.* **65:**905–910.

Burton, H. and R. P. Bunge (1975). A comparison of the uptake and release of[^{3}H]norepinephrine in rat autonomic and sensory ganglia in tissue culture, *Brain Res.* **97:**157–162.

Furshpan, E. J., P. R. MacLeish, P. H. O'Lague, and D. D. Potter (1976). Chemical transmission between rat sympathetic neurons and cardiac myocytes developing in microcultures: evidence for cholinergic, adrenergic and dual-function neurons, *Proc. Natl. Acad. Sci. U.S.A.* **73:**4225–4229.

Johnson, M., D. Ross, M. Meyers, R. Rees, R. Bunge, E. Wakshull, and H. Burton (1976). Synaptic vesicle cytochemistry changes when cultured sympathetic neurones develop cholinergic interactions, *Nature (London)* **262:**308–310.

Landis, S. C. (1976). Rat sympathetic neurons and cardiac myocytes developing in microculture: correlation of the fine structure of endings with neurotransmitter function in single neurons, *Proc. Natl. Acad. Sci. U.S.A.* **73:** 4220–4224.

Landis, S. C., P. R. MacLeish, D. D. Potter, E. J. Furshpan, and P. H. Patterson (1976). Synapses formed between dissociated sympathetic neurons: the influence of conditioned medium, *Abstr. Annu. Meet. Soc. Neurosci.*, 6th, Toronto, p. 197.

LeDouarin, N. M., D. Renaud, M. A. Teillet, and G. H. LeDouarin (1975). Cholinergic differentiation of presumptive adrenergic neuroblasts in interspecific chimeras after heterotopic transplanations, *Proc. Natl. Acad. Sci. U.S.A.* **72**:728–732.

Levi-Montalcini, R. and P. U. Angeletti (1963). Essential role of the nerve growth factor in the survival and maintenance of dissociated sensory and sympathetic embryonic nerve cells in vitro, *Dev. Biol.* **7**:653–659.

Levi-Montalcini, R. and B. Booker (1960). Destruction of the sympathetic ganglia in mammals by an antiserum to a nerve-growth protein, *Proc. Natl. Acad. Sci. U.S.A.* **46**:384–391.

Mains, R. E. and P. H. Patterson (1973a). Primary cultures of dissociated sympathetic neurons. I. Establishment of long-term growth in culture and studies of differentiated properties, *J. Cell Biol.* **59**:329–345.

Mains, R. E. and P. H. Patterson (1973b). Primary cultures of dissociated sympathetic neurons. III. Changes in metabolism with age in culture, *J. Cell Biol.* **59**:361–366.

Nurse, C. A. and P. H. O'Lague (1975). Formation of cholinergic synapses between dissociated sympathetic neurons and skeletal myotubes of the rat in cell culture, *Proc. Natl. Acad. Sci. U.S.A.* **72**:1955–1959.

O'Lague, P. H., P. R. MacLeish, C. A. Nurse, P. Claude, E. J. Furshpan, and D. D. Potter (1975). Physiological and morphological studies on developing sympathetic neurons in dissociated cell culture, *Cold Spring Harbor Symp. Quant. Biol.* **40**:399–407.

O'Lague, P. H., K. Obata, P. Claude, E. J. Furshpan, and D. D. Potter (1974). Evidence for cholinergic synapses between dissociated rat sympathetic neurons in cell culture, *Proc. Natl. Acad. Sci. U.S.A.* **71**:3602–3606.

Olson, L. and T. Malmfors (1970). Growth characteristics of adrenergic nerves in the adult rat, *Acta Physiol. Scand. Suppl.* **348**:1–112.

Patterson, P. H. and L. L. Y. Chun (1974). The influence of non-neuronal cells on catecholamine and acetylcholine synthesis and accumulation in cultures of dissociated sympathetic neurons, *Proc. Natl. Acad. Sci. U.S.A.* **71**:3607–3610.

Patterson, P. H. and L. L. Y. Chun (1977). The induction of acetylcholine synthesis in primary cultures of dissociated rat sympathetic neurons. I. Effects of conditioned medium, *Devel. Biol.*, in press.

Patterson, P. H., L. F. Reichardt, and L. L. Y. Chun (1975). Biochemical studies on the development of primary sympathetic neurons in cell culture, *Cold Spring Harbor Symp. Quant. Biol.* **40**:389–397.

Rees, R. and R. P. Bunge (1974). Morphological and cytochemical studies of synapses formed in culture between isolated rat superior cervical ganglion neurons, *J. Comp. Neurol.* **157**:1–11.

Reichardt, L. F., P. H. Patterson, and L. L. Y. Chun (1976). Norepinephrine and acetylcholine synthesis by individual sympathetic neurons under various culture conditions, *Abstr. Annu. Meet. Soc. Neurosci.*, 6th, Toronto, p. 225.

Yamauchi, A., J. Lever, and K. Kemp (1973). Catecholamine loading and depletion in the rat superior cervical ganglion, *J. Anat.* **114**:271–282.

DEVELOPMENT OF NEURONAL CIRCUITRY IN THE INSECT OPTIC LOBE

I. A. Meinertzhagen

Dalhousie University, Halifax, Nova Scotia

The optic neuropils of insects are impeccable examples of neuronal architecture by any standard, yet their anatomical intricacies are little known except to the few who study them. Patterns of neuronal interconnection in one of the best-studied examples, the first optic neuropil or lamina of the fly, are arguably the most completely described of any neuropil in any nervous system. These patterns have been defined at the level of individual, uniquely identifiable neurons, and the orderliness of their construction naturally provokes questions about the ontogenetic events that generate them (Meinertzhagen, 1973, 1975; Shelton, 1976; see also Bate, 1977, for an accomplished review of wider content). Within the context of the present symposium, studies on morphogenesis in the compound eye and optic neuropils provide some general principles of neurogenesis that may be valid outside their phyletic group. Especially is this instructive where fixity in features of neuronal morphology might a priori be considered the consequence of the action of largely intrinsic cellular mechanisms during development. The paucity of evidence on many points makes essential the pooling of data from different insect or arthropod groups. A comparative approach is in any case recommended by the obvious advantage that it allows each problem to be addressed to the species most suited to its solution.

We shall, therefore, adopt the pragmatic standpoint of regarding the insect optic lobe as a model piece of nervous tissue, which may be reduced to a few basic circuits in which morphological complexity is redeemed by the ability to characterize the constituent elements uniquely, and for which morphogenesis involves crucial interactions between relatively few cell classes.

Anatomy of the Adult System

To set the scene for questions of development, a minimal account of the adult structural organization will be provided. Arthropod visual systems in general are replete with structurally regular features, arrangements, and patterns that deserve more than cursory treatment here. A comprehensive account has recently appeared in Strausfeld (1976); some other details about cell patterns and fiber pathways also appear in the papers by Meinertzhagen (1975, 1976).

The eye is composed of a geometrically regular array of ommatidia; each ommatidium contains, in addition to various accessory cells, a retinula of photoreceptors, usually eight in number. For a particular species, the number, pattern, and orientation of photoreceptive retinular cells is in general constant such that each cell may be uniquely identified within the retinula. Among different species of insect, one distinction that may be recognized is between those with retinulae having their photoreceptor rhabdomeres, one from each receptor, united axially in a common or fused rhabdome, and those with retinulae in which the receptors each have a separate rhabdomere, the so-called open rhabdomere arrangement. The former arrangement is found in most insect groups, while the latter is found only in various Hemiptera, some Coleoptera, and in Diptera, best characterized in the fly. In the fly, the characterization of receptors by their position is possible because of the asymmetry of the retinular pattern; this is all the more remarkable because of a mirror-image inversion in the cellular arrangement of dorsal and ventral ommatidia (Dietrich, 1909). The asymmetrical retinular patterns of the two eye halves may be separated by an imaginary line, the equator, which is the interommatidial boundary between two regions of perfect mirror-image pattern duplication. Though most clearly revealed in the eye of the fly, retinular asymmetries and mirror-image inversions are nevertheless encountered in other insect retinae (Meinertzhagen, 1975).

Retinular axons connect centripetally with the optic lobe (Figure 1). Here they terminate either in the first optic neuropil or lamina (the short retinular axons) or in the second neuropil, the medulla (the long retinular axons or so-called long visual fibers). In these neuropils, the two respective axon types establish synaptic connections with higher-order interneurons, of which we will single out only lamina monopolar cells, the chief output neuron of the lamina. Retinular axon terminals and their associated interneurons are grouped in the lamina and medulla neuropils into arrays of cylindrical synaptic cartridges, or columns,

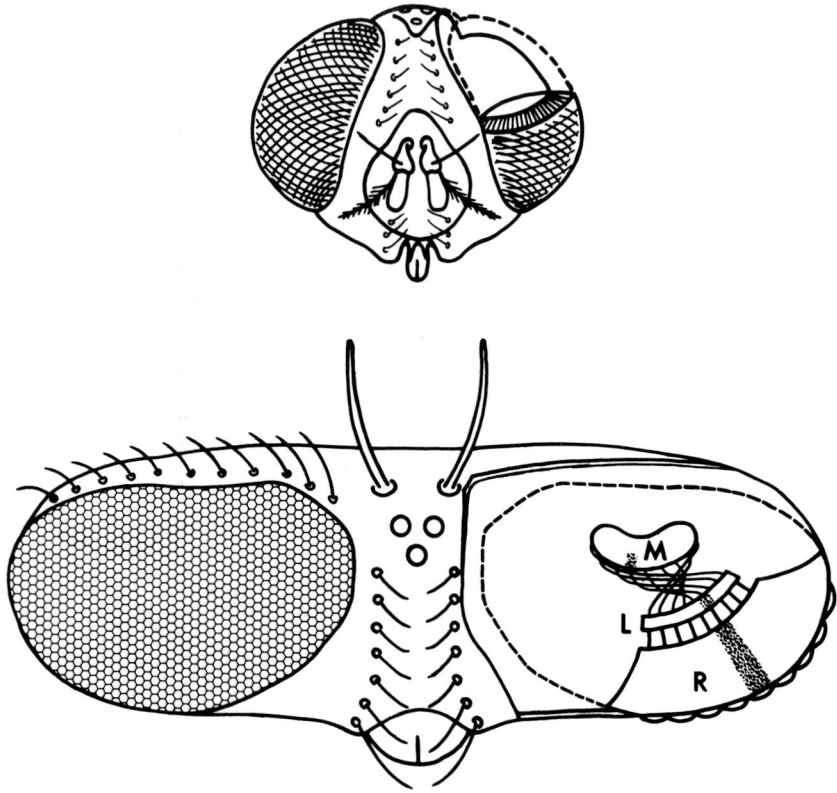

FIGURE 1. Morphology of the compound eye of a fly, in frontal view (top) and in greater detail from the dorsal aspect (bottom). The dorsal halves of the left eye and optic lobe are removed to reveal a horizontal section plane. Within this plane, bottom Figure, the topography of the two outermost optic neuropils, lamina (L) and medulla (M), is shown in relation to the overlying retina (R) together with the form of the fiber pathways that connect these three regions. One spatially corresponding set of an ommatidium, lamina cartridge, and medulla cartridge so connected is shown by the stippled areas.

corresponding in number and arrangement to the overlying ommatidial array of the retina. Each cartridge is therefore a unit compartment of the neuropil comprising the processes of a fixed number of neural elements, each with a distinctive morphology and predictable location within the cartridge cross section. The somata of a cartridge interneuron group are located in the cortex distal to their cartridge in spatially cohesive groups (Strausfeld, 1976, and personal communication). In the fly, processes of eleven interneurons, including five monopolar cells, are associated with each lamina cartridge (Strausfeld, 1971). Grossly simplified, these are the elements and their organization within the optic neuropils. Although the lamina is more nearly described by the summed organization of its component cartridges than is the medulla, in both there are additional cell types that do not have a periodic distribution, and wide-field interconnections exist between cartridges that do not fit so neatly the preceding account. Nevertheless, for present purposes we may regard the neuropil organization as fundamentally periodic, with many elements having demonstrable stereotypy in their connections identical to those of their congeners within all cartridges. The way in which axons project between the retina, lamina, and medulla demonstrates this stereotypy convincingly (Horridge and Meinertzhagen, 1970). Each telodendritic terminal has one predictable location within the neuropil, and in general that is where it is found.

The projection pattern from the retina upon its two outermost visual neuropils shows both striking uniformity and great precision when revealed in different insect groups (Figure 1). In all cases examined, axon bundles *between* these layers preserve both the retinotopic order between ommatidial and cartridge groupings and the point-for-point distribution of elements between a single ommatidium-lamina cartridge-medulla cartridge pathway, i.e., no lateral interweaving occurs between adjacent axon bundles. In the case of the retina-to-lamina connections, there is a direct projection of the visual field, while between lamina and medulla neuropils, the visual field is inverted about the vertical axis by the interpolation of a decussation, the external chiasma, in each optic lobe.

The projection patterns of short retinular axons between retina and lamina reveal, in different insect groups, two types of organization that differ in the lateral connections of terminals within the neuropil (Figure 2). In all insects examined with fused rhabdome ommatidia the receptor terminals derived from a single ommatidium are all located within a single cartridge (Figure 2A), while in those with open-rhabdomere ommatidia the receptor terminals of a single ommatidium are distributed among a number of cartridges (Figure 2B). The projection patterns differ between the two types only in the axon trajectories at the distal face of the lamina neuropil (Meinertzhagen, 1976). In both types, the spatial distribution of terminals within their cartridge reflects the intraommatidial pattern of their cell bodies in the overlying ommatidium, although in the first type (fused rhabdome) this distribution

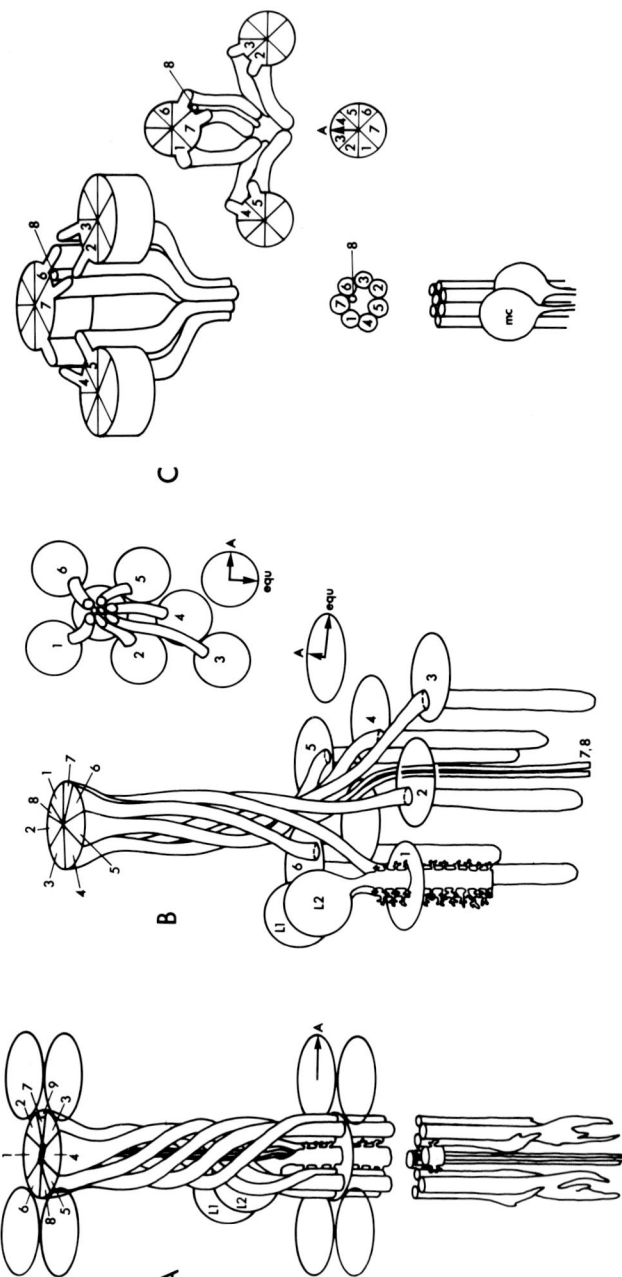

is entirely within a single cartridge, while in the second (open rhabdomere) it is among a group of cartridges. In the fly, the receptors of a single ommatidium all have divergent optical axes, each of which is coincident with a unique set of receptors located in adjacent ommatidia, a different one in each (Kirschfeld, 1967). The consequence of the distributed pattern of short retinular terminal connection patterns among a group of cartridges is to recombine at one lamina cartridge those receptor inputs which exclusively view one point in space (Braitenberg, 1967; Kirschfeld, 1967). Although not traced completely between retina and lamina, an interesting comparison emerges from studies of the retinular projection in various decapod Crustacea (Kunze, 1967; Nässel, 1976). It appears that the axon bundle of each fused rhabdome ommatidium also has a divergent projection, as in the open rhabdomere ommatidia of the fly, but in this case the lateral trajectories are established at the retina itself and, as the result of this, each ommatidium projects upon three neighboring cartridges and not upon a single one. The axons of an ommatidium segregate into four smaller

---

FIGURE 2. The retinular projection patterns of three representative arthropods, the bee, fly, and crayfish, shown in elevation and plan. Retinular cells are identified by the extant numbering conventions. (A) Projection from the retinula of the bee ommatidium characteristic of fused rhabdome ommatidia in which all retinular terminals of one ommatidium are associated with one lamina cartridge (Meinertzhagen, 1976). Short retinular terminals (cells 1 through 6) surround the axons of the long visual fibers, together with those of a group of monopolar cells, of which L1 and L2 are representative. From each lamina cartridge, long visual fibers and monopolar axons project as a single bundle upon a cartridge of the medulla. Four surrounding retinulae project upon each of four surrounding cartridges to complete the array indicated by the vacant elipses. Further details of cell types, their morphology, and projections are found in Ribi (1975). (B) Ommatidial projection of the fly, which, unlike that of the bee, results in the distribution of each of six short retinular axons to a separate cartridge where each terminates in a predictable circumferential position (see plan). Each lamina cartridge has an associated group of monopolar cells, of which only two (L1 and L2) are shown associated with the cartridge of terminal 1. The long visual fibers (7 and 8) alone project to the cartridge, which underlies their ommatidium of origin. Neighboring ommatidia project in identical fashion upon the array of cartridges, resulting in a complex interweaving of retinular axons at the distal face of the lamina neuropil. For further details, see text. (C) Projection of decapod crustacean retinulae (after Kunze, 1967, and Nässel, 1976) in which adjacent cells of three ommatidia form a single axon bundle that presumably projects upon a single lamina cartridge. Each ommatidium cooperates in this way with two others, different cells of the retinula joining with axons from different neighboring ommatidia. The pattern of convergence is shown in the plan. Abbreviations: A, anterior; equ, equator; mc, monopolar cell.

subgroups, each subgroup uniting with the closest subgroup of an adjacent ommatidium with which, as a reconstituted bundle of eight axons, it passes to the lamina (Figure 2C).

Some Implications from the Study of Adult Connection Patterns

A brief introductory review will be given of the adult projection patterns of fly short retinular axons, since they serve both as the neural substrate of vision (Trujillo-Cenóz and Melamed, 1966; Braitenberg, 1967) and, from a theoretical standpoint, as an example of precision in morphogenesis (Wolpert, 1971). Each ommatidium gives rise to six short retinular axons that are distributed among a trapezoidal array of underlying cartridges, each cartridge collecting the converging axons of six ommatidia as shown in Figure 2B. In the normal pattern, therefore, no two axons of the same ommatidium converge upon the same cartridge. Axon trajectories are repetitive, axons of each cell class being located in a predictable position at the circumference of their cartridge, each cartridge being related to the ommatidium of origin by the same spatial transposition (Trujillo-Cenóz and Melamed, 1966; Braitenberg, 1967). Because of their physical dimensions, axon trajectories and the location of retinular terminals can be traced in high-resolution serial photomicrographs and catalogued to reveal consistencies and inconsistencies; inconsistent connections reveal the nature of growth rules by which consistent connections are generated. Moreover, comparison of connection patterns from retinulae immediately dorsal and ventral to the equator of the eye reveals what happens when axons spread into a cellular matrix that is the mirror image of that which they might expect to encounter in any other region of the eye. The equator therefore models in a general way neuronal growth at the midline between left- and right-hand sides of the brain. Occasionally, too, nature performs an experiment for us in the form of irregularities, or dislocations, in the discontinuity of pattern symmetry at the equator; at these, axons have an additional complexity in which to express their growth tendencies.

Two such extensive catalogues have been prepared, sampling a total of approximately 1,000 retinular axons (still only a small, if selected, portion of two eyes) either in a region incorporating the retinal equator (Horridge and Meinertzhagen, 1970) or in a region incorporating part of the equator that was dislocated (Meinertzhagen, 1972) (Figure 3). The first general conclusion which bears emphasis is the very high

DEVELOPMENT OF INSECT OPTIC LOBE NEURONS

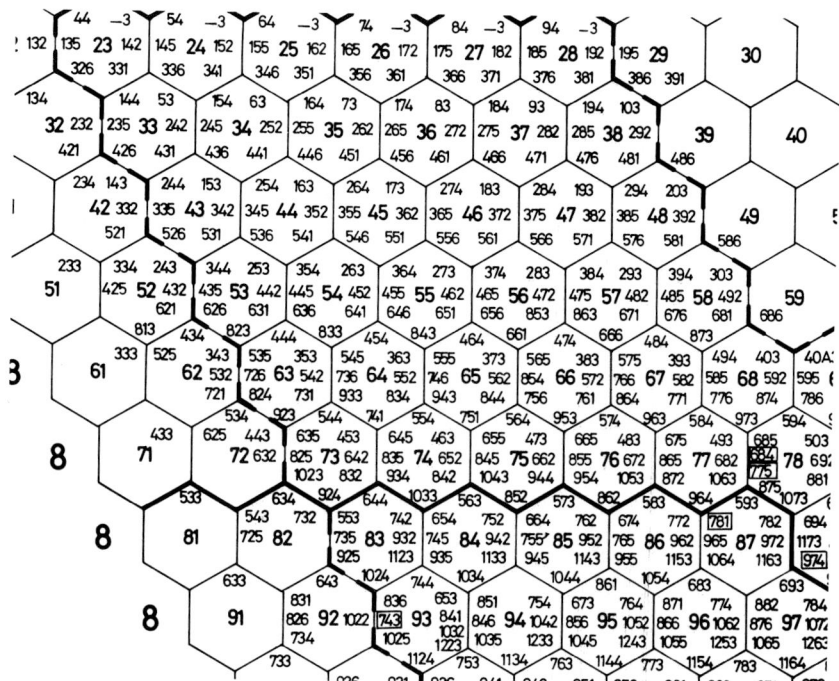

FIGURE 3. Part of an exactly reconstructed map of retinular terminals in the fly lamina (from Meinertzhagen, 1972) reveals the extraordinary spatial precision with which ommatidia become represented in the lamina neuropil during morphogenesis. Each hexagon is a cartridge numbered for the ommatidium overlying it; index numbers arranged within the hexagons are retinular terminals, numbered for their cell (last digit) and ommatidium (preceding digits) of origin. All positions exactly conform to the pattern illustrated in Figure 2B with the exception of the five shown here enclosed in a box, which terminate in unpredictable positions. The heavy line drawn between cartridges starting at the left of the map between cartridges 71 and 81 corresponds to the position of the equator in the retina. Note, in the three cartridge rows dorsal and ventral to the equator, the extra numbers of terminals formed by axons crossing the equator to terminate, as well as the variation in these numbers of terminals introduced by the location of terminals in incorrect cartridges.

degree of accuracy of connections even for axons which cross the equator to terminate. Where inconsistencies in the projection pattern were found, they were, with one exception, associated with the region of equatorial dislocation. A somewhat larger number of trivial mistakes occurred when the terminals were located out of their normal circumferential sequence around the cartridge periphery, usually being transposed with their neighbors, and these occurred more frequently at the equator than away from it. Cell classes 3 and 4, which normally travel farthest in the latticework of interweaving axons, account for most of the inconsistent projections and also for most of the transpositions in terminal sequence around the cartridge (presumably because these have the smallest angular separation when converging upon their normal cartridge). In addition, axons behave conservatively and, if they err, travel no farther in the lattice than they would normally. In general, axon trajectories in the lamina behave as if they had been drawn individually by a patient but rather lazy draughtsman, as straight lines between origin and anticipated termination. (Incidentally, it might be claimed that it was not the patient, lazy draughtsman who drew the lines in a real fly, but rather, an observer who later incorrectly traced out the axon pathways in a perfect fly. This would be countered with the claim that far greater care was taken in checking inconsistent connection patterns than in checking consistent ones; nevertheless, erroneous observation remains a possible objection.)

Errors are found in proportion to the difficulty one might intuitively anticipate the draughtsman would encounter in calculating the correct termination spot. The analogy holds true for the second general conclusion. Inconsistent connections are autonomous; they are not propagated like a fault in a crystal as they might be if a mechanism requiring cueing were involved in their formation, nor do they depend upon the connections made by the other axons of the same ommatidium. In short, there is no particular pattern of inconsistent projection; the errors merely introduce a small level of disorder into an otherwise perfect system of connections in a way that is both autonomous and probabilistic for all axons. Last, if inconsistent connections truly represent loopholes in the normal growth rules, there seems no reason to endow the cartridge as an entity with discriminative capacities. The cartridge appears to accept passively the growing terminals that it receives, even though the total complement of terminals may vary or though two terminals may arise from the same ommatidium. We will see later how well the ideas of autonomy and probability agree with the cytokinetic events by which the lateral excursions of axons are produced within the neuropil.

Fiber Growth Patterns Between Consecutive Cell Layers

To reemphasize the major features of the fiber pathway in the adult between retina and lamina cortex and in the chiasma between the

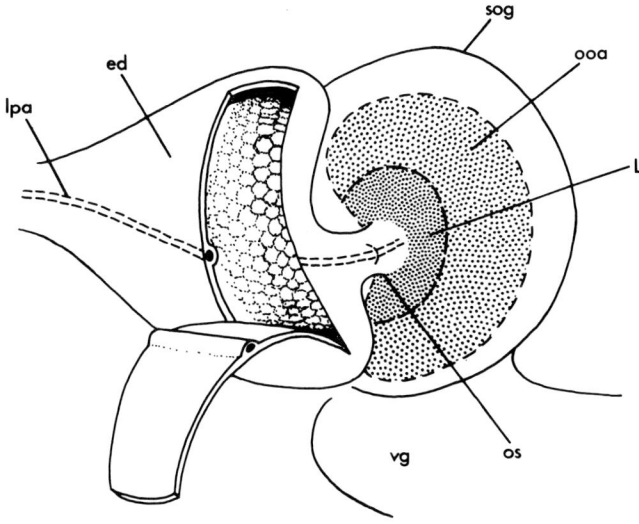

FIGURE 4. The connection between the retina developing within the eye imaginal disc (ed) and the visual neuropils developing within the larval supraesophageal ganglion (sog) is formed by the optic stalk (os) through which, down the path of the primitive larval photoreceptor axon bundle (lpa), grow retinular axons to innervate the lamina (L).

lamina and the medulla cortex: their essential similarity is that retinotopic order is faithfully preserved; their major difference is that the former is a direct, uncrossed projection, whereas the latter involves a decussation in the horizontal plane. This difference is, in theory, trivial: it represents merely an inversion in anteroposterior polarity with which spatially ordered fiber bundles stack up against each other in retinotopic sequence. Both features are the outcome of guided axon growth between the different cell layers.

In the fly eye, development occurs in the imaginal disc, while the two optic neuropils develop within the larval supraesophageal hemispheres. The two structures are connected through an optic stalk (Figure 4). The fiber pathways between the retina and the first two optic neuropils are laid down around a preexisting visual pathway, that of the larval photoreceptor axon bundle, or nerve of Bolwig (1946), which extends along the peripodial membrane of the eye disc and thence to the supraesophageal hemisphere through the optic stalk (Roberts, 1971). Outgrowth of retinular axon bundles occurs in a spatiotemporal sequence initiated in the sequence of ommatidial differentiation, which transfers retinal pattern centrally to the lamina cortex. Lamina and medulla cortices are proliferated from a population of neuroblasts (in invertebrates, these are generative cells whose progeny become neurons), the outer optic *anlage*. Each cortex expands with continued proliferation, and the two cortices are oriented orthogonally. Incoming waves of retinular axons innervate neurons closest to, and most recently proliferated from, the neuroblast group, penetrating the lamina cortex perpendicularly but (in the case of the long visual fibers that grow through the lamina) passing along the surface parallel to the medulla cortex (Figure 5). Each successive wave of innervation contributes to

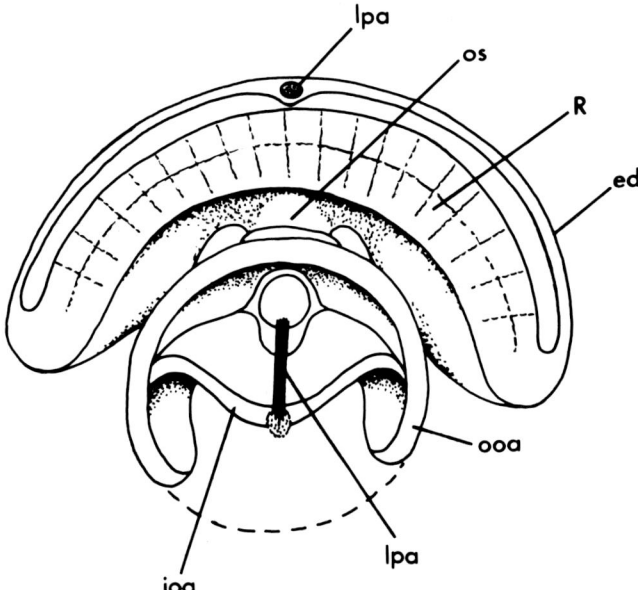

FIGURE 5. The relationship between the internal morphology of eye disc and optic *anlagen* of the supraesophageal ganglion, shown from the anterior aspect of the sectioned face of both structures (compare with Figure 4). The eye disc is a saclike pattern formation of the retina (R) occurring among cells of the inner face. The optic neuropils are laid down by progeny of two neuroblast plates, the inner and outer optic *anlagen* (ioa and ooa, respectively), which meet orthogonally at every point, the latter encircling the former. An orifice between the two provides entrance from the eye disc for the larval photoreceptor nerve that has its own neuropil at its central end. In growing down this nerve, imaginal retinular axons lay down the medulla neuropil along the face of the inner optic *anlage* and the lamina neuropil at the inner margin of the outer optic *anlage*, building up these two regions in the manner of a floor and a wall, respectively. Abbreviations are the same as in Figure 4.

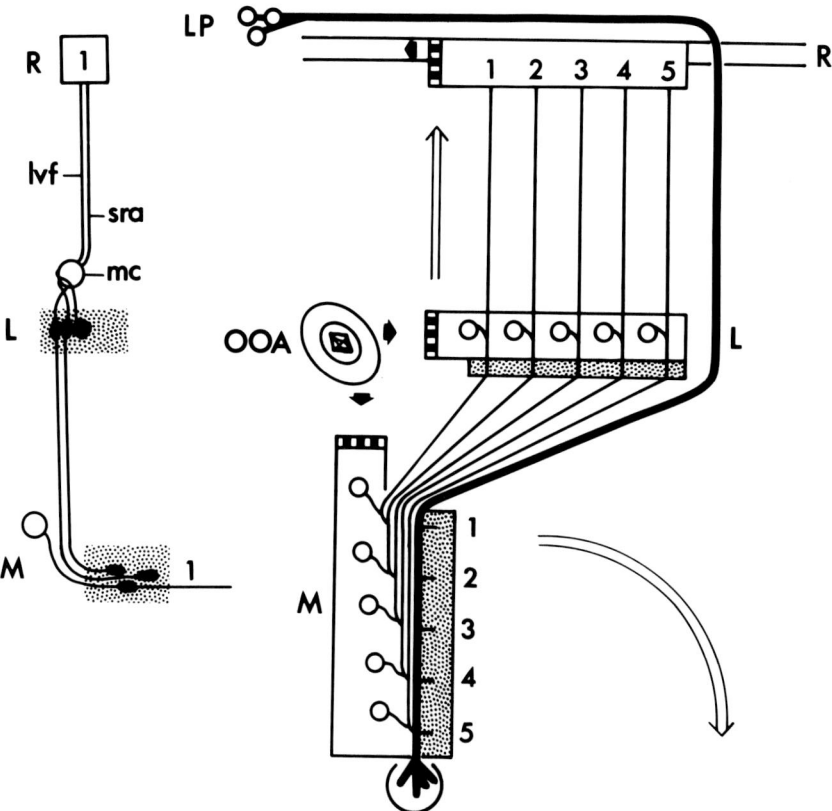

FIGURE 6. Right: schematic representation of the fiber growth patterns between retina (R), lamina (L), and medulla (M) summarizes the essential features involved in guided axon growth in a section plane at right angles to the growing front and containing the path of the pioneer axons of a group of anteriorly placed larval photoreceptors (LP). Neuroblast proliferation from the outer optic *anlage* (ooa) results in the accumulation of cells in two orthogonal directions into the cortices of lamina and medulla, while the invasive wave of retinal development spreads across the head epidermis. In all three zones, a chequered border indicates the margin of cellular accretion, and a solid arrow indicates the nature of this accretion, i.e., whether by invasion or addition. The growing edge of the neuropil zone (stippled) lies back a little from the growing edge of its respective cortex. Fiber bundles grow in the temporal sequence 5 (oldest, against LP nerve) to 1 (newest), with subsequent fiber bundles always feeding into the conveyor belt at a position corresponding to bundle 1. Open arrows indicate the direction of alteration in path length during subsequent development (see text). Left: the elements of fiber bundle 1 in the right-hand side of the Figure. Each element represents a class and is depicted with an expanded-growth cone within the appropriate neuropil. Abbreviations: lvf, long visual fiber; sra, short retinular axon; mc, monopolar cell.

the leading edge of the two neuropil regions; the fiber pathways between these are short and lay down the tract destined to become the chiasma. By continued accretion of new fiber bundles, older fibers lengthen as they become displaced further from the site of innervation. As a simple consequence of the direction that new fiber bundles approach the neuropil to which they will contribute (lamina, perpendicular to; medulla, parallel to), there develops a direct projection between the retina and the lamina and a chiasma between the lamina and the medulla. These features are illustrated schematically in Figure 6, and are discussed at greater length in Meinertzhagen (1973). The retina-lamina projection is initially long, but later shortens considerably (Shatoury, 1956), perhaps by the same (glial) mechanism by which certain interganglionic nerve cord connectives shorten in insects (Pipa, 1973). In shortening, the lamina is drawn up under the retinal basement membrane, and this extends the chiasmal pathway, subjecting the medulla neuropil to torsion and so revealing more conspicuously the nature of its decussation (Figure 6).

The intimate association between the first imaginal (adult) retinular axons to grow down the optic stalk and the larval photoreceptor axon bundle already there has led to the obvious ascription of a pioneer or pathfinder role to the former (Meinertzhagen, 1973; Trujillo-Cenóz and Melamed, 1973). Similarly, imaginal fibers that have already grown continue the process, laying down a path for those yet to grow. Each pathway heralds the next as new structures are laid down on old in what Bate (1977) has evocatively described as a refined game of "follow my leader." Recent studies emphasize, in various systems, a guiding role for other precociously differentiating pathways (the stemmatal nerve in the development of the butterfly visual system, Nordlander and Edwards, 1969; in the moth antenna, Sanes and Hildebrand, 1975; and in the locust thoracic ganglion, Bate, 1976), and all reiterate a general principle of developmental mechanics as applied to neuronal morphogenesis. These principles (Weiss, 1941) stress both the importance of surfaces and interfaces in the determination of axon trajectories by contact guidance forces and the modifiability of the length of the trajectory by subsequent stretching or shortening. These features, as we have seen, are all revealed in the events that lay down the fiber tracts between cell body populations in the optic lobe, but at a new level of resolution, characteristic of invertebrate studies, that of single identified cells.

In vitro studies on the pattern and speed of progression of individual growth cones across artificial substrates (reviewed in Letourneau, this volume) provide evidence for the importance of the relative adhesion of the substrate, regardless of its specific chemical nature. Progression occurs, in much the same way as a pedestrian on ice, in proportion to the growth cone's ability to cling to the substrate; we might therefore suppose that guided growth of retinular innervation in the insect optic lobe proceeds because existing axons offer a pathway of higher adhesiveness than other boundaries and interfaces in the developing system.

The Onset of Differentiation in Monopolar Neurons

The patterns of fiber growth through the optic stalk result in the guided delivery of axon bundles to the developing optic lobe in a precise spatial order, initiated peripherally by the temporal pattern of ommatidial differentiation. At the lamina cortex, new axon bundles innervate newly proliferated monopolar cell bodies and in this way write their ommatidium into the structure of the associated neuropil. But what of the monopolar cells themselves? Cytodifferentiation proceeds in the receptor groups independently of any connection with the brain (Chevais, 1937), but a complex (and for various reasons indecisive) literature has been interpreted to indicate that differentiation in the cells of the lamina cortex depends upon receipt of retinular innervation (the evidence is less clear for the medulla cortex) (Meinertzhagen, 1973). It is, in fact, extremely difficult to gain critical evidence for a morphogenetic dependence of visual interneurons upon their input neurons. The differentiative step that is critical to observe is neurite extension into the chiasma, by which the monopolar cell becomes itself written into the fabric of the next neuropil, the medulla. One needs at least to observe first, that this neutrite extension occurs after retinular innervation, and second, that cells of the lamina cortex deprived of access to such innervation never extend a neurite. This evidence is not yet available at an appropriate level of resolution for any insect because of the large number of elements that would need to be reconstructed from serial electronmicrographs. To elaborate, many retinular axon bundles are added over a short time interval (in the locust, up to 3,000 retinular terminals become accurately located in the lamina every day [Shelton, 1976]; in the fly *Calliphora*, one new row of up to approximately 50 ommatidia, or 300 terminals, adds its axons approximately every 3 h). This must mean that many retinular-lamina interactions are at a critical stage of innervation at any one time, so one might suppose that the search for these critical innervation stages should be feasible. The problem is that in a given preparation one has no way of knowing which of many retinular axon-monopolar cell interactions is doing something interesting. What is needed is an eye with very few elements, all of which may be accounted for in time-lapse serial electron microscopy. This may be possible in certain species, for example in primitive insect orders (Paulus, 1975) or dragonflies (Ando, 1957), which hatch postembryonically as diminutive adults with very few ommatidia.

For the time being, relevant observations come from another arthropod visual system, that of the crustacean water flea *Daphnia*, which has few ommatidia and embryos that may be precisely staged. In the development of retinular connections with the visual ganglion in *Daphnia*, the lead or pioneer growth cone of an axon bundle contacts a group of uninnervated, undifferentiated cell bodies, each of which in turn responds by a short-lived perikaryal envelopment of the pioneer axon after the growth cone of the relevant fiber has passed (Lopresti, Macagno, and Levinthal, 1973). The envelopment has been seen for at least four of the five cells of a cartridge (Lopresti, Macagno and Levinthal, 1974). The cells in the ganglion subsequently differentiate in the sequence in which they are contacted. Differentiation is manifested by the commencement of neurite extension, again within a period of a few hours, and this sequence is highly suggestive of a mechanism in which the stimulus for axon outgrowth from the visual interneurons is the receipt of retinular innervation. If this view is substantiated, then the envelopment process by the perikaryon would be the likely morphological correlate of the triggering process, an idea that is further strengthened by the formation of transient gap junctions between the contacting and contacted plasmalemmata (Lopresti et al., 1974). Further discussion centering around the nature of the transmitted signal, whether it be inductive (a nonspecific signal to commence differentiation) or instructive (controlling the developmental fate of the contacted cell), addresses the issue of the acquisition of a distinctive morphological phenotype by the second-order cells (Lopresti et al., 1974).

Development of the Retina

The preceding analysis of fiber growth patterns between retina, lamina, and medulla attributes retinotopic ordering of fiber bundle projections between the three layers to the autonomously differentiated patterns of photoreceptor development and suggests the requirement of retinal innervation as the stimulus for axon outgrowth in lamina monopolar cells. It is therefore particularly germane to uncover those patterning forces that control the construction of ommatidial receptor groupings, since retinal pattern formation is, indirectly, impressed upon the underlying neuropils by the exactly timed delivery of axon bundles to particular locations in the neuropil.

An understanding of the patterning forces at work during eye development in insects has moved in the last five years from being almost entirely misunderstood to being but poorly understood. Current ideas on retinal pattern formation stem from recent evidence in which cell phenotypes within the ommatidium are examined histologically and scored in eyes that contain portions of dissimilar genotype, constructed either by genetic (Ready, Hanson, and Benzer, 1976; Hofbauer and Campos-Ortega, 1976) or surgical (Shelton and Lawrence, 1974; Lawrence and Shelton, 1975) manipulation. A few critical observations are selected here that impute the existence of patterning forces during retinal pattern formation by which the developmental fate of a cell is influenced through the cells with which it is in contact or communication. More detailed reviews of descriptive observations have appeared elsewhere (Meinertzhagen, 1973; Shelton, 1976).

Ommatidia are laid down as cell clusters after a wavelike mitotic invasion among the cells of the head epidermis. The wave spreads in an approximately posteroanterior direction, and comprises two fronts, as revealed by tritiated thymidine incorporation (Egelhaaf, Berndt, and Kuthe, 1975; Campos-Ortega and Hofbauer, 1977; Ready et al., 1976). The first (anterior) front is wider and, in *Drosophila*, produces the progenitors of all retinular cell types, as well as cells 2–5 and 8 (Campos-Ortega and Hofbauer, 1977; Ready et al., 1976). The second front is narrow (2–3 ommatidial rows wide) and gives rise to the remaining cells (numbers 1, 6, and 7), which exclusively occupy equatorial positions in the retinula. Within these two waves, mitotic products of labeled mitoses are distributed among many ommatidia; the formation of cell clusters thus involves the recruitment of cells in two stages (Ready et al., 1976). Within a single ommatidium, however, there is no fixed lineage between the cells added from either or both mitotic waves. In particular there is no simple clonal relationship by which a single progenitor proliferates all or any fixed group of the cells of the ommatidium. This has been revealed both by scoring the phenotypes of small mosaic clones of dissimiliar genotype induced by somatic crossover in *Drosophila* (Campos-Ortega and Hofbauer, 1977; Ready et al.,

1976) and by scoring phenotypes at the borders of genetically distinct surgical implants in the bug *Oncopeltus* (Shelton and Lawrence, 1974; Lawrence and Shelton, 1975). This is not to say that regularities in lineage do not occur. A single progenitor seems to give rise always to certain cells of the retinula (in *Drosophila*, cell 7 and either cell 1 or 6), the remainder developing as some of cells 1–6 (Campos-Ortega and Hofbauer, 1977). It is merely that such lineage regularities as have been revealed do not respect ommatidial boundaries, and clonal descendants are often located in different ommatidia.

The central problem, at present, is to distinguish: (1) whether the lineage of a cell has any direct influence on the restriction of that cell to a particular phenotype, regardless of the ommatidium in which it is finally located, i.e., whether mitoses are themselves differentiative (as they are for the constitutent cells of other epidermally derived insect sensory organules [Lawrence, 1966]); or (2) whether the genealogy of a cell merely determines the time and place at which a pluripotent cell becomes incorporated into an ommatidial cluster, morphological phenotype being subsequently acquired by some interactive mechanism involving the other cells of the cluster, e.g., by the cell's position, as suggested by Lawrence and Shelton (1975) or more explicitly by the area of membrane contact formed by each cell, as suggested by Ready et al. (1976). These two alternatives (lineage versus position) would be indistinguishable in the formation of a normal ommatidium if the mitotic activity of progenitor cells had sufficient regularity always to deliver some cells to particular positions in the cluster, while the remaining progeny came to occupy positions in the cluster on a probabilistic basis.

Once constituted in a cluster, the spatial arrangement of its component cells confers polarity upon the ommatidium. This polarity is inherited from the epidermis that gives rise to the ommatidium, since in the bug *Oncopeltus*, 90° rotations of head epidermis lying in the path of retinal development produce, at the margins of the graft, ommatidia with an alignment intermediate between that of host and graft (Lawrence and Shelton, 1975). Epidermal transplants between dorsal and ventral head regions produce, after retinal invasion, no alteration in ommatidial polarity, indicating that the patterning force in the epidermis to which the cells respond when clustering is aligned in an anteroposterior direction and may be analogous to, if not identical with, the segmental gradient manifest throughout the insect integument as a whole (Lawrence, 1973).

The initiation of the sequence of patterned mitoses that generate ommatidial clusters has its origin at or near the posterodorsal eye margin in an autonomous region of the eye field that functions as a differentiation center (see, e.g., White, 1961, 1963; Wachmann, 1965). Eye development is propagated in wavelike fashion from this point, but precisely what influence spreads from a transformed region of head epidermis undergoing retinal development to an untransformed region is still obscure. It may be solely a stimulus for cells to commence mitosis, cell products undergoing differentiation according to an intrinsic timetable that starts at the cessation of mitosis, or alternatively, ommatidial differentiation itself may be propagated inductively from older to young cell clusters. Evidence against the latter alternative, i.e., in favor of an intrinsically determined timetable of differentiation, is provided by the observation of Sprengart, Cölln and Egelhaaf (1976). After an injection of ethidium bromide in the developing moth *Ephestia*, an undifferentiated band of retina conforming in curvature to the developmental wavefront is formed, separating on either side regions of more advanced retinal differentiation. The results warrant closer histological examination, but seem to indicate that the state of ommatidial differentiation does not depend upon that of neighboring ommatidia. Still remaining is the question of whether ommatidia develop as a whole, their cellular complement being in synchrony, or whether cells commence differentiation in accordance with their own intrinsic timetable, i.e., in the sequence of the two groups that are added to the retinular cluster at different times.

Growth Cone Morphologies

It is a rather telling comment on our state of knowledge that the best cytokinetic indication of the cellular and supracellular forces to which neurons react during development is the morphology of the growth cones at their extending neurite tips; yet at one level of analysis, this is the only account one can provide of morphogenesis, since the morphology of a neuron is in all important respects merely a cumulative log of selected growth cone excursions. Were we to know all the factors to which a growth cone responds at all stages of development, and in particular how certain excursions are selected over others, then we could arrive at a model of adult neuronal morphology.

The early observations of Sánchez (1919) on growth cones in the developing optic lobe of the butterfly *Pieris* described two basic types of cone morphology (Figure 7) that are apparently interconvertible.

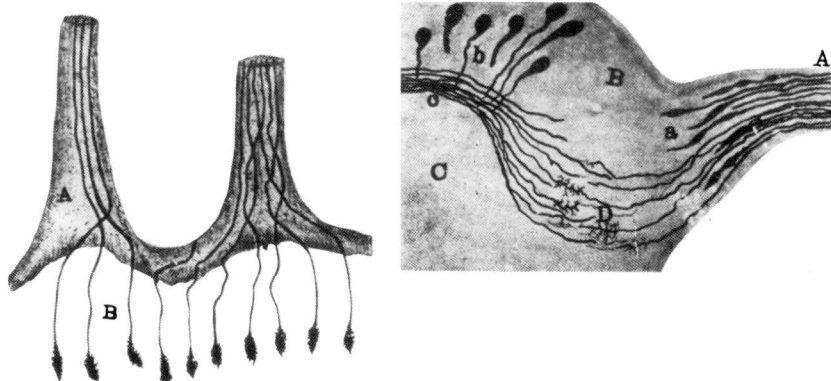

FIGURE 7. Morphology of growth cones revealed by Golgi impregnation of neurons in the developing optic lobe of the butterfly *Pieris* (from Sánchez, 1919). Right: the smooth, slender growth cone found in guided growth in the fiber tracts of retinular axons. Left: the expanded retinular growth cones, invested with numerous filopodia formed in the lamina.

They are revealed by Golgi impregnation with a frequency in approximate proportion to the time the cone spends in either state. The first type of smooth cone is the only form of terminal specialization reported at neurite tips undergoing guided growth in the fiber tracts between the retina and neuropil layers. It is slender, elongate, and relatively devoid of filopodia. It is also rarely impregnated in Golgi preparations (Sánchez 1919), perhaps because any one brain contains relatively few, since neurite extension occurs rapidly along the fiber tracts and is complete in the fly within the interval of a few hours growth in the optic stalk (Meinertzhagen, 1973). Within the neuropil, the slender growth cone expands and becomes invested with filopodia. Expanded growth cones are frequently impregnated in Golgi preparations and always found in a neuropil location, unless the cone is impeded ectopically, for example in passage through the retinal basement membrane (Sánchez, 1919). Frequency of impregnation, again, probably reflects simply the relatively protracted period of time the cone spends in this particular morphological configuration during progressive maturation. Expanded growth cones from different species (*Pieris*: Sánchez, 1919; the fly: Figure 8; the locust: Shelton, 1976) have a similar appearance, even though the adult morphology to which they give rise differs. This broad distinction between growth cone morphologies prompts various questions of their control at different growth stages. These will be considered under two separate headings: the factors that control linear progression of the cone (what starts it, what stops it, and in particular what controls the transition between slender and expanded growth cone or vice versa), and the factors that control lateral progression of the cone. This should not be taken to imply a separation of the factors influencing one vector of growth over those involved in the control of its orthogonal partner.

Control of linear progression

The initiation of outgrowth is, for the retinular cell, part of the autonomous program of retinal differentiation. There is still no decisive evidence on whether neurite extension from an ommatidial cluster occurs synchronously from all cells or whether in a temporal sequence

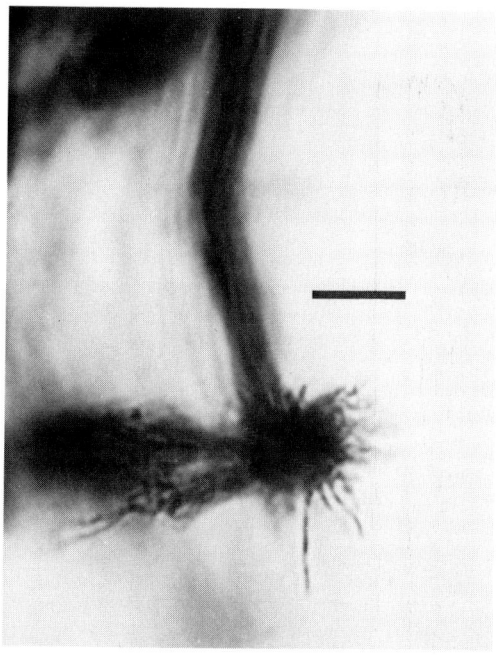

FIGURE 8. Morphology of the expanded-growth cone of a short retinular axon of the fly *Calliphora* impregnated by the rapid Golgi method. The cone at an immature stage is indistinguishable from those of *Pieris* (Figure 7) and is one of a cluster of elements impregnated, the remainder lying out of the plane of focus. Note the diameter of the expanded cone and the numerous straight, slender filopodia. Scale: 5 μm.

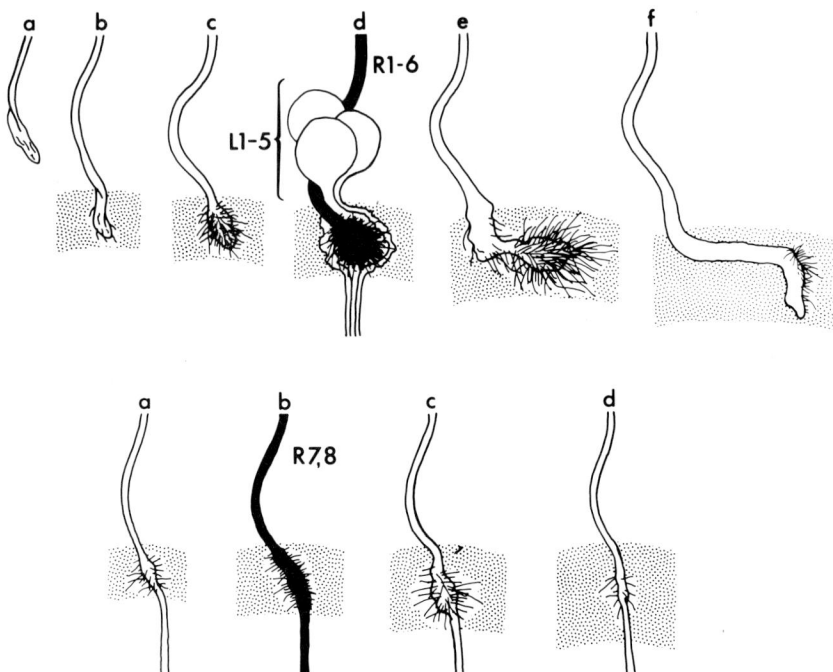

FIGURE 9. Summary diagrams of the maturative transition of expanded growth cone morphology in the fly lamina neuropil (stippled). The morphologies are based upon the combined evidence of serial electron microscope reconstruction and Golgi impregnation (Meinertzhagen, 1973; Trujillo-Cenóz and Melamed, 1973), but in some cases they are still tentative. Inherent indeterminancy of the shape of terminals is one outcome of the probabilistic nature of growth cone expansion: this contrasts with the invariance of mature neuronal morphology. Top: a series representing the short retinular axons (R1-6) at different stages, from the arrival of a postulated slender growth cone at the lamina (a) through its progressive expansion and later lateral migration (b through e), to the point at which the cone has reached a terminal locus associated with a different group of neurons from those that it initially innervated and commences centripetal growth of the telodendritic terminal (f). Stage d shows some of the constellation of elements of one ommatidial group, all of which show expanded growth cones. Bottom: a series representing the initial expansion and later regression of a long visual fiber (R7,8) within the lamina, which proceeds concomitantly with growth cone expansion in all elements.

reflecting the sequence of acquisition of cells by the cluster. One report describes bundles of five axons in the developing fly eye disc (Trujillo-Cenóz and Melamed, 1973) which could correspond with neurite extension from an immature cluster before the addition of the three remaining cells of the cluster. This would be consonant with retinular cell neurite extension occurring in a cell-autonomous fashion after a time period initiated either by the clustering of cells or by the mitoses preceding it. In the case of lamina monopolar cells, initiation of neurite extension is known only from the studies of Lopresti et al. (1973) (see previous section), and is non-autonomous, requiring retinular innervation, but again, occurring after a time period apparently initiated at the moment of innervation.

The transition between smooth and expanded growth cone occurs when the neurite encounters a neuropil layer and, for most cell types, spells an end to further linear progression. It would be difficult to imagine how this transition might be brought about by a totally intrinsic mechanism such as after a defined length of neurite extension had occurred. It is in fact not necessary to think that the growth cone changes in any way, rather that the cellular context, in which it finds itself in the neuropil, changes. The transition between smooth and expanded growth cone has previously been thought of as an impedance phenomenon (Meinertzhagen, 1973), but this is apparently not the case for the long visual fibers that form expanded growth cones in the lamina after their neurite has passed through its neuropil into the chiasma (Figure 9). It seems most likely that for these, as for all retinular elements, the formation of expanded growth cones is induced by the cellular elements encountered in the lamina. The long visual fibers, which go on to form an expanded growth cone in the medulla with a different pattern and timetable of morphogenesis, provide good evidence for the autonomous local control of growth cone behavior at two sites along the axon.

Control of lateral progression

Different motile behavior appears to mediate growth cone progression during guided growth and during growth within the neuropil.

During guided growth between the neuropil layers, the substrate of elongation is established by the pathways already laid down. Spatio-temporal sequences of axon outgrowth from the retina provide a mechanism by which the possibility of projection upon most lamina or medulla cartridge loci is denied to the developing ommatidium during the course of normal development. Nevertheless, many ommatidia distributed across an approximately dorsoventral wavefront must be at equivalent stages of neurite extension, and each new wave of innervation, arranged in the optic stalk cross section in a curvilinear sheet, contains fiber bundles that scrupulously maintain their retinotopic sequence. If the fiber bundles of any such wavefront actively assess their retinotopic sequence, then they can only do so by sampling the fiber bundles on either side of their own (correct) trajectory, and this should be evident in lateral excursions of the growth cone at their tips. Sánchez' descriptions often, in fact, refer to the slender growth cone having an undulatory, sinusoidal or lamelliform morphology, all of which are suggestive of lateral sampling, but confirmation would require that the relationship between the growth cone and the fiber substrate on which it travels be examined electron microscopically. It is not yet clear whether retinotopic ordering results from active sorting out among this population of axon bundles, although at a descriptive level evidence on this point will come when the morphology of growth cones during guided growth is adequately described. The precision with which a bundle is able to hold its station in the array is also important. If retinotopy is preserved by fiber bundles assessing their position by some locus-specific mechanism, e.g., within a gradient of information extending across the whole eye, as explicitly suggested by Bate and Lawrence (1973), then the wider the linear array of fiber bundles, the greater the magnitude of anticipated lateral excursions necessary to detect a change in the gradient. If, on the other hand, fiber bundles sort out with references only to their immediate neighbors, i.e., without access to information about all other fiber bundles, then excursionist cone behavior should involve sampling from a fixed number of fiber bundles only. These examples are considered in detail because they illustrate how descriptions of cellular behavior more precise than currently available permit inferences distinguishing between categories of mechanism.

During growth within the neuropil the mode of growth cone progression alters as the cones expand. They cease rapid extension and undergo a protracted phase of growth that is mediated in a probabilistic fashion by the exploration of filopodia. The diameter of the cone approximates 5 μm (Figure 8), and numerous straight filopodia are put forth, usually up to an equivalent length. Since all surrounding elements also have expanded growth cones behaving similarly, the surface of any one cone becomes highly convoluted, riddled with the filopodia from adjacent and subjacent elements. Any filopodial exploration is therefore made at the expense of an invagination into another cone. Glial cells are also invaginated superficially. The expanded growth cones of one retinular axon bundle initially are closely adherent and have symmetrical junctions between their apposed membranes (Trujillo-Cenóz and Melamed, 1973), but apparently as the result of their filopodial explorations, each cone gradually draws away from its parent axon bundle (Figure 9), diverging toward an adjacent monopolar cell group located within an arc of explored lamina. The convergence of groups of terminals upon appropriate monopolar cell groups converts the organization of the lamina from an ommatidial matrix to a cartridge matrix and also coincides with the transfer of cone-cone junctions, from between intraommatidial retinular growth cone neighbors to between intracartridge retinular growth cone neighbors (Trujillo-Cenóz and Melamed, 1973). The mechanism by which the direction of lateral divergence is attained is no less obscure now than when previously discussed (Meinertzhagen, 1973, 1975), and all shades of mechanism can still be entertained, from a complex map-reading of local gradients to simple mechanical models relying upon spatial geometry and the frequency of filopod-cone interaction. There is even a discrepancy, pointed out by Bate (1977), in the reported events of cytokinesis, i.e., between polarized outgrowth of a collateral from the expanded growth cone (Trujillo-Cenóz and Melamed, 1973) and the gradual condensation of the growth cone from behind its laterally advancing tip, as illustrated in Figure 9. Clearly more extensive description is needed.

Synaptogenesis

The events by which cone-cone junctions in the lamina give way to definitive synaptic connections are not reported, but one issue may be raised for conjecture. Adult synapses reveal dyadic and triadic arrangements of their postsynaptic elements (in the fly: Strausfeld and Campos-Ortega, 1976; Braitenberg and Burkhardt, 1976; in the dragonfly: Armett-Kibel et al., 1977). The numbers and proportions of each type of synapse vary with the identity of the presynaptic element and of the postsynaptic elements with which it is in contact. For a particular class of presynaptic element and combination of postsynaptic elements a characteristic synapse forms, dyad or triad. At some such synapses, glial elements take the place of neuronal processes, even though not apparently as synaptic communicants (Boschek, 1971; Armett-Kibel et al., 1977). In the dragonfly, retinular elements exclusively form triads, even though in the case of one long retinular fiber two of the postsynaptic elements may be glial. Moreover, in the fly, glial elements take the place of L3 (one of the monopolar cells) at a level where that neuron does not have processes

(Braitenberg and Burkhardt, 1976). These two findings, it has been suggested (Armett-Kibel et al., 1977), implicate the presynaptic element as the determinant of synapse type, dyad or triad.

CONCLUSIONS

It has been the intention of this review to illustrate the importance of detailed anatomical descriptions in sorting out the ways by which complex assemblages of neurons result during development from relatively few categories of cellular interaction. Those singled out have been: mitotic and clustering interactions which produce retinal pattern in a two-dimensional field of head epidermal cells; selectivity in guided axon growth between cell populations by which that pattern becomes transmitted to the underlying neuropils; retinular-monopolar interactions by which neurite extension from second-order neurons is controlled; filopod-growth cone interactions in the neuropil by which growth cones gradually acquire their characteristic telodendritic morphology. Each aspect of such a componential analysis needs further documentation, especially at a level of description which accounts for all cells uniquely. Description is a necessary prelude to perturbations in which the behavior of neurons may be observed in situations of abnormal growth. It is not sufficient merely to observe the adult patterns resulting from abnormal growth or the in vitro behavior of isolated growth cones; what is really needed is an ethological approach to the behavior of growth cones, in which the responses of individual cones are studied in the context of all other growth cones with which they interact. This of course needs a striking improvement in the temporal resolution with which descriptive studies on either normal or perturbed systems may be made.

ACKNOWLEDGMENTS

Supported by Canadian National Research Council grant, A-0065.

REFERENCES

Ando, H. (1957). A comparative study on the development of ommatidia in Odonata, *Sci. Rep. Tokyo Kyoiku Daigaku, Sect. B* **8**:174–216.
Armett-Kibel, C., I. A. Meinertzhagen, and J. E. Dowling (1977). Cellular and synaptic organisation in the lamina of the dragon-fly *Sympetrum rubicundulum, Proc. R. Soc. London, Ser. B*, in press.
Bate, C. M. (1977). The development of sensory systems in arthropods, in *Handbook of Sensory Physiology, Vol. 9, Development of Sensory Systems*, Jacobson, M., ed. Springer-Verlag, New York, in press.

Bate, C. M. (1976). Pioneer neurones in an insect embryo, *Nature (London)* **260**:54–56.
Bate, C. M. and P. A. Lawrence (1973). Gradients and the developing nervous system, pp. 37–49 in *Developmental Neurobiology of Arthropods*, Young, D., ed. Cambridge University Press, Cambridge.
Bolwig, N. (1946). Senses and sense organs of the anterior end of the house fly larvae, *Vidensk. Medd. Dan. Naturhist Foren.* **109**:81–217.
Boschek, C. B. (1971). On the fine structure of the peripheral retina and lamina ganglionaris of the fly, *Musca domestica*, *Z. Zellforsch. Mikrosk. Anat.* **118**:369–409.
Braitenberg, V. (1967). Patterns of projection in the visual system of the fly. I. Retina-lamina projections, *Exp. Brain Res.* **3**:271–298.
Braitenberg, V. and W. Burkhardt (1976). Beyond the wiring diagram of the lamina ganglionaris of the fly, in *Neural Principles of Vision*, Zettler, F. and R. Weiler, eds. Springer-Verlag, New York.
Campos-Ortega, J. A. and A. Hofbauer (1977). Cell clones and pattern formation: on the lineage of photoreceptor cells in the compound eye of *Drosophila*, *Wilhelm Roux Arch. Dev. Biol.*, in press.
Chevais, S. (1937). Sur la structure des yeux implantés de *Drosophila melanogaster*, *Arch. Anat. Microsc. Morphol. Exp.* **33**:107–112.
Dietrich, W. (1909). Die Facettenaugen der Dipteren, *Z. Wiss. Zool.* **92**:465–539.
Egelhaaf, A., P. Berndt, and H.-W. Küthe (1975). Mitosenverteilung und ^{3}H-Thymidin-Einbau in der Proliferie renden Augenanlage von *Ephestia kuehniella* Zeller, *Wilhelm Roux Arch. Entwicklungsmech. Org.* **178**:185–202.
Hofbauer, A. and J. A. Campos-Ortega (1976). Cell clones and pattern formation: genetic eye mosaics in *Drosophila melanogaster*, *Wilhelm Roux Arch. Dev. Biol.* **179**:275–289.
Horridge, G. A. and I. A. Meinertzhagen (1970). The accuracy of the patterns of connexions of the first- and second-order neurons of the visual system of *Calliphora*, *Proc. R. Soc. London, Ser. B* **175**:69–82.
Kirschfeld, K. (1967). Die Projektion der optischen Umwelt auf das Raster der Rhabdomere im Komplexauge von *Musca*, *Exp. Brain Res.* **3**:248–270.
Kunze, P. (1967). Histologische Untersuchungen zum Bau des Auges von *Ocypode cursor* (Brachyura), *Z. Zellforsch. Mikrosk. Anat.* **86**:466–478.
Lawrence, P. A. (1966). Development and determination of hairs and bristles in the milkweed bug, *Oncopeltus fasciatus* (Lygaidae, Hemiptera), *J. Cell Sci.* **1**:475–498.
Lawrence, P. A. (1973). The development of spatial patterns in the integument of insects, pp. 157–209 in *Developmental Systems: Insects*, Vol. 2, Counce, S. J. and C. H. Waddington, eds. Academic Press, London.
Lawrence, P. A. and P. M. J. Shelton (1975). The determination of polarity in the developing insect retina, *J. Embryol. Exp. Morphol.* **33**:471–486.
Lopresti, V. A., E. R. Macagno, and C. Levinthal (1973). Structure and development of neuronal connections in isogenic organisms: cellular interactions in the development of the optic lamina of *Daphnia*, *Proc. Natl. Acad. Sci. U.S.A.* **70**:433–437.

Lopresti, V. A., E. R. Macagno, and C. Levinthal (1974). Structure and development of neuronal connections in isogenic organisms: transient gap junctions between growing optic axons and lamina neuroblasts, *Proc. Natl. Acad. Sci. U.S.A.* **71**:1098–1102.

Meinertzhagen, I. A. (1972). Erroneous projection of retinula axons beneath a dislocation in the retinal equator of *Calliphora*, *Brain Res.* **41**:39–49.

Meinertzhagen, I. A. (1973). Development of the compound eye and optic lobe of insects, pp. 51–104 in *Developmental Neurobiology of Arthropods*, Young, D., ed. Cambridge University Press, Cambridge.

Meinertzhagen, I. A. (1975). The development of neuronal connection patterns in the visual systems of insects, pp. 265–288 in *Cell Patterning: Ciba Foundation Symposium 29*, Porter, R. and J. Rivers, eds. Excerpta Medica, Amsterdam.

Meinertzhagen, I. A. (1976). The organization of perpendicular fibre pathways in the insect optic lobe, *Phil. Trans. R. Soc. London, Ser. B* **274**:555–596.

Nässel, D. R. (1976). The retina and retinal projection on the lamina ganglionaris of the crayfish *Pacifastacus leniusculus* (Dana), *J. Comp. Neurol.* **167**:341–360.

Nordlander, R. H. and J. S. Edwards (1969). Postembryonic brain development in the monarch butterfly *Danaus plexippus plexippus*, L. II. The optic lobes, *Wilhelm Roux Arch. Entwicklungsmech. Org.* **163**:197–220.

Paulus, H. F. (1975). The compound eyes of apterygote insects, pp. 3–19 in *The Compound Eye and Vision of Insects*, Horridge, G. A., ed. Clarendon Press, Oxford.

Pipa, R. L. (1973). Proliferation, movement and regression of neurons during the postembryonic development of insects, pp. 105–129 in *Developmental Neurobiology of Arthropods*, Young, D., ed. Cambridge University Press, Cambridge.

Ready, D. F., T. E. Hanson, and S. Benzer (1976). Development of the *Drosophila* retina, a neurocrystalline lattice, *Dev. Biol.* **53**:217–240.

Ribi, W. A. (1975). The first optic ganglion of the bee. I. Correlation between visual cell types and their terminals in the lamina and medulla, *Cell Tissue Res.* **165**:103–111.

Roberts, M. J. (1971). The structure of the mouthparts of some calypterate dipteran larvae in relation to their feeding habits, *Acta Zool. (Stockholm)* **52**:171–188.

Sánchez, D. S. (1919). Sobre el desarollo de los elementos nerviosos en la retina del *Pieris brassicae* L. (continuación), *Trab. Inst. Cajal Invest. Biol.* **17**:1–63.

Sanes, J. R. and J. G. Hildebrand (1975). Nerves in the antennae of pupal *Manduca sexta* Johannsen (Lepidoptera: Sphingidae), *Wilhelm Roux Arch. Entwicklungsmech. Org.* **178**:71–78.

Shatoury, H. H. El (1956). Differentiation and metamorphosis of the imaginal optic glomeruli in *Drosophila*, *J. Embryol. Exp. Morphol.* **4**:240–247.

Shelton, P. M. J. (1976). The development of the insect compound eye, *Symp. R. Entomol. Soc. London* **8**:152–169.

Shelton, P. M. J. and P. A. Lawrence (1974). Structure and development of ommatidia in *Oncopeltus fasciatus*, *J. Embryol. Exp. Morphol.* **32**:337–353.

Sprengart, M., K. Cölln, and A. Egelhaaf (1976). Die Wirkung von Ethidium-

bromid auf die Ommatidienentwicklung bei *Ephestia kühniella* Zeller, *Wilhelm Roux Arch. Dev. Biol.* **179**:19–31.
Strausfeld, N. J. (1971). The organization of the insect visual system (light microscopy). II. The projection of fibres across the first optic chiasma, *Z. Zellforsch. Mikrosk. Anat.* **121**:442–454.
Strausfeld, N. J. (1976). *Atlas of an Insect Brain.* Springer-Verlag, New York.
Strausfeld, N. J. and J. A. Campos-Ortega (1977). Vision in insects: pathways possibly underlying neural adaptation and lateral inhibition, *Science* **195**: 894–897.
Trujillo-Cenóz, O. and J. Melamed (1966). Compound eye of dipterans: anatomical basis for integration—an electron microscope study, *J. Ultrastruct. Res.* **16**:395–398.
Trujillo-Cenóz, O. and J. Melamed (1973). The development of the retina-lamina complex in muscoid flies, *J. Ultrastruct. Res.* **42**:554–581.
Wachmann, E. (1965). Untersuchungen zur Entwicklungsphysiologie des Komplexauges der Wachsmotte *Galleria mellonella* L., *Wilhelm Roux Arch. Entwicklungsmech. Org.* **156**:145–183.
Weiss, P. (1941). Nerve patterns: the mechanics of nerve growth, *Growth (Suppl.)* **5**:163–203.
White, R. H. (1961). Analysis of the development of the compound eye in the mosquito *Aedes aegypti, J. Exp. Zool.* **148**:223–240.
White, R. H. (1963). Evidence for the existence of a differentiation center in the developing eye of the mosquito, *J. Exp. Zool.* **152**:139–148.
Wolpert, L. (1971). Positional information and pattern formation, *Curr. Top. Dev. Biol.* **6**:1–47.

Control of Mechanosensory Nerve Sprouting in Salamander Skin

Ellis Cooper, Sheryl A. Scott, and Jack Diamond

*M.R.C. (Canada) Group in Developmental Neurobiology
McMaster University, Hamilton, Ontario*

INTRODUCTION

The terminal field of a neuron is defined by two parameters, the number of endings that the axon develops at the target it innervates, and the area of the target over which these are distributed. The magnitude of this field is a significant measure of the influence that a neuron can exert in its particular circuit. The development of the terminal field of an axon occurs when the outgrowing axons sprout collaterals at their target; however, very little is known about the mechanisms involved. As Ramón y Cajal pointed out in 1919 (1960), axonal sprouting occurs only in the immediate vicinity of the target, and at some stage this sprouting appears to stop. The terminal field thus achieved could be regulated by mechanisms entirely intrinsic to the neuron. However, there are indications that the target tissue itself may play a role in the initiation of the sprouting (Ramón y Cajal, 1960; Fitzgerald, 1961; Olson and Malmfors, 1970; Landmesser and Pilar, 1976), for example, by producing an appropriate growth-promoting substance (Levi-Montalcini and Angeletti, 1968). However, the reason why nerves apparently stop sprouting is more obscure, because the neuron retains the ability to make more branches, as shown by partial denervation of a target, which almost invariably leads to collateral sprouting of the remaining undamaged nerve fibers (reviewed in Diamond, Cooper, Turner, and Macintyre, 1976).

Given the ubiquity and potential importance of sprouting in the nervous system, we have asked ourselves the following questions. What initiates sprouting? How is this sprouting regulated? And, in addition, do the mechanisms controlling the development of terminal fields persist in the mature animal?

Study of Nerve Sprouting and Its Regulation

The occurrence of sprouting in a variety of situations, both during development and in the mature animal, has recently been reviewed by Diamond et al. (1976). Their review focused on the problems concerned with the area of nerve fields, and we will not deal with that topic specifically in this presentation. Here, we discuss some preliminary findings on the possible involvement of specific target cells in the initiation and regulation of sprouting.

Aguilar, Bisby, Cooper, and Diamond (1973) showed by physiological means that when colchicine was used to interfere with neuronal transport in one of the nerves supplying the salamander hind limb, the other nerves (both motor and sensory) sprouted collaterals and hyperinnervated the skin and muscle supplied by the treated nerve. The treated nerve, however, conducted action potentials quite normally, and we could detect no axonal degeneration. More recently it has been shown not only that the area of the cutaneous mechanosensory field of the treated nerve is unaffected, but that the density and threshold of its endings in the skin (see below) can be quantitatively unchanged at a time when adjacent nerves sprout to hyperinnervate the same region of skin (Cooper, Diamond, and Turner, 1977). The hypothesis that was proposed for nerve sprouting (Aguilar et al., 1973) not only accounted for the results mentioned above, but could also explain most, if not all, other instances of collateral nerve sprouting, both during development and in the mature animal. In essence, this hypothesis states that target tissues continually release substances that initiate nerve sprouting, and that the effects of this sprouting stimulus are neutralized by the action of factors brought to the nerve terminals by axoplasmic transport; the extent of sprouting then is determined by the equilibrium reached between the effects of the two postulated factors.

In our studies on the salamander skin we found that partial denervation does not always lead to increases in areas of the terminal fields of the remaining mechanosensory nerves (Diamond et al., 1976). Nevertheless, we suspected that sprouting of new endings occurred *within* the terminal fields. In addition, our understanding of the mechanisms involved in the proposed neuron-target interaction regulating nerve sprouting required a quantitative description of this phenomenon. For these reasons it became necessary to have a measure of the density of the mechanosensory nerve endings in the skin.

The salamander skin (Figure 1) displays no characteristic sensory

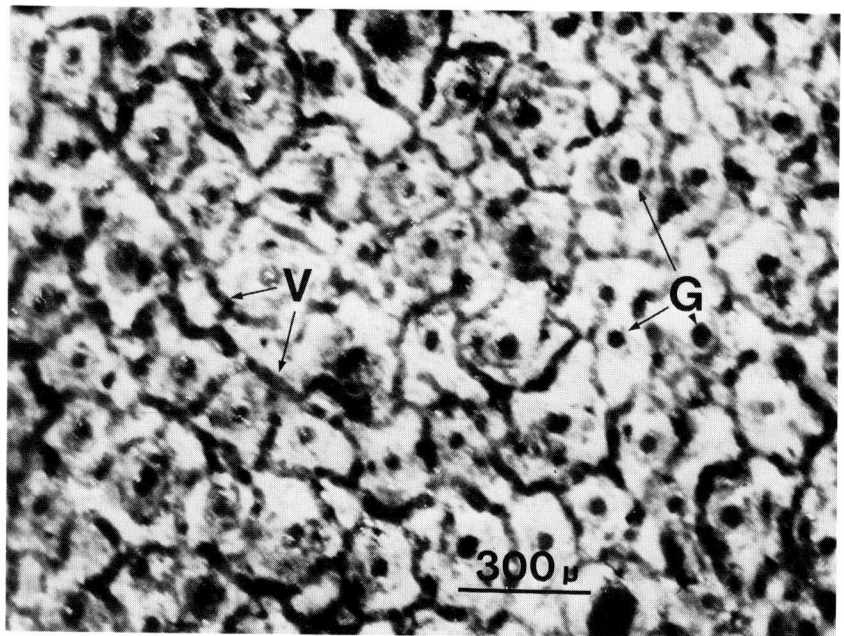

FIGURE 1. Surface of salamander skin as viewed through the dissecting microscope. The blood vessels (V) lie in the dermis and are seen through the transparent epidermis. G: Some of the openings of the secretory gland ducts. The physiological mapping with the 10-μm prodder is carried out at a magnification about four times that of this view.

structures on its surface, such as the touch domes of the mammal or the lateral line organs of many aquatic vertebrates. Furthermore, we could not readily identify any sensory structures in histological sections (Figure 2), such as those often visible in the skin of other vertebrates (Andres and Düring, 1973). Although we have stained cutaneous nerve axons, we were not sure that we could resolve the actual nerve endings without ultrastructural studies.

One likely problem we anticipated in doing such studies was the difficulty in distinguishing the mechanosensory nerve endings from those that might subserve other modalities, which we have shown (unpublished observations) are represented in salamander skin, or from efferent nerve endings to the skin. Moreover, we were especially interested in measuring the number of functional mechanosensory endings that could have newly sprouted in various experimental

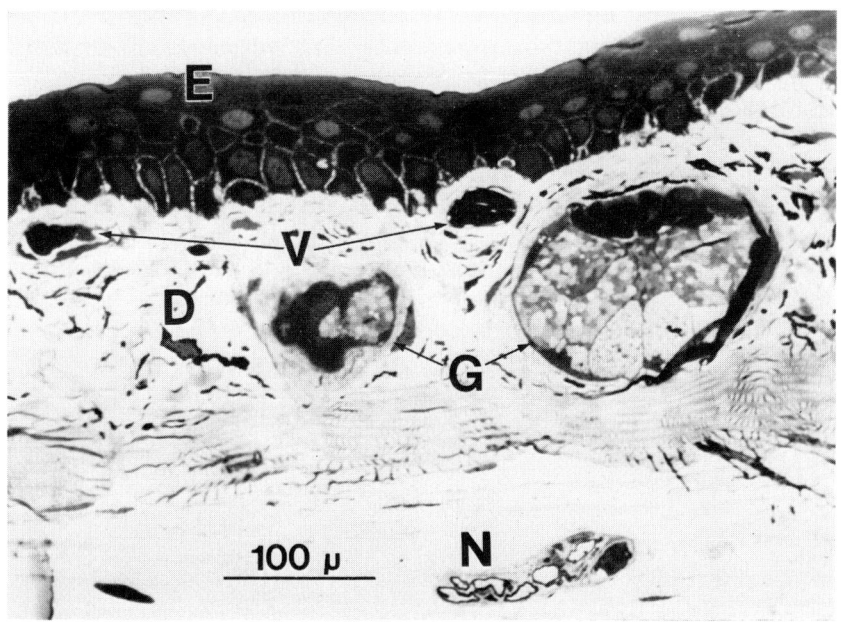

FIGURE 2. Light micrograph of salamander skin. No recognizable sensory structures are found in the epidermis (E) or dermis (D). Merkel cells identified with the electron microscope were found near the basal layer of epidermis. Abbreviations: V, blood vessels; G, secretory glands. Immediately beneath the dermis is a myelinated nerve bundle (N).

situations. As a first approach, therefore, we attempted to make a physiological analysis of the fine organization of the cutaneous touch receptors, which, aside from its own intrinsic interest, could help us in our ultrastructural investigations.

Physiological Analysis of the Mechanosensory Innervation

We have described our method of mechanical stimulation in detail elsewhere (Cooper and Diamond, 1977). Briefly, we use a stimulator consisting of a 10-μm diameter prodder attached to a piezo-electric crystal, which allows the delivery of mechanical stimuli whose rate of rise can be accurately controlled by the applied voltage pulse. The stimulator movement is monitored with a photoelectric device. We record the afferent impulses from whole spinal nerve trunks, and in this way measure the total mechanosensory output from the skin.

Interestingly, we found no slowly adapting mechanoreceptors in the skin, despite stimulation procedures that varied from sustained suprathreshold pulses with the fine-tip prodder, to large maintained deformations with prodders of many millimeters diameter.

By using these techniques we were able to activate single sensory units that were always rapidly adapting (Figure 3). It was clear that some spots were very much more sensitive to touch than others. An analysis of the frequency distributions of touch thresholds across the skin indicated the presence of a single population of low-threshold mechanoreceptors, distributed fairly uniformly across the skin, far enough apart for a randomly located small-diameter prodder frequently

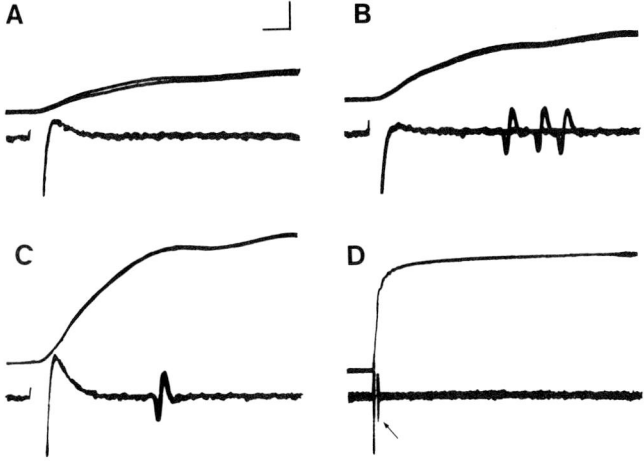

FIGURE 3. Response of rapidly adapting mechanoreceptors. Top trace of each pair shows the photocell output that monitors the prodder movement. Bottom trace shows extracellular recording from the nerve trunk. In (A) the applied stimulus was subthreshold; three traces are superimposed. In (B) the stimulus intensity was increased to just-threshold. Three traces are superimposed, and one spike occurred in each. The variation in the latencies of the spikes is typical with a just-threshold stimulus. (C) Response to a suprathreshold stimulus, which elicited one spike of constant latency; three traces are superimposed. (D) Single sweep with the same stimulus as in (C); the sweep speed was slowed to show that these rapidly adapting mechanoreceptors respond to a suprathreshold-sustained stimulus with a single spike (arrow). Horizontal calibration is 2 msec in (A), (B), and (C), and 50 msec in (D). Vertical calibration is $7\mu m$ for prodder movement, and 20 μV for extracellular records. In other experiments, the amplitude of prodder movement was held constant while its rate of rise was varied. The results showed that these rapidly adapting mechanoreceptors respond to the velocity of the applied stimulus, and not to its amplitude. From Parducz et al. (1977).

to be positioned between them. In the latter cases, higher stimuli (i.e., faster rising pulses) were needed to fire off the nearest receptor than when the prodder was positioned directly over a sensitive spot. We were naturally interested in the possibility that individual mechanosensory nerve endings are located at the highly sensitive spots. In the first instance we attempted to resolve the individual receptive fields of these receptors by making detailed systematic surveys of the skin. Briefly, we sampled about 200 spots on a selected region of skin, moving the prodder in 50-μm steps over a square grid, while testing the mechanosensitivity at each spot. The smallest mechanical stimulus needed to excite an impulse was recorded for each location, and the results were plotted in the form of histograms. These apparent thresholds were divided into three categories—low, medium, and high—in a way that took account both of the resolution of the technique, and of a predicted relationship between stimulus strength and skin deformation under these conditions of stimulation (Cooper and Diamond, 1977; Parducz, Leslie, Cooper, Turner, and Diamond, 1977).

The results of such a systematic survey were then plotted in a two-dimensional array corresponding to the original array of sampled locations on the skin. There was a clear tendency for the low-threshold spots to occur in groups; these were enclosed by lines drawn by eye, as in Figure 4. Our interpretation of these findings is that each of the small discrete sensitive areas represents the functional receptive field of a single-touch receptor. This view is based upon the results of the analysis of the frequency distribution of touch thresholds across the skin (Cooper and Diamond, 1977), which predicts that the receptors occur some 150 μm apart. The sensitive areas vary in size (Figure 4) and we presume that the larger ones represent a few individual receptive fields that were too close to be resolved by our physiological technique. One result of importance is that the highly localized sensitive areas, including the larger ones, were almost always innervated by only one axon, although one axon could innervate many such sensitive areas (usually grouped within one gross axonal field). By using two prodders in an occlusion technique, we have been able to measure the sizes of individual axonal fields, which range from 0.05–2.5 mm^2. If, indeed, individual branches of the parent axons end in the identified sensitive areas, then it can be calculated that each axon branches from as few as 4 to as many as 100 times, depending upon the size of the axonal field.

This pattern of branching of an individual mechanosensory nerve axon could have developed as a consequence of mechanisms intrinsic to the nerve, as we have pointed out above. However, our hypothesis for

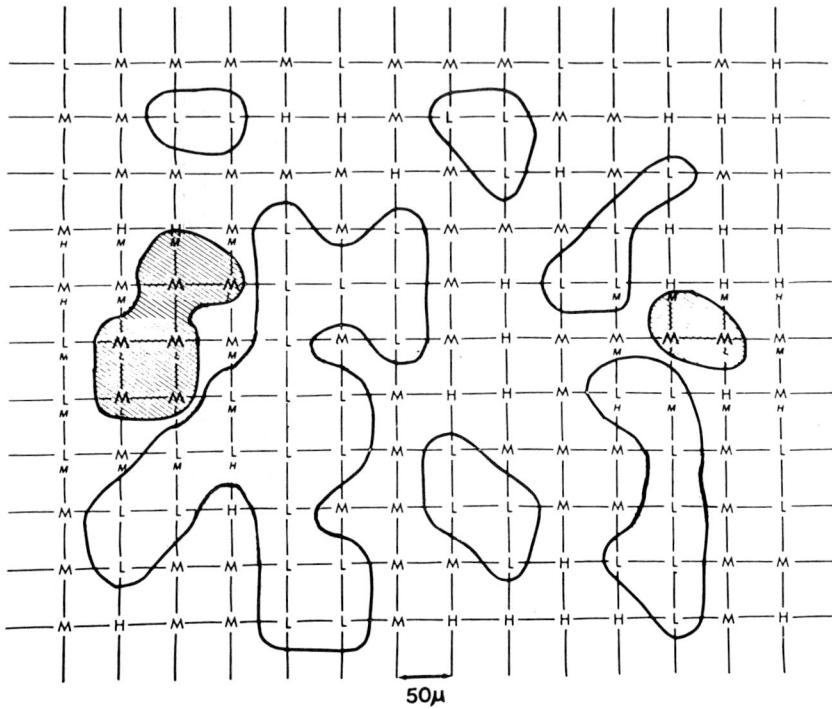

FIGURE 4. Receptive fields of touch receptors: the critical thresholds of approximately 200 points were determined in a systematic survey of the skin, and the values of critical stimuli were plotted as a histogram, which indicated their grouping into low- (L), medium- (M), and high- (H) threshold ranges. Each experimentally investigated point is represented on a scale map of the skin by a letter showing the threshold range in which it occurred; this figure thus shows the array of thresholds as found on the skin. The points in the low-threshold range (L) were found to occur in groups; these have been enclosed by a line, drawn by eye. The two hatched areas represent regions of low threshold supplied by a second nerve.

the regulation of nerve sprouting implicates the target as being responsible for stimulating the axons to sprout collaterals. Our ultrastructural studies, therefore, were especially concerned with the relationship of the nerve endings to the target tissue, and the possible existence of identifiable target cells.

Ultrastructural Investigations

The touch-sensitive regions were not related to the presence of any of the morphological features, such as gland openings or blood vessels, which were clearly visible through the transparent epidermis. It seemed, therefore, that the receptors might be located in the epidermis, and their high sensitivity to the applied mechanical pulse, which was lost or greatly reduced after epidermal scraping (Cooper and Diamond, 1977), further suggested an epidermal location for the touch receptors. We were intrigued to discover with the electron microscope that the epidermis of the salamander skin contains Merkel cells.

Merkel cells have been well described in vertebrates (see review by Winkelmann and Breathnach, 1973), and are usually found grouped in histologically identified structures that are commonly accepted as having a sensory function. For example, the domes of the mammalian skin, each of which contains a cluster of Merkel cells, have been clearly shown to function as mechanoreceptors (Iggo and Muir, 1969). It has not yet been established whether this mechanosensory function is attributable to the Merkel cell itself. Merkel cells have been reported almost always to occur close to the basal layer of the epidermis, and the most characteristic feature that distinguishes them from other epidermal cells is the presence of dense-core granules that are largely concentrated in the cytoplasm on the dermal side of the cell. Nerve fibers are usually found in close association with the Merkel cell, also on the dermal side. Interestingly, we find in the salamander skin only isolated Merkel cells, sparsely located in the epidermis (Figure 5), and, indeed, we estimate that approximately one epidermal cell in a thousand is a Merkel cell. These salamander Merkel cells display all the characteristic features mentioned above, and, in addition, the terminals of the associated nerve fibers always seem to contain clear vesicles (Figure 6) (Mustakallio and Kiistala, 1967; Smith, 1967; Kurosumi, Kurosumi, and Suzuki, 1969; Winkelmann and Breathnach, 1973; Düring, 1974; Düring and Andres, 1976; also see Iggo and Muir, 1969; Smith, 1970; Munger, Pubols, and Pubols, 1971; Andres and Düring, 1973). We have also occasionally seen suggestions of membrane specialization between Merkel cells and the nerve endings (Iggo and Muir, 1969; Andres and Düring, 1973; Chen, Gerson, and Meyer, 1973; Düring, 1974; English, 1974; Düring and Andres, 1976; also see Munger, 1965; Smith, 1967; Smith, 1970; Munger et al., 1971; Hashimoto, 1972a,b; Winkelmann and Breathnach, 1973). We were curious to see whether the location of the isolated Merkel cells in the epidermis correlated with the locations of the physiologically identified mechanosensitive areas. We were further interested in the possibility that the Merkel cell might function in the control of the skin innervation (see Munger, 1965).

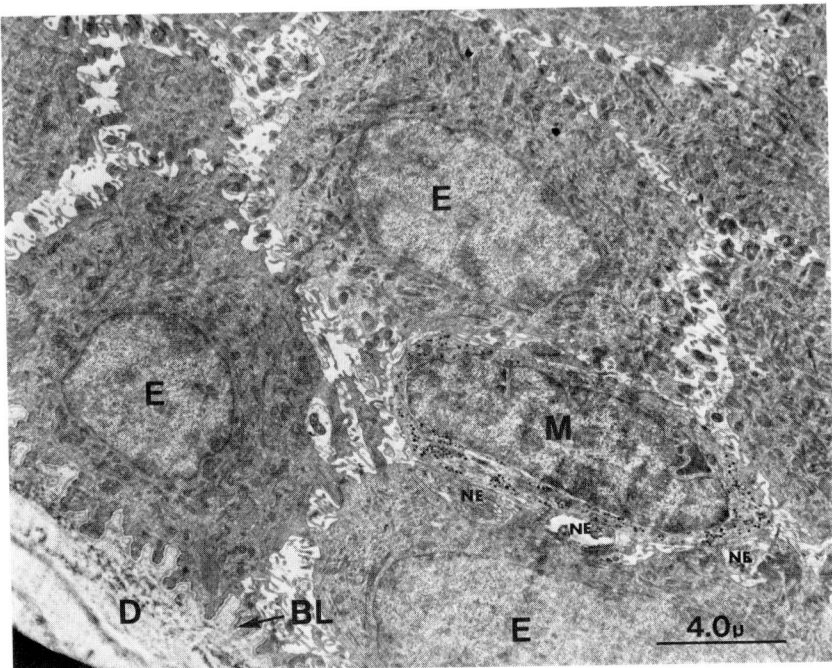

FIGURE 5. Low-power electron micrograph of salamander skin. The Merkel cell (M) and its associated nerve endings (NE) are located in the epidermis near the basal lamina (BL). It can be distinguished from other epidermal cells (E) by the presence of dense-core granules in its cytoplasm. D indicates dermis.

Relationship of Mechanosensory Nerve Endings to Merkel Cells

The possibility that the Merkel cells occurred in the regions of high sensitivity to touch was investigated by a combined physiological and morphological study of the skin. Regions of the skin, approximately 1.5 mm^2, were mapped physiologically, as described above, in order to define the localized touch-sensitive areas, and then the same regions were examined with the electron microscope to determine the location of Merkel cells within them. Our objective was subsequently to superimpose the physiological and morphological maps to see the relationship of the distribution of the Merkel cells to that of the touch spots.

Because shrinkage of the skin sample during fixation would distort the

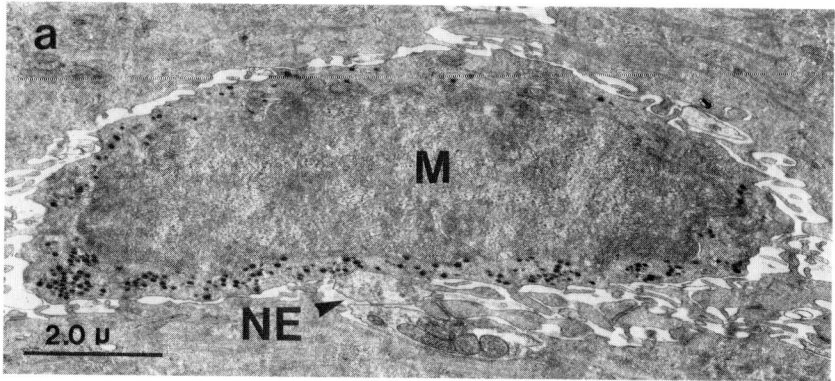
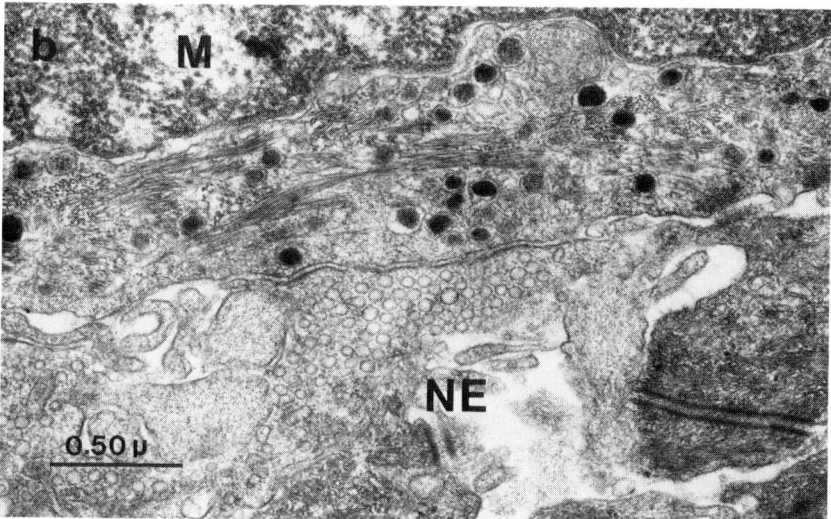

FIGURE 6. (a) Merkel cell (M) and an associated nerve ending (NE). Note the accumulation of dense-core granules on the dermal side of the cell. (b) Higher-power view of another Merkel cell and nerve ending, the former showing dense-core granules, the latter showing clear vesicles. From Parducz et al. (1977).

morphological map, we recorded the location of the Merkel cells and touch spots with reference to "internal markers" in the skin, namely the gland openings (see Figure 1), which we could readily identify on both maps. In making the physiological map, the sensitivity to touch was tested every 50 μm and recorded on a photograph of the skin that clearly showed the gland openings. The region of skin that had been mapped was then removed, fixed, and prepared for sectioning (Parducz et al., 1977).

We cut semi-thin transverse sections serially through the skin, and at a spacing of every 8 to 10-μm, we cut ultrathin sections until the whole block was surveyed. Each ultrathin section was scanned in the electron microscope for the presence of Merkel cells. The position of each Merkel cell was then located with reference to nearest gland openings and to the edges of the skin sample. From these results we made a map of the actual distribution of the Merkel cells in the examined skin.

The two independently obtained maps of the same skin, i.e., the morphological one showing Merkel cells, and the physiological one showing the sensitive touch spots, were then superimposed so that the gland openings were coincident. Figure 7 shows the results of three such investigations (from three different animals). The correlation between the sensitive areas and the presence of Merkel cells is quite clear, and equally important is the virtual absence of Merkel cells from the regions of skin that were relatively insensitive to touch. There are inevitable

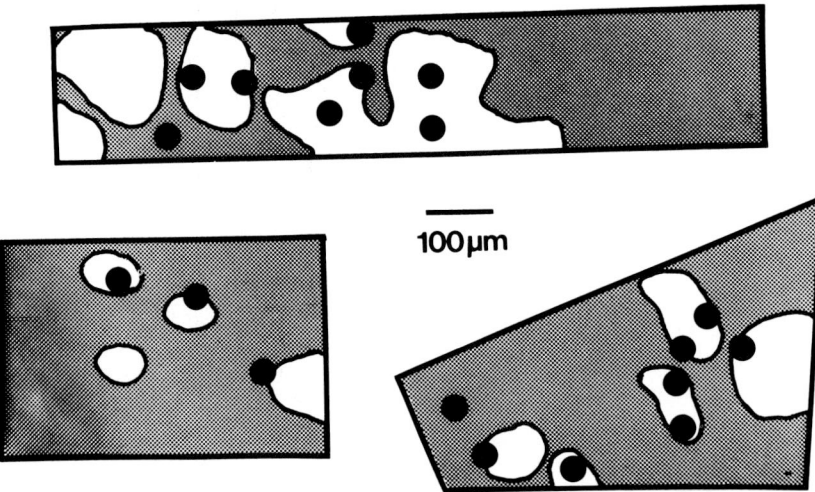

FIGURE 7. Relationship between Merkel cells (black spots) whose distribution was obtained from the morphological study, and the regions (white areas) that were found to be highly sensitive to mechanical stimulation in the physiological study (cf. Figure 4). The three samples of skin were from three different animals. In each case the correlation between Merkel cells and sensitive areas was highly significant ($P < 0.001$, Chi^2 test). From Parducz et al. (1977).

uncertainties in experiments of this sort: the unambiguous identification of the Merkel cell required the visualization of the dense-core granules in its cytoplasm, and it is possible that an occasional Merkel cell was missed. In addition, there are limitations in the resolution of the physiological mapping in which the smallest "steps" were 50 μm. These difficulties probably explain why two of the sensitive areas are apparently not associated with Merkel cells, and why one Merkel cell is apparently not associated with a sensitive area (Figure 7). However, when we examined the correlation of Merkel cells and sensitive spots statistically, it was highly significant ($P < 0.001$, Chi^2 test) for each skin sample.

On the basis of these results we propose that there is indeed a specific association between the touch-sensitive spots and the Merkel cells. Because nerve endings are associated with each Merkel cell, we can assume that they are mechanosensory. It follows then that there is a specific association between the Merkel cell and the mechanosensory nerve terminals. If the Merkel cells were the actual targets of the mechanosensory nerves, then according to our hypothesis they could play a role in the elaboration of the proposed stimulus which causes the nerves to sprout.

Trophic Relationships Between Merkel Cells and Nerve Endings

Some sensory structures disappear when their nerve supply is cut (Werner, 1974). Is the maintainance of the Merkel cell in salamander skin also dependent on an intact innervation? To answer this we have looked for Merkel cells in skin that was denervated by removing all of the dorsal root ganglia supplying the limb. Often the ventral roots were also sectioned. Before fixation we used electrophysiological techniques to check for the possibility that nerves had regenerated to the skin. We examined the skin morphologically at various times after denervation, for periods up to six months. In all skins we found Merkel cells. These Merkel cells were virtually identical to those in normal skin. However, there were no nerves associated with them (Figure 8). Clearly, therefore, the Merkel cell in salamander skin is not dependent on its nerve to survive. (Smith [1967] described a similar result for Merkel cells in the rat; however, there may be species differences among mammals in this regard. See Palmer [1965]; Burgess, English, Horch, and Stensaas [1974].) Further studies are underway to establish quantitatively the survival of Merkel cells in the salamander.

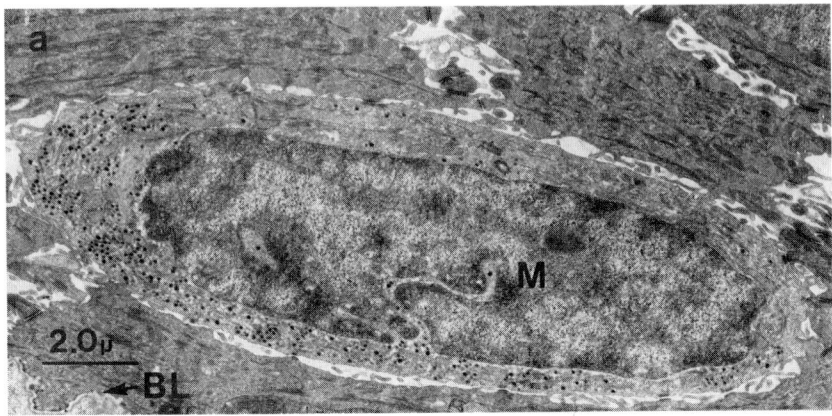

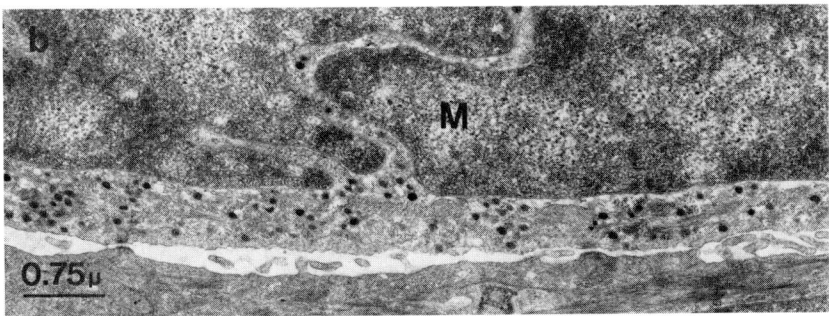

FIGURE 8. Merkel cell in skin six months after total denervation of the limb. (a) Low-power view of Merkel cell (M), which is normal in appearance and located near the basal lamina (BL). (b) Higher-power view of the same cell showing absence of nerve endings (cf. Figure 6).

How does the specific association between the mechanosensory nerve endings and the Merkel cells come about? Does the nerve induce the differentiation of the Merkel cell during development, or is it possible that the Merkel cells originate independently, and that the association with the nerve develops later? We are not dealing with primary innervation in the salamander, but as a model we have studied the development of regenerated skin, and of its innervation, in the mature animal.

We removed a portion of skin (up to 25 mm²) from a limb, and allowed new skin to regenerate in its place. We found that skin regeneration would occur even in the total absence of any nerves, both motor and sensory, from the limb. The obvious question was—would Merkel cells be present in such skin? This indeed proved to be the case. These Merkel cells are apparently quite normal in all respects, but of course there are no nerves associated with them. We have not yet done quantitative studies, but the frequency with which we find Merkel cells in nerve-free regenerated skin is approximately the same as that found normally. We do not yet know the origin of these Merkel cells; they could have migrated into the regenerating skin or differentiated within it. In some experiments, however, they were present in the new epidermis before any obvious dermis had formed (Hashimoto, 1972a; Breathnach, 1971), and Merkel cells were identified in 1- to 2-week-old regenerated skin; we are still investigating the time course of their appearance. In these experimental situations it is clear that the appearance of Merkel cells in regenerating skin does not require the presence of nerves (Lyne and Hollis, 1971).

Innervation of Regenerated Skin

What are the consequences when nerves are allowed to grow into the regenerated skin? In these experiments we removed skin patches from normally innervated limbs, and allowed time for innervation of the newly regenerated skin to occur. This skin was then mapped physiologically to determine its mechanosensitivity, as mentioned earlier (see above). Examples of the results from two animals are shown in Figure 9. The characteristics and distribution of the sensitive areas were essentially similar to those of normal skin. Furthermore, as in normal skin, a single sensitive spot was innervated almost invariably by only one axon. This skin was further investigated ultrastructurally. Although we have not yet completed a combined study of physiological and morphological maps, such as that done for normal skin, we have found that the regenerated skin contained Merkel cells, and in this situation those Merkel cells were found to be associated with nerve endings as they are in normal skin (Figure 10). Indeed, the morphological appearance was indistinguishable from normal. Although these experiments are still in progress, we would like to suggest that a specific association becomes established between the newly innervating sensory nerves and the apparently independently developing Merkel cells.

DISCUSSION AND CONCLUSIONS

The accuracy with which the incoming nerve becomes intimately associated with the Merkel cell in these experiments is remarkable,

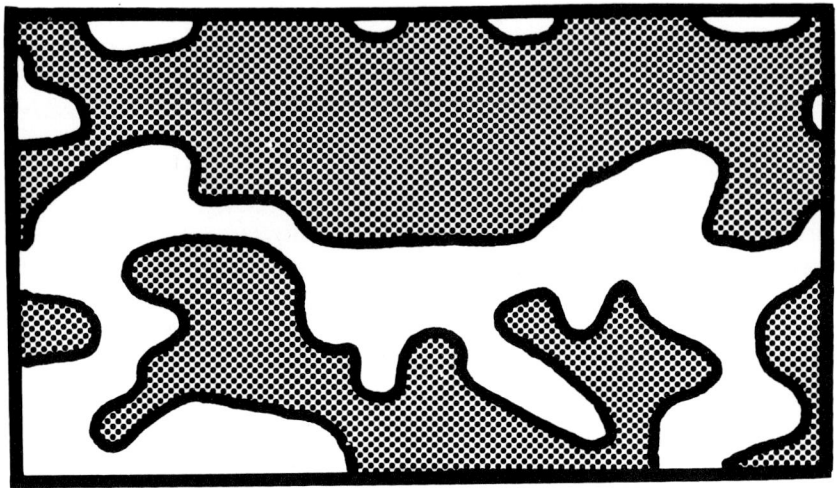

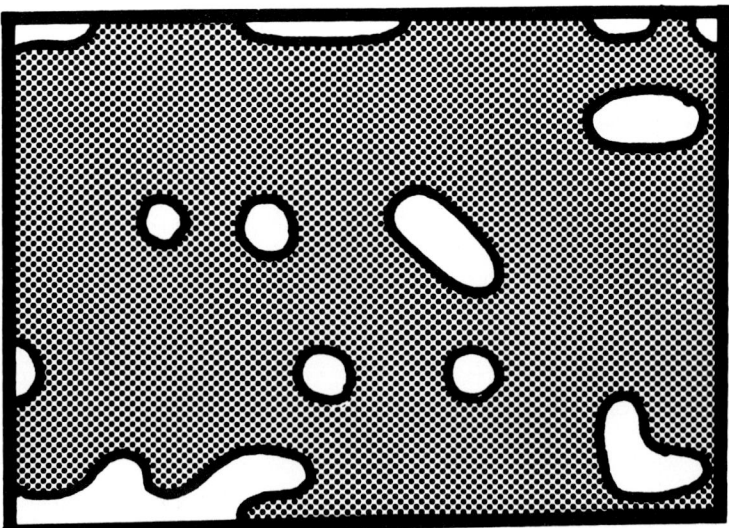

FIGURE 9. Distribution of mechanosensitive areas (white) in regenerated salamander skin from two animals. The size and distribution of sensitive areas were similar to those in normal skin (cf. Figures 4 and 7).

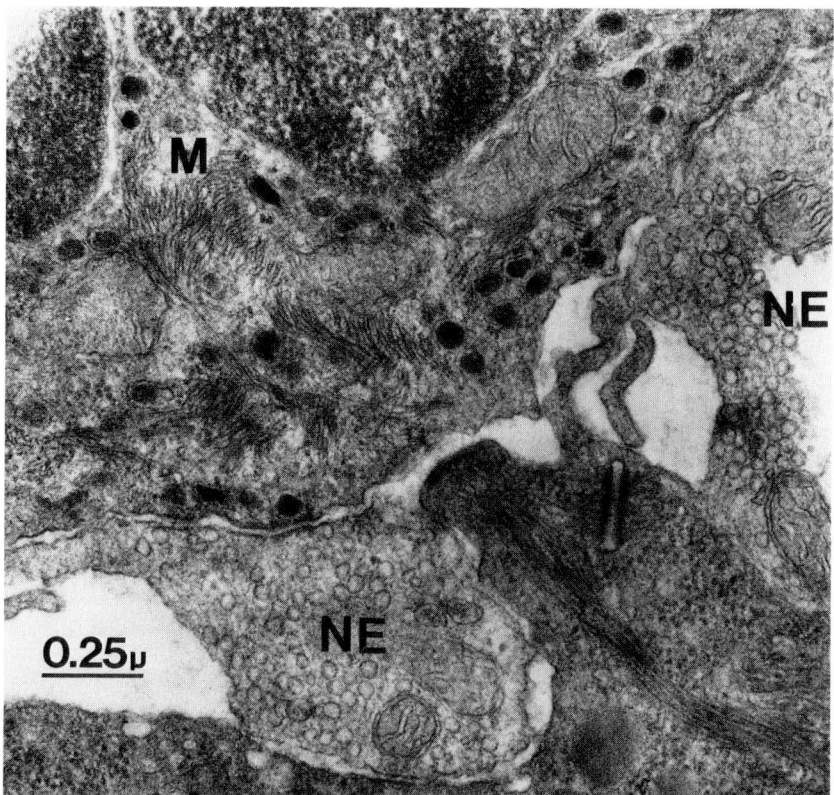

FIGURE 10. High-power view of Merkel cell in regenerated skin that physiological examination showed had become normally innervated. Nerve endings (NE) were found in association with the Merkel cells (M) in such preparations.

since the ratio of Merkel cells to all other cells in the epidermis is about 1:1,000. From these results it would seem reasonable to postulate that the Merkel cells are the true targets of the mechanosensory nerves, certainly in newly regenerating skin. Of course, we cannot say whether or not the nerve grows more or less randomly until it encounters a Merkel cell, which it then "recognizes" and with which it then develops an intimate association. We do know, however, that, in contrast to other situations (e.g., Weddell, 1942; Horch, 1976), the nerves in the newly regenerated skin cannot have been guided to the Merkel cells along pathways formed by degenerating nerves. Possibly the Merkel cell induces the nerve to sprout toward it by releasing some diffusable factor.

It is intriguing to note in the context of our hypothesis for nerve sprouting the presence in the Merkel cell of dense-core granules whose function is unknown, and the presence in the nerve endings of the clear vesicles, whose function is similarily unknown.

We have shown (Cooper et al., 1977) that after partial denervation of salamander skin, the sprouting of the remaining intact nerves to form new mechanosensory endings ceases when the original density of endings is restored. If all the Merkel cells survive the loss of their nerves, as our new findings suggest, then the new sprouts would presumably end at the "vacant" Merkel cells, as occurs in the regenerated skin. This indicates, then, that sprouting to form functional mechanoreceptors ceases when all the Merkel cells are occupied. Certainly our physiological results show that once the endings of one mechanosensory nerve axon become functionally established at a Merkel cell, the branches of other axons fail to achieve a similar association with that cell. The situation resembles that of an innervated skeletal muscle fiber, which will not normally accept another nerve, and that of the fertilized egg, which will not accept another sperm.

Because the pattern of the mechanosensory innervation of newly regenerated skin is normal, we are led to wonder whether the primary event in the development of the terminal field is the differentiation of Merkel cells; the branching pattern of the mechanosensory nerves would then be determined by the ensuing distribution of Merkel cells, whose influence, according to our hypothesis (Aguilar et al., 1973), would eventually become neutralized by neural factors.

REFERENCES

Aguilar, C. E., M. A. Bisby, E. Cooper, and J. Diamond (1973). Evidence that axoplasmic transport of trophic factors is involved in the regulation of peripheral nerve fields in salamanders, *J. Physiol. (London)* **234**:449–464.

Andres, K. H. and M. von Düring (1973). Morphology of cutaneous receptors, pp. 3–28 in *Handbook of Sensory Physiology*, Vol II, Iggo, A., ed. Springer-Verlag, New York.

Breathnach, A. S. (1971). Embryology of human skin. A review of ultrastructural studies, *J. Invest. Dermatol.* **57**:133–143.

Burgess, P. R., R. B. English, K. W. Horch, and L. J. Stensaas (1974). Patterning in the regeneration of type I cutaneous receptors, *J. Physiol. (London)* **236**:57–82.

Chen, S., S. Gerson, and J. Meyer (1973). The fusion of Merkel cell granules with a synapse-like structure, *J. Invest. Dermatol.* **61**:290–292.

Cooper, E. and J. Diamond (1977). A quantitative study of the mechanosensory innervation of the salamander skin, *J. Physiol. (London)* **264**:695–723.

Cooper, E., J. Diamond, and C. Turner (1977). The effects of nerve section and of colchicine treatment on the density of mechanosensory nerve endings in salamander skin, *J. Physiol. (London)* **264**:725–749.
Diamond, J., E. Cooper, C. Turner, and L. Macintyre (1976). Trophic regulation of nerve sprouting, *Science* **193**:371–377.
Düring, M. von (1974). The ultrastructure of cutaneous receptors in the skin of *Caiman crocodilus*. Symposium Mechanoreception. *Abh. Rhein Westfalen Akad. Wiss.* **53**:123–134.
Düring, M. von and K. H. Andres (1976). The ultrastructure of taste and touch receptors of the frog's taste organ, *Cell Tissue Res.* **165**:185–198.
English, K. B. (1974). Cell types in cutaneous type I mechanoreceptors (Haarscheibe) and their alterations with injury. *Am. J. Anat.* **141**:105–126.
Fitzgerald, M. J. T. (1961). Developmental changes in epidermal innervation, *J. Anat.* **95**:495–514.
Hashimoto, K. (1972a). The ultrastructure of human embryos. X. Merkel tactile cells in the finger and nail, *J. Anat.* **111**:99–120.
Hashimoto, K. (1972b). Fine structure of Merkel cells in human oral mucosa, *J. Invest. Dermatol.* **58**:381–387.
Horch, K. W. (1976). Specific conduit guidance after nerve crush and its absence after peripheral nerve transection in the cat, *Abstr. Annu. Meet. Soc. Neurosci.*, 6th, Toronto, p. 1042.
Iggo, A. and A. R. Muir (1969). The structure and function of a slowly adapting touch corpuscle in hairy skin, *J. Physiol. (London)* **200**:763–796.
Kurosumi, K., U. Kurosumi, and H. Suzuki (1969). Fine structure of Merkel cells and associated nerve fibers in the epidermis of certain mammalian species, *Arch. Histol. Jpn. (Okayama, Jpn.)* **30**:295–313.
Landmesser, L. and G. Pilar (1976). Fate of ganglionic synapses and ganglion cell axons during normal and induced cell death, *J. Cell Biol.* **68**:357–374.
Levi-Montalcini, R. and P. U. Angeletti (1968). Nerve growth factor, *Physiol. Rev.* **48**:534–569.
Lyne, A. G. and D. E. Hollis (1971). Merkel cells in sheep during fetal development, *J. Ultrastruct. Res.* **34**:464–472.
Munger, B. L. (1965). The intraepidermal innervation of the snout skin of the opossum, *J. Cell Biol.* **26**:79–97.
Munger, B. L., L. M. Pubols, and B. H. Pubols (1971). A slowly adapting sensory receptor in mammalian glabrous skin, *Brain Res.* **29**:47–61.
Mustakallio, K. K. and U. Kiistala (1967). Electron microscopy of Merkel's "tastzelle", a potential monoamine storing cell in human epidermis, *Acta Derm. Venereol.* **47**:323–326.
Olson, L. and T. Malmfors (1970). Growth characteristics of adrenergic nerves in the adult rat, *Acta Physiol. Scand. Suppl.* **348**:1–112.
Palmer, P. (1965). Ultrastructural alterations of Merkel cells following denervation, *Anat. Rec.* **151**:396–397.
Parducz, A., R. Leslie, E. Cooper, C. Turner, and J. Diamond (1977). The Merkel cells and the rapidly adapting mechanoreceptors in salamander skin, *Neuroscience*, in press.
Ramón y Cajal, S. (1960). Accion neurotropica de las epitelios (1919), pp. 149–200 (in English [Guth, L., trans.]) in *Studies on Vertebrate Neurogenesis*. Charles C. Thomas, Springfield, Ill.

Smith, K. R., Jr. (1967). The structure and function of the Haarscheibe, *J. Comp. Neurol.* **131**:459–474.

Smith, K. R. (1970). The ultrastructure of the human Haarscheibe and Merkel cell, *J. Invest. Dermatol.* **54**:150–159.

Weddell, G. (1942). Axonal regeneration in cutaneous nerve plexuses, *J. Anat.* **77**:49–62.

Werner, J. K. (1974). Trophic influence of nerves on the development and maintenance of sensory receptors, *Am. J. Phys. Med.* **53**:127–142.

Winkelmann, R. K. and A. S. Breathnach (1973). The Merkel cell, *J. Invest. Dermatol.* **60**:2–15.

ROLE OF CALCIUM IN SYNAPTIC TRANSMITTER RELEASE

Calcium and Transmitter Release in Squid Synapse

Rodolfo R. Llinás

New York University School of Medicine, New York, New York

The central theme of the present symposium concerns the role of Ca^{2+} in secretory phenomena. It is now agreed that many forms of cellular secretion are subserved by a general exocytotic mechanism most possibly triggered by a transient increase in intracellular Ca^{2+} concentration $[Ca^{2+}]_i$ (Smith, 1971; Rubin, 1975; Llinás and Heuser, 1977). According to this view, synaptic transmission may be considered a specialized variation of this secretion theme, such that (1) the transient increase in $[Ca^{2+}]_i$ is brought about by a voltage-dependent Ca^{2+} conductance change across the plasma membrane, and (2) the release occurs in the fraction of a millisecond-to-millisecond range after the onset of the stimulus (i.e., much faster than the usual secretory processes in other cells). A further point of specialization unrelated to the secretory theme is, of course, that the receptor sites for transmitter action must be located very near the point of release, since speed of transmission is of crucial importance.

Calcium and Synaptic Transmission

That extracellular Ca^{2+} is required for synaptic transmission was originally discovered in 1894 by Locke. He observed that nerve excitation was not followed by muscular contraction in frog neuromuscular preparations bathed in a calcium-free solution, but that contraction could occur if the muscle was stimulated directly. More importantly, he demonstrated that after the reintroduction of Ca^{2+} to the medium, the muscle responded once again to nervous stimulation. Similar observations were reported by Overton in 1904. The next level of investigation is represented by papers in the late 1930's and early 1940's (cf. Harvey and MacIntosh, 1940). The investigators demonstrated that extracellular Ca^{2+} was required for the actual release of acetylcholine (ACh), well known at the time as a synaptic transmitter substance. However, because at that time the chemical nature of synaptic transmission had not yet been strongly voiced, these observations are rarely quoted.

In more recent years it has been the work of Bernard Katz and his collaborators, using the frog neuromuscular junction, that has helped to provide a clearly stated hypothesis concerning the role of Ca^{2+} in synaptic transmission. In the neuromuscular junction, del Castillo and Stark (1952) reported that the amount of transmitter liberated with each nerve impulse (as measured by the size of the endplate potential [epp]) varied with the log of the external Ca^{2+} concentration. The size of the miniature epp (mepp), however, was not affected (Fatt and Katz, 1952). Moreover, the frequency of the mepp was controlled directly by the terminal's membrane potential and increased non-monotonically with membrane depolarization (del Castillo and Katz, 1954). Acting presynaptically, Ca^{2+} was envisioned as increasing the "effectiveness" of a given level of depolarization.

Later, during an investigation on the time course of Ca^{2+} action on transmitter release, Katz and Miledi (1967a) reported that hyperpolarizing or depolarizing pulses applied near the terminal during the falling phase of a presynaptic action potential decreased or increased, respectively, the amount of transmitter released. These results indicated that although the release process was initiated by the presynaptic spike, release continues to operate during the falling phase and perhaps even beyond the duration of the action potential itself.

Squid Synapse

Valuable information greatly expanding the work on the neuromuscular junction was provided by the study of the giant synapse in the squid stellate ganglion. Among other giant synapses where simultaneous pre- and postsynaptic recordings may be obtained, such as the chick ciliary ganglion (Martin and Pilar, 1963) and the hatchet fish Mauthner cell system (Auerbach and Bennett, 1969), the synapse in the squid ganglion remains one of the best preparations in which to study the presynaptic release phenomena. This is, of course, due to the size of the pre- and postsynaptic terminals that allows impalement with several electrodes under direct vision. The giant synapse is formed at the junction between the second order giant fiber that runs in the pallialis nerve from the palleovisceral ganglion and the third order giant motor axon that innervates the squid mantle (Young, 1939). A major advantage of this preparation is the accessibility and size of its pre- and postfibers, which allow simultaneous microelectrode penetration of both elements without significant damage to synaptic transmission (Bullock and Hagiwara, 1957; Hagiwara and Tasaki, 1958; Takeuchi and Takeuchi, 1962). In this manner the presynaptic electrical events leading to transmitter release can be recorded, and polarizing current can be applied directly across the membrane of this terminal.

When action potential invasion of the presynaptic terminal is prevented with tetrodotoxin (TTX), known to specifically block Na^+ conductance (Narahashi, Moore, and Scott, 1964), graded depolarization of this terminal leads to graded transmitter release, as evidenced by graded EPSPs recorded in the postsynaptic fiber (Bloedel, Gage, Llinás, and Quastel, 1966; Katz and Miledi, 1967b; Kusano, Livengood, and Werman, 1967; Kusano, 1968).

If the terminal is further treated with tetraethylammonium (TEA) to block K^+ conductance (Armstrong and Binstock, 1965), the presynaptic fiber can be polarized to potentials on the order of +200 mV (Katz and Miledi, 1967c; Kusano, 1968; Llinás and Nicholson, 1975). As the terminal is depolarized in graded steps up to approximately 60 to 80 mV from resting, the amplitude of the EPSP increases rapidly. At more positive presynaptic membrane potentials, the size of the EPSP decreases until a potential is reached at which no EPSP is recorded (Figure 1F)—that is, no transmitter is released (Katz and Miledi, 1967c; Kusano et al., 1967; Kusano, 1970; Llinás and Nicholson, 1975). However, after the end of the current pulse, an EPSP is observed; this is called the "off response." The lack of transmitter release by a large presynaptic depolarization was originally named "suppression," and the level of depolarization at which suppression occurred was called the "suppression potential" (Katz and Miledi, 1967c).

These results were interpreted as indicating that (1) depolarization increases the presynaptic membrane conductance to Ca^{2+} or to a Ca^{2+} complex that enters the terminal, and (2) the suppression potential corresponds to the equilibrium potential for Ca^{2+} (E_{Ca}) or the Ca^{2+} complex. This hypothesis was supported by the observation that Ca^{2+} spikes similar to those reported in other nerve cells (cf. Hagiwara, 1973) could be detected in the presynaptic terminal under appropriate conditions, and that such prolonged spikes were followed by large postsynap-

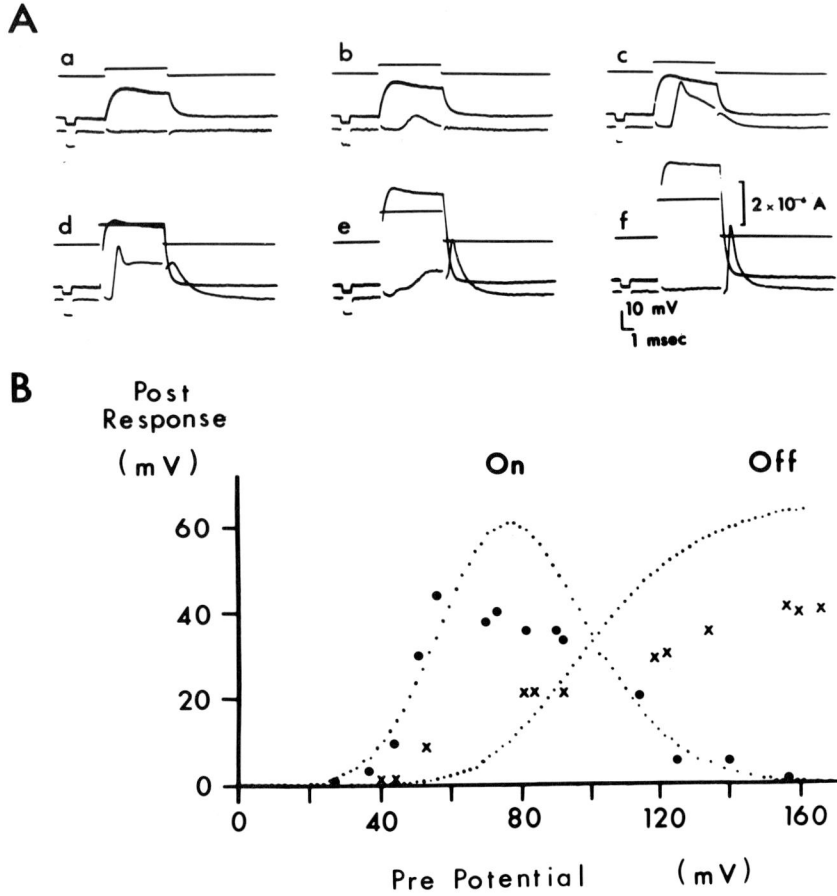

FIGURE 1. Synaptic transmission after blockage of voltage-dependent Na^+ and K^+ conductances. In (A), release of transmitter is evoked by direct depolarization of presynaptic terminal after blockage of Na^+ and K^+ conductance with TTX and TEA, respectively. (a) Presynaptic depolarization (middle trace) is obtained by current injection through a second intracellular presynaptic electrode. Postsynaptic response is shown in lower trace. As amplitude of the current injection increases, presynaptic depolarization and postsynaptic response increase (b to d). Further presynaptic depolarization is accompanied by a decrease (e) and final blockage (f) of the postsynaptic response during depolarization, with a reappearance of the postsynaptic response at the end of the current pulse (off response). Calibration pulses from pre- and postsynaptic pulse 10 mV in 1 msec. From Llinás and Nicholson (1975). (B) plot of relationship between presynaptic depolarization (abscissa) against postsynaptic response (ordinate) from the records shown in (A). Symbols: ●, on response; ×, off response, ···, numerical solutions for mathematical model of synaptic transmission. Modified from Llinás et al. (1976a).

tic potentials (Katz and Miledi, 1967b; Llinás, Walton, and Bohr, 1976b).

The first direct demonstration that the release of transmitter is accompanied by an increase in $[Ca^{2+}]_i$ was obtained through the use of the bioluminescent protein aequorin in squid presynaptic terminal (Llinás, Blinks, and Nicholson, 1972). Aequorin reacts with very small quantities of Ca^{2+} (as low as 10^{-8} M) to produce light—the binding of two Ca^{2+} ions to an aequorin molecule producing one photon (cf. Blinks, Prendergast, and Allen, 1976). Following presynaptic intracellular injection of this protein depolarization and subsequent transmitter release was accompanied by light emission, thus directly demonstrating an increase in $[Ca^{2+}]_i$. Further, in the absence of extracellular Ca^{2+} or in the presence of Ca^{2+} blocking agents, light emission and synaptic release were simultaneously blocked. The converse, that an increase in intracellular Ca^{2+} is an effective stimulus for release, was shown by Miledi (1973). He found that injection of Ca^{2+} into the presynaptic terminal caused a noticeable increase of synaptic noise in the postsynaptic terminal.

After the above results were obtained, it was generally accepted that if the presynaptic terminal is depolarized, Ca^{2+} enters and initiates the transmitter release sequence. However, there was no direct evidence that the inward movement of Ca^{2+} was itself necessary and sufficient to release transmitter and that the suppression potential was indeed E_{Ca}. This was provided by subsequent work of Llinás and Nicholson (1975) with aequorin. After the aequorin injection into the presynaptic terminal of a TEA-treated preparation, single action potentials elicited light pulses concomitant with transmitter release. More to the point, however, in a TEA- and TTX-treated preparation, graded depolarization led to a graded synaptic release and light emission only to about 90 mV deplarization. Beyond this level, light and transmitter output decreased gradually until the suppression potential was reached. At the suppression potential, both transmitter release and light emission disappeared simultaneously, only to reappear at the end of the pulse. These experiments provided, therefore, a direct demonstration that transmitter release is correlated with a Ca^{2+} influx into the terminal and that no inward Ca^{2+} current (I_{Ca}) is present at the suppression potential.

Presynaptic Voltage Clamp

Over the last two summers my colleagues and I, working at the Marine Biological Laboratory at Woods Hole, Massachusetts, have attempted to voltage clamp the presynaptic terminal in squid stellate ganglion (Llinás, Walton, and Hess, 1976c; Llinás, Steinberg, and Walton, 1976a). The experiment was designed to determine whether I_{Ca} could be observed at the presynaptic terminal after pharmacological blockage of the voltage-dependent permeability to Na^+ and K^+.

The obvious difficulties of obtaining a presynaptic terminal in good condition after double or triple microelectrode penetration were seriously compounded by the painstaking technique of iontophoretic intracellular injection of TEA to block the K^+ current (Katz and Miledi, 1967c; Kusano et al., 1967; Kusano, 1970; Llinás and Nicholson, 1975). This step, which may take 3 to 4 h of injection, was necessary because delayed rectification in this terminal is large enough to make a microelectrode voltage clamp approach impractical, besides the fact that it obscures I_{Ca}, which has a time course similar to I_K. For this reason we decided to use a combination of TTX and 3-aminopyridine (3-AmP) (Pelhate and Pichon, 1974; Yeh, Oxford, Wu, and Narahashi, 1976) to block the Na^+ and K^+ currents, respectively. We found that the addition of 3-AmP could produce a good blockage of K^+ current if the depolarizing levels were not larger than 60 or 70 mV from resting and if the repetition rate was no faster than one every 15 sec (Llinás et al., 1976b).

The voltage clamp techniques used for this study are illustrated in Figure 2. In the first case, total I_{Ca} was measured under clamp conditions. It was assumed that most of the I_{Ca} measured was flowing at the terminal under study. However, because the length constant of the presynaptic terminal is rather longer in the absence of delayed rectification (Katz and Miledi, 1971), it was conceivable that inward current, other than that generated at the terminal studied, could also be triggered by the depolarizing pulse. To determine the magnitude of this extra current, the triple electrode technique developed by Adrian, Chandler, and Hodgkin (1970) was used to measure transmembrane current at a single terminal (Figure 2B). The use of this technique demonstrated that the total current measured with the first method had an amplitude 20 to 30% larger than that measured with the triple electrode technique, but that the latency and time course were quite comparable.

Examples of presynaptic voltage clamp results are shown in Figure 3. Figure 3A shows a set of responses consisting of inward current (uppermost trace), postsynaptic potential (middle record), and presynaptic transmembrane potential (lower record) that illustrate the type of recordings obtained with the first clamp method. It is interesting to note

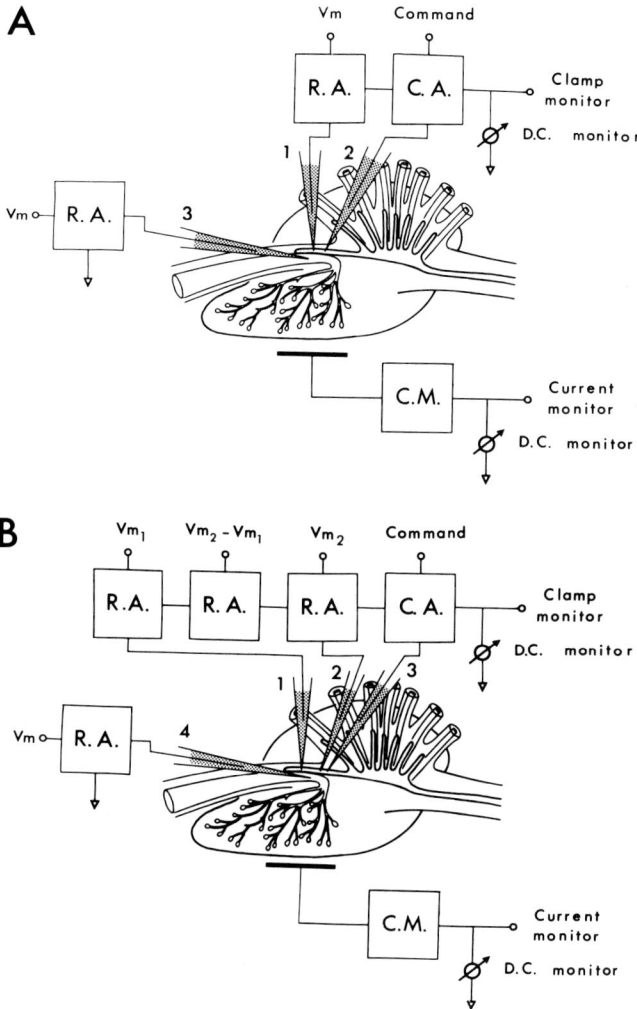

FIGURE 2. Voltage clamp techniques. In (A), presynaptic terminal is impaled with two electrodes (1 and 2), one to record potential (R.A.) and one to inject current via a feedback command amplifier (C.A.). Postsynaptic response is recorded through R.A. in electrode 3. Total current is measured at the indifferent electrode. In (B), the second voltage clamp technique is shown. Total current can be measured in the same manner as in (A), and the presynaptic terminal current can be measured by recording the difference between electrodes 1 and 2 ($V_{m_2} - V_{m_1}$) after current injection through a third presynaptic electrode (3). Postsynaptic response is recorded as in (A).

that the synaptic potential increases almost linearly with time for the first three levels of depolarization shown. It is also significant to show that the onset of the "off" response (marked with an arrow) has a very short latency compared with that of the "on," and lasts approximately as long as the tail current. Presynaptic depolarizations beyond this level produce EPSPs with increasing early peaks and faster rising phases that are then followed by a rapid decay. The results, which were obtained with apparent voltage clamp control, suggest that a transmitter depletion phenomenon takes place if release is large. This finding is to be expected if the transmitter released is limited by the amount of immediately available transmitter and by the rate of repletion of this immediately available store, especially in such a "phasic" type synapse (Hubbard, et al., 1969).

Details of the voltage clamp results at faster sweep speed are shown (Figure 3B) to illustrate the temporal relationship between presynaptic inward current and postsynaptic response. Four trials were superimposed at a frequency of one every 15 sec. It is noticeable that even at this

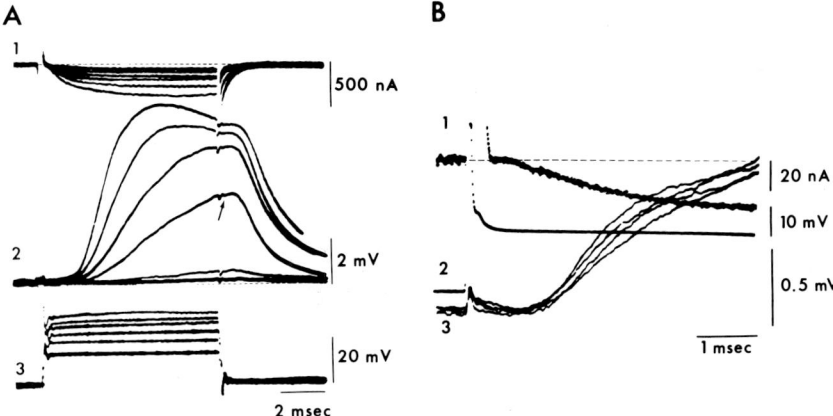

FIGURE 3. Voltage clamp of the presynaptic terminal and responses evoked postsynaptically. In (A), six levels of presynaptic depolarization are illustrated (third trace). These presynaptic depolarizations are accompanied by an inward current shown in the first trace (1). The postsynaptic responses evoked by the presynaptic depolarization are illustrated in the second trace (2). Note that the delay for on response is longer than that for the off response, which comes immediately after the end of the depolarization pulse. In (B), voltage clamp similar to that in (A) is shown at higher magnification and sweep speed. Inward current, uppermost trace (1); presynaptic potential, trace 2; postsynaptic response, trace 3. Time and voltage calibrations are as indicated.

frequency the amount of transmitter release decreases slightly with each successive stimulation, although the amount of inward current is the same for each pulse.

Voltage clamp results obtained with the Adrian method are illustrated in Figure 4A. In this case a certain amount of capacitative artifact was observed with injections in the hyperpolarizing direction (Figure 4B). To obtain the time course for the true ionic currents, the current generated by similar voltage steps in different directions (Figure 4B) was subtracted to give the records shown in Figure 4A. The time course and general amplitude of the inward current under these conditions were found to be similar to those measured with the double-microelectrode technique. Note once again the difference between the latency of the on and the off postsynaptic responses and their correspondence to the onset and the tail current, respectively. That the above currents are related to an inward movement of Ca^{2+} ions was determined by removing Ca^{2+} from the bath in the presence of normal Mg^{2+} (55 mM) or by blocking the late Ca^{2+} channel with Co^{2+} (Hagiwara, 1973; Baker, 1972) or Cd^{2+} in the bathing solution. The absence of inward current and transmitter release under such conditions provided the necessary indication that Ca^{2+} carried the inward current.

The actual relationship between the peak of the presynaptic depolarization and the I_{Ca} is illustrated in Figure 5A. The first discernible inward current determined with the present technique could be seen at approximately 18 to 20 mV from the holding potential level (-70 mV). From this point, I_{Ca} increases in an S-shaped manner and reaches maximum level at about 60 to 80 mV depolarization from the holding potential. Above this level, K^+ activation due to the voltage dependence of the 3-AmP blockage prevented us from studying larger presynaptic depolarization. It is immediately apparent that the shape of this plot is, in many ways, similar to that observed for the relation between presynaptic deplarization and transmitter release (Figure 1B). Finally, the slope for an e-fold change in I_{Ca} at the 40 to 45 mV level was calculated to be 6.5 mV, indicating properties similar to those found by Baker, Hodgkin, and Ridgway (1971) for the postfiber.

The relationship between amplitude of the Ca^{2+} current and the amount of transmitter released are illustrated in Figure 5B. The relation that was found to be linear (Llinás et al., 1976a,c) has been corroborated in over 20 voltage clamp experiments successfully done at $[Ca^{2+}]_0$ of 40, 11, and 5 mM. These results are in agreement with the almost linear rate of rise of the EPSP at low presynaptic depolarization.

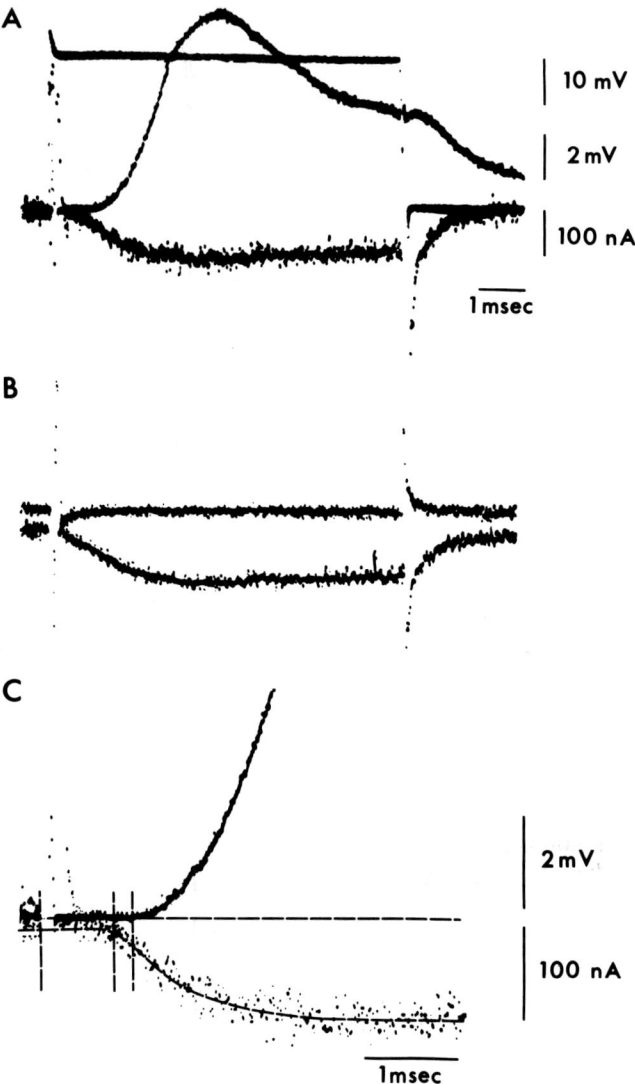

At first approximation it appears that, at the $[Ca^{2+}]_o$ concentrations studied, transmitter release seems to be a linear integration of I_{Ca}. This point shall be discussed later in this paper.

Regarding synaptic delay, our results suggested that it may be subdivided into two components, a and b. Thus, as may be seen from the records in Figures 3 and 4, the onset of the Ca^{2+} current is rather slow and comprises approximately 70% of the total synaptic delay in the present set of experiments. This seems to imply that, as suggested previously (Llinás et al., 1976a,c), the nature of the synaptic delay is related, for the most part, to the time-dependent properties of the opening of the Ca^{2+} gates (component a), the actual delay between onset of I_{Ca} and that of the EPSP being of the order of 200 μsec (component b). This delay component (b) has been consistently found in our results and has a duration similar to the synaptic delay observed for the off response (Figure 1), especially at the lower depolarization levels. The short latency for the off response is due to the fact that Ca^{2+} gates remain open for the full duration of the current pulse (no inactivation), and thus Ca^{2+} begins to enter as soon as the potential moves from E_{Ca}. The difference in latency between on and off release further supports the view that most of the synaptic delay is related to the onset of the Ca^{2+} conductance (component a). It is probable that the actual time required between the Ca^{2+} entry and the transmitter release may be much shorter in other synapses. This is clear from results such as those of Hubbard and Schmidt (1963), where the synaptic delay in rat neuromuscular junction was found to be 217 ± 4 μsec, a good part of which is probably taken by the activation of the Ca^{2+} channels.

Mathematical Model of the Ca^{2+} Gate and Synaptic Transmission

The kind of measurements illustrated above, and a study of the kinetics of the onset of the Ca^{2+} currents, were recently used to develop

---

FIGURE 4. Examples of voltage clamp using the three-microelectrode technique. In (A), presynaptic voltage trace (square pulse), postsynaptic response, and presynaptic current are superimposed. Inward current (downgoing trace) has been obtained by subtracting the current produced by a depolarizing pulse from that produced by a hyperpolarizing pulse of the same amplitude (B). Details of the delay between inward current and postsynaptic response are shown in (C). The upper trace is postsynaptic response; lower record retraced by broken line indicates time course of inward current. The first vertical line marks the onset of the depolarizing potential, the second line indicates the onset of the inward current, and the third line markes the onset of the postsynaptic response.

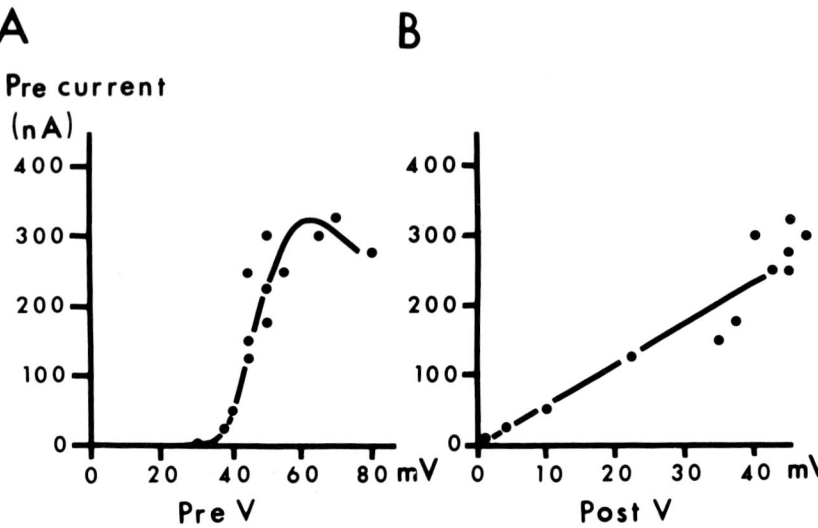

FIGURE 5. (A) Plot of the relationship between presynaptic depolarization and presynaptic calcium current (I_{Ca}). (B) Relationship between amplitude of presynaptic calcium current and amplitude of postsynaptic response.

a mathematical model in collaboration with Dr. Izchak Steinberg of the Weizmann Institute of Science (cf. Llinás et al., 1976a). The model related presynaptic depolarization to I_{Ca}, and I_{Ca} to transmitter release, and suggested that a fifth order kinetic process may be operant in the activation of the Ca^{2+} gate. The basic formula was derived from the assumption that the Ca^{2+} gate (G) may consist of several subunits (S), which may be separated in two states, S and S'. When n S' units are simultaneously present, a G is opened. The rate of change of state between S and S' is given by two time- and voltage-dependent rate constants, k_1 and k_2, for the forward and backward reactions, respectively (Llinas et al., 1976a), the probability $[G]/[G_o]$ that a given gate is open being

$$\frac{[G]}{[G_o]} = \left(\frac{k_1}{k_1 + k_2} [1 - \exp\{-(k_1 + k_2)t\}] \right)^5 \qquad (1)$$

where $[G_o]$ is the total number of gates (regardless of state) and t is time. Assuming constant field condition, the amount of I_{Ca} per channel (j) is given by

$$j = -\left[\frac{C_i - C_o\exp(-2\epsilon V/kT)}{1 - \exp(-2\epsilon V/kT)} \cdot \frac{2D\epsilon}{kT} \cdot \frac{A}{\ell}V\right] \quad (2)$$

where ϵ is the (positive) elementary electric charge, V is the membrane potential, k is Boltzmann's constant, T is absolute temperature, D is the diffusion coefficient, A is the cross-sectional area of the channel, and ℓ is the thickness of the membrane. Given these two equations, the total I_{Ca} must be the total number of gates open [G] times the ionic flow per channel unit time j:

$$I_{Ca} = [G] \cdot j$$

To calculate I_{Ca} to depolarization, other than step function, equation 3 was derived (Llinás et al., 1976a):

$$\frac{d[\tilde{G}]}{dt} = -5(k_1 + k_2)[\tilde{G}] + 5k_1[\tilde{G}]^{4/5} \quad (3)$$

By combining equations 2 and 3, the solution of I_{Ca} for a changing membrane potential may be obtained. The numerical solution for these equations and the assumptions (a) that Ca^{2+} current and transmitter release are related linearly and (b) that a synaptic delay close to 200 μsec is operant in the synapse allow two sets of results to be generated by the model. First, the voltage clamp simulation was computed using

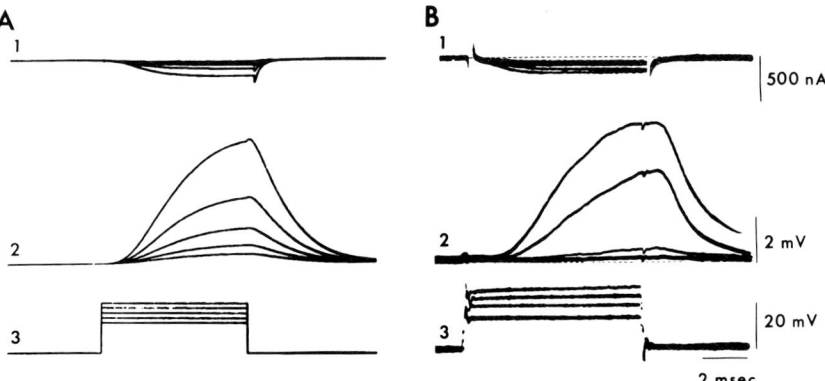

FIGURE 6. Comparison of numerical solutions for pre- and postsynaptic response produced by square voltage steps, using the model and actual responses obtained experimentally. Records 1, 2, and 3 respond to presynaptic current, postsynaptic response, and presynaptic potential, respectively. Similarities between these two are evident.

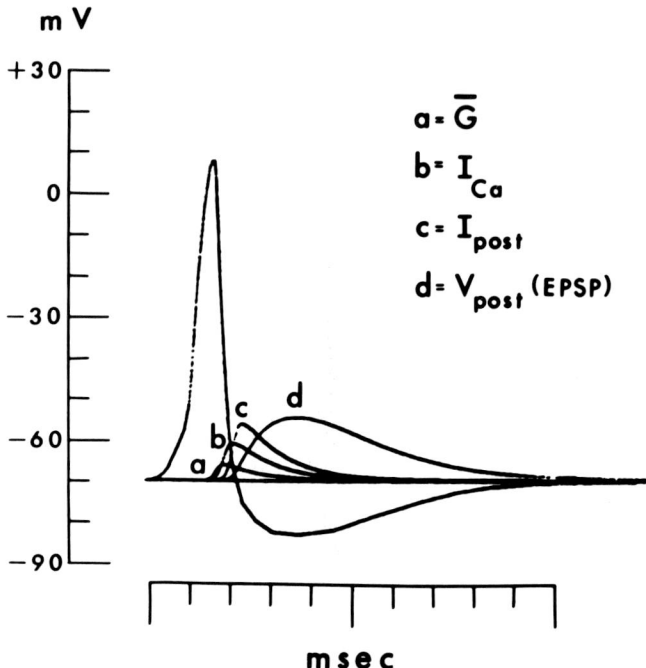

FIGURE 7. Reconstruction of events during synaptic transmission by solving equations 2 and 3. Presynaptic action potential was experimentally obtained. The four curves illustrated represent (a) time course for calcium gate formation [$\bar{G}$], (b) time course for I_{Ca}, (c) time course for the postsynaptic current, and (d) postsynaptic potential. The ordinate in mV corresponds to amplitude of the presynaptic action potential and the resting membrane potential level. Amplitude for (a) through (d) is in arbitrary units. Time calibration refers to all curves.

equations 1 and 2 and compared with the actual results for the pre- and postsynaptic potentials and their relation to I_{Ca}. As seen in Figure 6, the results of the numerical calculation (A) resemble closely those obtained experimentally (B). They also fit well the on and off properties seen in current clamp conditions (Figure 1B dot plot).

More specifically, however, the model could be tested by introducing a presynaptic action potential obtained experimentally by combining equations 2 and 3. The results obtained (Figure 7) offer, according to the model, an estimate of the onset, time course, and duration for channel formation (a), total Ca^{2+} current (b), synaptic current (c), and synaptic potential (d) during synaptic transmission. (A comparison of the numerical solution and the experimental results shown in

Figure 6 allowed a calibration of the current amplitude. With this calibration, an estimate of 550 nA peak current was calculated for I_{Ca} in Figure 7). A direct comparison of the numerical solution to these equations (Figure 8A) with the actual latency and time course of an experimentally obtained response (Figure 8B) offers further support to the model. The significant point is that the latency and time course for I_{Ca} during an action potential may be estimated. According to the present model, I_{Ca} begins to flow at approximately the peak of the presynaptic action potential, attains maximum amplitude during the falling phase, and lasts close to 4 msec after the termination of the spike (the initiation of the after-hyperpolarization, Figure 8A). Another test for the model was to compare the relationship between presynaptic spike and the postsynaptic response generated by the model to that observed

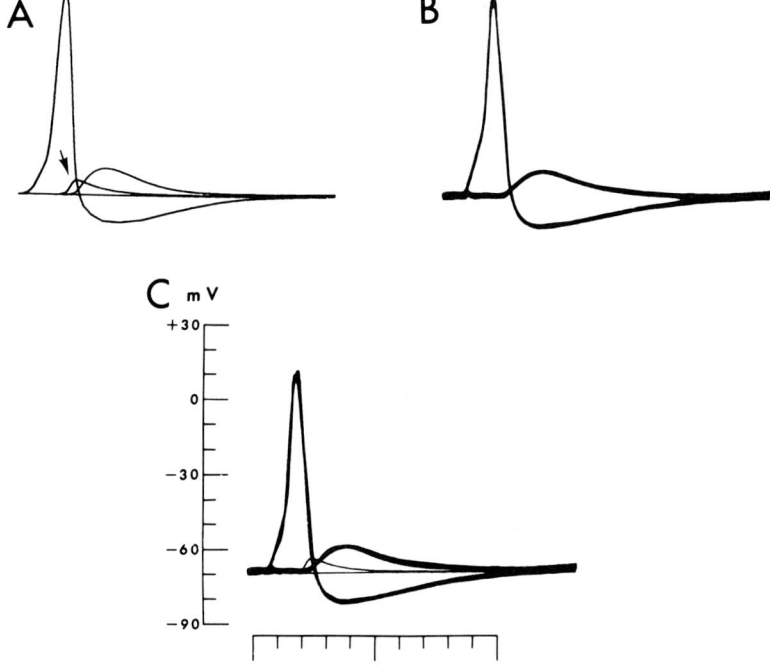

FIGURE 8. Comparison of numerical solution of equation and experimentally observed synaptic transmission. (A) Presynaptic action potential plus calculated I_{Ca} (arrow) and EPSP. (B) Actual recording of pre- and postsynaptic response from synapse. (C) Superposition of (A) and (B). Note that the Ca^{2+} current has a late onset and a rather prolonged time course.

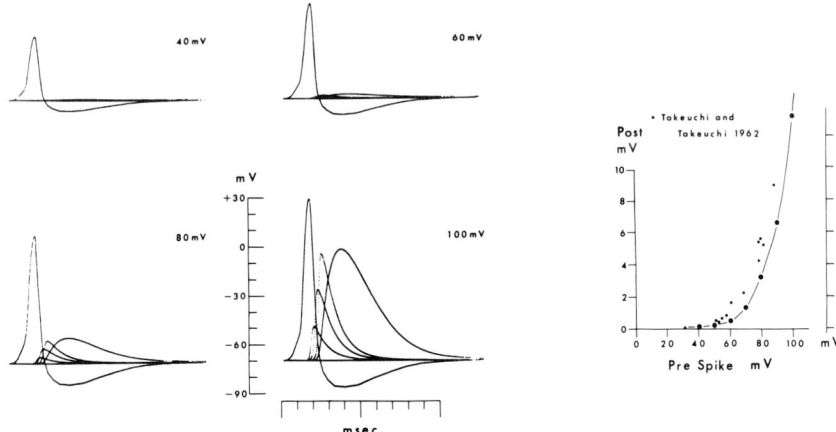

FIGURE 9. Relationship between amplitude of the presynaptic action potential and the different variables in synaptic transmission. The amplitude of the presynaptic spike is shown to the right of each figure (40, 60, 80, and 100 mV). The curves illustrated correspond to those shown in Figure 7. To the right, direct comparison of results obtained with the mathematical model (●) and those obtained experimentally (···). From Takeuchi and Takeuchi (1962).

experimentally (Hagiwara and Tasaki, 1958; Takeuchi and Takeuchi, 1962; and Miledi and Slater, 1966).

The degree to which the variables of Figure 6 change with amplitude of the presynaptic spike is shown for four spike amplitudes in Figure 9. The actual plot of the change of response with increasing prespike amplitudes matches well with the experimental results (Figure 9) of Takeuchi and Takeuchi (1962).

DISCUSSION

The present set of measurements indicates that under normal circumstances I_{Ca} across the presynaptic membrane may be correlated with the amount of transmitter release. Three general points may be considered regarding the results obtained after voltage clamp of the squid presynaptic terminal.

Relationship Between Presynaptic Potentials and Inward Ca^{2+} Current

The present results indicate that, as seen in other systems (Keynes, Rojas, Taylor, and Vergara, 1973; Reuter, 1973; Hagiwara, Fukuda, and Eaton, 1974; Meech and Standen, 1975; Eckert and Lux, 1976; Heyer and Lux, 1976), voltage-dependent I_{Ca} can be measured by using either the two or three electrode voltage clamp technique outlined above. Early measurement of Ca^{2+} currents in the squid giant axon using radioactive Ca^{2+} suggested that after spike activation there was an increase of $[Ca^{2+}]_i$ of up to 0.06 pmol/cm^2 per impulse (approximately 38 ions/μm^2 per impulse) (Hodgkin and Keynes, 1957). The permeability of Ca^{2+} to Na^+ ($^pCa/^pNa$) was estimated by them to be approximately 0.01, and the bulk Ca^{2+} diffusion coefficient in cytoplasm is approximately 6×10^{-7} cm^2/sec. They further suggest that this Ca^{2+} probably entered through the Na^+ channel, and that such Ca^{2+} entering at the nerve terminal could be related to transmitter release. The level of ionized $[Ca^{2+}]_i$ was calculated by them to be less than 0.01 mM. Recent calculations have set this value to between 10^{-7} M (Blaustein, 1974) and 10^{-8} M (Di polo, Requena, Brinley, Mullins, Scarpa, and Tiffert, 1976). In a second set of experiments, Baker et al. (1971) demonstrated, with the use of aequorin, that Ca^{2+} crosses the membrane through two different paths. The early current was confirmed to move through the Na^+ channel; however, a secondary voltage-dependent Ca^{2+} conductance was discovered. This "late Ca^{2+} channel" was found to be separable from the early Na^+ channel by several criteria. It was not blocked by TTX or TEA, but could be affected by manganese and magnesium, as well as by cobalt (Baker et al., 1971). From these experiments it was determined that the rate of Ca^{2+} entry is maximum at 35 to 45 mV depolarization from resting, with an increase of e-fold for 6 mV depolarization. These findings have been confirmed by Rojas and Taylor (1975), using radioactive tracers.

One of the limiting factors in studying the kinetics of I_{Ca} in the tertiary giant axon has been the lack of observable late inward currents with voltage clamp techniques. The consensus has been that the current is far too small to be seen with the usual techniques (Meves and Vogel, 1973). In the presynaptic terminal, on the other hand, an inward current should be observed, since it has been shown that after Na^+ and K^+ blockage, I_{Ca} may be large enough to generate spikes (Katz and Miledi, 1969; Llinás et al., 1976b). The present voltage clamp experiments indicate inward current on the order of 300 nA (i.e., $\frac{1}{10}$ to $\frac{1}{20}$ of the Na^+ current). Based on our mathematical model and assuming a presynaptic terminal area of 150,000 μm^2, a Ca^{2+} current density of 35 μA/cm^2 or $.17 \times 10^9$ Ca^{2+} ions is calculated to flow per spike. (This gives a total Ca^{2+} ion density of 1.14×10^3 ions/μm^2 per spike at 40 mM $[Ca^{2+}]_o$ as opposed to 500 ions/impulse for the giant axon at 112 mM $[Ca^{2+}]_o$; cf. Baker et al., 1971.)

Exactly how this increase of Ca^{2+} current is to release transmitter is unclear at present. Calculations by V. A. Parsegian (personal communication) indicate that given a 200 μsec free-moving path, the actual probability of collision between the Ca^{2+} ion and a vesicle "site" (a 100 $Å^2$ patch) is such that only on the order of one Ca^{2+} in 1,000 entering at one point would be likely to collide with such an area if the distance between the point of entry and the point of vesicle contact is on the order of 100 Å. This basically suggests that in order to ensure a collision between at least one Ca^{2+} ion and a vesicle, a rather sizeable Ca^{2+} current must flow. Conversely, the present set of assumptions also imply that only a small proportion of the Ca^{2+} ions that enter during the presynaptic depolarization are actually effective in releasing transmitter. In fact, a recent study of Mann and Joyner (1976) on miniature EPSP in this synapse indicates an average size of 10 to 20 μV (depending on the input impedance of the postfiber). Assuming about a 200-μm diameter for our postfibers, a quantal content of approximately 5,000 may be calculated for an EPSP of 40 mV amplitude (R. W. Joyner, personal communication). Given that 5,000 vesicles must be released and that a minimum of one Ca^{2+} ion must be required to release a vesicle, at least 5×10^6 ions must flow. The actual number obtained by our calculations ($.17 \times 10^9$) Ca^{2+}/impulse) indicates a great excess beyond this number. Finally, our present findings indicate that the S-shaped curve relating presynaptic depolarization to postsynaptic response (Katz and Miledi, 1967c; Kusano et al., 1967; Llinás and Nicholson, 1975) reflects mainly the nonlinear relationship between voltage and Ca^{2+} conductance change and that, at least at the levels of Ca^{2+} current used, the relationship between transmitter release and I_{Ca} is linear. Although these results are in apparent discord with the Dodge and Rahamimoff (1967) hypothesis regarding the number of Ca^{2+} ions required for a vesicular release, the final resolution of this problem requires further voltage clamp analysis at different Ca^{2+} concentrations.

Synaptic Delay

The question of synaptic delay bears centrally on the mechanism underlying transmitter release. The 200-μsec delay observed for the onset of transmitter release (component b) was obtained directly from the voltage clamp experiments, as well as in the measurement of the "off"

EPSP in nonvoltage clamped synapse. This result is of interest because it gives the minimum latency required for the initiation of transmitter release after the initiation of Ca^{2+} entry; its small value indicates that the point of Ca^{2+} entry must be very close to the site of transmitter release. Assuming that the ions radiate in a straight path, Parsegian has calculated that the ions could move 1,500 Å in 200 μsec (1977). This, of course, suggests that the actual point of Ca^{2+} entry must be very near the site of release (i.e., the site where the vesicles are located). In fact, as shown by Heuser in this symposium (1977), rows of membrane-bound particles are present in the vicinity of the release site for synaptic vesicles. Although the function of these particles is not clear, it is interesting to speculate, given the short latency for the release, that they may represent Ca^{2+} channels (cf. Llinás and Heuser, 1977). If this were to be the case, and given a particle density of $150/\mu m^2$ (Heuser, personal communication), a total of approximately 8 Ca^{2+} ions would enter, per impulse, through each channel.

Another implication of these findings, as pointed out previously (Llinás et al., 1976a), is that Ca^{2+} entry may in fact initiate release of transmitter from only those vesicles that are at or near the site of transmitter release. The action of Ca^{2+}, however, need not be limited to this site. One can thus imagine that besides exercising an immediate action on transmitter release, the presence of Ca^{2+} may facilitate the mobilization of vesicles to the release sites by changing the physical properties of the axoplasm in the presynaptic terminal. A further possibility, of course, as mentioned by Blaustein in this symposium (Blaustein, Kendrick, Fried, and Ratzlaff, 1977), is that Ca^{2+} itself may facilitate transmission by triggering Ca^{2+} release from intracellular stores.

In conclusion, the present results strongly suggest that the I_{Ca} in the presynaptic terminal triggers the release of synaptic transmitter release. Also, as indicated by the Blaustein and Kater talks in this symposium (Blaustein et al., 1977; Kater, 1977), such Ca^{2+} currents are probably present in central synapses, as well as in non-neurosecretory systems.

ACKNOWLEDGMENTS

Support was provided by Public Health Service grant NS-13742 from the National Institute of Neurological and Communicative Disorders and Stroke.

REFERENCES

Adrian, R. H., W. K. Chandler, and A. L. Hodgkin (1970). Voltage clamp experiments in striated muscle fibers, *J. Physiol. (London)* **208**:607–644.

Armstrong, C. M., and L. Binstock (1965). Anomalous rectification in the squid giant axon injected with tetraethylammonium chloride, *J. Gen. Physiol.* **48:** 859–872.

Auerbach, A. A. and M. V. L. Bennett (1969). Chemically mediated transmission at a giant fiber synapse in the central nervous system of a vertebrate, *J. Gen. Physiol.* **53:**183–210.

Baker, P. F. (1972). Transport and metabolism of calcium ions in nerve, *Prog. Biophys. Mol. Biol.* **24:**177–223.

Baker, P. F., A. L. Hodgkin, and E. B. Ridgway (1971). Depolarization and calcium entry in squid giant axons, *J. Physiol. (London)* **218:**709–755.

Blaustein, M. P. (1974). The interrelationship between sodium and calcium fluxes across cell membranes, *Rev. Physiol. Biochem. Pharmacol.* **70:**33–82.

Blaustein, M. P., N. C. Kendrick, R. C. Fried, and R. W. Ratzlaff (1977). Calcium metabolism at the mammalian presynaptic nerve terminal: lessons from the synaptosome, pp. 172–194 in *Society for Neuroscience Symposia*, Vol. 2, Cowan, W. M. and J. A. Ferrendelli, eds. Society for Neuroscience, Bethesda, Md.

Blinks, J. R., F. G. Prendergast, and D. G. Allen (1976). Photoproteins as biological calcium indicators, *Pharmacol. Rev.* **28:**1–93.

Bloedel, J. R., P. W. Gage, R. Llinás, and D. M. J. Quastel (1966). Transmission across the squid giant synapse in the presence of tetrodotoxin, *J. Physiol. (London)* **188:**52–53.

Bullock, T. H. and S. Hagiwara (1957). Intracellular recording from the giant synapse of the squid, *J. Gen. Physiol.* **40:**565–577.

del Castillo, J. and B. Katz (1954). Changes in end-plate activity produced by presynaptic polarization, *J. Physiol. (London)* **124:**586–604.

del Castillo, J. and L. Stark (1952). The effect of calcium ions on the motor end-plate potential, *J. Physiol. (London)* **116:**507–515.

Di polo, R., J. Requena, F. J. Brinley, Jr., L. J. Mullins, A. Scarpa, and T. Tiffert (1976). Ionized calcium concentration in squid axons, *J. Gen. Physiol.* **67:**433–467.

Dodge, F. A. and R. Rahamimoff (1967). Cooperative action of calcium ions in transmitter release at the nuclear junction, *J. Physiol. (London)* **193:** 419–432.

Eckert, R. and H. D. Lux (1976). A voltage-sensitive persistent calcium conductance in neuronal somata of Helix, *J. Physiol. (London)* **254:**129–151.

Fatt, P. and B. Katz (1952). Spontaneous subthreshold activity at motor nerve endings, *J. Physiol. (London)* **117:**109–128.

Hagiwara, S. (1973). Ca spike, *Adv. Biophys.* **4:**71–102.

Hagiwara, S., J. Fukuda, and D. C. Eaton (1974). Membrane currents carried by Ca, Sr and Ba in barnacle muscle fiber during voltage clamp, *J. Gen. Physiol.* **63:**564–578.

Hagiwara, S. and I. Tasaki (1958). A study of the mechanism of impulse transmission across the giant synapse of the squid, *J. Physiol. (London)* **143:** 114–137.

Harvey, A. M. and F. C. MacIntosh (1940). Calcium and synaptic transmission in a sympathetic ganglion, *J. Physiol. (London)* **97:**408–416.

Heuser, J. E. (1977). Synaptic vesicle exocytosis revealed in quick-frozen frog neuromuscular junctions treated with 4-aminopyridine and given a single electrical shock, pp. 215–239 in *Society for Neuroscience Symposia*, Vol. 2,

Cowan, W. M. and J. A. Ferrendelli, eds. Society for Neuroscience, Bethesda, Md.

Heyer, C. B. and H. D. Lux (1976). Properties of a facilitating calcium current in bursting pacemaker neurons of the snail, *Helix pomatia, J. Physiol. (London)* **262**:319–348.

Hodgkin, A. L. and R. D. Keynes (1957). Movements of labelled calcium in squid giant axon, *J. Physiol. (London)* **138**:253–281.

Hubbard, J. I., R. Llinás, and D. M. J. Quastel (1969). *Electrophysiological Analysis of Synaptic Transmission.* Edward Arnold, London.

Hubbard, J. I. and R. F. Schmidt (1963). An electrophysiological investigation of mammalian motor nerve terminals, *J. Physiol. (London)* **166**:145–167.

Kater, S. B. (1977). Calcium electroresponsiveness and its relationship to secretion in molluscan exocrine gland cells, pp. 195–214 in *Society for Neuroscience Symposia,* Vol. 2, Cowan, W. M. and J. A. Ferrendelli, eds. Society for Neuroscience, Bethesda, Md.

Katz, B. and R. Miledi (1967a). Modification of transmitter release by electrical interference with motor nerve endings, *Proc. R. Soc. London Ser. B* **167**:1–7.

Katz, B. and R. Miledi (1967b). The release of acetylcholine from nerve endings by graded electric pulses, *Proc. R. Soc. London Ser. B* **167**:23–38.

Katz, B. and R. Miledi (1967c). A study of synaptic transmission in the absence of nerve impulses, *J. Physiol. (London)* **192**:407–436.

Katz, B. and R. Miledi (1969). Tetrodotoxin-resistant electric activity in presynaptic terminals, *J. Physiol. (London)* **203**:459–487.

Katz, B. and R. Miledi (1971). The effect of prolonged depolarization on synaptic transfer in the stellate ganglion of the squid, *J. Physiol. (London)* **216**: 503–512.

Keynes, A. D., E. Rojas, R. E. Taylor, and J. Vergara (1973). Calcium and potassium systems of a giant barnacle muscle fiber under membrane potential control, *J. Physiol. (London)* **229**:409–455.

Kusano, K. (1968). Further study of the relationship between pre- and postsynaptic potentials in the squid giant synapse, *J. Gen. Physiol.* **52**:326–345.

Kusano, K. (1970). Influence of ionic environment on the relationship between pre- and postsynaptic potentials, *J. Neurobiol.* **1**:437–457.

Kusano, K., D. R. Livengood, and R. Werman (1967). Correlation of transmitter release with membrane properties of the presynaptic fiber of the squid giant synapse, *J. Gen. Physiol.* **50**:2579–2601.

Llinás, R., J. R. Blinks, and C. Nicholson (1972). Calcium transient in presynaptic terminal of squid giant synapse: detection with aequorin, *Science* **176**:1127–1129.

Llinás, R. and J. E. Heuser (1977). Depolarization-release coupling systems in neurons, *Neurosci. Res. Prog. Bull.*, in press.

Llinás, R. and C. Nicholson (1975). Calcium role in depolarization-secretion coupling: an aequorin study in squid giant synapse *Proc. Natl. Acad. Sci. U.S.A.* **72**:187–190.

Llinás, R., I. Z. Steinberg, and K. Walton (1976a). Presynaptic calcium currents and their relation to synaptic transmission: voltage clamp study in squid giant synapse and theoretical model for the calcium gate, *Proc. Natl. Acad. Sci. U.S.A.* **73**:2918–2922.

Llinás, R., K. Walton, and V. Bohr (1976b). Synaptic transmission in squid giant synapse after potassium conductance blockage with external 3- and 4-aminopyridine, *Biophys. J.* **16**:83–86.

Llinás, R., K. Walton, and R. Hess (1976c). Voltage clamp study of presynaptic calcium current in squid giant synapse, *Fed. Proc.* **35**:696.

Locke, F. S. (1894). Notiz ueber den Einfluss physiologischer Kochsalzloesung auf die elektrische Erregbarkeit von Muskel und Nerve, *Zentralbl. Physiol.* **8**:166.

Mann, D. M. and R. W. Joyner (1976). Quantal transmission at the squid giant synapse, *Abstr. Annu. Meet. Soc. Neurosci.*, 6th, Toronto, p. 1008.

Martin, A. R. and G. Pilar (1963). Transmission through the ciliary ganglion of the chick, *J. Physiol. (London)* **168**:464–478.

Meech, R. W. and N. B. Standen (1975). Potassium activation in *Helix aspersa* neurones under voltage clamp: a component mediated by calcium influx, *J. Physiol. (London)* **249**:211–239.

Meves, H. and W. Vogel (1973). Calcium inward currents in internally perfused giant axons, *J. Physiol. (London)* **235**:225–265.

Miledi, R. (1973). Transmitter release induced by injection of calcium ions into nerve terminals, *Proc. R. Soc. London Ser. B* **183**:421–425.

Miledi, R. and C. R. Slater (1966). The action of calcium on neuronal synapses in the squid, *J. Physiol. (London)* **184**:473–498.

Narahashi, T., J. W. Moore, and W. R. Scott (1964). Tetrodotoxin blockage of sodium conductance increase on lobster giant axons, *J. Gen. Physiol.* **47**: 965–974.

Overton, E. (1904). Beitraege zur allgemeinen Muskel und Nerven physiologie, *Pflugers Arch. Gesamte Physiol. Menschen Tiere* **105**:176–290.

Parsegian, V. A. (1977). Considerations in determining the mode of influence of calcium on vesicle-membrane interaction, pp. 161–171 in *Society for Neuroscience Symposia*, Vol. 2, Cowan, W. M. and J. A. Ferrendelli, eds. Society for Neuroscience, Bethesda, Md.

Pelhate, M. and Y. Pichon (1974). Selective-inhibition of potassium current in giant-axon of cockroach, *J. Physiol. (London)* **242**:P90–91.

Reuter, H. (1973). Divalent cations as charge carriers in excitable membranes, *Prog. Biophys. Molec. Biol.* **26**:1–43.

Rojas, E. and R. E. Taylor (1975). Simultaneous measurements of magnesium, calcium and sodium influxes in perfused squid giant axons under membrane potential control, *J. Physiol. (London)* **252**:1–27.

Rubin, R. P. (1975). *Calcium and the Secretory Process*. Plenum Press, New York.

Smith, A. D. (1971). Summing up: some implications of the neuron as a secreting cell, *Phil. Trans. R. Soc. London Ser. B* **261**:423–437.

Takeuchi, A. and N. Takeuchi (1962). Electrical changes in pre- and postsynaptic axons of the giant synapse of Loligo, *J. Gen. Physiol.* **45**:1181–1193.

Yeh, J. Z., G. S. Oxford, C. H. Wu, and T. Narahashi (1976). Interactions of aminopyridines with potassium channels of squid axon membranes, *Biophys. J.* **16**:77–81.

Young, J. Z. (1939). Fused neurons and synaptic contacts in the giant nerve fibres of cephalopods, *Phil. Trans. R. Soc. London Ser. B* **229**:465–503.

Considerations in Determining the Mode of Influence of Calcium on Vesicle-Membrane Interaction

V. A. Parsegian

National Institutes of Health, Bethesda, Maryland

We know from the electrical measurements of Llinás and his co-workers (Llinás, 1977) that calcium ions take at most only 200 μsec from the time of their entry into a nerve to effect the release of neurotransmitter. The present paper suggests that little vesicular movement—random or directed movement—can occur in such a short time. Calcium is probably acting within a few tens of Angstroms from its point of entry.

Measurement of repulsive forces between membranes gives some idea of what calcium can do to bring together vesicle and presynaptic membrane. Below about 30 Å separation, phospholipid membranes repel with a force that is only weakly dependent on membrane charge (Cowley, Fuller, Rand, and Parsegian, 1977). The force one encounters in pushing the membranes together is the work of transfer of water from the water-soluble polar groups that stabilize the membrane surface. Biochemical rather than physical chemical models for the action of Ca^{2+} better recognize the need to move or remove such hydrophilic groups to allow very rapid approach of membranes and subsequent membrane fusion without internal loss of vesicle contents.

In the general scheme used by Heuser (Llinás and Heuser, 1977) for discussing depolarization-release coupling (Figure 1), there are four stages in the life of a vesicle on its way to release of its contents at the presynaptic membrane. The first two, "approach" and "contact," involve translation of the vesicle up to some finite minimum energy separation from the nerve membrane, whereas "fusion" and "release" envisage rearrangement of membrane components. In the next three

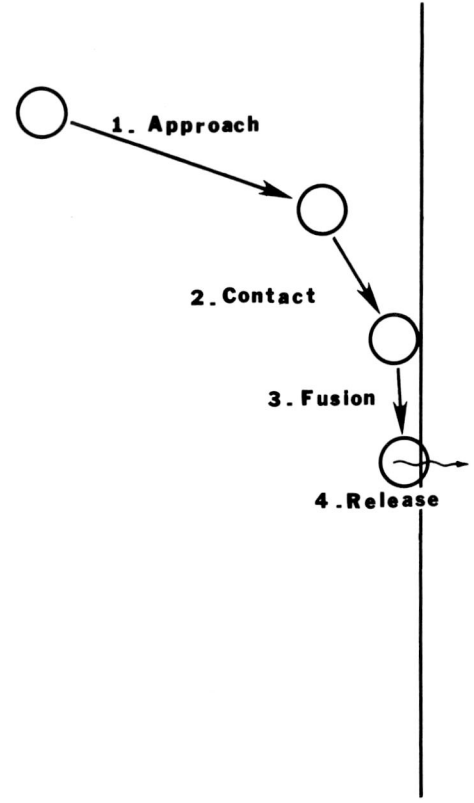

FIGURE 1. Stages in vesicle-presynaptic membrane interaction. The result of contact in this nomenclature is two membranes closely opposed, but remaining structurally distinct, with a separation of the order of a few nanometers. Steps 3 and 4 imply rearrangement and redistribution of membrane components.

sections, I will consider vesicle displacement, Ca^{2+} movement, and intermembrane forces; the final discussion will use these considerations to suggest that Ca^{2+} acts to provoke enzymatic activity destabilizing membranes prior to neurotransmitter release.

Vesicle Movement

Two distinctly different kinds of movement can be imagined for vesicles. The first is random or Brownian motion that can occur during the interval between depolarization and release. The second type of movement is sustained displacement that results from an applied force dragging the vesicle through a viscous medium.

For diffusion we use the Stokes-Einstein relation (Einstein, 1956) for the mean square displacement $\overline{(\Delta x)^2}$ in one direction

$$\overline{(\Delta x)^2} = 2Dt.$$

Here t is the time elapsed, and D the diffusion constant

$$D = \frac{kT}{6\pi a \eta}$$

where k is Boltzmann's constant, T the absolute temperature, a the vesicle radius, and η the viscosity of the medium. The validity of these expressions applied to vesicle-sized spheres has been verified from light-scattering studies (Dubin, Lunacek, and Benedek, 1967).

We take

$$kT = 4 \times 10^{-14} \text{ erg}$$
$$a = 250 \text{ Å} = 2.5 \times 10^{-6} \text{ cm}$$
$$\eta = 10^{-2} \text{ poise}$$

to get

$$D = 8.5 \times 10^{-8} \text{ cm}^2/\text{sec}.$$

The consequent estimate for mean displacement $\sqrt{\overline{(\Delta x)^2}}$ in 200 μsec is then roughly 580 Å. This is a shift of about one vesicle diameter. Morphologically it looks as though random motion creates a relatively small change in position, enough only to accomplish step 2 in Figure 1.

Alternatively, one may assume that the vesicle is moved by an imposed force, but the expected displacement is smaller than from random motion. We let

$$\text{force} = 6\pi a \eta v$$

where v is the vesicle velocity $d\ell/dt$ and ℓ is the distance between surfaces of membranes. As a representative force we use the electrostatic interaction between a sphere and a wall (Bell, Levine, and McCartney, 1970),

$$\text{force} = \epsilon \psi_m \psi_v \kappa a e^{-\kappa \ell}.$$

Here we use

$$\epsilon = 80$$

for the dielectric constant of the medium,

$$\psi_m = +10 \text{ mV}$$

for the (transient) presynaptic membrane potential,

$$\psi_v = -80 \text{ mV}$$

for the vesicle surface potential,

$$\kappa = 1(/10 \text{ Å})$$

for the Debye screening constant (cf., e.g., Parsegian, 1973) and again

$$\eta = 10^{-2} \text{ poise.}$$

The numbers for ψ_m, ψ_v are not based on any experiment, but are chosen to make an electrostatic force as sharply attractive as possible. Because it still leads to forces too weak and displacements too small to be of consequence, use of these number is permissible.

The momentary velocity of the vesicle is then

$$v = \frac{d\ell}{dt} = \frac{\epsilon \psi_m \psi_v \kappa e^{-\kappa \ell}}{6\pi\eta}.$$

We ask how long a time, T, it takes to move from an initial position $\ell = L$ to "contact" $\ell = 0$ (Gingell and Parsegian, unpublished observations,

$$T = \int_0^T dt = \frac{6\pi\eta}{\epsilon \psi_m \psi_v \kappa} \int_L^0 e^{\kappa \ell} d\ell$$

$$= \frac{6\pi\eta}{\epsilon \psi_m \psi_v \kappa^2} (1 - e^{\kappa L}) \cong - \frac{6\pi\eta}{\epsilon \psi_m \psi_v \kappa^2} e^{\kappa L}.$$

For the numbers assumed, we find that for T equals 200 μsec, L is only about 112 Å. This is less than the root mean square displacement from random motion. And this is probably an overestimate. The frictional drag will be greater than that of the Stokes law assumed here when the particle approaches a wall. The electrostatic attraction used here is probably too strong. The vesicle will encounter additional very strong repulsion from the presynaptic membrane, as will be described below.

Either by random motion or long-range attraction, a vesicle cannot move very far in 200 μsec. In the scheme of Figure 1, neither step 1 nor step 2 is likely to occur during the action potential.

CA^{2+} Diffusion

Calcium ions move fast in comparison to a 250Å radius vesicle. Presynaptic vesicles near contact (cf. Figure 1) are probably enveloped in a cloud of calcium during the early moments of depolarization and release. The diffusion constant of calcium determined by radiotracer movement in an axon (Hodgkin and Keynes, 1957) is of the order of 6×10^{-7} cm^2/sec (compared with 6×10^{-6} cm^2/sec in free solution). In a 200-μsec period, the mean square displacement in one dimension is $\sqrt{2Dt} > 1500$ Å. One can expect that Ca^{2+} ions easily diffuse several hundreds, and even thousands, of Angstroms during the period between Ca^{2+} entry in depolarization and the release of neurotransmitter.

Judging from Llinás' (1977) estimates of calcium current during depolarization, massive numbers of ions flow in to stimulate the release of relatively few vesicles. He infers that about 1.7×10^9 ions flow into the presynaptic terminal during an action potential that causes the release of the contents of 5×10^3 vesicles. It appears that some 3.4×10^5 Ca^{2+} ions are used per vesicle released. Taking the 1.7×10^9 ions and imagining them to be uniformly distributed over the presynaptic terminal of area 150×10^3 μm^2 = 1.50×10^{-3} cm^2 and in a layer 2,000 Å = 2×10^{-5} cm thick, the density of ions in this cloud is about 5.7×10^{17} ions/cc or about 1.0 mM, much higher than the background Ca^{2+} of the presynaptic nerve (cf. Llinás, 1977, for numerical data).

It is unlikely that calcium acts only, or primarily, by screening electrostatic repulsion forces between vesicle and presynaptic membrane. A vesicle of 250 Å radius has an area of about 8×10^5 Å^2. If it bears as much as one unit negative ionic charge per 100 Å^2, 4,000 Ca^{2+} ions would be required to neutralize the vesicle area. There are probably enough Ca^{2+} ions released to do this.

But note that charge neutralization by divalent cations may not be enough to cause transmitter release. Heuser (1977; see also Llinás and Heuser, 1977) has shown that very high concentrations of Mg^{2+} cause the vesicle to appear to push against the presynaptic membrane after depolarization and fixation in a Mg^{2+}-containing medium. Assuming that Mg^{2+} actually enters the presynaptic cell (Miledi, 1973), this behavior seems to show that a repulsive force between them is being annulled (probably in its competition with a long-range van der Waals attractive force [Parsegian, 1973]) to allow the membranes to come close to each other. But there is no transmitter release. Electrostatic repulsion may have prevented approach to contact (step 2, Figure 1), but its electrical neutralization does not allow fusion. In fact, morphologically, the two contacting membranes remain distinct. Ca^{2+} must have more than electrostatic activity to allow the vesicles to undergo steps 3 and 4

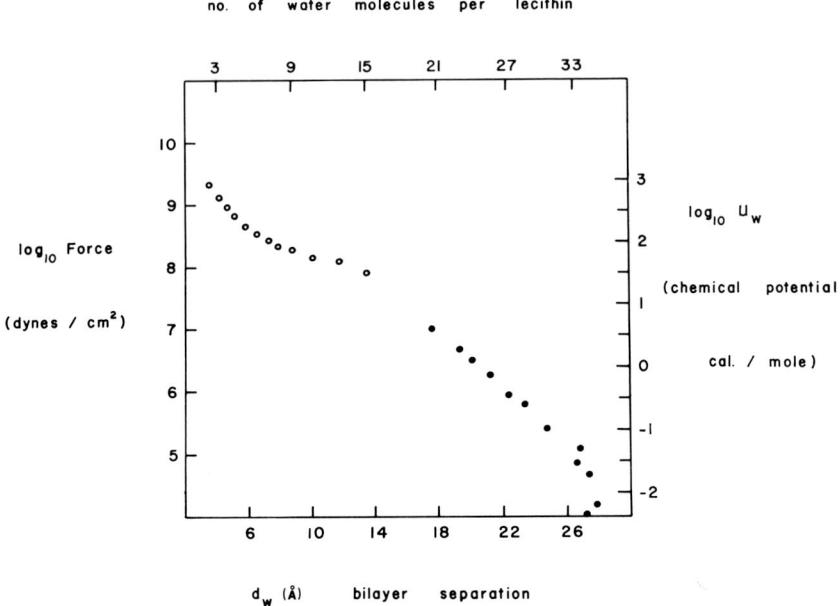

FIGURE 2. Repulsive force versus separation of phospholipid egg lecithin bilayers. From LeNeveu et al. (1976).

(Figure 1). The reasons for this become clear when we take note of the forces between membranes separated by a few tens of Angstroms.

Membrane Interactions

At separations of a few tens of Angstroms, even electrically neutral membranes feel a very strong repulsion. Figure 2 shows the measured force per unit area between bilayers of the zwitterionic phospholipid lecithin from LeNeveu, Rand, and Parsegian (1976). Below 27 Å separations, the force seems to grow exponentially, at least until an interbilayer distance of about 15 Å. LeNeveu et al. (1976) pointed out that this force measured between planar membranes can be restated as one between a spherical vesicle and planar bilayer. In thermal units, it takes about 15 kT of work to bring a 500 Å diameter vesicle of lecithin to within 15 Å of a lecithin bilayer. This force presupposes no significant redistribution of the phospholipid polar groups upon vesicle approach. On this supposition, the probability of a vesicle making a 15 Å approach is about one in three million.

Somewhat surprisingly, the interaction between charged lipids at these separations is little different from that between egg lecithin bilayers. Cowley et al. (1977) have reported measurements between several charged lipid membranes. These repulsive forces show two distinct regimes (Figure 3): above approximately 30 Å separation, the force is sensitive to membrane charge and varies (comparatively) slowly, as expected from the theory of electrostatic double layers; below about 30 Å, all membranes show the repulsion first observed between lecithins. We have chosen to refer to the latter interaction as a hydration force because it is by its very nature a work of removal of water from between bilayers (an operational definition made explicit in the right-hand ordinate of Figure 2).

Cowley et al. (1977) have observed the behavior schematically represented in Figure 3 for several phospholipid bilayers: pure phosphatidyl glycerol, egg lecithin mixed (1) with 3, 5, or 10% sodium oleate, (2) with 10% phosphatidyl inositol, and (3) with 5 or 50% phosphatidyl glycerol. Clearly, much remains to be measured as model systems are developed to mimic real membranes. Nevertheless, the available force measurements give a broad hint as to what is going on between vesicle and presynaptic membrane.

All membranes are stabilized by highly polar water-soluble moieties anchored to a lipid interior. It will always require work to remove water from these moieties. Membranes that are not so covered would

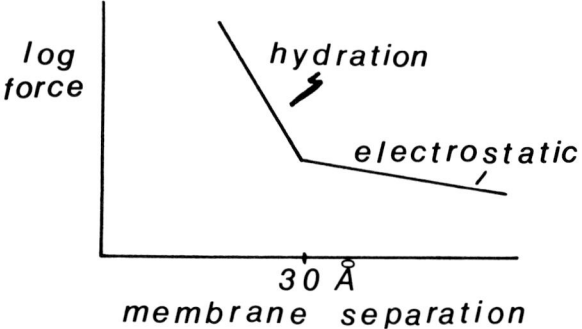

FIGURE 3. Qualitative behavior of repulsion between charged phospholipid membranes (Cowley et al., 1977). Above 30 Å separation, the force depends on electrostatic charge density and ion concentration in the suspending medium; below this distance, the repulsion closely resembles that of electrically neutral egg lecithin (Figure 2).

in effect be oil drops that are always unstable in water. The water-soluble group on zwitterionic lecithin is small, as membrane polar groups go; the work of removal of water from larger soluble species should be even greater than the forces demonstrated in Figure 2. There is also some evidence that the regions of contact between vesicle and presynaptic membrane are clear of intramembrane particles (Heuser, 1977), so that their interaction may further resemble that between model phospholipid membranes.

Actually, the main point does not depend on such speculation. One need only recognize that the energies of hydration translate into very large physical forces when the act of dehydration involves movement together of membranes. It is the very presence of groups that stabilize membranes that prevents their being pushed together. Remler (1973) and Bass and Moore (1966) have considered the role a monolayer of hydrating water might play in vesicle movement.

DISCUSSION

Even very rough computations of vesicle movement tell us that calcium must act near its site of entry into the cell. The vesicles that respond to its entry are likely to be those that appear under the electron microscope to be nearly in contact with the presynaptic membrane (Figure 1). Measurements of forces between phospholipid bilayers show that strong repulsion is encountered by membranes closer together than 30 Å. This repulsion is apparently independent of electrostatic charge on the membranes and is probably best described as a work of removal of water from water-soluble groups stabilizing the membrane surface.

What, then, can calcium be doing to hasten or allow membrane contact during the 200 μsec delay? It seems most likely that the mode of action is to move or remove the membranes' water-soluble groups that cling to water between the membranes.

One should not expect that Ca^{2+} acts only by screening negative electrostatic charges attached to the membranes; otherwise, very high concentrations of internal Mg^{2+} would also enhance neurotransmitter release. On the contrary, Mg^{2+} inhibits release (del Castillo and Engback, 1954; Muller and Finkelstein, 1974) and, morphologically, seems to help vesicles stick near membranes without allowing fusion or transmitter release (Heuser, 1977). The apparent antagonism of Mg^{2+} and Ca^{2+} also suggests that they are not acting in the same manner as in those model systems where their comparative effect on fusion is not one of kind but of degree. (See, e.g., Miller and Racker, 1976; and Papadjopoulous, Vail, Pangborn, and Postep, 1976). Nowhere in the large and confusing literature concerning vesicle fusion in model systems have I found any indication that fusion rates can approach 100 μsec or shorter relaxation times. If purely physical-chemical systems can show (1) 100 μsec rates, (2) strong Ca^{2+} versus Mg^{2+} specificity, and (3) high efficiency against loss of vesicle contents to the wrong medium, then they might be relevant to synaptic depolarization-release coupling.

It is probably more fruitful to look to biochemistry rather than physical chemistry to describe the molecular details of the very rapid release of transmitter. Two kinds of reaction immediately come to mind. One is phospholipase activity, which allows removal of polar groups. The second (envisaging displacement) is the action of the actomyosin analogue neurostenin (Llinás and Heuser, 1977).

If there were some means of removing whole polar groups at a region of membrane repulsion, the barrier to mutual approach toward fusion would disappear. For example, a phospholipase, on or next to a membrane triggered specifically by calcium, should have time to detach a dozen polar groups within hundreds of microseconds. This would suffice to allow controlled fusion at the shaven spots. According to Mahler (Llinás and Heuser, 1977), Ca^{2+}- or Mg^{2+}-dependent enzymes may exist in both vesicle and presynaptic membranes.

Alternatively, the stabilizing polar groups could be pulled away from the place of membrane confrontation to allow merger of the lipid membrane interior. Again, membrane areas of the order of 1,000 $Å^2$ need be cleared to allow contact leading to fusion. The necessary lateral displacements are of the order of tens of Angstroms; this movement is possible when driven by contractile proteins working for hundreds of microseconds. (At their fastest, muscle proteins contract at 7 μm/sec per sarcomere [Wolpert, 1965; Lowy, Millman, and Hanson, 1964] or 7 Å in 100 μsec.)

In either case, displacement or removal, one expects that biochemical activity is necessary for the rapid membrane fusion implied by Llinás' measurements. I suggest the following elaboration of the general scheme (Figure 1) as a working hypothesis: (1) Ca^{2+} ions enter the presynaptic nerve and diffuse rapidly to surround those vesicles very near the presynaptic membrane; (2) the water-soluble components on both vesicular and cell membranes are rapidly detached or pulled aside in a Ca^{2+}-specific process that may consume energy; (3) the two membranes then fuse spontaneously; and (4) the vesicular membrane merges with the presynaptic membrane as vesicle contents are released.

ACKNOWLEDGMENTS

I am indebted to Francis O. Schmitt and the members of the Neurosciences Research Program for making possible several stimulating discussions introducing me to recent experimental work in this area. I have also enjoyed helpful informal discussions with Rodolfo Llinás, John Heuser, and Arthur Forer. I thank Stephen Brenner for a careful reading of the text.

REFERENCES

Bass, L. and W. J. Moore (1966). Electrokinetic mechanism of miniature post synaptic potentials, *Proc. Natl. Acad. Sci. U.S.A.* **55**:1214–1217.

Bell, G. M., S. Levine, and L. N. McCartney (1970). Approximate methods of determining the double-layer free energy of interaction between two charged colloidal spheres, *J. Coll. Int. Sci.* **33**:335–359.

Cowley, S., N. Fuller, R. P. Rand, and V. A. Parsegian (1977). Measurement of repulsion between charged phospholipid bilayers, *Biophys. J.* **17**: 85a.

del Castillo, J. and L. Engback (1954). The nature of the neuromuscular block produced by magnesium, *J. Physiol.* **124**:370–384.

Dubin, S. B., J. H. Lunacek, and G. B. Benedek (1967). Observation of the spectrum of light scattered by solutions of biological macromolecules, *Proc. Natl. Acad. Sci. U.S.A.* **57**:1164–1171.

Einstein, A. (1956). *Investigations of the Theory of Brownian Movement.* Dover Publications, New York.

Heuser, J. E. (1977). Synaptic vesicle exocytosis revealed in quick-frozen frog neuromuscular junctions treated with 4-aminopyridine and given a single electrical shock, pp. 215–239 in *Society for Neuroscience Symposia*, Vol. 2, Cowan, W. M. and J. A. Ferrendelli, eds. Society for Neuroscience, Bethesda, Md.

Hodgkin, A. L. and R. D. Keynes (1957). Movements of labelled calcium in squid giant axon, *J. Physiol. (London)* **138**:253–281.

LeNeveu, D. M., R. P. Rand, and V. A. Parsegian (1976). Measurement of forces between lecithin bilayers, *Nature (London)* **259**:601–603.

Llinás, R. (1977). Calcium and transmitter release in squid synapse, pp. 139–160 in *Society for Neuroscience Symposia*, Vol. 2, Cowan, W. M. and J. A. Ferrendelli, eds. Society for Neuroscience, Bethesda, Md.

Llinás, R. and J. E. Heuser (1977). Depolarization-release coupling systems in neurons, *Neurosci. Res. Prog. Bull.*, in press.

Lowy, J., B. M. Millman, and J. Hanson (1964). Structure and function in smooth tonic muscles of lamelli branch molluscs, *Proc. R. Soc. London Ser. B* **160**:525.

Miledi, R. (1973). Transmitter release induced by injection of calcium ions into nerve terminals, *Proc. R. Soc. London Ser. B* **183**:421–425.

Miller, C. and E. Racker (1976). Fusion of phospholipid vesicles reconstituted with cytochrome c oxidase and mitochondrial hydrophobic protein, *J. Membr. Biol.* **26**:319–333.

Muller, R. U. and A. Finkelstein (1974). The electrostatic basis of Mg^{++} inhibition of transmitter release, *Proc. Natl. Acad. Sci. U.S.A.* **71**:923–926.

Papadjopoulous, D., W. J. Vail, W. A. Pangborn, and G. Postep (1976). Studies on membrane fusion, II. Induction of fusion in pure phospholipid membranes by calcium ions and other divalent metals, *Biochim. Biophys. Acta* **448**:265–283.

Parsegian, V. A. (1973). Long-range physical forces in the biological milieu, *Ann. Rev. Biophys. Bioeng.* **2**:221–255.

Remler, M. P. (1973). A semi-quantitative theory of synaptic vesicle movements, *Biophys. J.* **13**:104–117.

Wolpert, L. (1965). Cytoplasmic streaming and amoeboid movement, pp. 270–293 in *Society for General Microbiology, 15th Symposium*. Function and Structure in Microorganisms: Proceedings. Polleck, M. R. and M. H. Richmond, eds. Cambridge University Press, New York.

Calcium Metabolism at the Mammalian Presynaptic Nerve Terminal: Lessons from the Synaptosome

M. P. Blaustein, N. C. Kendrick, R. C. Fried, and R. W. Ratzlaff

Washington University School of Medicine, St. Louis, Missouri

Synaptosomes as Functional Units

Membrane potentials

Our present knowledge of the cellular basis of synaptic transmission has been derived primarily from a variety of very elegant experiments on the frog neuromuscular junction and the squid giant synapse. With respect to neurotransmitter release, the fundamental notion, derived from the seminal work of Katz and Miledi and their collaborators (see Katz, 1969), is that depolarization increases (transiently) the calcium conductance of the presynaptic nerve terminals; Ca enters the terminals, moving down an electrochemical gradient, and the consequent rise in intraterminal ionized Ca^{2+} concentration ($[Ca^{2+}]_i$) somehow triggers transmitter release (cf. Miledi, 1973; Llinás and Nicholson, 1975). The central role of the Ca ion in this process provides ample justification for carefully examining the factors that control $[Ca^{2+}]_i$. Moreover, it would be useful to know whether or not these concepts, garnered from studies on squid and frog synapses, can be extrapolated to synapses in the mammalian CNS.

Information about the mechanism of transmitter release in the mammalian CNS was more difficult to obtain because of the lack of preparations amenable to the appropriate physiological manipulations. However, in 1962, Gray and Whittaker, and De Robertis and his colleagues prepared fractions from rat brain homogenates that were enriched with pinched-off presynaptic nerve terminals, "synaptosomes." Many of these terminals appeared to have resealed, in that they retained ("occluded") soluble cytoplasmic proteins and small ions (e.g., potassium) that could be released by osmotic shock (Marchbanks, 1967). Early studies also suggested that the synaptosomes retained some functional integrity (see the reviews by De Robertis, 1972; Bradford, 1975): they had intact glycolytic and oxidative metabolic pathways, and could accumulate K and extrude Na at the expense of ATP. This ion transport (cardiac glycoside-inhibitable Na-K exchange) was confirmed in our laboratory. It implied that the synaptosomes, like intact neurons, might develop K^+ diffusion potentials across their plasma membranes. With the advent of fluorometric dye methods for measuring membrane potentials (Cohen, Salzberg, Davilla, Ross, Landowne, Waggoner, and Wang, 1974), it became possible to test this hypothesis; the experimental results (Blaustein and Goldring, 1975) strongly supported the view that synaptosomes, incubated in physiological saline, do have membrane potentials that respond to depolarizing agents in a manner comparable to those of intact neurons.

Calcium conductance

In view of the evidence that synaptosome membranes can maintain ion gradients and transmembrane electrical potentials, it seemed appropriate to test for further evidence of functional integrity. If synaptosomes are to be useful preparations for the study of presynaptic physiology and pharmacology, they must be capable of carrying out at least some of those functions that are peculiar to the terminals.

Katz and Miledi (see Katz, 1969) had shown that the initial stage of neurotransmitter release at the squid giant synapse and frog neuromuscular junction involves depolarization of the presynaptic terminal. This induces a voltage-dependent increase in the Ca conductance of the terminal, thereby allowing Ca to enter (Llinás, 1977). To determine whether or not a similar Ca conductance change occurs at the mammalian central synapse, various depolarizing agents (K, Rb, veratridine, scorpion [*Leiurus quinquestriatus*] venom, and gramicidin-D) were tested for their effects on the rate of ^{45}Ca accumulation by synaptosomes. Synaptosomes, incubated in standard physiological saline (with 5 mM K), take up a small amount of ^{45}Ca—presumably due to Ca-Ca exchange, because there is no net change in Ca content (Blaustein, 1975). When exposed to the depolarizing agents, the rate of ^{45}Ca uptake is increased three- to sixfold (Figure 1; Blaustein and Wiesmann, 1970; Blaustein, 1975; Blaustein and Ector, 1975), and,

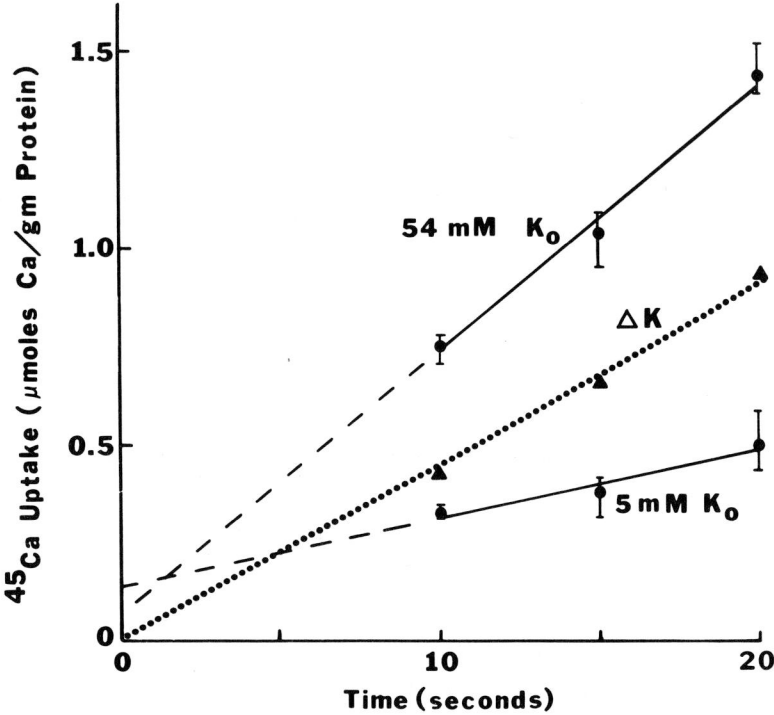

FIGURE 1. Time course of ^{45}Ca uptake by synaptosomes incubated in media containing 5 mM K + 132 mM Na or 54 mM K + 83 mM Na. The K-stimulated Ca uptake is indicated by the dotted line. The abscissa indicates the period of incubation with ^{45}Ca. The $[Ca]_o$ was 1.2 mM in all preincubation and incubation solutions. Each symbol indicates the mean of three determinations; the bars show the range of the individual values. From Blaustein (1975).

under these circumstances, there is a net gain of Ca (Blaustein, 1975). Although these data imply that the Ca conductance of the synaptosome membranes is increased by "depolarization," it should be recognized that the Ca conductance change associated with a normal action potential may last only for a few milliseconds (Llinás, 1977). However, Katz and Miledi (1971) have shown that, at the squid giant synapse, the Ca conductance increase may last for at least 1 to 2 sec, with minimal inactivation, in response to prolonged current pulses. Our data from the synaptosomes (Blaustein, 1975) suggest that there may be a *slow* inactivation, measured on a time scale of minutes. The conclusion is that the increased Ca entry into synapto-

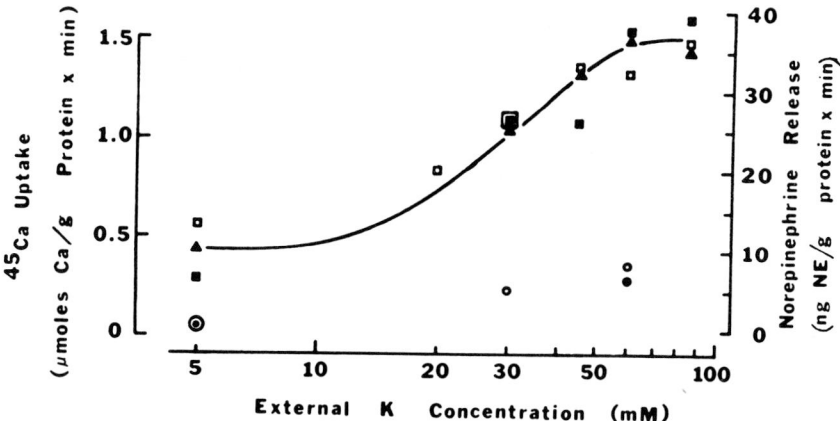

FIGURE. 2. ^{45}Ca uptake and norepinephrine release by samples of crude mitochondrial P$_2$ fraction. For the ^{45}Ca curve (▲), samples were incubated in the ^{45}Ca containing physiological salt solution for 1 min. Each point represents the mean of three determinations, and the solid curve has been drawn through these points. Norepinephrine release data are shown for two experiments (open versus solid symbols): the P$_2$ preparation represented by the solid symbols is the same as that used for the ^{45}Ca uptake curve. To obtain sufficient norepinephrine for assay, a 10-min incubation period was used to measure norepinephrine release. Incubation was in Ca-free medium containing 2 mM EGTA (○,●) or in the presence of 1.2 mM Ca (□,■); each square or circle represents the mean of four determinations. The amount of norepinephrine released into the Ca-free Na + 5 mM K medium (23.2 ± 1.3 and 28.7 ± 1.5 ng of norepinephrine per g of protein × min, in the experiments represented by the solid and open symbols, respectively) was substracted from all other values, as a "baseline." Cocaine (165 µM) and pargyline (260 µM) were present in all media. The similarity of the K-stimulated ^{45}Ca accumulation and the Ca-dependent norepinephrine release curves do not necessarily imply a linear relationship between these two parameters. From Blaustein et al. (1972).

somes, observed in the presence of depolarizing agents, probably does represent a Ca conductance increase, indicating that mammalian central presynaptic terminals are, in this respect, similar to those of the squid synapse and frog neuromuscular junction.

An interesting corollary is the fact that veratridine and scorpion venom depolarize the presynaptic terminals and allow Ca to enter by a tetrodotoxin (TTX)-sensitive mechanism (Blaustein and Goldring, 1975; Blaustein, 1975). This implies that the terminals have sodium channels similar to those of the axon. It therefore seems likely that action potentials, propagated down the axons of intact neurons, actually invade the terminals.

Transmitter release

The next step was to determine whether or not the pinched-off nerve terminals could be triggered to release neurotransmitter substances when treated with depolarizing agents. The synaptosome preparations from mammalian brain are, of course, a heterogeneous population in terms of their transmitter content: some of the terminals are cholinergic, some are noradrenergic, some are GABA-nergic, etc. We tested for the release of endogenous norepinephrine and acetylcholine, using K-rich media, veratridine, and scorpion venom as depolarizing agents. The results were affirmative: the depolarizing agents stimulated transmitter release, and the release was external Ca dependent (Figure 2; Blaustein, Johnson, and Needleman, 1972; Blaustein, 1975). Moreover, TTX, which specifically blocks the depolarization and Ca uptake induced by veratridine and scorpion venom, also prevented these agents from triggering transmitter release. Similar observations on the Ca-dependent release of acetylcholine and GABA have been made in other laboratories (De Belleroche and Bradford, 1972; Levy, Redburn, and Cotman, 1973; Cotman, Haycock, and White, 1976). These data support the view that some of the nerve terminals in the synaptosome preparations are resealed and can function in a manner comparable to intact terminals.

Electrophysiological studies on the frog neuromuscular junction and squid synapse provide convincing evidence that the transmitter molecules are released in packets or "quanta" (Katz, 1969). There is also evidence for quantal transmitter release at synapses in the mammalian spinal cord (Kuno, 1971). This type of release can be accounted for if the transmitters are "packaged," presumably in synaptic vesicles, within the presynaptic terminals, and if release occurs by a process of exocytosis (e.g., Heuser, 1977). Direct evidence of exocytosis has not yet been obtained in synaptosome preparations, but we have found that extracellular markers (horseradish peroxidase or colloidal thorium dioxide) are taken up and appear within the synaptic vesicles after depolarization with veratridine or K-rich media (Figure 3; Fried and Blaustein, 1976). This uptake of extracellular marker may represent retrieval and recycling of vesicle membrane after exocytosis and fusion of the vesicle and plasma membranes. The uptake of marker was greatly reduced or abolished by omitting Ca from the medium or, in the case of the veratridine-depolarized synaptosomes, by adding TTX prior to the veratridine. As already noted, transmitter release is inhibited under these circumstances.

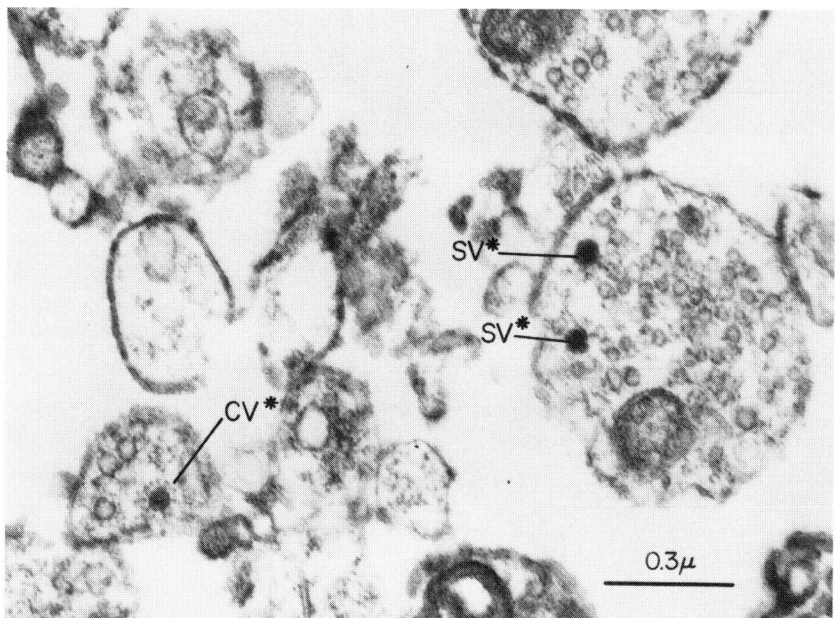

FIGURE 3. Morphology of synaptosomes incubated in K-rich media. The synaptosomes were incubated in a solution containing 100 mM Na + 50 mM K and 5 mg of horseradish peroxidase (HRP) per ml for 30 min. Note the HRP-labeled synaptic vesicles (SV*) and coated vesicle (CV*). Bar represents 0.3 µm. From Fried and Blaustein (1976).

The conditions that promoted transmitter release and uptake of the morphological markers were also associated with the appearance of many coated vesicles (Heuser and Reese, 1973) within the terminals. When colloidal thorium dioxide or horseradish peroxidase was present in the incubation medium, the coated vesicles frequently were labeled with these markers (Figure 3). These observations are consistent with the view (Gray and Willis, 1970; Heuser and Reese, 1973) that one of the early steps in the vesicle retrieval process may involve coated vesicles.

The main conclusion from the experiments mentioned above is that many of the presynaptic terminals obtained in synaptosome preparations from rat brain homogenates are resealed and retain considerable functional integrity. However, interpretation of data from studies using these preparations must be tempered by the recognition of three facts. (1) The synaptosome preparations are not "pure" nerve terminals. Some free mitochondria, myelin, fragmented membranes, small vesicles, and other cellular debris are also present. (2) Not all terminals in the preparation are resealed and functional. (3) The terminals obtained from brain (or ganglion) homogenates are very heterogeneous in terms of the types of transmitters they contain. Problems (1) and (2) may not be a serious handicap for physiological studies if properties specific to nerve terminals are being assessed. However, with regard to problem (3), the data on, for example, membrane potentials and Ca transport must simply represent an average of all the functional elements in the preparations.

With this caveat in mind, we may now examine some additional aspects of Ca metabolism in the presynaptic terminals.

Calcium extrusion: the role of Na-Ca exchange

As mentioned earlier, the Ca that enters the terminals during depolarization is net Ca entry (Blaustein, 1975); the Ca moves into the terminals down an electrochemical gradient. Although the concentration of ionized Ca^{2+} in the cytoplasm ($[Ca^{2+}]_i$) is not known, indirect evidence (to be presented below) indicates that it is probably less than 10^{-6}M. For comparative purposes, it should be noted that several types of experiments indicate that the level of ionized Ca^{2+} in the axoplasm of squid giant axons is on the order of 10^{-7}M (Baker, 1972; Blaustein, 1974; Di Polo, Requena, Brinley, Mullins, Scarpa, and Tiffert, 1976). Calcium is not distributed at "equilibrium" across the nerve terminal plasma membrane; however, with an external Ca^{2+} concentration ($[Ca^{2+}]_o$) of about 1 mM (10^{-3}M), and a (resting) membrane potential of about -60 mV (cytoplasm negative), according to the Nernst equation,

$$E_{Ca} = \frac{RT}{2F} \ln \frac{[Ca^{2+}]_o}{[Ca^{2+}]_i} \qquad (1)$$

$[Ca^{2+}]_i$ would have to be about 100 mM if the Ca equilibrium potential (E_{Ca}) were to equal the resting potential. This distribution certainly does not fit with experimental observation: even total cell Ca is far less than that predicted from equilibrium considerations. The obvious conclusion is that the Ca that enters the nerve terminals during depolarization must subsequently be extruded against a large electrochemical gradient, in order for the terminals to return to a physiological steady state. Clearly, an energy-utilizing transport system is required to extrude Ca against the Ca electrochemical gradient. An important clue to the underlying mechanism is illustrated in Figure 4. These data show that ^{45}Ca exits quite rapidly from ^{45}Ca-loaded synaptosomes when Na is present in the bathing medium; the efflux is markedly reduced when the NaCl is replaced, isomotically, by LiCl or by sucrose. This raises the possibility that Ca extrusion may involve an exchange of Na for Ca, and that some of the energy for this transport process may be supplied by the Na electrochemical gradient.

Additional data on the influence of external cations on Ca efflux are shown in Figure 5. These data indicate that the efflux of Ca into choline- and, especially, into Li-based solutions is promoted by external Ca. Similar observations on Ca fluxes in squid axons (Blaustein and Russell, 1975) can be accounted for by an exchange of internal Ca for external Ca; thus, net Ca efflux may involve, primarily, Na-Ca exchange. The relationship between the (external) Na concentration and the Ca efflux is sigmoid (Figure 6), and suggests that two or more Na^+ ions (perhaps three, as in the squid axon; Blaustein, Russell, and De Weer, 1974; Blaustein and Russell, 1975) enter in exchange for each exiting Ca^{2+} ion. A simple model of such a counterflow mechanism, involving an exchange of 3 Na^+ for 1 Ca^{2+}, is illustrated in Figure 7; although the model is based primarily on Ca flux studies in squid axons (Blaustein, 1976), it is also compatible with the synaptosome Ca flux data (Blaustein and Oborn, 1975; Blaustein and Ector, 1976). The model represents a simultaneous (as opposed to a sequential or shuttle) transport mechanism, which can move 1 Ca^{2+} in either direction across the plasma membrane, in exchange for 3 Na^+ moving in the opposite direction (Blaustein, 1976). With counterflow coupling, the downhill movement of Na into the neuron could supply energy to help power Ca extrusion. With a stoichiometry of 3 Na^+ for 1 Ca^{2+}, a resting membrane potential (V_M) of about -60 mV, and an external/ internal Na concentration ratio $[Na^+]_o/[Na^+]_i$ of about 10, the mechanism illustrated in Figure 7 could, in principle, maintain a Ca concentration ratio ($[Ca^{2+}]_o/[Ca^{2+}]_i$) of about 10^4 as given by (Blaustein and Hodgkin, 1969):

$$\frac{[Ca^{2+}]_o}{[Ca^{2+}]_i} = \frac{[Na^+]_o^3}{[Na^+]_i^3} \exp - \frac{V_M F}{RT} . \qquad (2)$$

Thus, if $[Ca^{2+}]_o$ is about 1 mM, sufficient energy would be available from the Na electrochemical gradient, alone, to maintain $[Ca^{2+}]_i$ at about 10^{-7}M (the Na electrochemical gradient is, of course, maintained by the

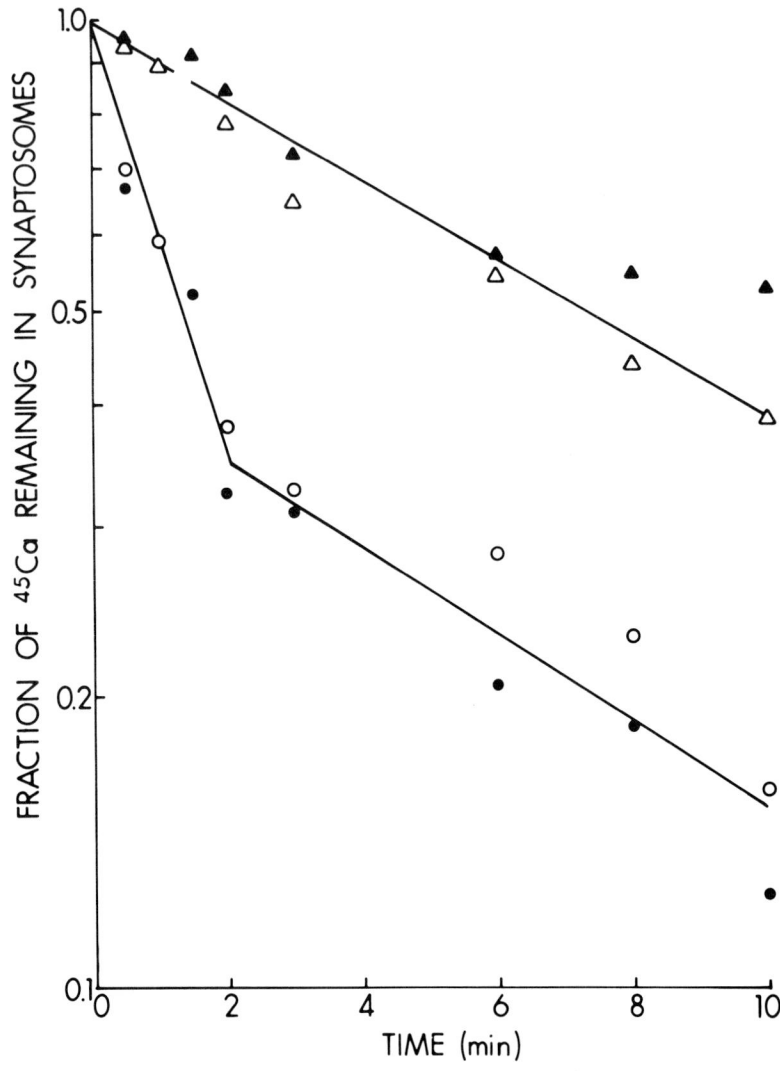

FIGURE 4. Time course of ^{45}Ca efflux from synaptosomes. Four synaptosome pellets (approximately 20 mg of protein) were each suspended in 0.7 ml of standard physiological saline (Na + 5 mM K) and preincubated for 15 min at 30°C. A 0.7-ml portion of the same solution, but including ^{45}Ca and 1.5×10^{-4}M veratridine (to stimulate Ca uptake; cf. Blaustein, 1975), was then added to each suspension, and incubation was continued for another 2 min. Ca uptake was then terminated by diluting the suspensions with 29 ml of Ca-free 132 mM Na + 5 mM K + 1 mM EGTA

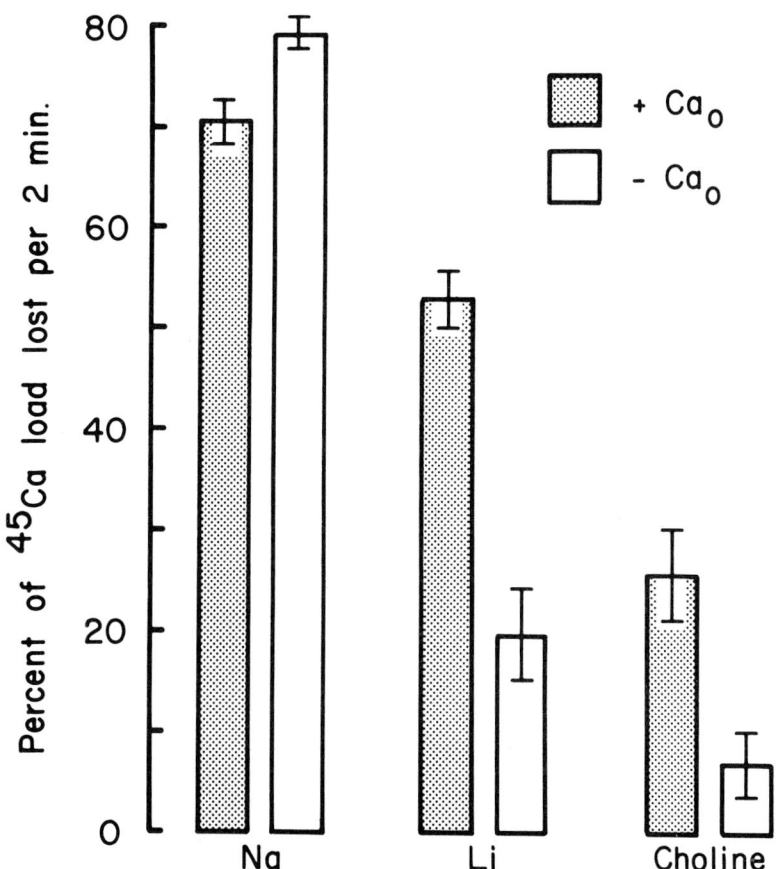

FIGURE 5. Effect of external cations on Ca efflux from ^{45}Ca-loaded synaptosomes. Open bars represent efflux in the absence of external Ca (0.5 mM EGTA present); stippled bars represent efflux with 1.2 mM ^{40}Ca present in the medium. The solutions contained 5 mM K and 132 mM Na, Li, or choline, as indicated below the bars; standard errors are indicated. Data from Table 2 of Blaustein and Ector (1976).

+ 2.5 × 10^{-7}M tetrodoxtoxin (○,●), Ca-free 132 mM Li + 5 mM K + EGTA + TTX (△), or Ca-free 264 mM sucrose + 5 mM K + TTX (▲). The suspensions were maintained at 30°C and were agitated by bubbling O$_2$ through the flasks. At the times indicated on the graph, 2.0-ml portions of the suspensions were filtered through glass fiber filters; the filters were washed with Na-free solution, and assayed for ^{45}Ca. The lines were drawn by eye. From Blaustein and Oborn (1975).

cardiac glycoside-sensitive Na-K exchange pump, at the expense of ATP; cf. De Weer, 1975).

The question of whether or not ATP or other energy-rich compounds participate directly in the Ca extrusion mechanism has been ignored in the preceding discussion, largely because there is no pertinent information available. Clearly, any metabolic inhibitors which, by

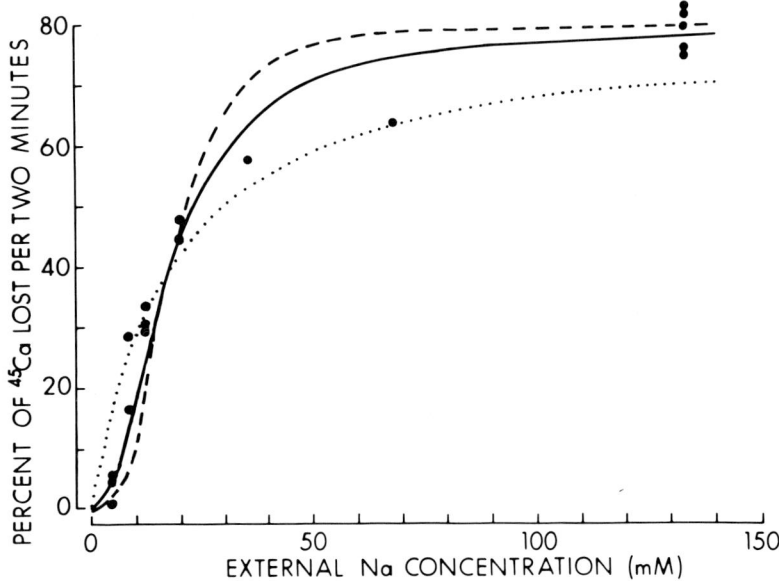

FIGURE 6. Effect of external Na concentration on ^{45}Ca efflux into Ca-free solutions. Na was replaced isomotically by choline. The ordinate shows the percentage of the ^{45}Ca load lost during a 2-min efflux period. Data from six synaptosome preparations are shown. Each point on the graph represents the mean of three Ca efflux determinations from one synaptosome preparation; two to four different external Na concentrations were tested in each experiment. The curves were calculated from the equation:

$$M_{Ca} = \frac{M^*_{Ca}}{1 + \left(\frac{\bar{K}_{Na}}{[Na]_o}\right)^n}$$

where M_{Ca} is the Ca efflux at any external Na concentration ($[Na]_o$). The maximal Ca efflux, M^*_{Ca}, is equal to 80% of the total Ca load lost per 2 min; $\bar{K}_{Na}$ is the apparent mean half-saturation constant for external Na, with a value of 18 mM. The exponent, n, has a value of 1 (· · ·), 2 (———), or 3 (– – –). From Blaustein and Ector (1976).

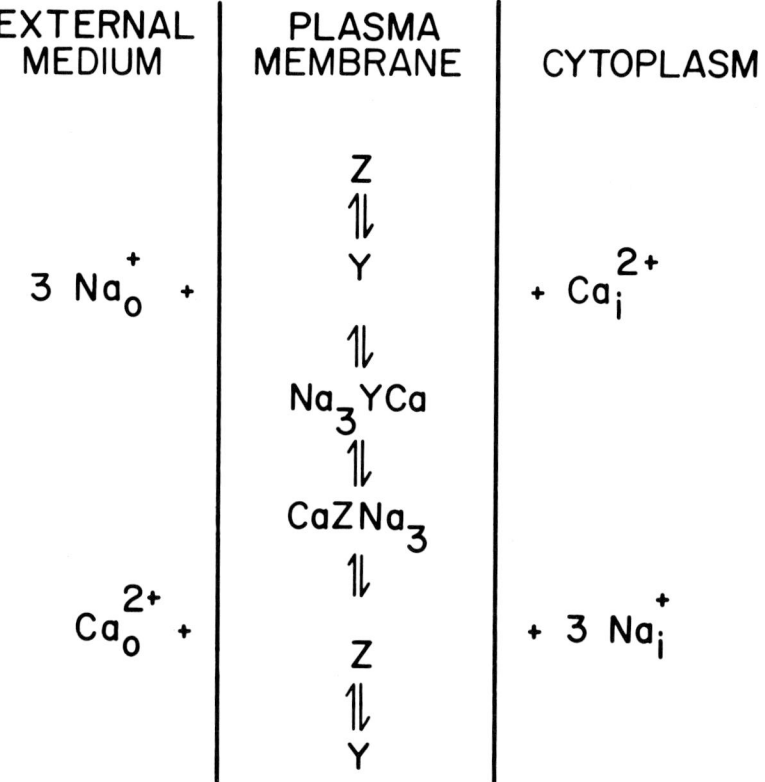

FIGURE 7. Model of a countertransport "carrier" mechanism that simultaneously exchanges 3 Na$^+$ for 1 Ca^{2+}. The "Y" form of the carrier denotes the configuration with Na-binding sites exposed to the external medium and the Ca-binding site exposed to the sarcoplasmic fluid; the "Z" form of the carrier has the Na sites on the sarcoplasmic side and the Ca site facing the external medium. The carriers can rotate through the plane of the membrane only when free (i.e., fully unloaded), as Y or Z, or when fully loaded, as Na$_3$YCa or CaZNa$_3$ (cf. Blaustein, 1976).

reducing ATP levels, lead to dissipation of the Na electrochemical gradient, would be expected, pari passu, to dissipate the Ca gradient, according to equation 2. And, although there is evidence that ATP does directly affect the Na-Ca exchange mechanism in squid axons, the question of whether or not it serves as a direct energy source for this exchange is unsettled (Blaustein, 1976).

The tentative conclusion from these studies is that net Ca extrusion from nerve terminals involves an Na-Ca exchange mechanism, although some of the details of this transport system are still unresolved.

Intraterminal Calcium Storage

The preceding discussion emphasizes the fact that the Ca that enters the terminals during depolarization must be extruded subsequently.

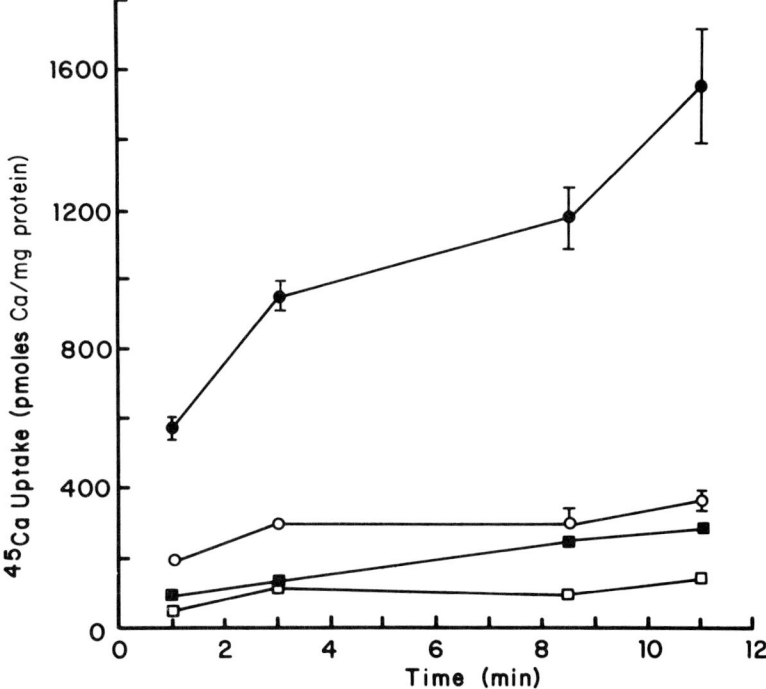

FIGURE 8. Time course of ^{45}Ca uptake by intact and disrupted synaptosomes in the presence and absence of ATP. The "intact" synaptosomes (□, ■) were incubated in 2 ml of a standard physiological salt solution containing 5 mM K, 145 mM Na, 1.3 mM Mg, and 10 μM CaCl$_2$ labeled with ^{45}Ca; the solution also contained 0.1 mM DNP, 0.1 mM Na azide, and 0.7 μg of oligomycin per ml. The "disrupted" synaptosomes (○, ●) were resuspended and incubated in 2 ml of a solution similar in composition except for the omission of all the NaCl; the sudden exposure to the markedly hypotonic media presumably induced lysis. When 2 mM ATP was present (●, ■), the MgCl$_2$ concentration in the incubation fluid was increased to 3 mM; open symbols refer to tissue incubated in ATP-free solutions. Incubations were carried out at 30°C; the protein concentration in the suspensions was 0.41 mg/ml. Each symbol represents the mean of three determinations; error bars are shown where the standard errors extend beyond the borders of the symbols. From Kendrick et al. (1977).

However, this extrusion may not occur as rapidly as the decline in transmitter release rate after repolarization. For example, some Ca-dependent postexcitation phenomena, such as facilitation (Katz and Miledi, 1968) and post-tetanic potentiation (Weinreich, 1971), may be the consequence of Ca retention within the terminals. The increased frequency of spontaneous miniature end plate potentials (i.e., spontaneous transmitter release) observed at the motor end plate after a period of activity may also be a manifestation of prolonged elevation of $[Ca^{2+}]_i$ (Miledi and Thies, 1971).

One possible explanation for this observation is that the Ca that enters terminals during depolarization is buffered by cytoplasmic proteins. Baker and Schlapfer (1975) have described a Ca^{2+} buffer with an apparent half-saturation constant for Ca (K_{Ca}) of about 0.5 μM, in squid axoplasm; however, although a similar buffer may be present in the cytoplasm of vertebrate neurons, none has yet been observed.

Energy-dependent mechanisms may also be involved in Ca sequestration within nerve terminals. Several investigators (Kraatz and Trautwein, 1957; Alnaes and Rahamimoff, 1975) have noted that mitochondrial poisons, such as 2,4-dinitrophenol (DNP) and ruthenium red, may induce spontaneous transmitter release, even in the absence of external Ca (Alnaes and Rahamimoff, 1975). These observations have led to the suggestion (Alnaes and Rahamimoff, 1975) that Ca may be sequestered in intraterminal mitochondria, and that inhibition of mitochondrial metabolism may cause the release of this stored Ca; the consequent rise in free $[Ca^{2+}]_i$ would then be responsible for the enhanced transmitter release. Although it is widely recognized that mitochondria can utilize energy from ATP or from electron transport to accumulate Ca, two observations tend to cast doubt on the idea that mitochondria are the main intraterminal Ca storage sites. (1) The apparent K_{Ca} for Ca uptake by mitochondria from K- and Mg-rich media (i.e., with ion concentrations similar to those of cytoplasm) is on the order of 10 to 50 μM (Hutson, Pfeiffer, and Lardy, 1976). (2) The mitochondria within nerve terminals are rarely observed close to the regions of synaptic contact (e.g., see the figures in Birks, Huxley, and Katz, 1960; Gray, 1963). It seems unlikely that organelles with a relatively low affinity for Ca could effectively buffer $[Ca^{2+}]_i$ over a distance of several tenths of a micrometer (Parsegian, 1977).

As an alternative to the hypothesis that mitochondria are the primary intraterminal Ca storage sites, we have recently obtained evidence (Kendrick, Blaustein, Ratzlaff and Fried, 1977) that another, as yet

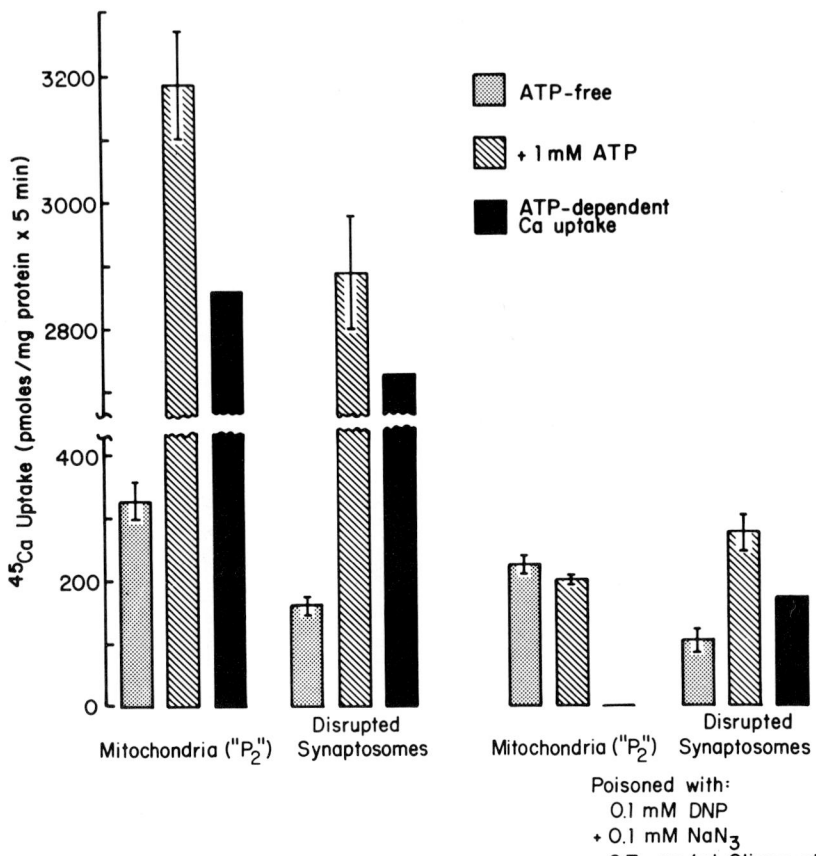

FIGURE 9. Comparison of ^{45}Ca uptake by mitochondria and disrupted synaptosomes. The "crude mitochondrial pellet" (P_2 of Gray and Whittaker, 1962) was suspended in about 30 ml of ice-cold 0.32 M sucrose. Half of the suspension was used to prepare a synaptosome-enriched fraction. The remainder of the suspension was immediately diluted with about 100 ml of ice-cold standard physiological saline; isotonic solutions were used to avoid lysis of the nerve terminals present in this fraction (cf. Figure 8). Aliquots (6 ml) were pipetted into centrifuge tubes and the particulate material was pelleted by centrifugation at 15,000 × g for 5 min at 5°C. The supernatant solutions were discarded, and the pellets (1.39 mg of protein) were suspended in 1.0 ml of physiological saline with all the NaCl replaced by KCl; the solution that was pipetted into some tubes also contained DNP, NaN$_3$, and oligomycin (to give final concentrations of 0.1 mM, 0.1 mM, and 0.7 μg/ml, respectively). After 1 min of incubation at 30°C, 1 ml of similar K-rich saline containing 10 μM Ca labeled with ^{45}Ca was added; the solution that was added to some tubes

unidentified, organelle may store Ca at the expense of ATP. The main observation is illustrated in Figure 8. The data show that ^{45}Ca uptake by synaptosomes incubated in an isotonic medium containing 10 µM Ca is only minimally enhanced by ATP; on the other hand, after disruption of the terminals by exposure to a hypotonic solution, ATP markedly stimulates Ca uptake. This latent ATP-dependent Ca uptake process is presumably not associated with the intraterminal mitochondria, because it is observed in the presence of two mitochondrial uncouplers, DNP (0.1 mM) and azide (0.1 mM), and a specific inhibitor of mitochondrial Ca transport, oligomycin (0.7 µg/ml).

Evidence that this combination of poisons is sufficient to virtually abolish mitochondrial Ca accumulation is presented in Figure 9, in which Ca uptake by brain mitochondria (the crude mitochondrial preparation; "P_2" of Gray and Whittaker, 1962) and by disrupted synaptosomes is compared in the absence and presence of the poisons. The P_2 fraction was suspended and incubated in isotonic solutions (osmolarity $\simeq$ 320 mosMol/kg) to avoid disrupting the synaptosomes and exposing the latent (intraterminal) ATP-stimulated Ca uptake activity; under these circumstances, the stimulatory effect of ATP was completely blocked in the presence of the DNP, azide, and oligomycin. In four such experiments, the mean stimulation by ATP, after poisoning, was only $1 \pm 1\%$ (SE) of the value in the unpoisoned controls. By way of comparison, a significant stimulation of Ca uptake by ATP was always observed in disrupted synaptosome preparations, even in the presence of the three mitochondrial poisons (Figure 9).

Preliminary experiments with Ca-EGTA (ethylene glycol-bis-[β-aminoethyl ether]-N,N'-tetraacetic acid) buffers indicate that the

---

(see graph) also contained ATP (final concentration equals 1 mM). After a 5-min incubation period at 30°C, portions of the suspensions were filtered; the filters were washed and counted.

The synaptosomes obtained by gradient centrifugation of the sucrose-suspended P_2 were diluted with saline and centrifuged. The resulting pellets (0.93 mg of protein) were suspended in 1 ml of "lysis solution" (standard physiological saline with all the NaCl omitted); the solution that was used to suspend some of the pellets also contained the three mitochondrial poisons. After 1 min of incubation at 30°C, 1 ml of buffered saline containing 290 mM KCl (and no NaCl) was added to each suspension; this solution contained 10 µM CaCl$_2$ labeled with ^{45}Ca and, where appropriate (see graph), ATP (final concentration equals 1 mM). After a 5-min incubation period at 30°C, portions of the suspensions were filtered; the filters were washed and counted. Each bar represents the mean of three determinations ± SEM. From Kendrick et al. (1977).

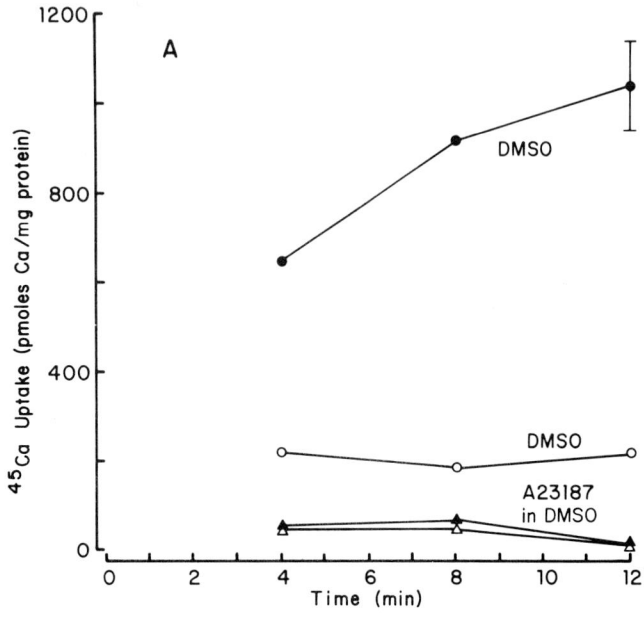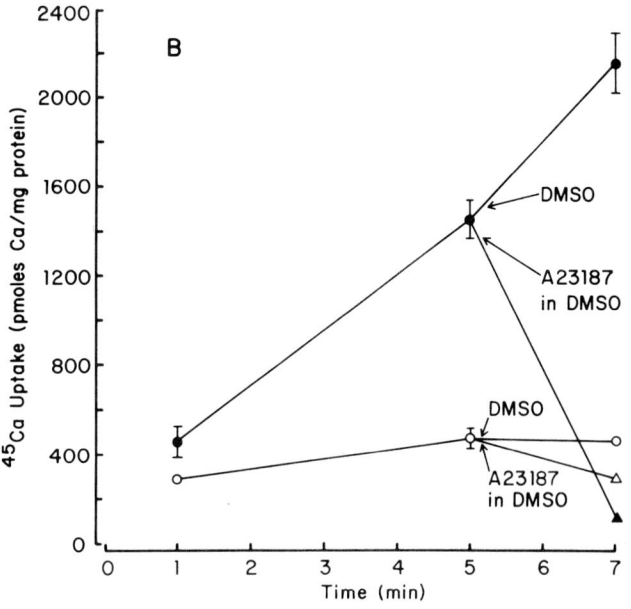

apparent half saturation (K_{Ca}) for the latent ATP-stimulated Ca uptake (in the presence of the poisons) is about 0.3 to 0.4 μM Ca^{2+}. Moreover, at this level of ionized Ca^{2+}, mitochondria (i.e., the P_2 fraction) do not accumulate Ca, and the ATP-stimulated uptake by disrupted synaptosomes is not further enhanced if the mitochondrial poisons are omitted from the medium. These observations are consistent with the idea that there are two ATP-stimulated Ca uptake mechanisms present within the nerve terminals: (1) a low-affinity system ($K_{Ca} > 10$ μM Ca^{2+}), presumably associated with mitochondria (Baker and Schlapfer, 1975; Hutson et al., 1976), and (2) a high-affinity system ($K_{Ca} < 0.5 \mu$M Ca^{2+}), which is insensitive to the mitochondrial poisons.

Several observations suggest that the high-affinity Ca uptake involves Ca transport into vesicular compartments rather than binding to membranes. (1) The divalent cation-specific ionophore A-23187, which is known to make vesicular systems leaky to Ca (Scarpa, Baldassare, and Inesi, 1972), abolishes the ATP-promoted Ca uptake (Figure 10A) and induces rapid release of previously accumulated Ca (Figure 10B). (2) Atomic absorption analyses of the particulate material and supernatant solutions indicate that the ATP-promoted uptake represents a net Ca accumulation by the intraterminal particles. Furthermore, as shown in Figure 11, the presence of 5 mM oxalate in the incubation medium

---

FIGURE 10. Effect of ionophore A-23187 on ^{45}Ca uptake by disrupted synaptosomes. Data in A and B are from different synaptosome preparations. In both experiments, the synaptosomes were disrupted by preincubating them for 1 min in 1 ml of standard physiological salt solution with the NaCl omitted. Incubation fluid (1 ml) was then added to provide a (final) composition similar to that of the standard solution, but with all of the NaCl (145 mM) replaced by KCl. In addition, the incubation fluid contained sufficient ^{45}Ca-labeled $CaCl_2$ to give a final concentration of 10 μM in Ca; when 2 mM ATP was present (●, ▲), the $MgCl_2$ concentration was increased to 3 mM. All lysis and incubation fluids contained 0.1 mM DNP, 0.1 mM Na azide, and 0.7 μg of oligomycin per ml. All incubations were carried out at 30°C. Each symbol represents the mean of three determinations; error bars are shown where the standard errors ranged beyond the borders of the symbols. (A) ^{45}Ca-labeled incubation fluids containing dimethylsulfoxide (DMSO; final concentration equals 4.2 μl/ml), without (○, ●) or with A-23187 (△, ▲; final concentration equals 10 μM), were added at 0 time; the DMSO was used as a solvent for the ionophore stock solution. The protein concentration in the suspensions was 0.51 mg/ml. (B) The ^{45}Ca-containing solutions were added at 0 time. As indicated on the graph, DMSO (final concentration equals 2.5 μl/ml), without or with A-23187 (final concentration = 10 μM), was added immediately after the 5-min samples were drawn. The protein concentration in the suspensions was 0.49 mg/ml. From Kendrick et al. (1977).

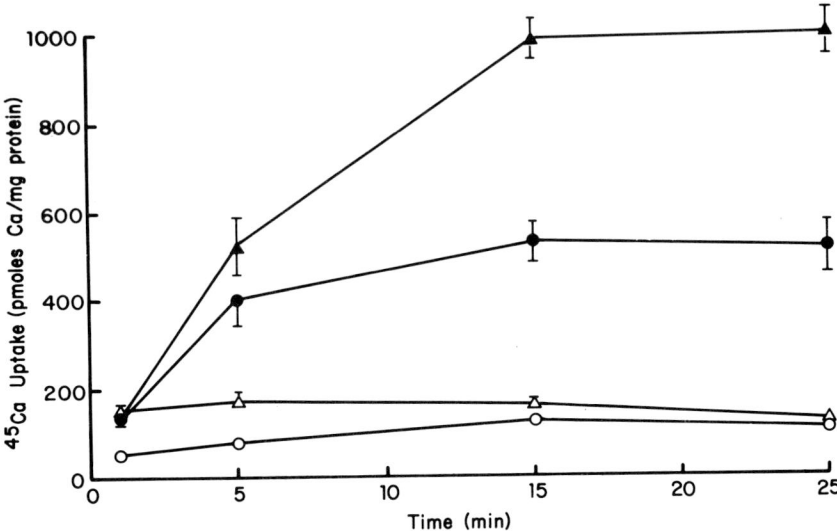

FIGURE 11. Effect of oxalate on the time course of ^{45}Ca uptake by disrupted synaptosomes. Synaptosomes were suspended in 1.0 ml of lysis fluid (standard salt solution with NaCl omitted); after 1 min (0 time on the graph), ^{45}Ca-containing solutions (1.0 ml) were added to give a final Ca concentration of 5 μM. The final composition of the incubation solutions was similar to the standard salt solution, except that all of the NaCl was replaced either by 145 mM KCl (oxalate-free solutions; ○, ●) or by 5 mM K oxalate plus 137.5 mM KCl (△, ▲); all solutions contained 0.1 mM DNP, 0.1 mM Na azide, and 0.7 μg of oligomycin per ml. When 2 mM ATP was present (●, ▲), the MgCl$_2$ concentration was raised to 3 mM. Incubations were carried out at 30°C; the protein concentration in the suspensions was 0.49 mg/ml. Each symbol is the mean of three determinations; error bars are shown where the standard errors range beyond the borders of the symbols. From Kendrick et al. (1977).

enhances ^{45}Ca uptake even though the Ca-oxalate solubility product was exceeded in the solutions. The data imply that the Ca is sequestered in a compartment whose limiting membrane is permeable to oxalate; thus, when Ca is transported into the compartment, some of it combines with oxalate, thereby lowering the intravesicular ionized Ca^{2+} concentration so that more Ca can be transported in. (3) The ATP-promoted Ca transport may involve a Mg-dependent ATPase because it is abolished in the absence of Mg, and because the uptake is very specific for ATP (apparent half-saturation constant, $K_{ATP} \simeq 25$ μM ATP) and deoxyATP; other nucleotide triphosphates, such as GTP, ITP, UTP, and CTP, are ineffective, as are ADP and cyclic 3′,5′-AMP. The properties of this intraterminal high-affinity Ca transport system resemble, in many ways, those of the Ca sequestration system in the sarcoplasmic reticulum of muscle (Hasselbach, Suko, Stromer and The, 1975). A similar Ca storage system has also been observed in "microsomal" fractions prepared from whole brain homogenates (de Meis, Rubin-Altschul, and Machado, 1970; Trotta and de Meis, 1975). We do not yet know which intraterminal organelles are associated with the high-affinity Ca uptake described above. One possibility is that the Ca is sequestered within the 400 to 500 Å diameter "synaptic vesicles," similar to those that store neurotransmitters (Whittaker, 1971). However, preliminary data from sucrose gradient subfractionation studies (employing the method of Whittaker, Michaelson, and Kirkland, 1964), indicate that most of the ATP-promoted Ca-accumulating activity is associated with the more dense particulate material. One possibility is that endoplasmic reticulum may serve as the Ca storage sites (Henkart, Landis, and Reese, 1976). Unfortunately, this remains an unsolved problem.

An even more important question concerns the role of this high-affinity Ca sequestration system in synaptic physiology. A reasonable hypothesis is that some of the Ca that enters the presynaptic terminals during depolarization is buffered by cytoplasmic proteins, and some is sequestered in the storage system described above (and, perhaps, in mitochondria, although these organelles may be more important as suppliers of ATP for the high-affinity Ca transport system). Then, as Ca gets "pumped" out of the terminals (via the Na-Ca exchange mechanism described earlier; see Figure 7), the transiently sequestered Ca will slowly leak out of the (vesicular) storage sites and help to buffer $[Ca^{2+}]_i$ at a level slightly above the normal resting level (about 10^{-7}M; see above). The elevated $[Ca^{2+}]_i$ would be expected to enhance transmitter release, and could account for the increased spontaneous transmitter release observed after periods of activity, and for the phenomena of facilitation and post-tetanic potentiation.

ACKNOWLEDGMENT

This research was supported by NIH grant NS-08442. Dr. Kendrick was supported by NIH postdoctoral fellowship 1 F22-NS01105 from the National Institute of Neurological and Communicative Disorders and Stroke.

REFERENCES

Alnaes, E. and R. Rahamimoff (1975). On the role of mitochondria in transmitter release from motor nerve terminals, *J. Physiol.* **248**:285–306.

Baker, P. F. (1972). Transport and metabolism of calcium ions in nerve, *Prog. Biophys. Mol. Biol.* **24**:177-223.

Baker, P. F. and W. Schlapfer (1975). Calcium uptake by axoplasm extruded from giant axons of *Loligo*, *J. Physiol.* **249**:37-38 P.

Birks, R. I., H. E. Huxley, and B. Katz (1960). The fine structure of the neuromuscular junction of the frog, *J. Physiol.* **150**:134-144.

Blaustein, M. P. (1974). The interrelationship between sodium and calcium fluxes across cell membranes, *Rev. Physiol. Biochem. Pharmacol.* **70**:33-82.

Blaustein, M. P. (1975). Effects of potassium, veratridine and scorpion venom on calcium accumulation and transmitter release by nerve terminals *in vitro*, *J. Physiol.* **247**:617-655.

Blaustein, M. P. (1976). The ins and outs of calcium transport in squid axons: internal and external ion activation of calcium efflux, *Fed. Proc.* **35**:2574-2578.

Blaustein, M. P. and A. C. Ector (1975). Barbiturate inhibition of calcium uptake by depolarized nerve terminals *in vitro*, *Mol. Pharmacol.* **11**:369-378.

Blaustein, M. P. and A. C. Ector (1976). Carrier-mediated sodium-dependent and calcium-dependent calcium efflux from pinched-off presynaptic nerve terminals (synaptosomes) *in vitro*, *Biochim. Biophys. Acta* **419**:295-308.

Blaustein, M. P. and J. M. Goldring (1975). Membrane potentials in pinched-off presynaptic nerve terminals monitored with a fluorescent probe: evidence that synaptosomes have potassium diffusion potentials, *J. Physiol.* **247**:589-615.

Blaustein, M. P. and A. L. Hodgkin (1969). The effect of cyanide on the efflux of calcium from squid axons, *J. Physiol.* **200**:497-527.

Blaustein, M. P., E. M. Johnson, Jr., and P. Needleman (1972). Calcium-dependent norepinephrine release from presynaptic nerve endings *in vitro*, *Proc. Natl. Acad. Sci. U.S.A.* **69**:2237-2240.

Blaustein, M. P. and C. J. Oborn (1975). The influence of sodium on calcium fluxes in pinched-off nerve terminals *in vitro*, *J. Physiol.* **247**:657-686.

Blaustein, M. P. and J. M. Russell (1975). Sodium-calcium and calcium-calcium exchange in internally dialyzed squid giant axons, *J. Membr. Biol.* **22**:285-312.

Blaustein, M. P., J. M. Russell, and P. De Weer (1974). Calcium efflux from internally dialyzed squid axons: the influence of external and internal cations, *J. Supramol. Struct.* **2**:558-581.

Blaustein, M. P. and W. P. Wiesmann (1970). Potassium ions and calcium ion fluxes in isolated nerve terminals, pp. 291-307 in *Drugs and Cholinergic Mechanisms in the CNS*, Heilbronn, E. and A. Winter, eds. Research Institute of National Defense, Stockholm.

Bradford, H. F. (1975). Isolated nerve terminals as an *in vitro* preparation for the study of dynamic aspects of transmitter metabolism and release, pp. 191-252 in *Handbook of Psychopharmacology*, Vol. 1, Iverson, L. L., S. D. Iverson, and S. H. Snyder, eds. Plenum Press, New York.

Cohen, L. B., B. M. Salzberg, H. V. Davilla, W. N. Ross, D. Landowne, A. S. Waggoner, and C.-H. Wang (1974). Changes in axon fluorescence during activity: a search for useful probes, *J. Membr. Biol.* **19**:1-36.

Cotman, C. W., J. W. Haycock, and W. F. White (1976). Stimulus-secretion coupling processes in brain: analysis of noradrenaline and gamma-aminobutyric acid release, *J. Physiol.* **254**:475–505.

De Belleroche, J. S. and H. F. Bradford (1972). The stimulus-induced release of acetylcholine from synaptosome beds and its calcium dependence, *J. Neurochem.* **19**:1817–1819.

de Meis, L., B. M. Rubin-Altschul, and R. D. Machado (1970). Comparative data of Ca^{2+} transport in brain and skeletal muscle microsomes, *J. Biol. Chem.* **245**:1183–1189.

De Robertis, E., A. Pellegrino de Iraldi, G. Rodriguez de Lores Arnaiz, and L. Salganicoff (1962). Cholinergic and non-cholinergic endings in rat brain. I. Isolation and subcellular distribution of acetylcholine and acetylcholinesterase, *J. Neurochem.* **9**:23–35.

De Weer, P. (1975). Aspects of the recovery processes in nerve, pp. 231–278 in *MTP International Review of Science, Physiology Series*, Vol. 3, Hunt, C. C., ed. Medical and Technical Publishing Co., Ltd., London.

Di Polo, R., J. Requena, F. J. Brinley, Jr., L. J. Mullins, A. Scarpa, and T. Tiffert (1976). Ionized calcium concentrations in squid axons, *J. Gen. Physiol.* **67**:433–467.

Fried, R. C. and M. P. Blaustein (1976). Synaptic vesicle recycling in synaptosomes *in vitro*, *Nature (London)* **261**:255–256.

Gray, E. G. (1963). Electron microscopy of presynaptic organelles of the spinal cord, *J. Anat.* **97**:101–106.

Gray, E. G. and V. P. Whittaker (1962). The isolation of nerve endings from brain: an electron-microscopic study of cell fragments derived by homogenization and centrifugation, *J. Anat.* **96**:79–88.

Gray, E. G. and R. A. Willis (1970). On synaptic vesicles, complex vesicles and dense projections, *Brain Res.* **24**:147–168.

Hasselbach, W., J. Suko, M. H. Stromer, and R. The (1975). Mechanism of calcium transport in sarcoplasmic reticulum, *Ann. N.Y. Acad. Sci.* **264**:335–349.

Henkart, M., D. M. Landis, and T. S. Reese (1976). Similarity of junctions between plasma membranes and endoplasmic reticulum in muscle and neurons, *J. Cell Biol.* **70**:338–347.

Heuser, J. E. (1977). Synaptic vesicle exocytosis revealed in quick-frozen frog neuromuscular junctions treated with 4-aminopyridine and given a single electrical shock, pp. 215–239 in *Society for Neuroscience Symposia*, Vol. 2, Cowan, W. M. and J. A. Ferrendelli, eds. Society for Neuroscience, Bethesda, Md.

Heuser, J. and T. Reese (1973). Evidence for recycling of synaptic vesicle membrane during transmitter release at the frog neuromuscular junction, *J. Cell Biol.* **57**:315–344.

Hutson, S. M., D. R. Pfeiffer, and H. A. Lardy (1976). Effect of cations and anions on the steady state kinetics of energy-dependent Ca^{2+} transport in rat liver mitochondria, *J. Biol. Chem.* **251**:5251–5258.

Katz, B. (1969). *The Release of Neural Transmitter Substances*. Charles C. Thomas, Springfield, Ill.

Katz, B. and R. Miledi (1968). The role of calcium in neuromuscular facilitation, *J. Physiol.* **195**:481–492.

Katz, B. and R. Miledi (1971). The effect of prolonged depolarization on synaptic transfer in the stellate ganglion of the squid, *J. Physiol.* **216**:503–512.

Kendrick, N. C., M. P. Blaustein, R. W. Ratzlaff, and R. C. Fried (1977). ATP-dependent calcium storage in presynaptic nerve terminals, *Nature (London)* **265**:246–248.

Kraatz, H. G. and W. Trautwein (1957). Die Wirkung von 2,4-Dinitrophenol (DNP) auf die neuromuskulare Erregung subertragung, *Arch. Exp. Pathol. Pharmakol.* **231**:419–439.

Kuno, M. (1971). Quantum aspects of central and ganglionic synaptic transmission in vertebrates, *Physiol. Rev.* **51**:647–678.

Levy, W. B., D. A. Redburn, and C. W. Cotman (1973). Stimulus-coupled secretion of γ-aminobutyric acid from rat brain synaptosomes, *Science* **181**:676–678.

Llinás, R. (1977). Calcium and transmitter release in squid synapse, pp. 139–160 in *Society for Neuroscience Symposia*, Vol. 2, Cowan, W. M. and J. A. Ferrendelli, eds. Society for Neuroscience, Bethesda, Md.

Llinás, R. and C. Nicholson (1975). Calcium role in stimulus-secretion coupling: an aequorin study in squid giant synapse, *Proc. Natl. Acad. Sci. U.S.A.* **72**:187–190.

Marchbanks, R. M. (1967). The osmotically sensitive potassium and sodium compartments of synaptosomes, *Biochem. J.* **104**:148–157.

Miledi, R. (1973). Transmitter release induced by injection of calcium ions into nerve terminals, *Proc. R. Soc. London Ser. B* **183**:421–425.

Miledi, R. and R. Thies (1971). Tetanic and post-tetanic rise in frequency of miniature end-plate potentials in low-calcium solutions. *J. Physiol.* **212**:245–257.

Parsegian, V. A. (1977). Considerations in determining the mode of influence of calcium on vesicle-membrane interaction, pp. 161–171 in *Society for Neuroscience Symposia*, Vol. 2, Cowan, W. M. and J. A. Ferrendelli, eds. Society for Neuroscience, Bethesda, Md.

Rodriguez de Lores Arnaiz, G. and E. De Robertis (1972). Properties of the isolated nerve terminals, *Curr. Top. Membr. Transp.* **3**:237–272.

Scarpa, A., J. Baldassere, and G. Inesi (1972). The effect of calcium ionophores on fragmented sarcoplasmic reticulum, *J. Gen. Physiol.* **60**:735–749.

Trotta, E. E. and L. de Meis (1975). ATP-dependent calcium accumulation in brain microsomes enhanced by phosphate and oxalate, *Biochim. Biophys. Acta* **394**:239–247.

Weinreich, D. (1971). Ionic mechanism of post-tetanic potentiation at the neuromuscular junction of the frog, *J. Physiol.* **212**:431–446.

Whittaker, V. P. (1971). Subcellular localization of neurotransmitters, pp. 319–330 in *Advances in Cytopharmacology*, Vol. I. First International Symposium on Cell Biology and Cytopharmacology, Clementi, F., ed. Raven Press, New York.

Whittaker, V. P., I. A. Michaelson, and R. J. A. Kirkland (1964). The separation of synaptic vesicles from nerve-ending particles ("synaptosomes"), *Biochem. J.* **90**:293–303.

Calcium Electroresponsiveness and Its Relationship to Secretion in Molluscan Exocrine Gland Cells

Stanley B. Kater

University of Iowa, Iowa City, Iowa

Investigations of secretory mechanisms in non-neural cell types have paralleled developments in synaptic transmission by independently demonstrating the key role of calcium in secretion. By the early 1960's, Douglas and Rubin (1961) had implicated calcium as an indispensible component of stimulus-secretion coupling, a hypothesis that has been confirmed repeatedly. The important generality of calcium as an essential component in a wide spectrum of secretory processes is contrasted by the diversity of mechanisms suggested for increasing concentrations of this ion immediately before secretion. The essential division exists between the regenerative, voltage-dependent conductance changes of neural elements and the passive membrane characteristics of other types of cells. These apparent differences, however, may result from the fact that whereas the technically advantageous squid giant synapse has been available as a model for neural tissues, there have been no such preparations for electrophysiological investigations of endocrine and exocrine secretion. In many ways, the progress already made is remarkable in light of the formidable difficulty posed by preparations often composed of small cells, enmeshed in other tissue, and extensively electrically coupled to their neighbors. This communication introduces a technically favorable exocrine preparation that allows analyses like those performed on the giant synapse. The important and unexpected finding reported here is the striking similarity of the properties of these exocrine cells to those of classical synaptic transmission.

The early work of Lundberg (1955) demonstrated that mammalian salivary gland cells are electrically inexcitable. Similarly, the inferred increase in intracellular calcium concentration accompanying secretion from other exocrine cell types shows no sign of regenerative ionic currents (see review by Petersen, 1976). The effect of secretagogues on these cells is primarily to increase ion conductances, producing only local potential changes (hyperpolarizing, depolarizing, or biphasic, depending upon cell type). Two notable exceptions to the general case of non-neural secretion are the endocrine pancreatic islet cells (Dean and Matthews, 1968) and adrenocortical cells (Matthews and Saffran, 1973), both of which display electrical activity characteristic of neurons. In the islet cells, which have been more extensively studied, calcium is suggested as the major carrier of the inward current for the 20- to 25-mV spikes characteristic of these cells (Matthews and Sakamoto, 1975). It appears that the model provided by the squid giant synapse may be extended, in its general form, to endocrine secretion. The question that now arises is whether the ionic events underlying exocrine secretion are distinctly different. Evidence to be presented subsequently demonstrates that at least some classes of exocrine cells can support regenerative electrical activity.

The present investigation is derived from our studies of the neural mechanisms underlying the feeding behavior of the pulmonate snail, *Helisoma* (e.g., Kater and Rowell, 1973; Kater, 1974). In our survey of motoneurons to the feeding musculature, we located a pair of identified buccal ganglion neurons that could synaptically activate the salivary glands. We have now confirmed this observation on many species of pulmonate molluscs (Figure 1). The overall system, which is best known for *Helisoma*, is summarized in Figure 2 (Kater, Murphy, and Rued, 1977*a*; Kater, Rued, and Murphy, 1977*b*). Action potentials in identified buccal ganglion neurons 4R and 4L give rise to EPSPs in acinar cells of the proximal salivary gland. When suprathreshold, these depolarizations give rise to all-or-none, overshooting action potentials. These action potentials propagate through the extensive electrically coupled network, and action potentials are generated progressively in each acinar cell—presumably as the stimulus for secretion. The discovery of action potentials in these exocrine cells (e.g., Kater, 1974) was in marked contrast to all previous reports and prompted inquiry into the ionic bases of these events and the relationships of ionic currents to secretion. However, molluscan salivary gland cells are not particularly well

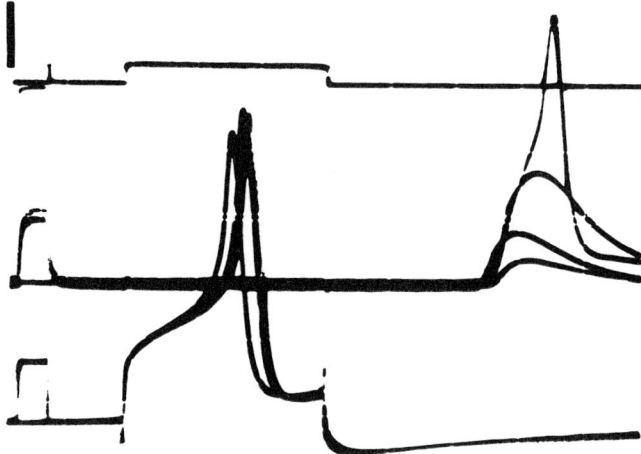

FIGURE 1. Neural control of the salivary glands of *Ariolimax*. Action potentials in a large, identified buccal ganglion neuron (lower trace) evoked by intracellular depolarizing current injection (upper trace, current monitor) give rise, in a salivary gland acinar cell, to one-for-one EPSPs, which, when suprathreshold, evoke action potentials from this secretory cell (middle trace). Calibrations:20 mV by 10 msec pulses at the onset of voltage trace; bar at onset of current trace equals 2×10^{-9} A. From Kater and Senseman (unpublished data).

suited for such studies because of their limited size (ca. 30 μm in diameter) and the extensive electrical coupling that makes it difficult to resolve electrical events. The present communication introduces an entirely different exocrine system composed of larger cells that show no intercellular coupling; this system has allowed us to begin a description of the ionic events underlying action potentials and exocrine secretion.

An important role for exocrine secretion in the behavior of our experimental animal is shown in Figure 3. The salient physical feature of *Ariolimax californicus* is that this slug covers everything contacted with mucous slime. In the course of traveling 1 mile, a 35-g animal could leave a mucous trail weighing 2,276 g. This copious secretion of mucus from the cells of the prominent pedal gland is the subject of the remainder of this paper.

The pedal gland is a tubular structure that runs nearly the entire length of the animal (Barr, 1926). Secretory cells, 100 to 200 μm in diameter (Figure 4), are arranged around the central lumen such that their secretion is swept along by cilia to the opening near the mouth.

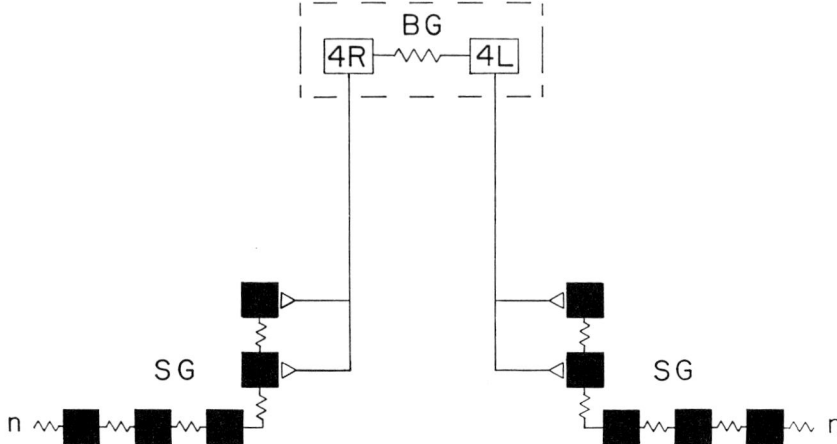

FIGURE 2. A schematic representation of the salivary gland neuro-effector system in *Helisoma*. A pair of bilaterally symmetrical, identified neurons, 4R and 4L, innervate the two halves of the salivary glands. These neurons are coactivated with motoneurons during the feeding cycle, and are further synchronized by electrical coupling between themselves. Chemical excitatory synapses are made between neuron 4 and proximal salivary gland acinar cells. A single EPSP usually evokes an all-or-none, overshooting action potential in these acinar cells. Salivary gland cells show a very high level of electrical coupling with their neighbors, with coupling coefficients of 0.8 being common. Action potentials generated in proximal acinar cells propagate via the electrotonic junctions and throughout each salivary gland. Summarized from Kater et al. (1977a,b).

Under Nomarski optics, individual cells are seen swollen with secretory granules of various sizes, up to several micrometers (Figure 4A). This is also evident in specimens that were cryofractured to expose inner cellular surfaces for scanning electron microscopy (Figures 4C, D). Our tentative view is that secretion is accomplished by a process of compound exocytosis (Horsfield, 1965; Röhlich, Anderson, and Uvnäs, 1971) involving the intermediate fusion of individual granules within the cell prior to secretion.

Intracellular microelectrode recordings from pedal gland cells are readily accomplished under visual control, employing the low-power optics of a dissecting microscope. A section of the gland 4 to 8 mm long was mounted in a chamber that allowed a rapid change in the composition of the continuously flowing saline solutions (Thomas, 1972; Partridge and Thomas, 1974). The composition of saline was that of Thomas (1972); sucrose was used for isosmotic replacement of

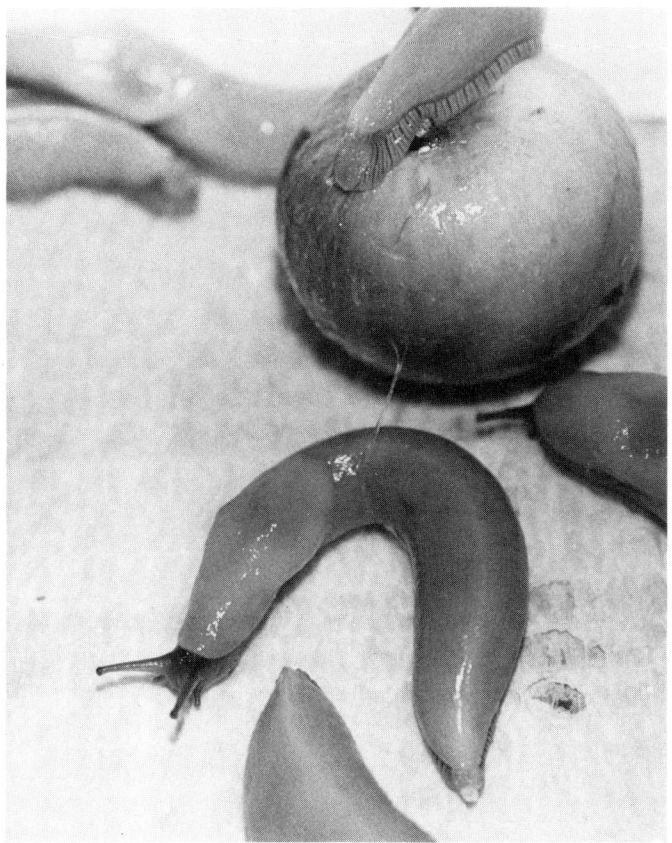

FIGURE 3. *Ariolimax californicus* in captivity, displaying the product of their sliming behavior.

sodium chloride in sodium-free solutions, and magnesium chloride replaced calcium chloride in calcium-free solutions. When employed, cobalt and manganese were added in 10 mM quantities as chloride salts to normal saline. Recordings were obtained either with one electrode and a bridge circuit for passing current, or, alternatively, a second current-passing electrode was inserted. Our electrodes, filled with 3 M potassium acetate, had a DC resistance of 20 to 50 MΩ.

Figure 5 shows typical responses of gland cells to depolarizing intracellular current injection. The usual response to long current pulses is a single action potential followed by subsequently dampening oscil-

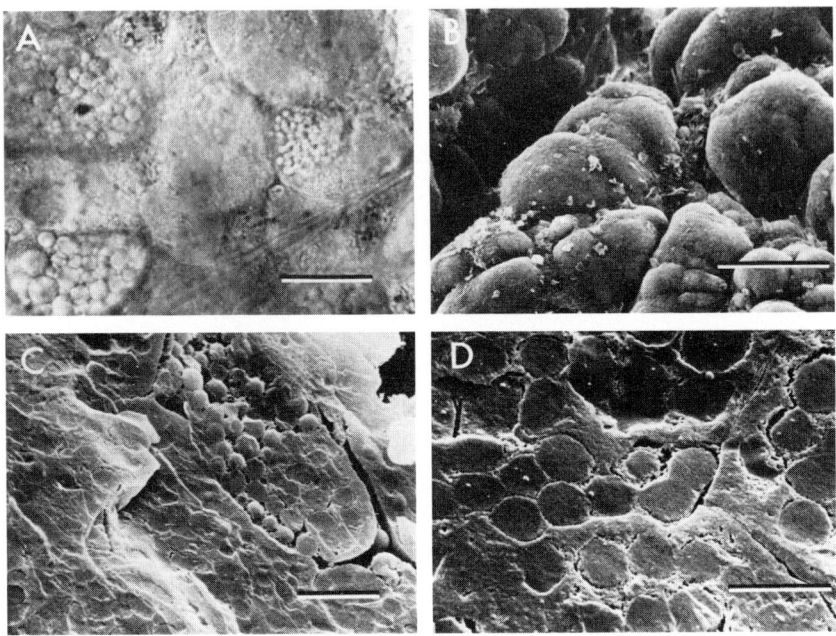

FIGURE 4. Cells of the mucus-secreting pedal gland of *Ariolimax*. (A) Living cells as viewed under Nomarski optics. Note the presence of cells with various sized inclusions, as well as cells that appear empty. (B) The surface of the pedal glands as viewed by the scanning electron microscope (SEM). (C) and (D) Cryofractured specimens of pedal gland viewed by SEM, showing secretory granules. Calibrations: A = 100 μm; B = 50 μm; C = 10 μm; D = 5 μm.

lations in membrane potential. Repetitive firing is not observed in response to sustained current injections. Short-duration pulses (Figure 5B) demonstrate the regenerative nature of the action potentials. Most cells display all-or-none action potentials overshooting the zero potential with a waveform like that of the squid axon. A variable percentage (20 to 50%) of the cells in a given pedal gland, however, display a more complex waveform (Figure 6) consisting of a shoulder on the rising phase of the action potential. Even in cells that normally show no shoulder, the two distinct phases can be detected and/or accentuated at threshold (Figure 7), after tetraethylammonium chloride (TEA) injection (Figure 11C), or by repetitive firing (Figure 11D).

Complex waveforms such as those in Figures 6 and 7 can result from compound ionic events and/or complex morphologies. Our histological studies have indicated that the large cells on the exterior of the gland are essentially spherical and are not likely sources of events

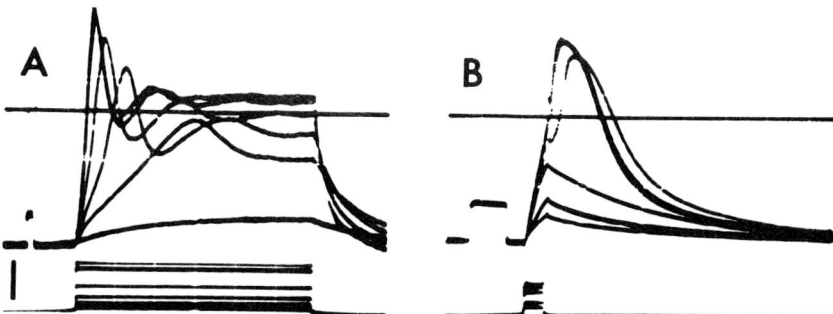

FIGURE 5. Intracellularly recorded responses of a pedal gland cell to depolarizing current injections. (A) Superimposed oscilloscope traces showing the effect of relatively long-duration current pulses of increasing magnitude. (B) Action potential evoked by short-duration pulses showing the all-or-none, regenerative nature of the response. Upper trace marks the zero potential, bottom trace indicates current injection. Calibrations: 20 mV by 10 msec pulse at the onset of each voltage trace; current bar for (A) = 2×10^{-9} A, for (B) = 1×10^{-9} A.

similar to the A and S spikes of neurons (Coombs, Curtis, and Eccles, 1957; Fuortes, Frank, and Becker, 1957; Tauc, 1962a, b). More direct evidence was obtained by recording intracellularly from cells displaying shoulders on evoked action potentials and then in-

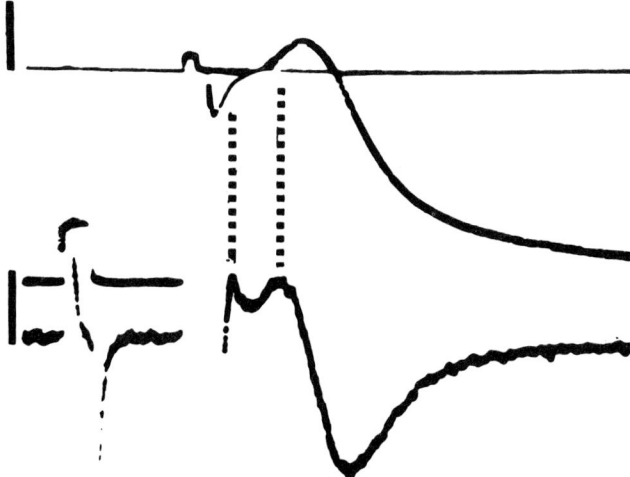

FIGURE 6. Intracellularly recorded action potential evoked by a brief depolarizing current injection. Upper trace indicates current injection and zero potential; lower trace, the first derivative (dVm/dt); center trace, Vm. Note two distinct rising components of the evoked action potential. Calibrations: 1×10^{-8} A; pulse at onset of Vm trace = 20 mV by 10 msec; dVm/dt = 2.5 V/sec.

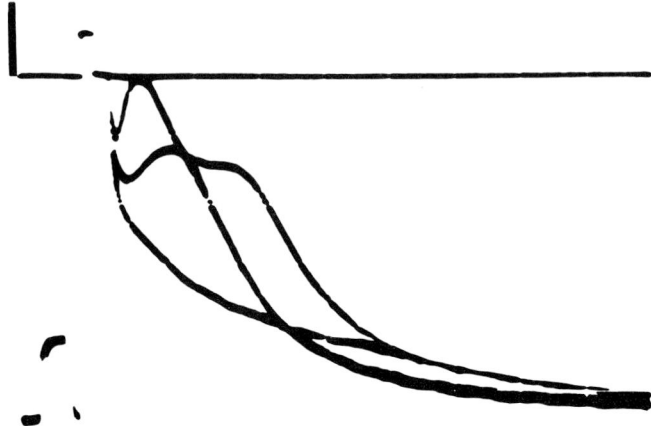

FIGURE 7. Threshold responses of a pedal gland cell. The four superimposed traces show two simple action potentials (superimposed), one failure, and one intermediate response with two distinct peaks. Calibrations: bar at onset of current trace equals 2.5×10^{-9} A; 20 mV by 10 msec pulse at onset of voltage traces.

jecting the dye Fast Green iontophoretically (Thomas and Wilson, 1966; Rovainen, 1967) to reveal the morphology of that specific cell (Figure 8). These experiments revealed only simple, essentially spherical, form and gave no indication of a morphological basis for complex action potential waveforms.

Examination of the ionic dependencies of these action potentials has shed some light on the basis of the complex waveforms (Figure 9). Removing all external sodium results in complete suppression of the regenerative event (Figure 9A). In addition, sodium-free saline always results in a 5 to 10 mV hyperpolarization, presumably due to a contribution of sodium conductance to the resting potential. Increasing intracellular current injections, to counter the hyperpolarization effect, reveals a graded regenerative potential in the absence of sodium (Figure 9B). The size of this regenerative potential is greatly reduced if calcium, in addition to sodium, is removed from the bathing medium (Figure 9C). The return of sodium to the bathing fluid restores an early peak in the regenerative event (Figure 9D), whereas reintroduction of calcium restores the overshooting characteristic of the potential (Figure 9E). Of further interest is the fact that the regenerative event in the absence of calcium is graded (Figure 9F). These findings suggest the hypothesis that the inward current for

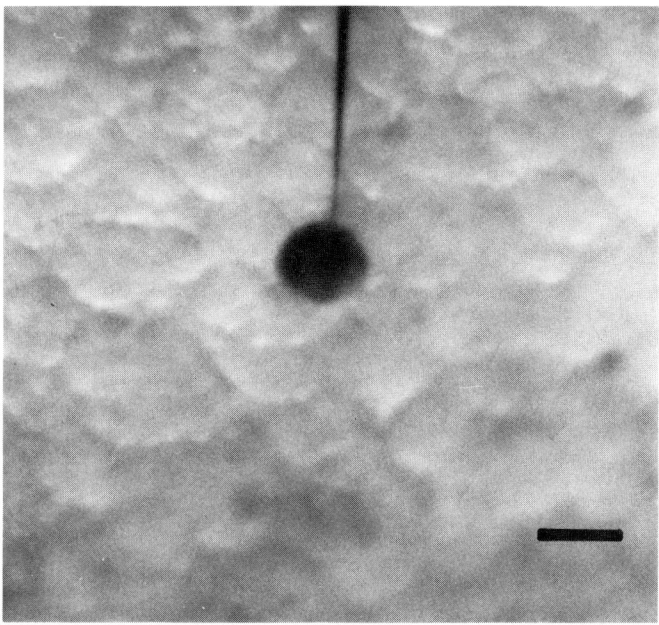

FIGURE 8. The morphology of a pedal gland cell that displayed a shoulder on the rising phase of evoked action potentials. Iontophoretic injection of the dye Fast Green revealed an essentially spherical form. Calibration: 100 μm.

the action potential is a composite of an early sodium entry and a delayed calcium entry.

The use of pharmacological agents has supported the suggestion of calcium's involvement. Treatment with cobalt ions suppresses action potentials previously evoked by slightly suprathreshold stimulation (Figure 10A), but a regenerative component can be restored by increasing the magnitude of the intracelluar current injection (Figure 10B). Some idea of the magnitude of the calcium component can be obtained by blocking calcium currents with cobalt or manganese at higher stimulus strengths. Cobalt (10 mM) diminishes the overall action potential amplitude by 15 to 20 mV (Figure 10C), whereas the equivalent concentration of manganese decreases the amplitude by 20 to 25 mV (Figure 10D).

The sodium component of the action potential, although highly sensitive to external bath concentrations of sodium, is insensitive to tetrodotoxin (TTX) even at concentrations as high as 10^{-5} M (Figure 11A).

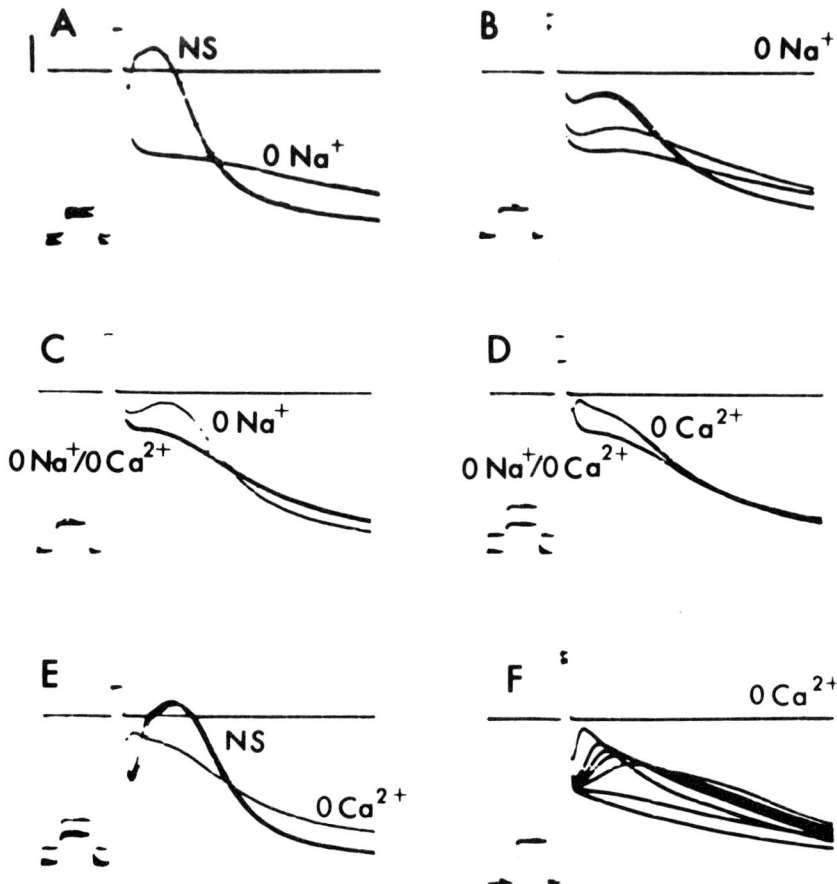

FIGURE 9. The effect of changes in the ionic composition of the bathing saline solution on the waveform of action potentials evoked by brief depolarizing current injections. The upper trace in each record is a current monitor and also indicates the zero potential. Records in (A) through (E) are from the same cell. Those in (F) are from an adjacent cell. Abbreviations: NS, normal saline; 0Na$^+$, sodium-free saline; 0Ca^{2+}, calcium-free saline; 0Na$^+$/0Ca^{2+}, sodium- and calcium-free saline. See text for details. Calibrations: 20 mV by 10 msec pulses at onset of traces; current bar shown in (A) equals 5×10^{-9} A for (A) through (E) and 1×10^{-8} A for (F).

The occurrence of a TTX-insensitive sodium current, however, seems to be a rather common feature in invertebrates (e.g., Wald, 1972; Standen, 1975).

TEA applied in the bathing medium has proved, in some prepara-

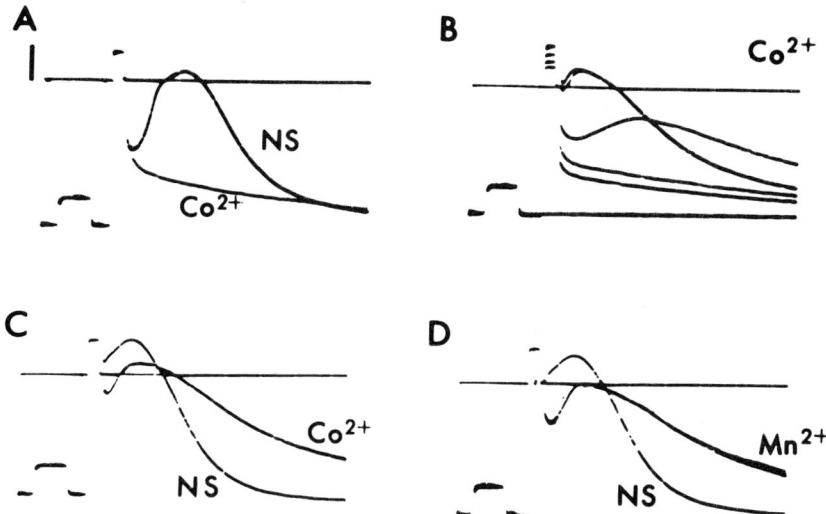

FIGURE 10. The effect of 10 mM cobalt (Co^{2+}) or manganese (Mn^{2+}) on evoked action potentials in a single pedal gland cell (for details, see text). Calibration: 20 mV by 10 msec pulses at onset of each trace; current bar shown in (A) equals 5×10^{-9} A for all records.

tions, a useful agent for blocking potassium activation (Kleinhaus and Prichard, 1975). Action potentials are significantly prolonged after a 30-sec treatment (Figure 11B). Important here is the fact that the shoulder is essentially unchanged by TEA treatment, indicating that delayed potassium activation is not producing this waveform in normal saline. Furthermore, in cells with action potentials that do not normally have a shoulder on the rising phase, TEA treatment reveals such an event (Figure 11C). It seems likely that TEA is acting here in a fashion analogous to its effect on the squid presynaptic terminal, namely, to unmask an additional depolarizing component of the action potential that is usually shunted by increased potassium conductance (Katz and Miledi, 1969).

We have examined the regenerative calcium potential in sodium-free, high-calcium TEA-containing saline solution (Figure 12). With threshold stimulation, changing from TEA saline to sodium-free, TEA, high-calcium saline results in a hyperpolarization due to the effect of sodium on the resting potential as discussed above (Figure 12A). Increasing current injection in this medium reveals a very large, graded, regenerative calcium response that is analogous to that produced in the presynaptic terminal of the squid giant synapse under similar con-

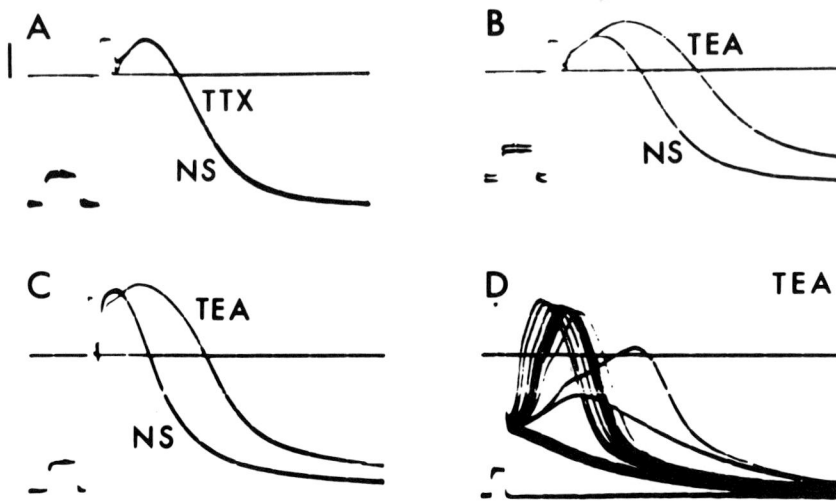

FIGURE 11. (A) Lack of effect of tetrodotoxin (10^{-5} M) on evoked action potentials. (B) Change of waveform 30 sec after transferring from normal saline (NS) to 30 mM TEA in the bathing saline. (C) As in (B), but note change in waveform from simple action potential to one having a shoulder after TEA treatment. (D) The effect of repetitive firing (in TEA) is frequently to dissociate two distinct components of the rising phase of the action potential. Calibration: 20 mV by 10 msec pulses at the onset of each trace; current bar shown in (A) equals 5×10^{-9} A for all traces.

ditions (Katz and Miledi, 1969). The graded nature of this response in both systems makes quantification difficult by any method short of voltage clamping. The elegant voltage clamp experiments described earlier in this symposium (Llinás, 1977) provide such clear data as to indicate the advantage of duplication on pedal gland cells. Such experiments will allow further comparison of both the magnitude and time course of inward current carried by calcium in the squid and slug systems.

With the data available, it appears that a considerable amount of calcium enters pedal gland cells with the generation of each action potential. Such a situation is entirely in accord with the specialized secretory role of these cells. In light of the fact that sodium entry has been implicated as a sufficient stimulus for secretion in some cell types, we wondered if a similar role might exist for the sodium component of pedal gland cell action potentials. For example, Lowe, Richardson, Taylor, and Donatsch (1976) recently have shown that

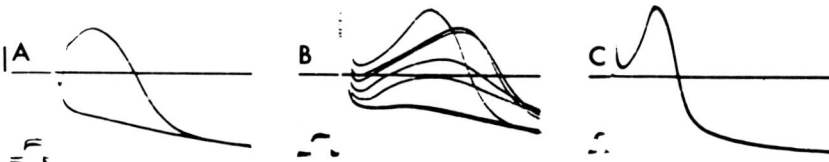

FIGURE 12. Action potentials produced in sodium-free, high-calcium (49 mM), TEA-containing saline solution. The action potential evoked in (A) is blocked by changing to sodium-free, high-calcium TEA saline, but in (B), graded increases in current injection resulted in a graded regenerative potential. (C) A single regenerative calcium potential as seen in (B), but in a compressed time base. In all records, the upper trace is both a current monitor and an indicator of the zero potential. Calibrations: 20 mV by 10 msec pulse at the onset of each trace; current bar in (A) equals 5×10^{-9} A for all records.

veratridine-induced sodium influx in calcium-free (plus 1 mM EGTA) saline solution can induce insulin release from pancreatic islet cells. Furthermore, this whole process is blocked by TTX. These are curious findings, because Matthews and Sakamoto (1975) found that action potentials in these cells were TTX insensitive, but were blocked by cobalt or manganese. Lowe et al. (1976) suggest that sodium influx results in the release of calcium from intracellular stores and thus triggers insulin release. We have been interested in whether the sodium component of pedal gland action potentials might have a similar function.

We have begun our investigation of the ionic requirements for secretion by initial experiments designed to measure the overall secretory capability of the pedal gland. The tubular morphology of the pedal gland facilitates quantitative analysis of mucous secretion, because ciliary motion sweeps mucus to the anterior opening of the gland, where it can be collected readily (Figure 13). For such experiments we pin a whole gland that has been slit open along its lumen into a Sylgard (Dow-Corning) chamber fitted with silver/silver chloride field stimulating electrodes at each end. Throughout the dissection and initial mounting, the gland is bathed in a high-magnesium (20 mM) saline solution to retard secretion. The protocol of a typical experiment calls for a series of incubations (10 or 15 min in duration) in either normal saline solution or one of the standard ionic substitutions employed in the electrophysiological studies presented above. Figure 14 shows an example of an experiment testing the effect of field stimulation on mucus secretion. Each bar in the histo-

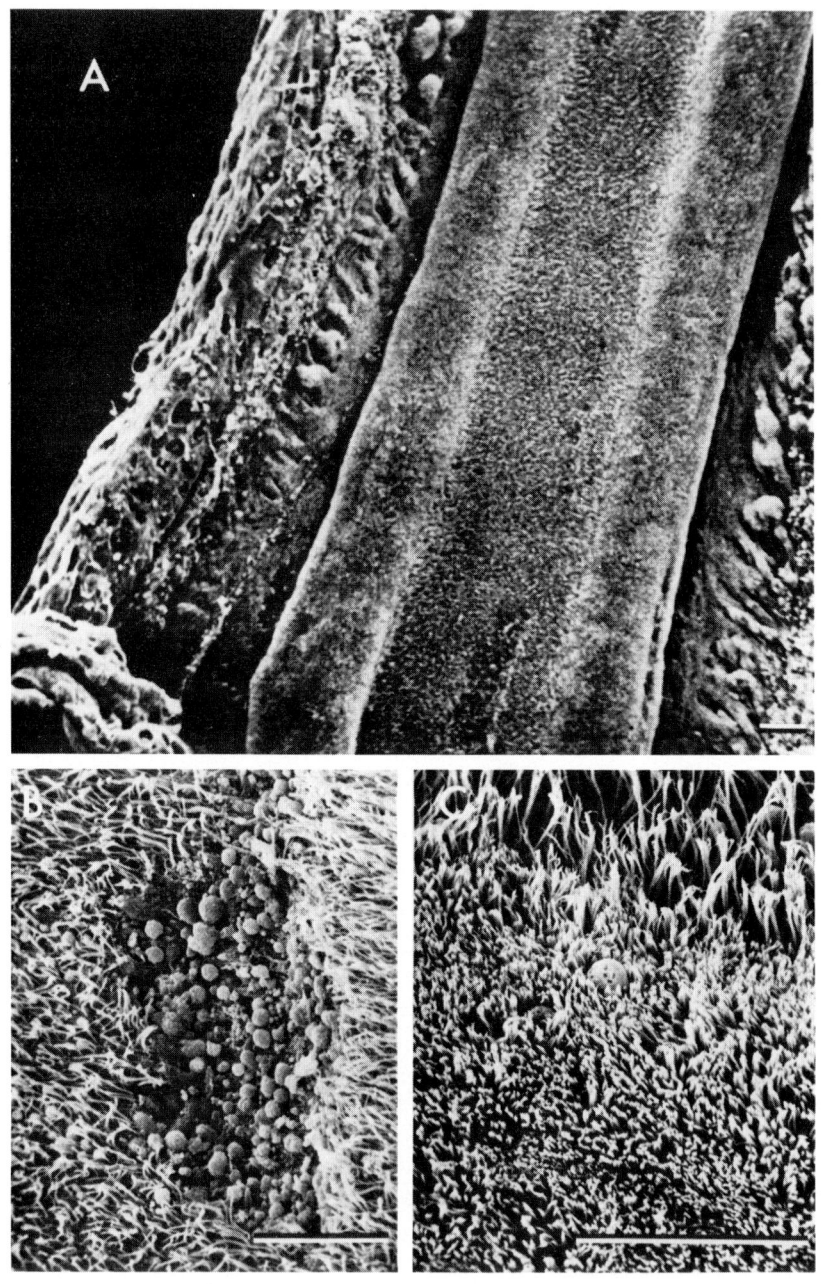

gram represents the dry weight of the total mucus secreted during a 15-min incubation period. During the 4- to 7-min interval between incubation periods, the 4 ml of bathing saline was collected, the gland was vigorously washed with an additional 5.7 ml of the same kind of saline, and finally the gland was rewashed twice in the type of saline specified for the subsequent incubation period. To each 4-ml bath sample, combined with its 5.7-ml wash solution, was added 0.5% cetylpyridinium chloride to precipitate the mucus. Mucus collected in this way from each incubation period was then placed on pre-weighed membrane filters (Millipore Corp.) and dried at 60°C for 1 h. The dry weight of mucus secreted during each incubation period was normalized to milligrams of mucus secreted per hour in order to allow some comparison between preparations.

The rest rate of mucous secretion from these glands can be quite constant (Figure 14). Electrical stimulation, as expected, markedly increased this basal secretion level. In various experiments, stimulation consisted of pulses 5 to 15 msec in duration occurring at frequencies ranging from 10 to 60 Hz, depending upon the specific experiment. In the experiment shown in Figure 14, the magnitude of stimulus employed in the first stimulation period was selected as that current strength required to elicit minimal visually detectable contraction of the muscular elements of the gland. This level of stimulation evoked several times the amount of secretion of the control period. Increasing the stimulus strength by a factor of three resulted in an approximately sixfold increase in mucous secretion as compared to controls. The effect of pulsed electrical field stimulation on mucous secretion is highly reproducible and can be observed during experiments lasting as long as 8 h. Over extended periods, however, it is necessary to control for possible depletion effects by replicating experiments periodically and comparing them with initial results.

The ability to stimulate mucous secretion has been tested under various ionic conditions (Figure 15). First, we examined the possibility that sodium entry into the cells might be required for secretion and found that secretion is not impaired by the absence of sodium

---

FIGURE 13. Scanning electron micrographs of the intralumenal morphology of the pedal gland. The gland has been slit open along the length of the duct, and a dense bed of cilia is revealed on the ventral inner surface. These cilia vigorously propel mucus (B and C) along the length of the gland to the anterior opening near the mouth. Calibration: 50 μm.

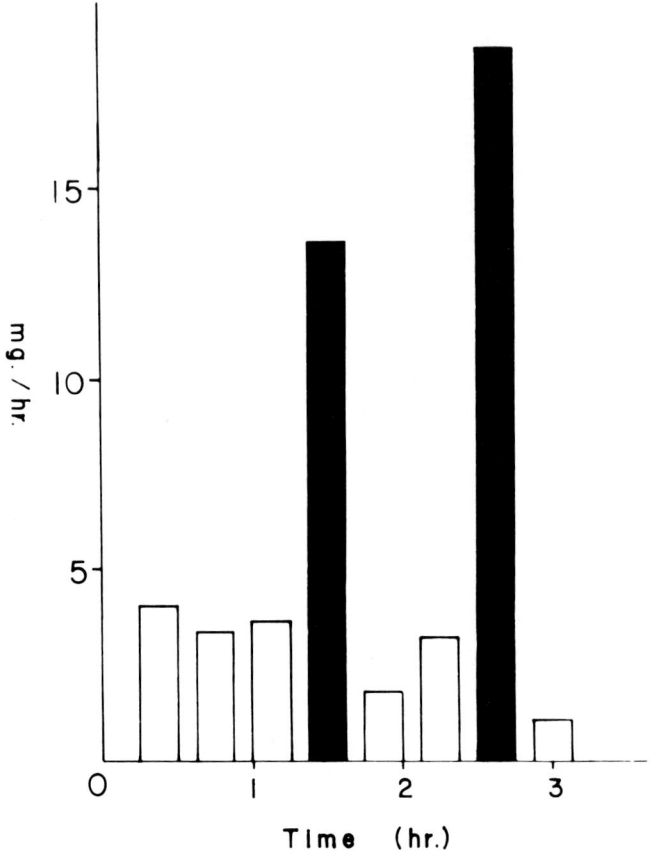

FIGURE 14. Pedal gland mucous secretion during quiescent periods (open bars) and stimulated periods (solid bars), expressed as the dry weight secreted per hour. Each bar represents mucous secretion during a 15-min incubation period. During the second stimulation period, the stimulus strength was increased by a factor of three. See text for details.

in the bathing fluid. On the contrary, both the unstimulated, basal secretion amounts and the stimulated secretion amounts were larger in zero-sodium saline than their respective controls. Although this clearly needs closer examination, such a result would not be surprising if the absence of sodium causes intracellular calcium build-up, as has been observed elsewhere (Baker, 1972; Douglas, 1976). We have found in other experiments that secretion is also possible in saline solutions from which calcium was omitted. We questioned

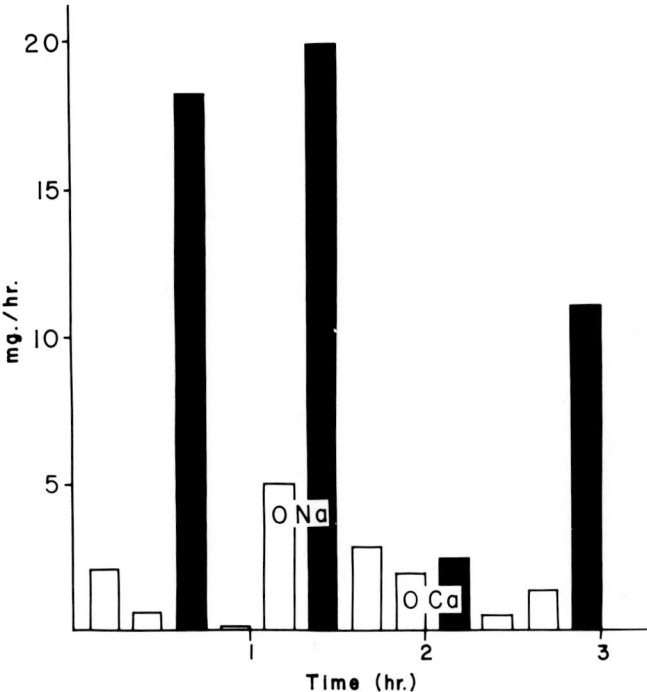

FIGURE 15. Pedal gland mucous secretion during quiescent (open bars) and stimulated (solid bars) periods in various ionic solutions. The gland was in normal saline solution during each of the 10-min incubation periods except those indicated "0Na" (sodium-free saline) or "0Ca" (calcium-free plus 1 mM EGTA saline). See text for details.

whether this really represented a zero-calcium situation, because our electrophysiological experiments suggest that calcium may be released to the bathing fluid from the tissue (Figure 9D). When the gland is bathed in zero-calcium saline containing 1 mM EGTA, stimulation fails to evoke mucous release (Figure 15, third stimulation period). That this is not due to prior depletion of mucus is demonstrated by the large amount of secretion evoked subsequently in normal saline.

These results help to clarify the roles of sodium and calcium influxes during action potentials. Calcium required for secretion comes from outside these cells. Apparently, sodium plays no role in releasing the bound calcium stores, but, rather, functions conjointly with calcium electroresponsiveness to produce the all-or-none character of the action potential. The regenerative events produced either by sodium in

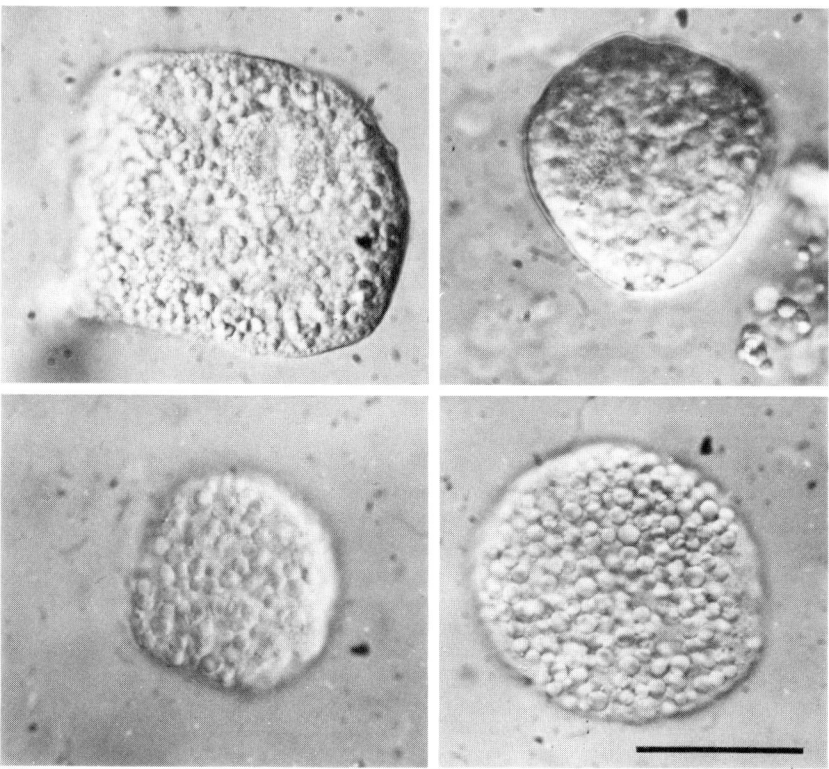

FIGURE 16. Individual pedal gland mucus-secreting cells obtained by enzymatic dissociation. Calibration:100 μm.

the absence of calcium, or by calcium in the absence of sodium, are graded in nature, but the synergistic effects of the two could guarantee a reproducible and fixed calcium entry with each neural input to these glands.

The ionic events underlying regenerative electrical activity in these exocrine cells correspond to the secretory characteristics of the gland as a whole. Further studies should examine secretion at the cellular level. Ideally, because the secretory granules are so large, we would like to visually monitor secretion from a single cell under voltage control. Such experiments seem feasible in isolated pedal gland cells. We have employed the cell isolation procedures developed by Kostenko, Geletyuk, and Veprintsev (1974) for use on molluscan neurons to isolate individual pedal gland cells. Results like those shown in Figure

16 have been encouraging. Such cells can be observed during secretion by means of Nomarski optics and should, by virtue of their simple geometry, be useful for questions as yet unanswered even in neural preparations.

At the outset of this work we asked about the *differences* between synaptic transmission and exocrine secretion. What we have found are *similarities*. Are these properties unique to exocrine cells in gastropods, or should we perhaps re-examine other less technically favorable exocrine tissues in light of the present findings? It would not be surprising to find conservative evolutionary processes at work, not only in the selection of calcium as a mediator of secretion, but also in the mechanisms regulating calcium entry into secretory cells.

ACKNOWLEDGMENTS

This research was supported by Public Health Service research grant 1 R01 NS09696. I thank Dr. D. Senseman for introducing us to *Ariolimax*, Drs. D. Soll and R. Thomas for their recommendations on methods, and Mr. J. Rued and Ms. J. Kater for their excellent technical assistance.

REFERENCES

Baker, P. F. (1972). Transport and metabolism of calcium ions in nerve, *Prog. Biophys. Mol. Biol.* **24**:177–223.

Barr, R. A. (1926). Some observations on the pedal gland of *Milax*, *Q. J. Microsc. Sci.* **70**:647–669.

Coombs, J. S., D. R. Curtis, and J. C. Eccles (1957). The generation of impulses in motoneurones, *J. Physiol. (London)* **139**:232–249.

Dean, P. M. and E. K. Matthews (1968). Electrical activity in pancreatic islet cells, *Nature (London)* **219**:389–390.

Douglas, W. W. (1976). The role of calcium in stimulus-secretion coupling, pp. 17–48 in *Stimulus-Secretion Coupling in the Gastrointestinal Tract*, Case, R. M. and H. Goebell, eds. University Park Press, Baltimore.

Douglas, W. W. and R. P. Rubin (1961). The role of calcium in the secretory response of the adrenal medulla to acetylcholine, *J. Physiol. (London)* **159**:40–57.

Fuortes, M. G. F., K. Frank, and M. C. Becker (1957). Steps in the production of motoneuron spikes, *J. Gen. Physiol.* **40**:735–752.

Horsfield, G. I. (1965). The effect of compound 40/80 on rat mast cells, *J. Pathol. Bacteriol.* **90**:599–605.

Kater, S. B. (1974). Feeding in *Helisoma trivolvis*: the morphological and physiological bases of a fixed action pattern, *Am. Zool.* **14**:1017–1036.

Kater, S. B., A. D. Murphy, and J. R. Rued (1977a). Neural control of the salivary glands of *Helisoma trivolvis*, in preparation.

Kater, S. B. and C. H. F. Rowell (1973). Integration of sensory and centrally programmed components in generation of cyclical feeding activity of *Helisoma trivolvis*, *J. Neurophysiol.* **36**:142–155.

Kater, S. B., J. R. Rued, and A. D. Murphy (1977*b*). Propagation of action potentials through electrotonic junctions in the salivary glands of the pulmonate mollusc *Helisoma trivolvis*, in preparation.

Katz, B. and R. Miledi (1969). Tetrodotoxin-resistant electric activity in presynaptic terminals, *J. Physiol. (London)* **203**:459–487.

Kleinhaus, A. L. and J. W. Prichard (1975). Calcium dependent action potentials in leech Retzius cells by tetraethylammonium chloride, *J. Physiol. (London)* **246**:351–361.

Kostenko, M. A., V. I. Geletyuk, and B. N. Veprintsev (1974). Completely isolated neurons in the mollusc, *Lymnaea stagnalis*. A new objective for nerve cell biology investigation, *Comp. Biochem. Physiol. A* **49**:80–100.

Llinás, R. (1977). Calcium and transmitter release in squid synapse, pp. 139–160 in *Society for Neuroscience Symposia*, Vol. 2, Cowan, W. M. and J. A. Ferrendelli, eds. Society for Neuroscience, Bethesda, Md.

Lowe, D. A., B. P. Richardson, P. Taylor, and P. Donatsch (1976). Increasing intracellular sodium triggers calcium release from bound pools, *Nature (London)* **260**:337–338.

Lundberg, A. (1955). The electrophysiology of the submaxillary gland of the cat, *Acta Physiol. Scand.* **35**:1–25.

Matthews, E. K. and M. Saffran (1973). Ionic dependence of adrenal steroidogenesis and ACTH-induced changes in the membrane potential of adrenocortical cells, *J. Physiol. (London)* **234**:43–64.

Matthews, E. K. and Y. Sakamoto (1975). Electrical characteristics of pancreatic islet cells, *J. Physiol. (London)* **246**:421–437.

Partridge, L. D. and R. C. Thomas (1974). A twelve-way rotary tap for changing physiological solutions, *J. Physiol. (London)* **245**:22–23P.

Petersen, O. H. (1976). Electrophysiology of mammalian gland cells, *Physiol. Rev.* **56**:535–577.

Röhlich, P., P. Anderson, and B. Uvnäs (1971). Electron microscope observations on compound 40/80-induced degranulation in rat mast cells. Evidence for sequential exocytosis of storage granules, *J. Cell Biol.* **51**:465–483.

Rovainen, C. M. (1967). Physiological and anatomical studies on large neurons of central nervous system of the sea lamprey (*Petromyzon marinus*). I. Müller and Mauthner cells, *J. Neurophysiol.* **30**:1000–1023.

Standen, N. B. (1975). Calcium and sodium ions as charge carriers in the action potential of an identified snail neurone, *J. Physiol. (London)* **249**:241–252.

Tauc, L. (1962*a*). Site of origin and propagation of spike in the giant neuron of *Aplysia*, *J. Gen. Physiol.* **45**:1077–1098.

Tauc, L. (1962*b*). Identification of active membrane areas in the giant neuron of *Aplysia*, *J. Gen. Physiol.* **45**:1099–1115.

Thomas, R. C. (1972). Intracellular sodium activity and the sodium pump in snail neurones, *J. Physiol. (London)* **220**:55–71.

Thomas, R. C. and V. J. Wilson (1966). Marking single neurons by staining with intracellular recording microelectrodes, *Science* **151**:1538–1539.

Wald, F. (1972). Ionic differences between somatic and axonal action potentials in snail giant neurons, *J. Physiol. (London)* **220**:267–281.

Synaptic Vesicle Exocytosis Revealed in Quick-Frozen Frog Neuromuscular Junctions Treated with 4-Aminopyridine and Given a Single Electrical Shock

J. E. Heuser

University of California, San Francisco, California

INTRODUCTION

Reese and I have proposed a hypothesis for the recycling of synaptic vesicles in frog neuromuscular junctions, illustrated in Figure 1, that may explain how neurosecretion is carried out by synapses in general. The hypothesis starts from the widely held premise that neurotransmitters are stored in synaptic vesicles and are discharged by exocytosis. It maintains that after exocytosis, synaptic vesicles merge fully into the presynaptic membrane and mix with it, as a natural consequence of its fluidity. The hypothesis further holds that such exocytosis is balanced by a compensatory endocytosis, and that this endocytosis is carried out primarily by coated vesicles that are capable of hauling back into the interior of the synapse specific components of synaptic vesicle membranes. The hypothesis concludes that such coated vesicles contribute what they have retrieved from the presynaptic membrane to the formation of a new generation of synaptic vesicles that can enter the cycle once again.

The evidence for this scheme of vesicle membrane recycling has been collected over the past several years from electron microscope studies of structural changes that occur during tetanic nerve stimulation, and from observations on the uptake of extracellular tracer into synaptic vesicles that result from nerve stimulation (Heuser and Reese, 1973). Our interpretation of this data can be distinguished from certain other proposals for how synaptic vesicles turn over, which argue that synaptic vesicles do not collapse into the presynaptic membrane and do not lose their integrity after exocytosis, but simply pinch off from the surface and refill with transmitter again and again (Ceccarelli, Hurlbut, and Mauro, 1972; Akert, Pfenninger, Sandri, and Moor, 1972). Such views do not attribute to coated vesicles the central role in the retrieval of synaptic vesicle membranes that we argue for.

In an effort to resolve these different views, Reese and I developed a freezing machine that we hoped would allow us to see directly the structural changes that occur during neurosecretion (Heuser, Reese, and Landis, 1974). In this neuroscience symposium lecture, we showed for the first time that our machine could freeze frog muscles fast enough to catch each stage of synaptic vesicle exocytosis as it appears at the neuromuscular junction. Electron micrographs were shown of each

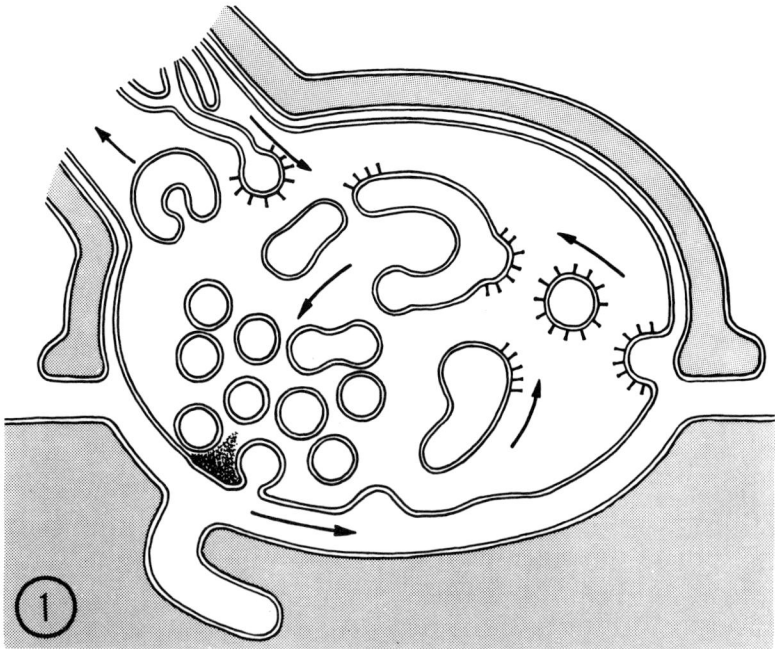

FIGURE 1. Our current view of synaptic vesicle recycling at the frog neuromuscular junction, supported by the new views shown here of synaptic vesicle exocytosis as it looks in quick-frozen frog neuromuscular junctions treated with 4-aminopyridine and given a single electrical shock. Each step is reviewed in the text.

stage in the sequence of synaptic vesicle exocytosis, collapse, and retrieval from the presynaptic membrane, all of which fit with the particular scheme of vesicle recycling we originally proposed.

METHODS

The basic experiment that was performed many times to reconstruct this whole sequence of structural changes was to apply one single electrical stimulus to the nerve leading into a frog cutaneous pectoris muscle, and then abruptly halt the secretion of acetylcholine from the nerve terminals in this muscle, to see what structural changes accompanied it, by quick freezing the muscle at preset short intervals after the electrical stimulus. To accomplish the freezing, the muscle was dissected from the frog and mounted in the freezing machine so that at the proper moment it could be smacked against a super-cold block of copper or silver of the purest type, most highly conductive of heat. I will explain later why this is the fastest possible way to freeze any sort of biological tissue.

It is worth pointing out that we were not attempting to stop membrane changes *directly* by this method, but rather *indirectly*, by trapping the membrane within a solidified matrix of water. We could not have hoped to arrest membrane changes by simply cooling the membrane until it became a gel of phospholipids, as Rash and his colleagues (1976) have claimed to do simply by pouring an ice-cold solution over a muscle. We could see quite clearly that nerve membranes remain pliant enough to accommodate all sorts of distortions produced by the ice crystals, which, unfortunately, grew quickly to visible proportions when the freezing was not quite fast enough. These membrane distortions appeared within milliseconds, even though the membrane must have been surrounded by ice-cold tissue water at the time. So it seems unlikely that it will ever be possible to cool a membrane fast enough to "gel" it, and in this way catch the phospholipid rearrangements involved in such fast changes as exocytosis, without at the same time freezing the water around the membrane. But then the freezing itself will have been sufficient to capture the event. Thus, the principle on which we have operated is that if we can make the freezing occur faster than the time it takes for a natural membrane change to occur, then we can efficiently trap this change within a matrix of frozen water, and we can obtain a view of it that is representative or true to nature.

The critical difficulty with the experiment we had in mind is that the membrane events that underlie neurosecretion are very fast. To capture an event that we think lasts no more than a few milliseconds, and that is preceded by a critical delay of a fraction of a millisecond, during which intracellular calcium is producing unknown molecular changes that lead to membrane fusion and exocytosis, we must freeze the muscle very fast. Indeed, we believe that freezing can be done this fast, in a small fraction of a millisecond, at least on the surface of the muscle that strikes the cold metal block. This we conclude not from direct measurement, which poses difficulties we have not so far overcome, but from inference from equations kindly provided by A. F. Huxley. If we interpret these equations correctly, they predict that the most superficial 15 μm of muscle tissue freezes in 0.3 msec or less (Figure 2). Deeper than 15 μm, we can see clearly, but with considerable regret, that freezing is not fast

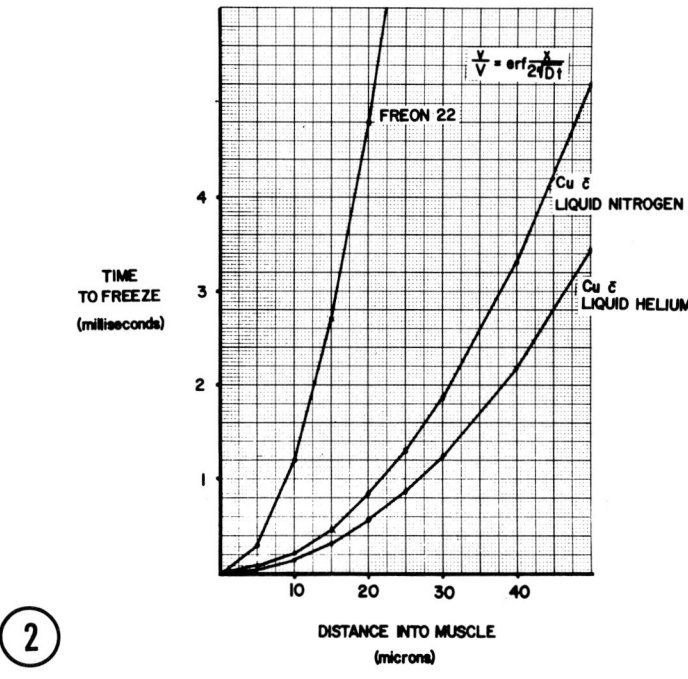

FIGURE 2. How fast the muscle freezes at various depths, calculated from equations provided by A. F. Huxley and based on the Carslaw and Jaeger (1947) mathematical model of the flow of heat out of a flat object (such as a frog cutaneous pectoris muscle) and into a cold surround (such as the ultracold copper block against which the muscle is frozen). The copper block is cooled with liquid helium to 4°K, so the appropriate curve is the lowest, which shows that the zone from 10 to 20 μm beneath the free surface of the muscle freezes in about 0.5 msec, more or less, depending on the exact depth. Such freezing should be fast enough to catch exocytosis, at least if it lasts more than a millisecond or so; and it does so, as the subsequent electron micrographs will show.

enough to prevent the formation of ice crystals that are just large enough to distort the membrane structure on the level we wish to study (100 to 500 Å). As a consequence, the only nerve terminals that we can study are those that happen to be located in the well-frozen zone, less than 15 μm from the surface, and it is these nerve terminals that are frozen in a small fraction of a millisecond.

To see nerve membranes in this zone, we have to remove the water overlying them without warming them significantly and without disturbing their shape and location. One way this can be done is by careful control of the freeze-fracture technique, in which we gingerly scrape away the overlying water with a sharp razor blade mounted in the accurate cryomicrotome designed by the Balzers Company. Then we make a carbon-platinum replica of the exposed membrane surface, or, more accurately, a replica of its fractured surface, while the membrane is still frozen solid. In fact, the membrane is not really dead at the time of replication. Cells can survive freezing and thawing, at least when it is done without forming large ice crystals within them. Indeed, some "life" is left in our muscles after fracturing and replication, as we learned the hard way when we found that cutaneous pectoris muscles inevitably contract violently when they thaw, and so destroy the delicate replicas on their surfaces. We now avoid this catastrophe by removing the muscles to a cold methanol slush and allowing them to thaw slowly. Then we dissolve away the underlying muscle in sodium hypochlorite and float the replicas onto grids for the standard transmission electron microscope.

Alternatively, the frozen water can be removed from around the trapped membranes by dissolving it out with organic solvents. When this is done at subzero temperatures, the membranes seem to be greatly stiffened, perhaps due to strengthened Van der Waal's forces and hydrogen bonds, because as one can clearly see in Figures 3a and 3b, they will stay put long enough for us to apply a subsequent chemical fixation with osmium tetroxide to cross-link them chemically. We assume that such cross-links, even though they are formed at reduced temperatures, are strong enough to hold the membranes in their true location during the subsequent steps of staining, embedding in plastic, and thin sectioning that one uses to see membranes in the traditional way in the electron microscope.

Thus, by the two approaches outlined above, we can preserve muscles in a state closer to nature, and can study the process of neurosecretion in either face-on views of nerve membranes (in replicas of freeze-fractured muscles), or in cross-sectioned views of nerve membrane (in thin sections of freeze-substituted muscle).

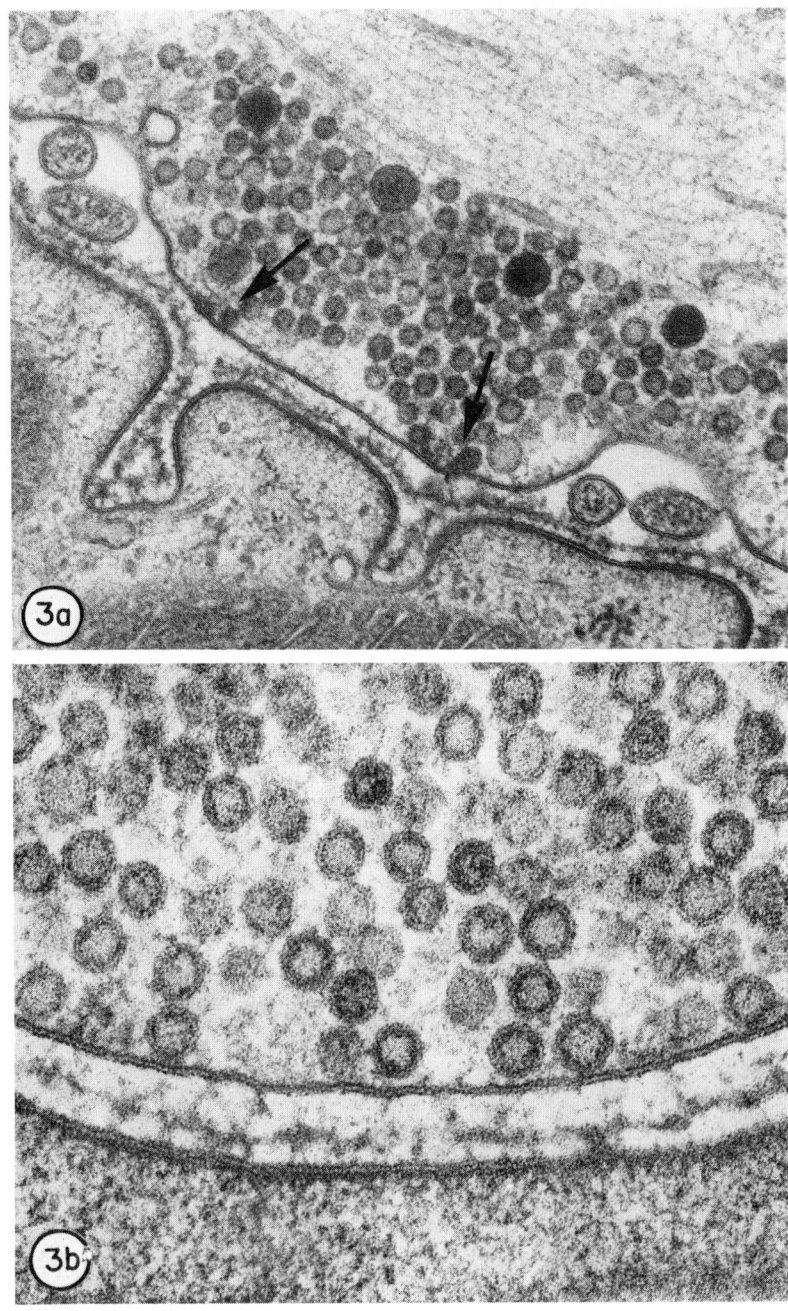

When Reese and I finally had all of these techniques working for frog muscles, we searched for images of synaptic vesicle exocytosis in several dozen muscles that we froze near the peak of the secretory response to one single nerve impulse; but, as Figure 5 illustrates, we found so few possible examples of exocytosis that we began to doubt that transmitter was discharged from synaptic vesicles at all (Heuser et al., 1974).

Exocytosis Caught with 4-Aminopyridine

We remained at this impasse until Lily and Yuh-nung Jan joined my laboratory to study the structural consequences of stimulating frog muscles in 4-aminopyridine. They had recently shown that 4-aminopyridine greatly increases the size of the postsynaptic end plate potential that follows each nerve impulse (Jan, Jan, and Dennis, 1977). They had reason to believe that 4-aminopyridine does this by blocking the voltage-sensitive K^+ channels in the nerve membrane and thus prolonging the duration of its action potential. This, in turn, prolongs the opening of Ca^{2+} channels that occurs in response to depolarization, thus allowing an unusually large amount of calcium to enter the nerve, which in turn triggers the discharge of more than the usual number of quanta of transmitter—in fact, nearly two orders of magnitude more than are usually discharged from the neuromuscular junction with each nerve impulse.

When we applied 2 mM of this cation to muscles during stimulation and freezing, we were immediately able to see abundant examples of synaptic vesicle exocytosis, so long as we looked at the appropriate times during neuromuscular transmission. Figure 6 is an example of one of our early views, which though not perfectly frozen, showed quite clearly several circular dimples in the presynaptic plasma membrane just outside the rows of particles that delineate the "active zones." Each of these dimples we presumed to be an opening or "pore" into an underlying synaptic vesicle fused with the plasma membrane, such as we could see quite clearly in thin sections of muscles that were freeze substituted in the same experiments, some examples of which are shown in Figures 4a through c.

FIGURE 3. The natural beauty of the thin-sectioned results obtained by the freeze substitution method we use, in neuromuscular junctions that are optimally frozen, is well illustrated by these two views of the active zone of the frog neuromuscular junction. The active zones may be recognized as the foci where synaptic vesicles collect just inside the presynaptic membrane, at the arrows in (a) ($\times 50{,}000$). The exact location of vesicles relative to the plasma membrane can be seen quite clearly, and presumably without significant alteration during freezing and fixation, at higher magnification in (b) ($\times 140{,}000$).

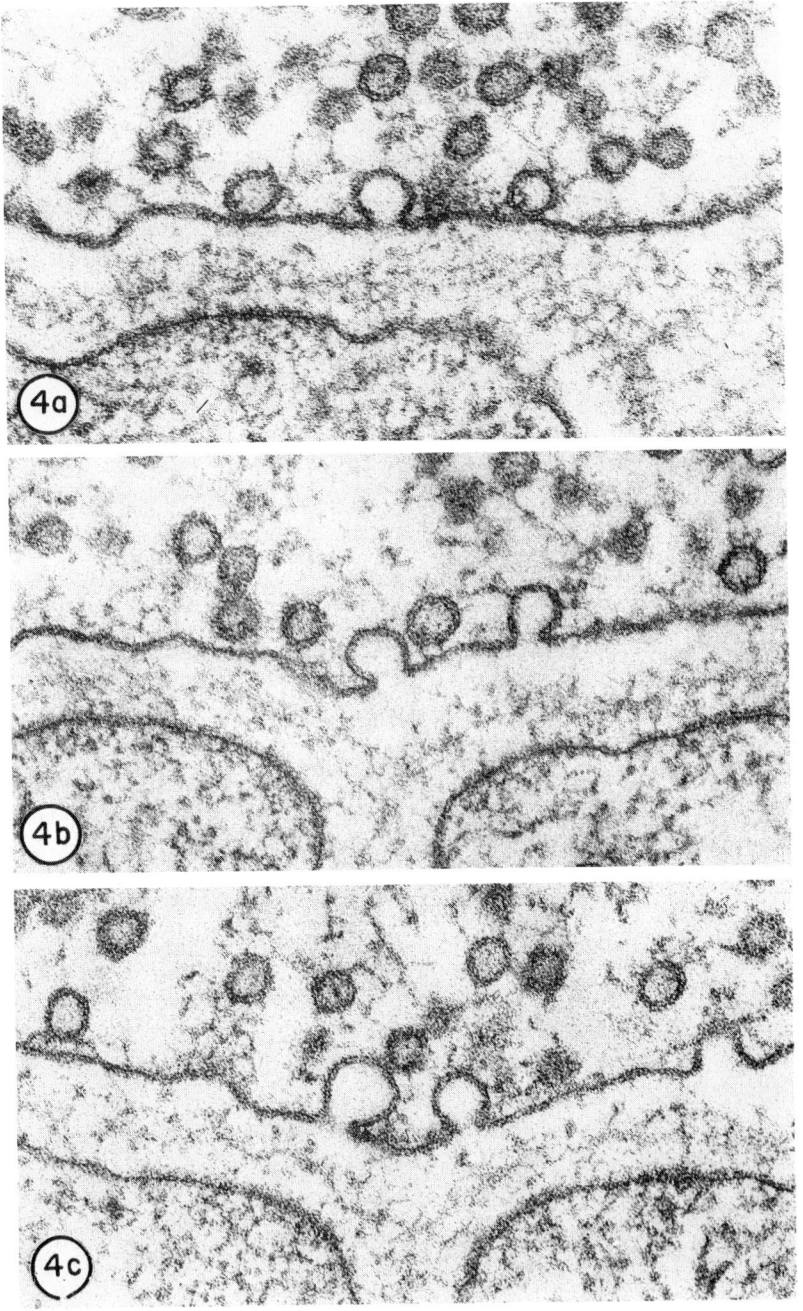

FIGURE 4. Three separate high-magnification (×145,000) views of freeze-substituted neuromuscular junctions in a muscle frozen during the abnormally large burst of acetylcholine release that is provoked by a single nerve stimulus in 2 mM 4-aminopyridine, in this case delivered 5.1 msec before the muscle was frozen. These sections were cut unusually thin (about 200 Å) in order to show quite clearly the fine structure of the presynaptic membrane, which, in all the nerves we saw, displayed many examples of synaptic vesicles apparently caught in the act of exocytosis. In all cases, these open vesicles were found just above the mouths of the postsynaptic folds, hence at the site of the presynaptic active zones.

FIGURE 5. The freeze-fracture appearance of adjacent active zones on a control nerve given one stimulus 6.5 msec before freezing, but not treated with 4-aminopyridine. The rows of large intramembranous particles that delineate the active zones in such "P-face" views are undisturbed by any signs of synaptic vesicle exocytosis. (Figures 5 through 9 are best viewed by turning the book sideways, so that the shadow angle—marked by the arrow—is aiming up.) We still do not know why we cannot find even one vesicle opening in each such view, at ×90,000, since it is highly probable that at least one quantum should have discharged from such an area even when the stimulus was in normal Ringer.

The first fact that we can note about these openings is that they occur in regularly repeating rows that are oriented perpendicular to the long axis of the nerve terminal. Couteaux has illustrated that the exocytosis he finds in thin sections is similarly distributed, and he has named the regions of abundant exocytosis the "active zones" of the nerve terminal (Couteaux and Pecot-Dechavassine, 1970). Peper and his collaborators were the first to see these rows of exocytosis in freeze-fracture views of the frog neuromuscular junction (Dreyer, Peper, Akert, Sandri, and Moor, 1973), and they correctly identified them as Couteaux's active zones. We then illustrated that this exocytosis was best caught by stimulating the nerve at the moment of fixation (Heuser et al., 1974). But we realized that the chemical fixation in aldehydes, which we all had to use at that time, was distorting the process of exocytosis in the act of catching it, and that the strict localization we all found after fixation might be an artifact. In fact, Pumplin and Reese (1976) have gone on to claim that exocytosis can be found far away from the active zones, at least under the abnormal stimulus of brown widow spider venom. Nevertheless, the vesicles that we are now able to freeze in the act of discharge in 4-aminopyridine-treated muscles after only one nerve stimulus (as shown in Figures 6 through 8) are just as strictly localized as those Couteaux originally saw, which were caught by aldehyde fixatives such as those in Figure 9. So the quick-freezing view of synaptic vesicle exocytosis strongly supports Couteaux's original claim that secretion is concentrated in the neuromuscular junction at discrete active zones along the nerve terminal surface.

As to the number of vesicle openings we see, and how that number compares with the number of quanta that ought to have been discharged by each nerve impulse in the presence of 4-aminopyridine, we only say, at the moment, that the two are within an order of magnitude of each other. We are now in the process of measuring the actual number of openings per nerve terminal, though we face a more difficult task when we wish to calculate the exact quantal content from EPP amplitude/ MEPP amplitude, because the 2 mM dose of 4-aminopyridine we used has a bad side effect, in that it depresses the action of secreted transmitter on the muscle to such an extent that miniature end plate potential amplitudes become unmanageably small. We cannot use the coefficient of variation method to estimate quantal content, either, because the effectiveness of 4-aminopyridine on stimulating release wears off when the nerve is stimulated repeatedly.

We still find it hard to understand why the images of synaptic vesicle exocytosis were so rare in the muscles that Reese and I froze out of normal Ringer. We should have been able to find a few vesicle openings,

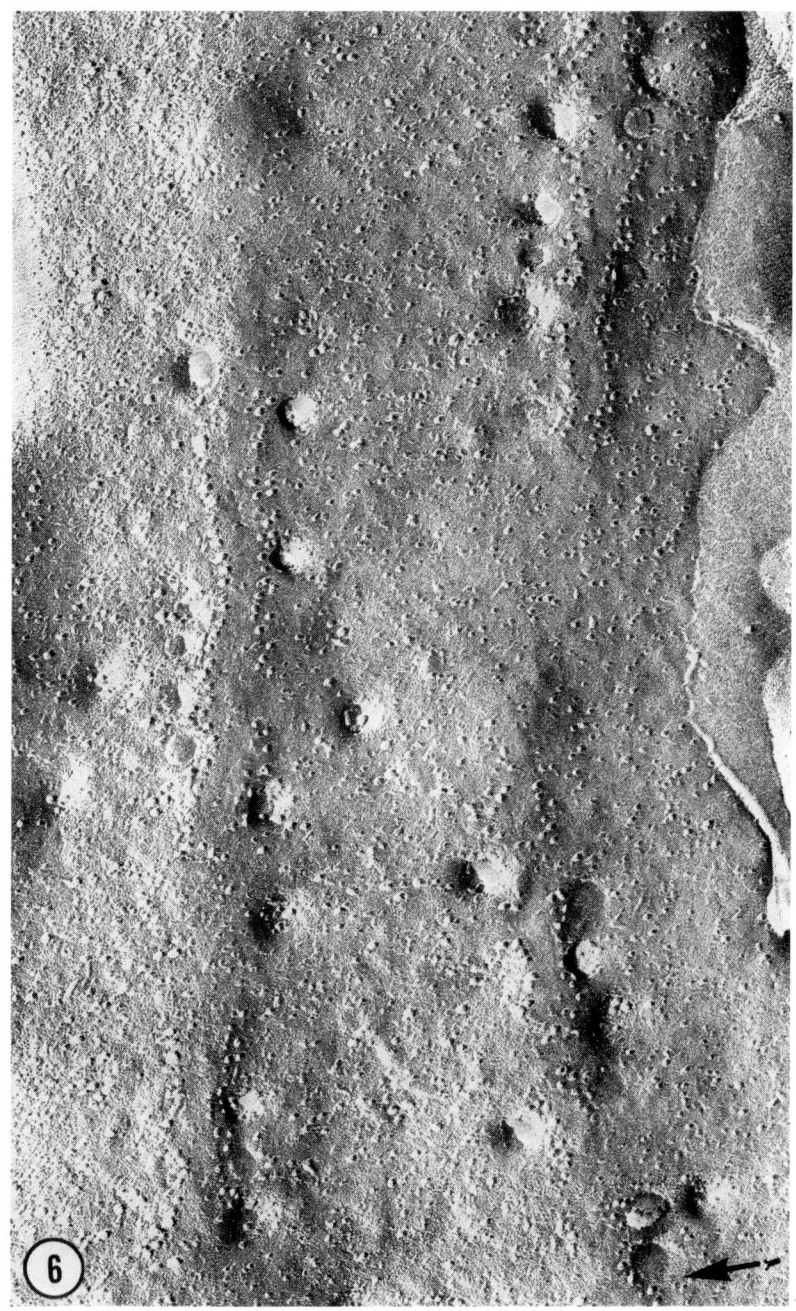

FIGURE 6. The freeze-fracture appearance of exocytosis as it looks from outside a nerve given one shock in 2 mM 4-aminopyridine, in this case 4.4 msec before freezing. Most of the plasmalemmal dimples present are of relatively uniform size, somewhat smaller than the size that a synaptic vesicle would be in this ×100,000 view, and most are located just beside the large particles that delineate the active zones. (The active zones are discontinuous in this field, but that is a natural variation unrelated to the stimulation. Also, the few "ectopic" openings are thought to be endocytotic, and a result of an earlier stimulus delivered inadvertently to this particular muscle.)

because even two orders of magnitude fewer than the number of exocytoses we now see in 4-aminopyridine would still have been 1 opening in about every 10 active zones; and yet we rarely found 1 in 100! Figure 10a is an example of one of the few vesicle openings that we were able to find. Possibly we found so few because the openings disappear very rapidly in normal Ringer, and so are harder to catch, but disappear more slowly in 4-aminopyridine (or more slowly when neighboring vesicles have just discharged in their immediate vicinity).

Mixing of Exocytosed Vesicles with the Presynaptic Membrane

We need to know whether the exocytosis we see in 4-aminopyridine-treated muscles is artificially prolonged in such a manner, because if it is, we will not be able to conclude much from the exact way that exocytosis appears to dissipate or resolve itself in these muscles. It looks as if most vesicles collapse into the presynaptic membrane completely after exocytosis, before their membrane can be retrieved by endocytosis from the presynaptic membrane elsewhere. For example, when we extend the intervals between stimulation and freezing to 20 or 50 msec, we find that many of the openings into vesicles at the active zones are replaced by gently curved pouches in the presynaptic membrane, of about twice the diameter of the original vesicles, which is what we should expect to see if synaptic vesicles flatten out into the presynaptic surface after exocytosis.

What is puzzling is why this process takes so long for some vesicles and happens so fast for others. Such a time disparity must be present, because we find that the total number of vesicle openings at the active zones declines progressively after one shock, and is already down to about 50% after only 20 msec; and yet we can see that several openings remain, and look as if they are at widely different stages of collapse, as long as 50 and 100 msec after the nerve impulse. Possibly we will learn that the vesicles that open first collapse fast, and that the later ones collapse more slowly, as they might if their collapse became retarded or blocked by the progressive development of a phospholipid excess or a

---

FIGURE 7. The appearance of synaptic vesicle exocytosis at the same magnification as in Figure 6 in a muscle frozen 50 msec after the nerve impulse is quite different, because many of the openings have broadened out into shallow depressions that are larger than one vesicle diameter. These must indicate that some vesicles collapse completely into the presynaptic membrane after exocytosis. There is a lower concentration of small openings, but many still do remain at this time, even though we know from physiological records that all measurable acetylcholine release stopped more than 40 msec earlier. ×100,000.

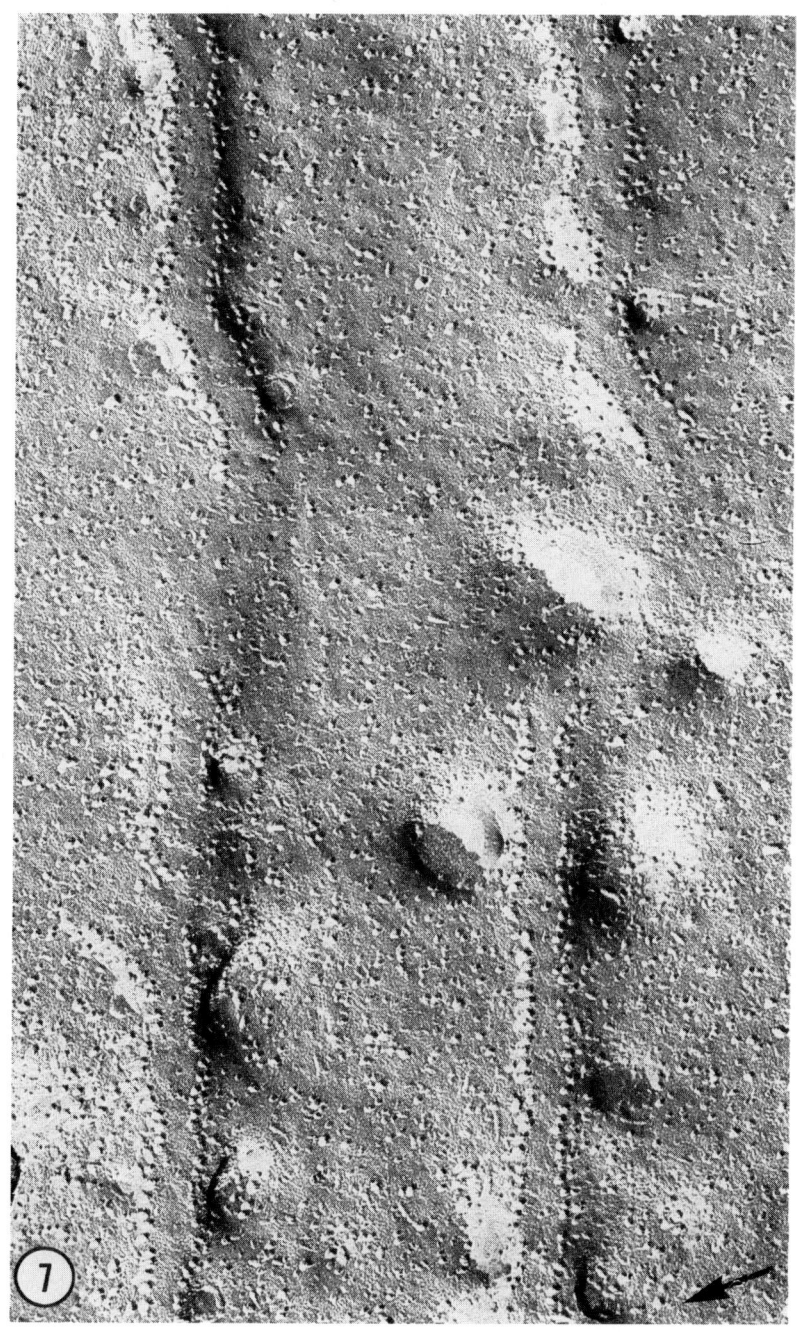

"compression" in the presynaptic membrane, from all the exocytosis going on around them. Reese and I have shown before, at a relatively gross level in fixed tissues, that massive exocytosis does produce an abnormal expansion of the presynaptic membrane, which often relieves itself by developing bizarre redundancies and infoldings (Heuser and Reese, 1973). Clearly, we have much to learn about the forces that govern vesicle collapse and formation in biological membranes. Both processes must be operating in some sort of balance during the secretion from motor nerve terminals that we are witnessing.

We are currently attempting to show that vesicle collapse can be slowed by shrinking nerve terminals osmotically, and producing plasma membrane compression in that way. Our preliminary results indicate that collapse can be slowed. Ordinarily, in 4-aminopyridine, there are no signs of vesicle exocytoses remaining at 1 sec after the nerve impulse; but we found many examples persisting on one muscle frozen 15 sec after the impulse (Figure 8), which was a muscle that we had reason to believe had dried out quite a bit before freezing. These vesicle openings were more variable in size and shape than the openings we usually saw in muscles frozen at earlier times after one stimulus in 4-aminopyridine; in fact, the openings in this "hypertonic" muscle looked more like the ones that are caught by chemical fixatives, shown in Figure 9, and, particularly by those slow-acting fixatives that take on the order of 15 sec to stop secretion.

Compensatory Retrieval of Vesicle Membrane After Exocytosis

Quick freezing has helped considerably to sort out the differences between exocytosis and endocytosis. By providing a new precision of timing, it has allowed us to distinguish the brief burst of exocytosis that we see in the short intervals after the nerve impulse from the more leisurely process of coated vesicle formation, which we find does not become abundant until several seconds after stimulation. When finally such endocytosis of coated vesicles does become abundant, it can be distinguished from exocytosis in two ways, as shown in Figures 10a and

---

FIGURE 8. The typical freeze-fracture appearance of active zones in a muscle in which signs of synaptic vesicle exocytosis persisted for more than 1 sec after a single nerve impulse, and which we inadvertently allowed to dry out a bit during mounting and stimulation. Its active zones were in many places undercut by broad, confluent deformities that matched in three dimensions the openings which Couteaux saw in chemically fixed muscles exposed to osmotic stress. The unusual number of tiny vesicle openings may have meant that many vesicles had no tendency to collapse under these conditions. The reason for this is discussed in the text. ×100,000.

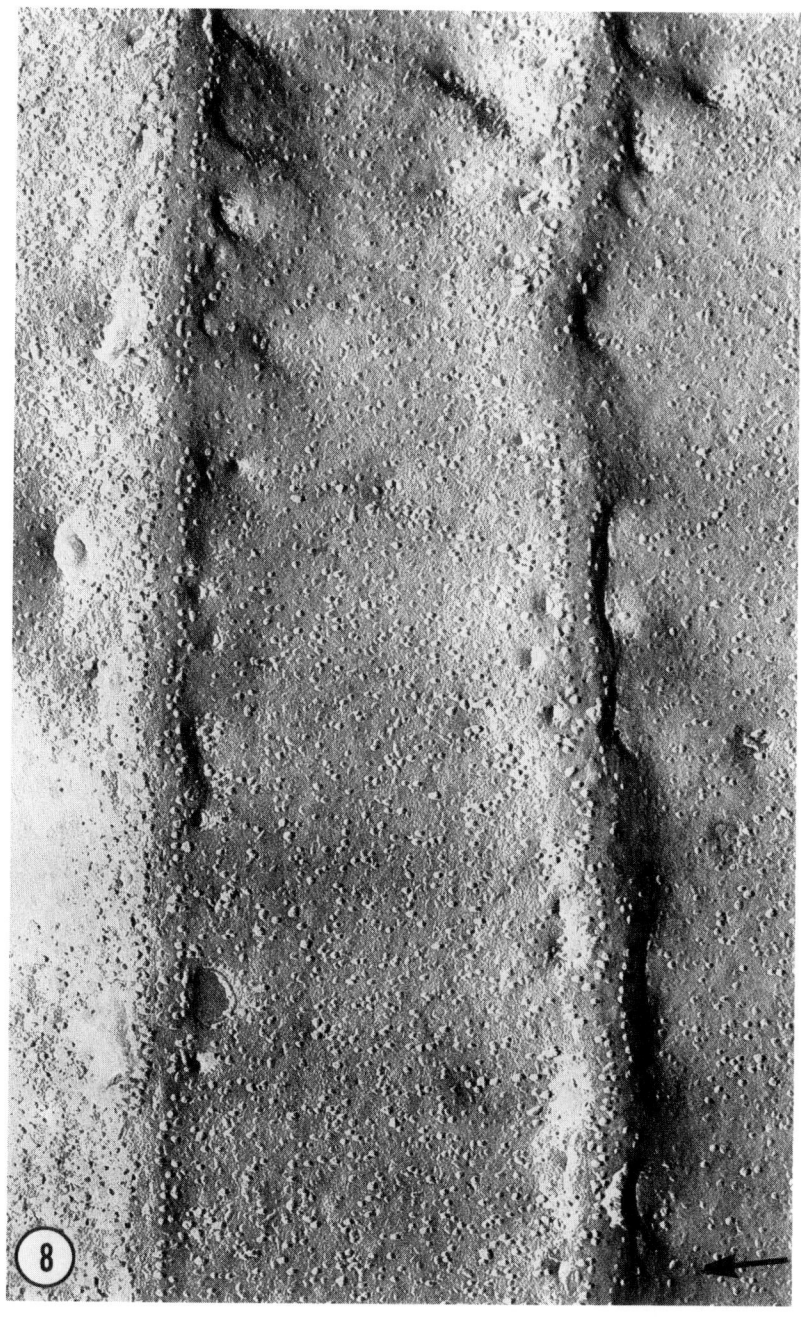

b. First, it has a distinct distribution, in that it can be found anywhere on the presynaptic membrane except at the active zones, which is exactly complementary to the distribution of exocytosis. Second, this sort of endocytosis has a distinct freeze-fracture appearance, in that the nascent coated vesicles invariably contain a cluster of 3 to 5 unusually large intramembranous particles. Reese and I have suggested before that these particles could be the same as synaptic vesicle particles, in which case their concentration in developing coated vesicles would illustrate that such endocytosis is able to retrieve from the presynaptic membrane specific components—probably proteins—that belong to the discharged synaptic vesicles (Heuser and Reese, 1975; Heuser, 1976).

It is worth pointing out that the quick-freezing technique establishes beyond any doubt that intramembranous particles do cluster in coated vesicles during life, since this technique is not subject to all the problems of particle clumping and redistribution that have plagued the earlier methods of fixation or treatment with antifreezes. (McIntyre, Gilula, and Karnovsky, 1974; Mandel, 1972; Verklej, Ververgaert, Van Deenen, and Elberts, 1972). These pretreatments were necessary when ice crystals had to be avoided during the relatively slow freezing by quenching in organic liquid that we used to use. With our new faster method of freezing against metal, no pretreatment or fixation need be applied to the muscle, and there is no time for the particles to redistribute artifactitiously at the moment of death. So we can catch their natural distribution, and can hope to see the mixing of large particles derived from synaptic vesicles into the presynaptic membrane, during the period of vesicle collapse or during the moments soon after.

Unfortunately, we must search for these large particles among a rich background of other particles in the presynaptic membrane, most of which are only slightly smaller in size, and some of which are even the same size, and can only be distinguished from vesicle particles by their fixed location along the inner margins of the active zones. Disregarding these particles, which we presume are something quite different, such as the calcium channels in the presynaptic membrane, we can see in micrographs of quick-frozen terminals, such as in Figures 6 and 7,

---

FIGURE 9. The appearance of synaptic vesicle exocytosis in a frog muscle stimulated tetanically as it was slowly fixed with formaldehyde. In such preparations, exocytosis is strictly localized to the active zones, but does not assume the same clear and circular shapes that it does in quick-frozen tissue, and looks in places rather more like the osmotically distorted forms shown in Figure 8. ×100,000.

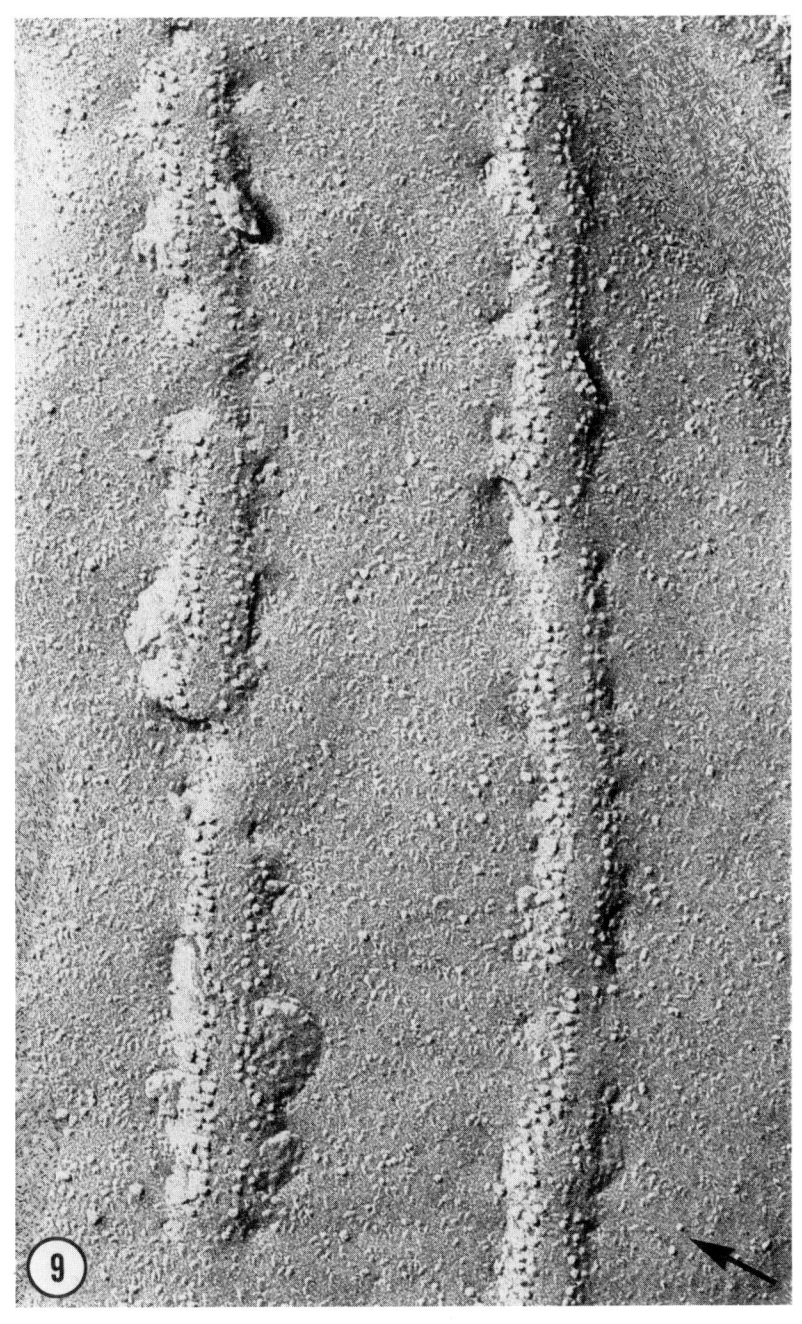

several hints of what appear to be intramembranous particles emerging from the mouths of the collapsing vesicles and spreading out onto the presynaptic membrane proper. We cannot be sure about this point, however, and must still rely on our earlier observation that the total number of such large particles in the presynaptic membrane increases several-fold during prolonged stimulation, at a time when vesicle membrane is being added to the surface more quickly than it is being retrieved (Heuser and Reese, 1975). Hopefully, by careful timing of the freezing we will be able to reconstruct the complete sequence by which these distinctive particulate components of the vesicle membrane mix with the plasma membrane after exocytosis and then are segregated into clusters and retrieved by coated vesicles.

Specific Versus Nonspecific Membrane Retrieval

Quick freezing also promises to clarify the other sort of endocytosis we find at nerve terminals during high rates of stimulation, namely the formation of vacuoles or cisternae. Miledi and I showed some time ago (1971) that such membrane compartments appear when synaptic vesicles disappear during prolonged lanthanum stimulation, and that they are endocytotic in the sense that they take up extracellular tracer from outside the nerve terminals. We presumed that they were formed by endocytosis of large bites of presynaptic membrane, in compensation for synaptic vesicle exocytosis. But how they formed has remained a puzzle. Reese and I thought that they were formed secondarily, by coalescence of newly formed coated vesicles; but we had a hard time explaining how they could appear as fast as they did during tetanic stimulation, whereas coated vesicle formation developed so leisurely (Heuser and Reese, 1973). We were forced to retract that idea completely when we saw in freeze fracture that the cisternae and vacuoles

---

FIGURE 10. (a) One of the rare instances in which vesicle openings were found in a muscle given one shock without 4-aminopyridine. The opening beside the active zone is like many in the 4-aminopyridine-treated muscle in Figure 6, but the other opening is different because it is located further away from the active zone and it contains three very large particles, in addition to the few smaller ones. This particle-laden dimple is like the many dimples that can be seen in (b), in each of which one can barely discern (in this less-than-ideal replica) a similar cluster of three to four large intramembranous particles. (Both views are ×130,000.) As explained in the text, such dimples are found in abundance on the surface of nerves that have been stimulated repeatedly, and that we know (from thin section and tracer studies) are engaged in pinching off coated vesicles from their plasma membranes. Thus we believe these dimples to be sites of coated vesicle formation, not sites of potential vesicle fusion as Akert and his collaborators believed (Llinás and Heuser, 1977).

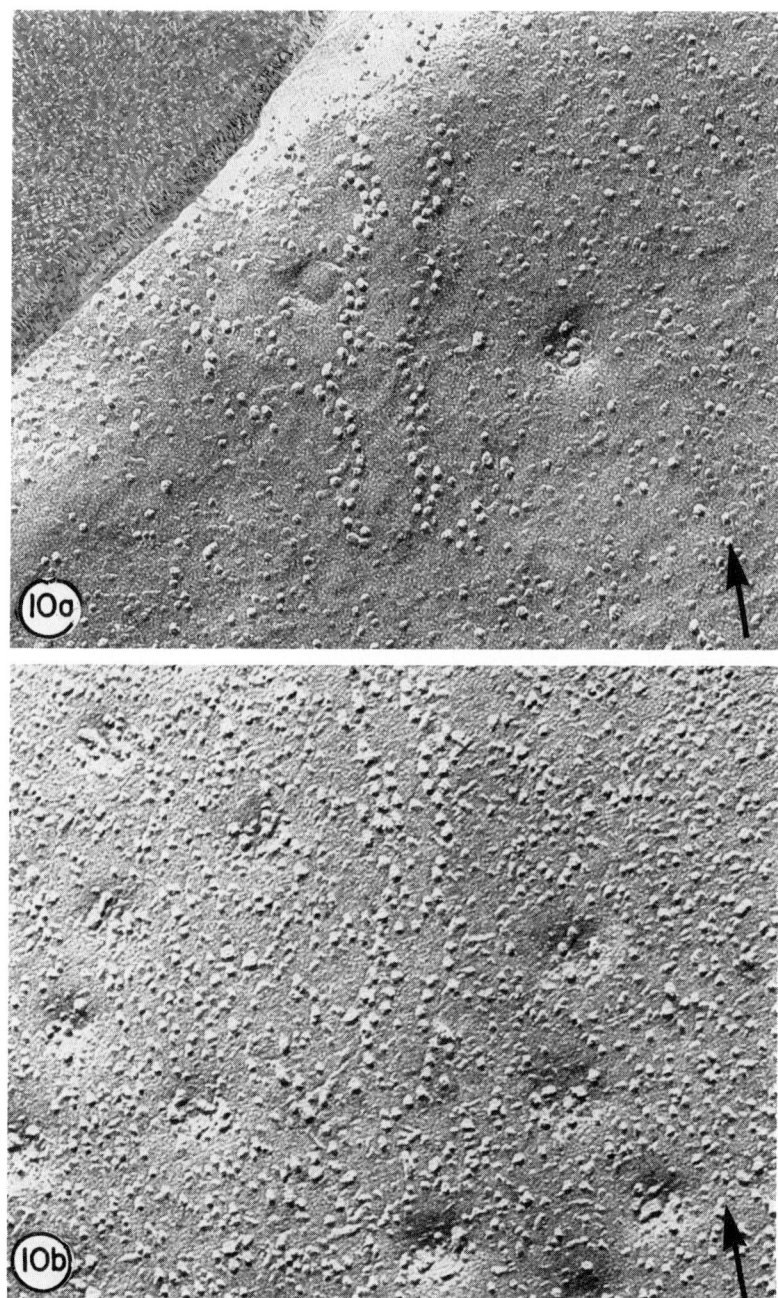

are composed of membrane that is totally unlike coated vesicle membrane with its high concentration of particles (Heuser, 1976). It began to seem more likely that cisternae formed by direct invagination of the presynaptic membrane, and we began to recognize possible examples of this process in freeze fractures of brown widow spider venom-stimulated nerves (Damassa, Davis, Shotten, Heuser, Pumplin, and Reese, 1976). But these tissues had again been chemically fixed, so we could conclude very little about the natural appearance and time course of such "bulk" endocytosis, if it did occur.

Quick freezing of 4-aminopyridine-treated terminals soaked in ferritin has very recently allowed Reese and me to see that such vacuoles and cisternae do indeed form directly from the surface, and do so with remarkable rapidity. We have examined freeze-substituted muscles, frozen at 250 msec and at 1 sec after a single nerve impulse in 4-aminopyridine *plus ferritin*, and find that by 1 sec there are already many ferritin-filled vacuoles present inside the nerve terminal! This is so soon after the nerve impulse that we must conclude that such vacuoles can form almost as soon as the synaptic vesicles collapse, and so we must begin to worry about how we are going to distinguish in static electron microscope images their stages of formation from the synaptic vesicles' stages of collapse.

At the moment, we presume that plasmalemmel deformities, which are broader or deeper than could be formed by a single collapsing synaptic vesicle (greater than 1,000 Å in diameter), logically must represent developing vacuoles or cisternae. It is interesting to note in Figure 7 that the membrane of these deformities, like the vacuoles that appear inside, have a particle complement in freeze fracture that is very much like the plasma membrane in general, in contrast to the high concentration of large particles in synaptic vesicles and coated vesicles. (Apparently, there is still sufficient time in this short period between exocytosis and endocytosis for vesicle membrane to mix with the plasma membrane.) This could explain why large particles accumulate in presynaptic membrane during stimulation: because the exocytosed vesicle membrane has more of these particles than the endocytosed cisternal membrane. From this we conclude that bulk endocytosis is not specific for vesicle membrane constituents, and that the burden for specific retrieval of vesicle particles falls on the coated vesicles. This is now only one example of a rapidly growing number of instances in which coated vesicles have been found to retrieve specific membrane molecules from the cell surface (Fawcett, 1965; Anderson, Goldstein, and Brown, 1976; Bretscher, 1976).

Structural Changes During the Synaptic Delay That Precedes Exocytosis

One final point worth discussing is that quick freezing offers the chance to see whether or not any presynaptic membrane changes *precede* synaptic vesicle exocytosis, during the critical "synaptic delay" period when calcium is entering the nerve. We would expect to see that during this period, synaptic vesicles come into contact with the presynaptic membrane before they fuse with it (Figure 11). Figure 12a illustrates that calcium can promote such contact between vesicle and plasma membrane. (So, also, can strontium or magnesium, from which we conclude that each of these divalent cations may be acting to reduce negative surface charges that normally keep vesicles and plasma membranes apart.) But we find such broad and bulging contacts only in fixed tissues or in tissues treated with high levels of magnesium before fixation. We have not found them in quick-frozen tissue during the

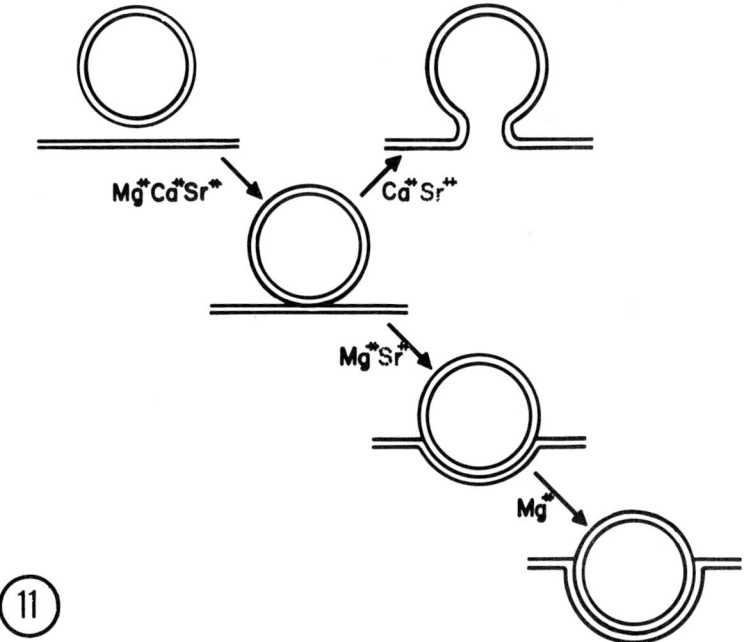

FIGURE 11. The way in which magnesium (and to some extent strontium) can be used to enlarge the zone of contact between synaptic vesicle and plasma membranes, to the extent seen in Figure 12, illustrates that neutralization of negative surface charge may be sufficient to bring about contact, but that something more is required to cause vesicle fusion, which magnesium for one cannot activate.

synaptic delay. We presume this is because the stages of membrane contact that are promoted by calcium proceed rapidly to vesicle fusion and exocytosis, before the contact can grow to such distorted proportions.

Nevertheless, the very breadth of such bulging contacts in chemically fixed nerves has allowed us to recognize an important feature of divalent cation-induced membrane contact. That is, intramembranous particles in both the synaptic vesicles and the plasma membrane are excluded from the regions of contact (Figure 12b). This illustrates that these are fluid membranes. With this in mind, we can examine nerves quick frozen during the synaptic delay for any signs of small "clear" patches immediately beside the active zones, where we would expect to find that synaptic vesicles come into contact with the presynaptic membrane. We do see such particle-free zones beside some active zones, but we have not yet been able to determine whether they develop during the synaptic delay or are present all the time. If we could show that the breadth of such zones varied under different conditions, we might have a structural basis for understanding how agents that affect membrane fluidity could alter the number of synaptic vesicles that could discharge with each nerve impulse and thus alter the effectiveness of synaptic transmission (Barondes, Schlapfer, and Woodson, 1977).

SUMMARY AND CONCLUSIONS

In summary, these new views of synaptic vesicle exocytosis in quick-frozen neuromuscular junctions treated with 4-aminopyridine and given a single electrical shock fit with the vesicle recycling scheme proposed by Heuser and Reese (1973) and updated recently by Heuser (1976). They showed that synaptic vesicles collapse after exocytosis and mix their membrane with the presynaptic membrane. Also, they showed that vesicle membrane is retrieved from the presynaptic membrane in a spatially and temporally distinct process of endocytosis. Furthermore, the quick-freezing technique allowed us to determine accurately the

---

FIGURE 12. (a) A lucky fracture through one of the plasmalemmal "domes" that can be found on nerves that have been chemically fixed in the presence of elevated divalent cation concentrations, which shows that the domes are areas where underlying synaptic vesicles form close contacts with the plasma membrane (×150,000). The obvious partitioning of intramembranous particles away from these zones of contact, which are seen so clearly in (b), is taken in the text as a sign of membrane fluidity and a clue of what to look for, albeit in less exaggerated form, in muscles quick frozen *just before* exocytosis, during the synaptic delay. ×120,000.

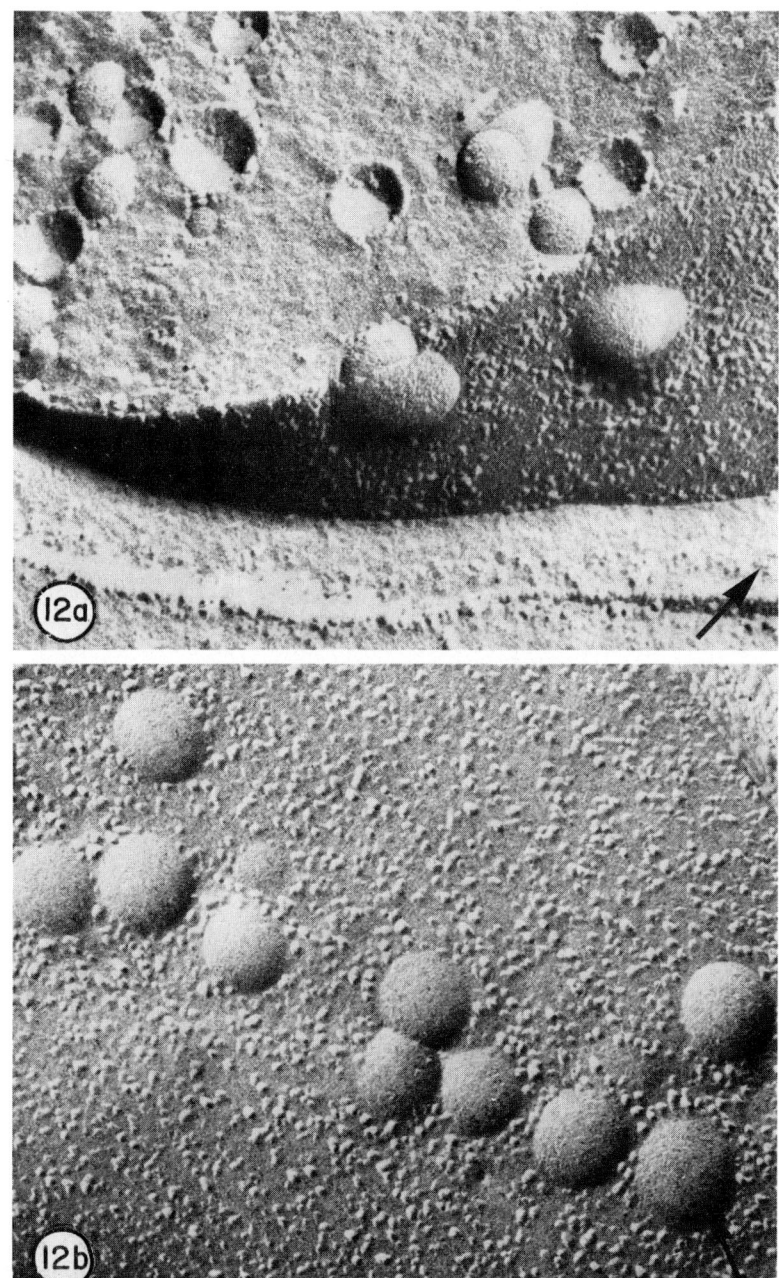

time course of these changes, at least as they occur in 4-aminopyridine. It showed that images of exocytosis appear within a millisecond after the arrival of the nerve impulse and last from 1 to 100 msec. Quick freezing at increasing times after the one shock revealed that many vesicles collapse into the presynaptic membrane within a few milliseconds after exocytosis, whereas others take up to 100 msec or more, possibly depending on the state of hydration of the terminal and the resulting amount of tension on the presynaptic membrane. The timing of ferritin uptake into intracellular vacuoles showed that such endocytotic structures begin to form inside the nerves terminal within 1 sec after the nerve impulse, presumably to compensate for the rapid membrane expansion provoked by the massive exocytosis that occurs in 4-aminopyridine. On the other hand, freeze fracture showed that coated vesicle formation does not become plentiful until several seconds later, and that when it does, it is structurally distinct from synaptic vesicle exocytosis.

ACKNOWLEDGMENTS

This lecture reviewed work that was done in close collaboration with Tom Reese, Mike Dennis, Lily Jan, and Yuh-nung Jan, which will be published in more complete form elsewhere. We wish to thank Ms. Louise Evans for her outstanding technical assistance, and the Muscular Dystrophy Association of America for its financial support. This work was also supported by National Institutes of Health (National Institute of Neurological and Communicative Disorders and Stroke) extramural grants awarded to J.E.H. and M.J.D., and by intramural funds given to T.S.R.

REFERENCES

Akert, K., K. Pfenninger, C. Sandri, and H. Moor (1972). Freeze-etching and cytochemistry of vesicles and membrane complexes in synapses of the central nervous system, pp. 67–86 in *Structure and Function of Synapses*, Pappas, G. D. and D. P. Purpura, eds. Raven Press, New York.

Anderson, R. G. W., J. L. Goldstein, and M. S. Brown (1976). Localization of low density lipoprotein receptors on plasma membrane of normal human fibroblasts and their absence in cells from a familiar hypercholesterolemia homozygote, *Proc. Natl. Acad. Sci. U.S.A.* **73**:2434–2438.

Barondes, S., W. T. Schlapfer, and P. B. J. Woodson (1977). Membrane fluidity implicated in the regulation of decay of post-tetanic potentiation, pp. 435–454 in *Society for Neuroscience Symposia*, Vol. 2, Cowan, W. M. and J. A. Ferrendelli, eds. Society for Neuroscience, Bethesda, Md.

Bretscher, M. S. (1976). Directed lipid flow in cell membranes, *Nature (London)* **260**:21–23.

Carslaw, H. S. and J. C. Jaeger (1947). *Conduction of Heat in Solids*. Clarendon Press, Oxford.

Ceccarelli, B., W. P. Hurlbut, and A. Mauro (1972). Depletion of vesicles from frog neuromuscular junctions by prolonged tetanic stimulation, *J. Cell Biol.* **54**:30–38.

Couteaux, R. and M. Pecot-Dechavassine (1970). Vesicules synaptiques et poches au viveau des zones actives de la junction neuromusculaire, *C. R. Acad. Sci. Ser. D* **271**:2346–2349.

Damassa, D. A., T. L. Davis, D. M. Shotten, J. E. Heuser, D. Pumplin, and T. S. Reese (1976). Structure of nerve terminals in frog muscle after prolonged treatment with brown widow spider venom, *Biol. Bull.* **151**:406–407.

Dreyer, F., K. Peper, K. Akert, C. Sandri, and H. Moor (1973). Ultrastructure of the "active zone" in the frog neuromuscular junction, *Brain Res.* **62**: 373–380.

Fawcett, D. W. (1965). Surface specializations of absorbing cells, *J. Histochem. Cytochem.* **13**:75–91.

Heuser, J. E. (1976). Morphology of synaptic vesicle discharge and reformation at the frog neuromuscular junction, pp. 51–115 in *Motor Innervation of Muscle*, Thesleff, S., ed. Academic Press, London.

Heuser, J. E. and R. Miledi (1971). Effects of lanthanum ions on function and structure of frog neuromuscular junction, *Proc. R. Soc. London Ser. B* **179**:247–260.

Heuser, J. E. and T. S. Reese (1973). Evidence for recycling of synaptic vesicle membrane during transmitter release at the frog neuromuscular junction, *J. Cell Biol.* **57**:315–344.

Heuser, J. E. and T. S. Reese (1975). Redistribution of intramembranous particles from synaptic vesicles: direct evidence for vesicle recycling, *Anat. Rec.* **181**:374.

Heuser, J. E., T. S. Reese, and D. M. D. Landis (1974). Functional changes in frog neuromuscular junctions studied with freeze-fracture, *J. Neurocytol.* **3**:109–131.

Jan, Y. N., L. Y. Jan, and M. J. Dennis (1977). Two mutations of synaptic transmission in *Drosophila, J. Physiol. (London)*, in press.

Llinás, R. and J. E. Heuser (1977). Depolarization-release coupling systems in neurons. *Neurosci. Res. Prog. Bull.*, in press.

Mandel, T. E. (1972). Intramembranous marker in T-lymphocytes, *Nature (London) New Biol.* **239**:112.

McIntyre, J. A., N. B. Gilula, and M. J. Karnovsky (1974). Cryoprotectant-induced redistribution of intramembranous particles in mouse lymphocytes, *J. Cell Biol.* **60**:192–203.

Pumplin, D. W. and T. S. Reese (1976). Freeze-fracture study of transmitter release at neuromuscular junctions treated with brown widow spider venom, Botulinum toxin, and cation ionophores, *Abstr. Annu. Meet. Soc. Neurosci.*, 6th, Toronto, p. 706.

Rash, J. E., J. E. Warnick, E. X. Albuquerque, and M. H. Ellisman (1976). Freeze-fracture studies of quiescent, stimulated, briefly rested, and toxin-activated rat neuromuscular junctions, *J. Cell Biol.* **70**:303a.

Verklej, A. J., P. H. L. Ververgaert, L. L. M. Van Deenen, and P. F. Elberts (1972). Phase transitions of phospholipid bilayers and membranes of Acholeplasma laidlawii B visualized by freeze-fracturing electron-microscopy, *Biochim. Biophys. Acta* **288**:326–332.

ROLE OF PEPTIDES IN NEURONAL FUNCTION

Substance P and Related Peptides

J. W. Phillis

*College of Medicine, University of Saskatchewan,
Saskatoon, Saskatchewan*

The CNS contains and is able to synthesize a number of pharmacologically active peptides (Zetler, 1970*b*; Barker, 1976). The term "peptidergic neuron" was first applied to the hypothalamic neurons that synthesize the peptides oxytocin and vasopressin (Bargmann, Lindner, and Andres, 1967). The investigators noted that the axons of these neurons not only released hormones into the bloodstream, but also possessed terminals forming specialized neurosecretomotor junctions with epithelial cells of the pars intermedia of the pituitary. Thus arose the concept of peptidergic neurons that could influence target cells through the release of polypeptides at "peptidergic" synapses.

It is now known that a number of active polypeptides are variously distributed throughout the CNS, particularly in neural tissues devoid of morphological evidence of neurosecretory activity (Zetler, 1970*b*). Consideration must therefore be given to extending the term peptidergic neuron to include not only neurosecretory cells, but also other neurons containing polypeptides that may serve either as actual neurotransmitters or as modulators of neuronal activity.

Until recently, little was known about the effects on single neurons of various polypeptides known to exist in the CNS. The recent availability of synthetic peptides, identical to the naturally occurring substances, has acted as a potent stimulus to pharmacological exploration, and this, in conjunction with immunofluorescent histochemical techniques for their localization, has precipitated a flurry of investigations into the biological role of centrally occurring polypeptides.

Substance P was discovered in 1931 by von Euler and Gaddum during a search for active principles in extracts of equine brain and intestine. Intravenous injection of the active material into anesthetized rabbits elicited a transient fall in blood pressure, and also caused contraction of isolated intestine. These actions were distinguishable from those of acetylcholine in that they were not inhibited by atropine. Further experiments revealed that the material was a peptide, and it was given the designation of "Substance P" (Gaddum and Schild, 1934; von Euler, 1936).

The distribution of substance P and its possible physiological role in the nervous system have attracted considerable attention. The work done prior to its final purification and characterization has been reviewed extensively (Zetler, 1970a; Lembeck and Zetler, 1971) and is only outlined briefly here.

A number of workers began attempting to isolate substance P, and considerable effort was directed toward the development of specific and sensitive assay techniques. The methods employed generally involved measurement of the fall in blood pressure in the rabbit or the contraction of isolated organs, such as the guinea pig ileum, rabbit jejunum, estrous uterus of the rat, or rectal cecum of the fowl (Lembeck and Zetler, 1971). Whereas the guinea pig ileum was considered to be the most specific assay, a micromethod using the isolated goldfish gut was particularly sensitive. Attempts to isolate substance P by using these assays yielded a considerable measure of success (Vogler, Haefely, Hürliman, Studer, Lergier, Strässle, and Berneis, 1963; Zuber, 1966; Meinardi and Craig, 1966), but prior to 1970, even the purest preparations were still not homogeneous.

Like its initial discovery, the first complete purification of substance P was fortuitous. While attempting to isolate a corticotropin-releasing factor from bovine hypothalamic extracts, Leeman and her colleagues discovered a peptide that stimulated salivation in anesthetized rats (Leeman and Hammerschlag, 1967). When this sialogogic peptide was purified, it proved to have many similarities to substance P. Lembeck and Starke (1968) had already suggested that the "sialogen" and substance P might be identical, and further studies by Chang and Leeman (1970) established this to be true.

The amino acid sequence in substance P was determined (Chang, Leeman, and Niall, 1971) and a synthetic substance P was prepared (Tregear, Niall, Potts, Leeman, and Chang, 1971). The synthetic peptide had properties identical to the naturally occurring peptide. Synthetic substance P has subsequently been prepared by other groups (Yajima and Kitagawa, 1973; Fisher, Humphries, Folkers, Pernow, and Bowers,

1974). Substance P's isolated from the equine intestine and bovine or feline dorsal roots are identical to the bovine hypothalamic peptide (Studer, Trzeciak, and Lergier, 1973; Takahashi, Konishi, Powell, Leeman, and Otsuka, 1974).

Crude extracts of mammalian tissue containing substance P can be separated into several fractions by aluminum oxide chromatography, each fraction containing biologically active polypeptide material (Zetler, 1961). One fraction, designated Fa, corresponds pharmacologically to substance P; another, designated Fb, can be converted to Fa. Zetler (1970a) has therefore suggested that substance P might be made up of a group of related peptides displaying similar biological activities.

Also present in brain tissue are bradykinin-like peptides, together with the enzymes for their liberation and catabolism (Hori, 1968; Shikimi and Iwata, 1970; Camargo, Ramalho-Pinto, and Greene, 1972; Camargo, Shapanka, and Greene, 1973). Kinin concentrations are highest in the hypothalamus and decrease markedly during fever induced by bacterial pyrogens (Pela, Gardey-Lavassort, Lechat, and Rocha e Silva, 1975). Bradykinin injected intraventricularly causes behavioral, electroencephalographic, and metabolic alterations in various species (Graeff, 1969; Pearson, Lambert, and Lang, 1969; Lambert and Lang, 1970; Corrêa and Graeff, 1974; Melo and Graeff, 1975).

Physalaemin and eledoisin, two peptides of nonmammalian origin, are of interest because of their structural similarities to substance P, which can be readily appreciated from Table 2. The three peptides share a common C-terminal amino acid sequence, -Phe-X-Gly-Leu-Met-NH$_2$, where X is Ile, Tyr, or Phe. Eledoisin was first isolated from the salivary glands of the Mediterranean octopod *Eledone moschata* (Anastasi and Erspamer, 1962), and physalaemin was isolated from skin extracts of various species of the amphibian genus *Physalaemus* (Anastasi, Erspamer, and Cei, 1964). Both peptides have potent hypotensive actions and stimulate contraction of intestinal muscle and salivation (Erspamer, 1971). Thus they share a common spectrum of pharmacological activity with substance P.

Bombesin is a tetradecapeptide from skin extracts of European discoglossid frogs of the genus *Bombina* (Anastasi, Erspamer, and Bucci, 1971). This peptide also has a potent hypotensive action and stimulates contraction of intestinal smooth muscle preparations (Erspamer, 1971).

Distribution of Substance P in the Nervous System

Substance P has been identified in the brain and is localized in the subcellular fraction containing synaptic vesicles (Inouye and Kataoka, 1962; Ryall, 1964; Powell, Leeman, Tregear, Niall, and Potts, 1973; Duffy, Mulhall, and Powell, 1975). An enzyme that inactivates substance P is present in rat brain (Benuck and Marks, 1975). The release of a substance P-like peptide from the feline cerebral cortex has been demonstrated, the rate of release being enhanced by the convulsants picrotoxin and leptazol (Shaw and Ramwell, 1968).

The development of a sensitive and specific radioimmunoassay for the detection and quantification of substance P levels (Powell et al., 1973) has facilitated studies on the distribution of this peptide in the central and peripheral nervous systems. Investigators using either this method or the more recently developed immunohistochemical techniques have confirmed earlier reports on the uneven distribution of substance P in the brain, with the concentrations highest in the basal ganglia, hypothalamus, and substantia nigra (Table 1; Powell et al., 1973; Duffy, Wong, and Powell, 1975; Duffy et al., 1975; Hökfelt, Kellerth, Nilsson, and Pernow, 1975a, b; Mroz, Brownstein, and Leeman, 1976; Hökfelt, Elde, Johansson, Luft, Nilsson, and Arimura, 1976; Hökfelt, Meyerson, Nilsson, Pernow, and Sachs, 1976).

Lembeck (1953) found higher concentrations of substance P in dorsal roots than in ventral roots, and he suggested that it might be the transmitter released at the central terminals of dorsal root fibers.

TABLE 1. *Substance P in human brain*[a]

Area of brain	Sp act μg/g (wet wt)
Frontal cortex	4
Precentral gyrus	3
Occipital cortex	6
Cingulate gyrus	8
Amygdaloid nucleus	18
Caudate nucleus	24
Putamen	36
Globus pallidus	28
Substantia nigra	145
Red nucleus	8
Thalamus	6
Hypothalamus	12
Medulla oblongata	5

[a] From Zetler (1970a).

Consistent with this suggestion is the finding that substance P levels are higher in the dorsal horn than in the ventral horn of rats and cats (Hökfelt et al., 1975a, b; Takahashi and Otsuka, 1975) and that a substance P-like material is released from the amphibian spinal cord by dorsal root stimulation (Angelucci, 1956). Immunohistochemical techniques have demonstrated that substance P-like material is present in small neuronal cell bodies in spinal ganglia and in fine dorsal root and peripheral nerve fibers of cats and rats (Figure 1; Hökfelt et al., 1975a, b). Substance P-positive fibers are also present in the spinal cord, with the highest concentration in laminae I and II of the dorsal horn (Figure 2). In lamina I, fibers run transversely and parallel to the border of the white matter. Some substance P-positive fibers are present in the Lissauer tract and the adjacent part of the lateral funiculus. The substance P in the spinal cord appears to be partly of dorsal root fiber origin, because cutting or constriction of the dorsal roots is followed by a reduction in the amount of peptide in the substantia gelatinosa, but not in the remainder of the spinal cord (Figure 3; Hökfelt et al., 1975a, b; Takahashi and Otsuka, 1975). This finding, taken in conjunction with the accumulation of substance P-like activity in the dorsal roots on the ganglionic side of the constriction (Figure 4), indicates that the material must be transported from the cell body to its terminals in the spinal cord. After ligation of the sciatic nerve, many substance P-positive swollen fibers can be seen central to the ligation, showing that the material is also transported out to the periphery (Hökfelt et al., 1975a, b). These fibers appear to be unmyelinated. In the skin, substance P is found in free nerve endings. Although the rate of transport has not been determined, the material accumulates within 24 h, suggesting that it is moved by a rapid transport mechanism. In peripheral nerves, unlike the brain, the peptide is most highly concentrated in the microsomal rather than the synaptic vesicle fraction (von Euler and Lishajko, 1961).

Actions of Substance P on Central Neurons

A functional role for substance P in the spinal cord is suggested by its pharmacological actions. Initially, a reduction in polysynaptic reflexes after intravenous administration of a substance P-containing preparation was reported (Stern and Dobrič, 1957). More recently, excitant actions of pure synthetic or extracted substance P have been described on in vitro amphibian or neonatal rat spinal cord preparations (Konishi and Otsuka, 1974a, b; Otsuka and Konishi, 1976). The excitatory effects

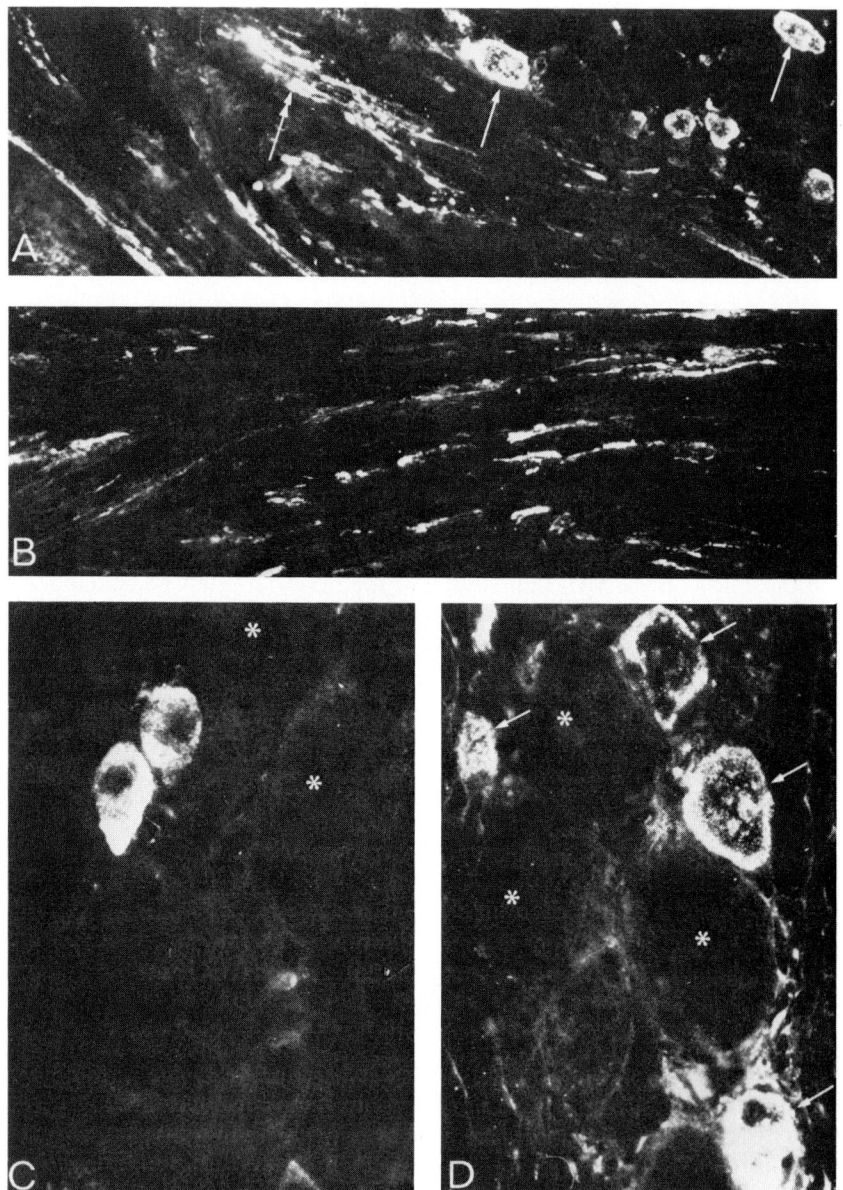

of topically applied substance P, physalaemin, and eledoisin were compared with those of L-glutamate, another putative neurotransmitter that has been proposed to mediate the primary afferent input. The three peptides depolarized spinal cord motor neurons (Figure 5), and their effects persisted when synaptic transmission in the spinal cord was blocked by reducing calcium in the perfusion medium or by tetrodotoxin, indicating that they act directly on the motoneurons rather than through a presynaptic mechanism that releases some other excitatory agent. Substance P was considerably more potent than glutamate as an excitant on a molar concentration basis (Konishi and Otsuka, 1974a).

Iontophoretically applied, substance P excited about 50% of the cells tested in the spinal cord and cuneate nucleus (Krnjević and Morris, 1974; Henry, Krnjević, and Morris, 1975). Typically, the discharge rate of the excited neurons began to accelerate 10 to 30 sec after the onset of the application of substance P, slowly reached maximum, and decayed slowly once the application had ceased. This was in marked contrast to the excitant action of glutamate, which had a short latency and which ceased within a few seconds of the termination of the application. Substance P excitation was observed with a variety of dorsal horn neurons, including many that responded with a short latency to cutaneous sensory activation. Depressant actions of substance P were also observed on non-spontaneously firing neurons activated by applications of glutamate.

Neurons that respond to noxious thermal cutaneous stimulation are excited by substance P or bradykinin, and it has been suggested that both peptides are involved in the transmission of nociceptive information (Henry, 1976; Randić and Yu, 1976).

Intracellular recordings from motoneurons during the extracellular ejection of substance P have shed some light on the mechanism of excitation by this agent. Substance P caused a progressive depolariza-

---

FIGURE 1. Substance P-like immunofluorescence micrographs of cat spinal ganglia (L7) after compression of the dorsal roots close to the ganglion (A through C) or after local application of colchicine (D). Some small-sized cell bodies exhibit a positive immunofluorescent reaction localized mainly in the peripheral part of the cytoplasm. Note that large-sized cell bodies (asterisks) are negative. Within the ganglion (A), and in the most proximal part of the dorsal root (B), accumulations of substance P-like immunofluorescence are found. (A) ×200; (B) ×250; (C) and (D) ×400. Reproduced with permission from Hökfelt et al. (1975b).

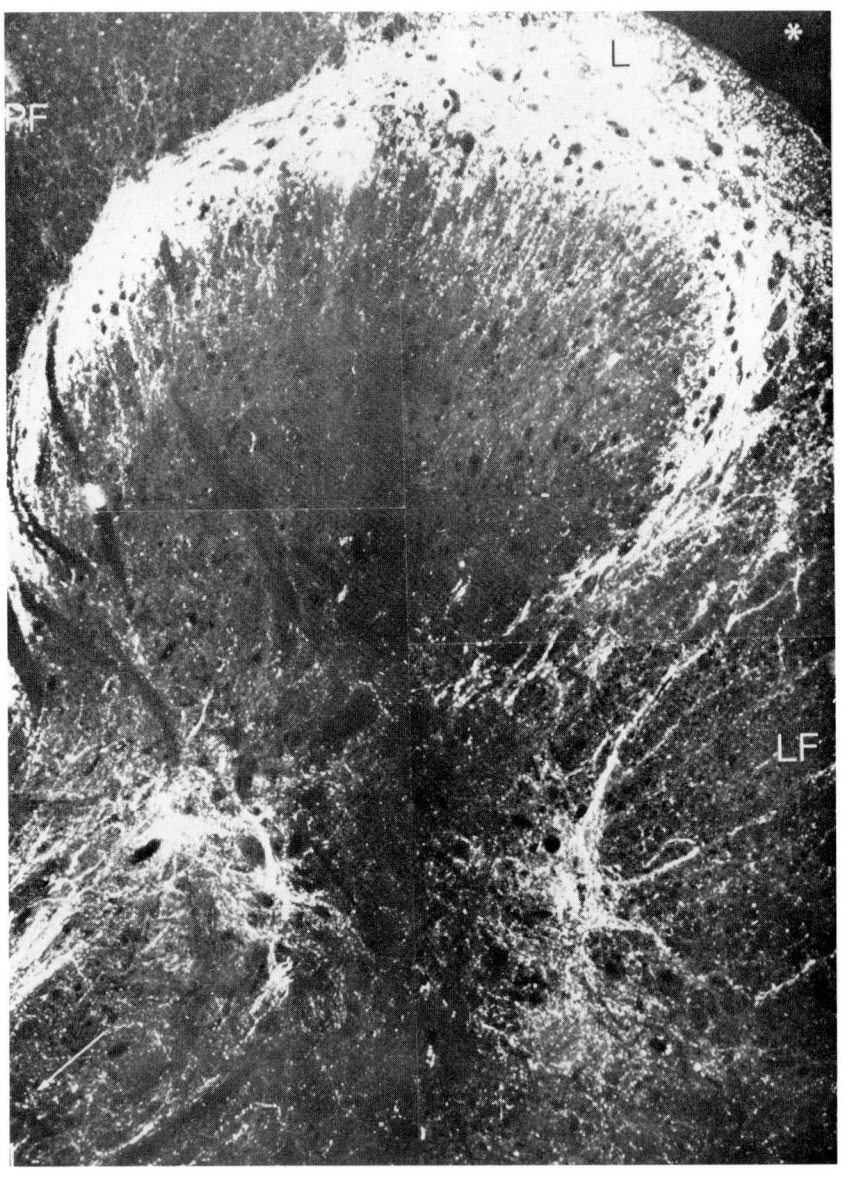

tion that was slowly reversed after cessation of the iontophoretic application pulse (Krnjević, 1976). The depolarization, which was associated with an increase in membrane resistance, had a reversal potential more negative than the resting potential, indicating that its generation may involve a reduction in membrane potassium conductance.

Iontophoretically applied substance P has been tested on neurons in the mesencephalic reticular formation, substantia nigra, and cerebral cortex (Walker, Kemp, Yajima, Kitagawa, and Woodruff, 1976; Davies and Dray, 1976a; Phillis and Limacher, 1974a, b). Excitation was the predominant response in each area, although some examples of depression were observed in the substantia nigra and cerebral cortex. The latencies for onset of excitation were frequently shorter than those reported in the spinal cord, although still greater than with glutamate.

Substance P is the most potent excitant polypeptide yet tested on cerebral cortical neurons. Excitation frequently occurred with a latency of 7 to 15 sec and often continued for 1 min or more after termination of the application (Phillis and Limacher, 1974a, b). Both identified (corticospinal) and unidentified neurons were found to be excited, but responsive neurons shared the common property of being spontaneously active. No excitant effects were seen on non-spontaneously active glutamate-fired cells. Many of the units that were excited by substance P were also excited by acetylcholine, prompting consideration of a possible relationship between peptide sensitivity and acetylcholine sensitivity, including the possibility that peptides have a presynaptic action evoking release of acetylcholine. Locally applied atropine abolished the actions of acetylcholine, but not those of the polypeptides (Figure 6), clearly establishing that the effects of the peptides are independent of an action either on cholinergic presynaptic terminals or on the acetylcholine receptors themselves. Nerve terminals containing a substance P-like peptide have been observed in the cerebral cortex

---

FIGURE 2. Substance P-like immunofluorescence in the dorsal horn of the spinal cord of a cat (S1). Note the dense fluorescent plexus in the Lissauer fasciculus and in laminae I through III, extending ventrally along the white matter and joining in the laminae V and VI (×160). Abbreviations: L, the Lissauer fasciculus; LF, lateral fasciculus; PF, posterior fasciculus. Asterisk indicates surface of the spinal cord. Arrow points to the central canal. Reproduced with permission from Hökfelt et al. (1975b).

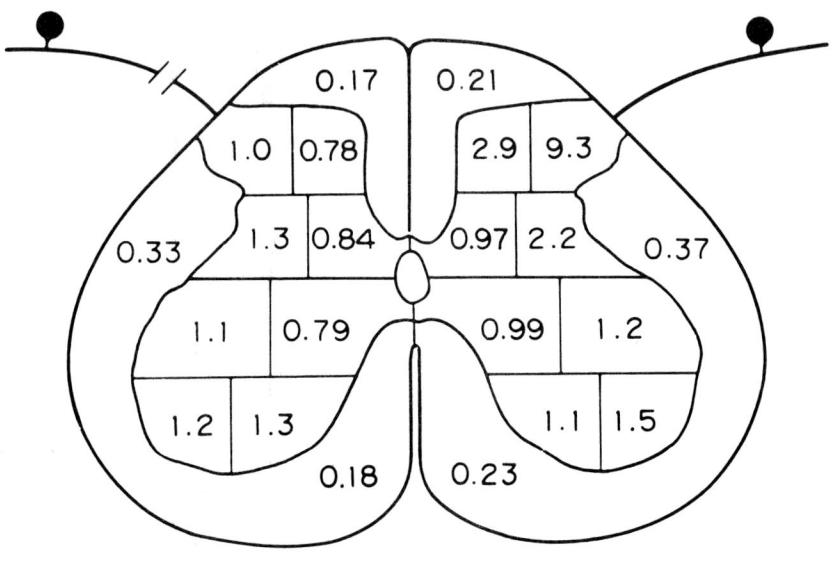

FIGURE 3. Distribution of substance P in the spinal cord (L5-S1) of a cat, 11 days after a unilateral section of the dorsal roots (below L5). Numbers in the figure indicate the concentration of substance P given in 10^{-10} mole/g (wet weight). Reproduced with permission from Takahashi and Otsuka (1975).

(Hökfelt et al., 1976). Substance P may therefore function as an excitatory transmitter or modulator on cerebral cortical neurons.

Actions of Other Peptides and Analogues of Substance P

Substance P was the most potent of the excitant polypeptides tested on cerebral cortical neurons, physalaemin (Figure 7) and bradykinin being next in potency, followed by eledoisin and bombesin (Table 2). Iontophoretically applied angiotensin II had only a weak excitant action (Phillis and Limacher, 1974a, b). Insulin, a polypeptide of far greater complexity, also had weak excitant actions on cerebral cortical neurons (Figure 8).

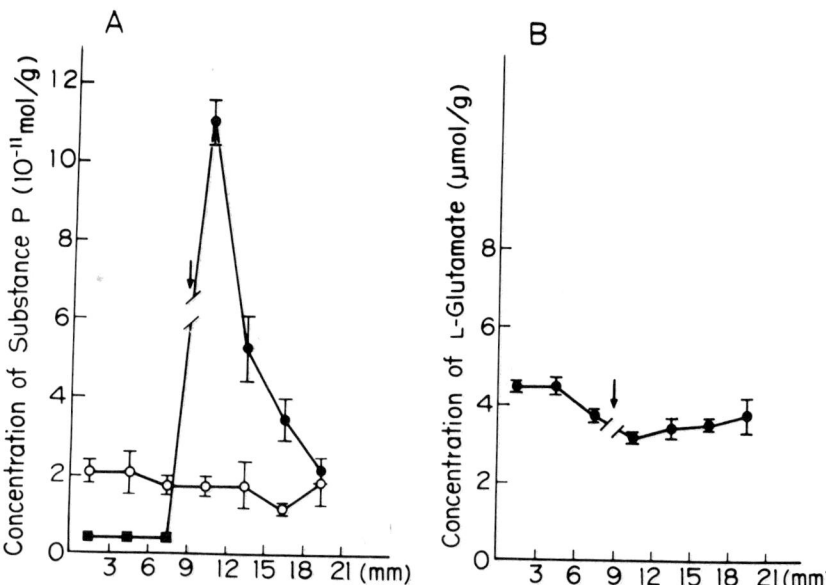

FIGURE 4. Distribution of substance P and L-glutamate in ligated and intact dorsal roots. Ordinate: concentration of substance P in (A), and that of glutamate in (B). Abscissa: distance from the entry of the dorsal root into the cord. Site of ligation is indicated by arrows. Each point and vertical line represents mean ± SEM obtained from three determinations derived from three animals in (A), and two determinations derived from two animals in (B). Symbols: ●, substance P and L-glutamate in the ligated dorsal roots; ○, substance P in the intact roots; and ■, threshold value of assay for substance P. Reproduced with permission from Takahashi and Otsuka (1975).

Physalaemin and eledoisin are the most potent excitants on the in vitro amphibian spinal cord, the latter being approximately one order of magnitude more active than substance P on a molar concentration ratio. Bradykinin and angiotensin are less potent than substance P (Konishi and Otsuka, 1974b, and their excitant action is abolished in a calcium-free perfusion solution or by tetrodotoxin (procedures that do not affect the depolarizations evoked by physalaemin, eledoisin, or substance P). It appears, therefore, that bradykinin and angiotensin have an indirect action on motoneurons: they probably function by activating interneurons, thus inducing the release of an excitatory transmitter from nerve terminals on the motoneurons.

These studies showed that the structural requirement for a motoneuron-depolarizing action of a peptide is especially rigorous at the

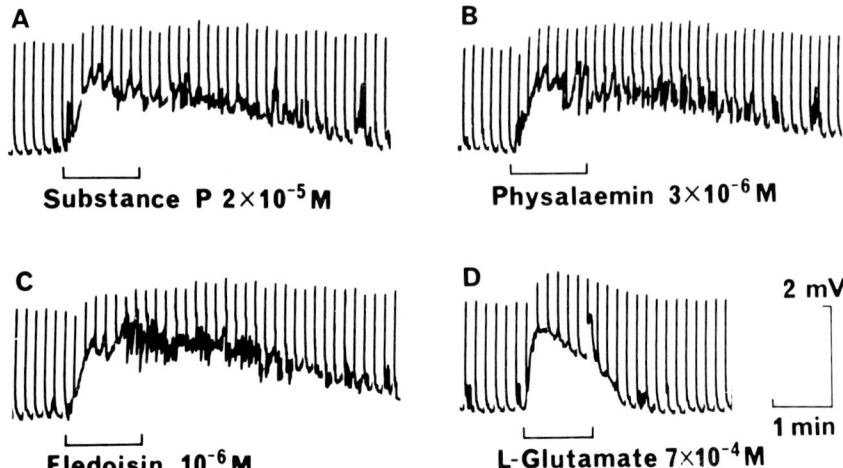

FIGURE 5. Effects of substance P, physalaemin, eledoisin, and L-glutamate on the isolated spinal cord of the frog (*Rana catesbeiana*). Potential changes generated in motoneurons were recorded from the eighth ventral root. Drugs were applied in the bath during the periods indicated in the figure. The corresponding dorsal root was stimulated maximally at the rate of 0.1 Hz. Direct current recording. Depolarization upwards. Reproduced with permission from Konishi and Otsuka (1974b).

C-terminal sequence of the peptide chain, raising the possibility that substance P might be only a precursor, which must first be transformed to an active peptide by removal of some N-terminal amino acids before it can have its excitatory effect. To test this hypothesis, Konishi and Otsuka (1974a) tested a series of shorter C-terminal substance P analogues for their depolarizing activities on in vitro rat spinal cords (Table 3). Deca-, nona-, and octapeptides were about as potent as the undecapeptide substance P. Penta-, tetra-, and tripeptides were practically inactive, but two analogues, a hepta- and hexapeptide, were several times more active than substance P. It is possible, therefore, that substance P may act at a receptor that is normally activated by an endogenously released hepta- or hexapeptide.

Antagonism of Substance P: Lioresal (Baclofen)

The centrally acting muscle relaxant Lioresal (Baclofen, β-chlorophenyl-GABA) has been reported by Saito, Konishi, and Otsuka (1975) to selectively antagonize the excitant effects of substance P in the rat spinal cord. Lioresal also blocks excitatory postsynaptic

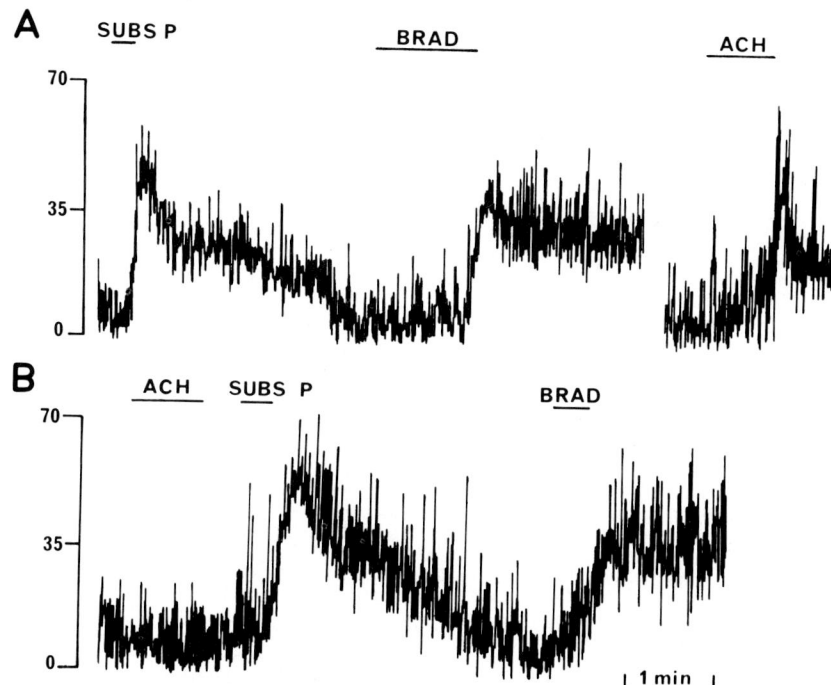

FIGURE 6. Ratemeter records from a cerebral cortical Betz cell (depth 1183 μm, antidromic invasion latency 1.8 msec). (A) Substance P (SUBS P; 50 nA), bradykinin (BRAD; 60 nA), and ACh (70 nA) excited the cell. Because of the very long duration of the excitation by bradykinin, the recording was interrupted for 7 min before testing the ACh. (B) After atropine (60 nA for 1 min), the action of ACh was abolished, but the actions of substance P and bradykinin were not. The ordinate shows firing rate in impulses per second, whereas the horizontal bars above the ratemeter tracings indicate the periods of drug application. Reproduced with permission from Phillis and Limacher (1974a).

potentials evoked by dorsal root stimulation, but the resting potential and antidromic action potential are not affected appreciably. This evidence was interpreted as support for the hypothesis that substance P or a closely related peptide is a sensory transmitter released by spinal dorsal root fibers.

Iontophoretic experiments have failed to provide support for the claim that Lioresal is a specific substance P antagonist. In experiments on cerebral cortical neurons, Lioresal antagonized substance P and acetylcholine-induced excitations to a comparable extent, although

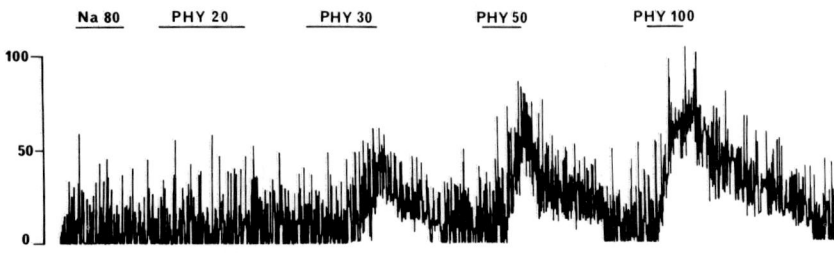

FIGURE 7. Excitation of a spontaneously active cortical neuron by increasing applications of physalaemin (PHY). Control current (80 nA) passed through a NaCl-containing barrel that had no effect. Reproduced with permission from Phillis and Limacher (1974a).

glutamate-evoked depolarizations were less affected (Figure 9). Spontaneous activity was also depressed (Phillis, 1976). The conclusion that Lioresal is not a specific substance P antagonist, but rather that it has a direct depressant action, is supported by iontophoretic

TABLE 2. *Responses of cortical neurons to various polypeptides*[a]

| | Unidentified cells | | | | | Betz cells | |
| | Non-spontaneously active | | Spontaneously active | | | | |
Polypeptide	Excitation	Nil	Excitation	Depression	Nil	Excitation	Nil
Angiotensin II	0	1	1 (7%)	0	13	4 (33%)	8
Bombesin	0	22	19 (56%)	3	12	11 (50%)	11
Bradykinin	0	35	47 (76%)	0	15	38 (91%)	4
Eledoisin	0	21	10 (26%)	6	22	29 (88%)	4
Eledoisin-related peptide	0	4	3 (30%)	0	7	14 (67%)	7
Physalaemin	0	37	59 (91%)	1	5	12 (71%)	5
Substance P	0	8	62 (91%)	0	6	29 (94%)	2

[a] Amino acid sequences:

Angiotensin II: Asp-Arg-Val-Tyr-Ile-His-Pro-Phe
Bombesin: Pyr-Glu-Arg-Leu-Gly-Asn-Gln-Trp-Ala-Gly-His-Leu-Met-NH_2
Bradykinin: Arg-Pro-Pro-Gly-Phe-Ser-Pro-Phe-Arg
Eledoisin: Pyr-Pro-Ser-Lys-Asp-Ala-Phe-Ile-Gly-Leu-Met-NH_2
Eledoisin-related peptide: Lys-Phe-Ile-Gly-Leu-Met-NH_2
Physalaemin: Pyr-Ala-Asp-Pro-Asn-Lys-Phe-Tyr-Gly-Leu-Met-NH_2
Substance P: Arg-Pro-Lys-Pro-Gln-Gln-Phe-Phe-Gly-Leu-Met-NH_2

From Phillis and Limacher (1974b).

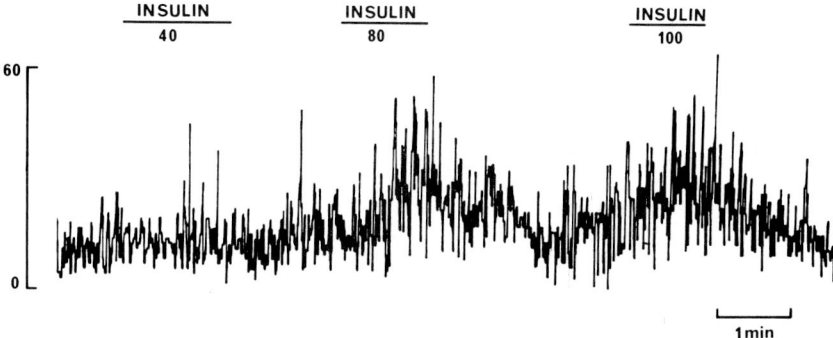

FIGURE 8. Ratemeter recording from a spontaneously active corticospinal neuron. Insulin applied by currents of 40, 80, and then 100 nA evoked increasing amounts of excitation. Control Na^+ expelling currents passed through a NaCl-containing barrel that did not affect the firing rate of this neuron.

experiments on neurons in the spinal cord and substantia nigra (Curtis, Game, Johnston, and McCulloch, 1974; Davies and Watkins, 1974; Davies and Dray, 1976a; Puil, Krnjević, and Werman, 1976). Experiments on ganglia and guinea pig ileum have also failed to reveal any specific antagonism of substance P by Lioresal (Fotherby, Morrish, and Ryall, 1976).

Substance P—Is It a Transmitter of Primary Sensory Neurons?

Substance P meets many of the requirements for consideration as a transmitter released by primary sensory neurons. It is present in higher

TABLE 3. *Relative potencies of substance P and its shorter analogues in depolarizing rat spinal motor neurons*[a]

Peptide	Relative potency (substance P = 1)
H-Arg-Pro-Lys-Pro-Gln-Gln-Phe-Phe-Gly-Leu-Met-NH_2	1
H———Pro-Lys-Pro-Gln-Gln-Phe-Phe-Gly-Leu-Met-NH_2	0.6–0.9
H————Lys-Pro-Gln-Gln-Phe-Phe-Gly-Leu-Met-NH_2	0.4–1
H—————Pro-Gln-Gln-Phe-Phe-Gly-Leu-Met-NH_2	0.8–1
H——————PCA^b-Gln-Phe-Phe-Gly-Leu-Met-NH_2	2–12
H———————PCA-Phe-Phe-Gly-Leu-Met-NH_2	5–12
H————————Phe-Phe-Gly-Leu-Met-NH_2	<0.02
H—————————Phe-Gly-Leu-Met-NH_2	<0.0002
H——————————Gly-Leu-Met-NH_2	<0.00008

[a] From Otsuka and Konishi (1976).
[b] PCA, Pyrrolidone carboxylic acid.

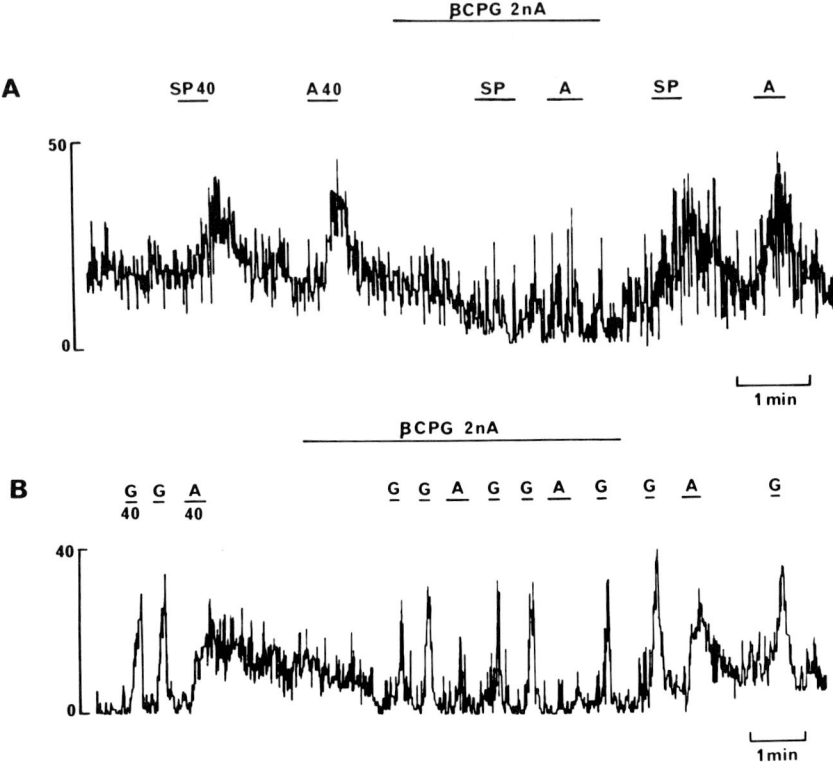

FIGURE 9. (A) Ratemeter recording of the firing of a single corticospinal neuron. Substance P (SP, 40 nA) and acetylcholine (A, 40 nA) excitation of this neuron, as well as its spontaneous discharge, were substantially depressed during the application of β-chlorophenyl-GABA (β-CPG, 2 nA). Recovery occurred rapidly once the β-CPG application was terminated. Periods of drug application are indicated by the horizontal bars above the trace. The ordinate is calibrated in spikes per second. (B) Ratemeter recording of an unidentified cortical neuron. Acetylcholine (A, 40 nA) and L-glutamate (G, 40 nA) excited this cell. During the application of β-CPG, ACh excitation, but not that evoked by L-glutamate, was antagonized. Recovery of the ACh response is apparent shortly after the termination of the β-CPG application. Reproduced with permission from Phillis (1976).

concentration (1,000 times) in dorsal root than in ventral root fibers, and in these roots it is present in unmyelinated fibers arising from small dorsal root ganglion cells. It is transported from these cells toward nerve terminals in the spinal cord, and after dorsal root transection or ligation, the levels of substance P in the spinal cord are markedly reduced.

Subcellular fractionation studies on CNS tissues have shown that it is concentrated in the nerve ending particles.

However, when applied iontophoretically onto neurons in the spinal cord, substance P has a rather prolonged action, with a slow onset of excitation, and studies on motoneurons have revealed that this is generated by a depolarization associated with a decrease in membrane conductance. These actions of substance P are rather different from those that characterize the monosynaptic depolarizing excitatory postsynaptic potential generated in spinal neurons by primary afferent fibers. In motoneurons, these EPSPs have an extremely brief time course, which is sometimes associated with an increase in membrane conductance and a reversal level that is more positive than the resting membrane potential (Rall, Burke, Smith, Nelson, and Frank, 1967; Jack, Miller, Porter, and Redman, 1971). (The lack of clear conductance changes or a reversal level for some EPSPs recorded from motoneurons has been ascribed to a possible component of electrical transmission.) Primary afferent activation of interneurons in the spinal cord has been less extensively explored, but the responses are also associated with a short-latency excitatory action of short duration.

Thus, the excitant action of substance P appears to have only a superficial resemblance to that of the synaptic transmitter released by the primary afferents. The excitatory amino acids, L-glutamic and L-aspartic acids, have actions that appear to be more comparable to those of the primary afferent transmitter.

If primary afferent fibers can release more than one transmitter, it is possible that substance P could be released in addition to the rapidly acting mediator. A system of dual transmitters could be of special significance in those pathways in which repetitive stimulation causes a slow increase in the level of excitability of the postsynaptic pool of neurons. Slowly increasing excitation and prolonged after-discharge are features of the excitation evoked by high-threshold (nociceptive) afferents to the spinal cord, and are characteristic of the changes in motoneuronal excitability during the flexor reflex (Hunt and Perl, 1960; Mendell, 1966; Handwerker, Iggo, and Zimmerman, 1975).

An involvement of substance P in transmission along nociceptive pathways is also suggested by behavioral studies on mice. Synthetic substance P was found to be a potent analgesic, and its action was abolished by the morphine antagonist naloxone (Stewart, Getto, Nelder, Reeve, Krivoy, and Zimmerman, 1976). Cross-tolerance with morphine was evident in these experiments. Stern and Hadzović (1973) had previously shown that synthetic substance P can abolish the abstinence syndrome in morphinized mice. A possible interpretation for these findings is that substance P (or a shorter-chain-length fragment) may activate a peptidergic receptor that also serves as the opiate receptor. Such a possibility is supported by the finding of a marked overlap in the distribution of immunohistochemical substance P-like activity (Hökfelt et al., 1975a,b) and opiate receptors (LaMotte, Pert, and Snyder, 1976) in the substantia gelatinosa. Opiate receptors are known to interact with the pentapeptides met- and leu-enkephalin, which are currently thought to act as endogenous morphinomimetic agents (Hughes, Smith, Kosterlitz, Fothergill, Morgan, and Morris, 1975; Kosterlitz and Hughes, 1975). Excitant actions of iontophoretically applied morphine and enkephalin on acetylcholine-excited neurons in the spinal cord, brain stem, and thalamus have been reported (Davies and Dray, 1976b; Duggan, Davies, and Hall, 1976). These excitant effects were reversibly reduced by the narcotic antagonist naloxone. Further investigation of the effects of substance P-like and enkephalin-like peptides on the same spinal neurons will be required to clarify the relationships between the actions of these two groups of compounds.

A further role for substance P in sensory transmission may be implied by its presence in peripheral nerve terminals. Lembeck (1953) proposed that substance P mediates the phenomenon of antidromic vasodilation, and more recently Juan and Lembeck (1974) have shown that extracted preparations of this peptide were the most potent agents tested in causing excitation of sensory afferents in an isolated perfused rabbit ear preparation. Synthetic substance P does not possess this algesic action (Juan and Lembeck, 1974; Stewart et al., 1976), which must therefore be attributed to the presence of other kinins in the extracted material.

The role of substance P at higher levels of the CNS is even less apparent than in the spinal cord. However, it is clear that substance P-like peptides are widely distributed throughout the brain, and these findings, in conjunction with numerous reports of pharmacological actions in the brain, indicate that peptides may act as transmitters or modulators of neuronal excitability at higher levels of the neural axis.

CONCLUSIONS

Substance P-like activity is found widely distributed in nerve fibers throughout the central and peripheral nervous systems. Small neurons in the dorsal root ganglia contain a substance P-like material that is transported away from the cell bodies along both the dorsal roots and peripheral nerves. The levels of substance P in the most dorsal laminae of the spinal grey matter are dependent on the integrity of the dorsal root afferents, and decrease quite markedly after section of the dorsal roots. Substance P-containing fibers have been visualized in higher centers of the neural axis, including the cerebral cortex.

Substance P and structurally related peptides have a potent excitant action on neurons in the spinal cord, cuneate nucleus, mesencephalon, and cerebral cortex. On motoneurons, the underlying depolarization is associated with an increase in membrane resistance, and may be due to a decrease in potassium permeability. It has been argued that the time course of the excitation makes it unlikely that substance P is the rapidly acting transmitter released by dorsal root afferents. It is possible, therefore, that substance P may be released together with a rapidly acting transmitter, and that its role may be to modulate cell excitability. An alternative possibility is that substance P released by a small proportion of dorsal root afferents may set the level of responsiveness of spinal neurons to more rapidly acting transmitters released by other afferents. This may also be the function of substance P-releasing neurons at higher levels of the neural axis.

Recent publications suggest that substance P may be able to activate opiate receptors in the CNS, and further experiments on the interrelationships between the substance P-like peptides and the newly discovered enkephalins are obviously needed.

ACKNOWLEDGMENTS

The support of the Canadian Medical Research Council is gratefully acknowledged.

REFERENCES

Anastasi, A. and V. Erspamer (1962). Occurrence and some properties of eledoisin in extracts of posterior salivary glands of *Eledone, Br. J. Pharmacol. Chemother.* **19**:326–336.

Anastasi, A., V. Erspamer, and M. Bucci (1971). Isolation and structure of bombesin and alytesin, two analogous active peptides from the skin of the European amphibians *Bombina* and *Alytes, Experientia* **27**:166–167.

Anastasi, A., V. Erspamer, and J. M. Cei (1964). Isolation and amino acid sequence of physalaemin, the main active polypeptide of the skin of *Physalaemus fuscumaculatus, Arch. Biochem. Biophys.* **108**:341–348.

Angelucci, L. (1956). Experiments with perfused frog's spinal cord, *Br. J. Pharmacol. Chemother.* **11**:161–170.

Bargmann, W., E. Lindner, and K. H. Andres (1967). Uber Synapsen an endokrinen Epithelzellen und die Definition sekretorischer Neurone. Untersuchungen am Zwischenlappen der Katzenhypophyse, *Z. Zellforsch.* **77**:282–298.

Barker, J. L. (1976). Peptides: roles in neuronal excitability, *Physiol. Rev.* **56**:435–452.

Benuck, M. and N. Marks (1975). Enzymatic inactivation of substance P by a partially purified enzyme from rat brain, *Biochem. Biophys. Res. Commun.* **65**:153–160.

Camargo, A. C. M., F. J. Ramalho-Pinto, and L. J. Greene (1972). Brain peptidases: conversion and inactivation of kinin hormones, *J. Neurochem.* **19**:37–49.

Camargo, A. C. M., R. Shapanka, and L. J. Greene (1973). Preparation, assay and partial characterization of a neutral endopeptidase from rabbit brain, *Biochemistry* **12**:1838–1844.

Chang, M. M. and S. E. Leeman (1970). Isolation of a sialogogic peptide from bovine hypothalamic tissue and its characterization as substance P, *J. Biol. Chem.* **245**:4784–4790.

Chang, M. M., S. E. Leeman, and H. D. Niall (1971). Amino acid sequence of substance P, *Nature (London) New Biol.* **232**:86–87.

Corrêa, F. M. A. and F. G. Graeff (1974). Central mechanism of the hypertensive action of intraventricular bradykinin in the unanaesthetized rat, *Neuropharmacology* **13**:65–76.

Curtis, D. R., C. J. A. Game, G. A. R. Johnston, and R. M. McCulloch (1974). Central effects of β-(p-chlorophenyl)-γ-aminobutyric acid, *Brain Res.* **70**:493–499.

Davies, J. and A. Dray (1976a). Substance P in the substantia nigra, *Brain Res.* **107**:623–627.

Davies, J. and A. Dray (1976b). Actions of enkephalin and morphine on spinal cord and brain stem neurones, *Br. J. Pharmacol.* **58**:458–459 P.

Davies, J. and J. C. Watkins (1974). The action of β-phenyl-GABA derivatives on neurones of the cat cerebral cortex, *Brain Res.* **70**:501–505.

Duffy, M. J., D. Mulhall, and D. Powell (1975). Subcellular distribution of substance P in bovine hypothalamus and substantia nigra, *J. Neurochem.* **25**:305–307.

Duffy, M. J., J. Wong, and D. Powell (1975). Stimulation of adenylate cyclase activity in different areas of human brain by substance P, *Neuropharmacology* **14**:615–618.

Duggan, A. W., J. Davies, and J. G. Hall (1976). Effects of opiate agonists and antagonists on central neurons of the cat, *J. Pharmacol. Exp. Ther.* **196**:107–120.

Erspamer, V. (1971). Biogenic amines and active polypeptides of the amphibian skin, *Annu. Rev. Pharmacol.* **11**:327–350.

Fisher, G. H., J. Humphries, K. Folkers, B. Pernow, and C. Y. Bowers (1974). Synthesis and some biological activities of substance P, *J. Med. Chem.* **17**:843–846.

Fotherby, K. J., N. J. Morrish, and R. W. Ryall (1976). Is Lioresal (Baclofen) an antagonist of substance P? *Brain Res.* **113**:210–213.

Gaddum, J. H. and H. Schild (1934). Depressor substances in extracts of intestine, *J. Physiol. (London)* **83**:1–14.

Graeff, F. G. (1969). Behavioural and somatic effects of bradykinin injected into the cerebral ventricles of unanaesthetized rabbits, *Br. J. Pharmacol.* **37**:723–732.

Handwerker, H. O., A. Iggo, and M. Zimmerman (1975). Segmental and supraspinal actions on dorsal horn neurons responding to noxious and non-noxious skin stimuli, *Pain* **1**:147–165.

Henry, J. L. (1976). Responses of dorsal horn units in cat spinal cord to some putative transmitters and to cutaneous stimulation, *Br. J. Pharmacol.* **57**:435P.

Henry, J. L., K. Krnjević, and M. E. Morris (1975). Substance P and spinal neurones, *Can. J. Physiol. Pharmacol.* **53**:423–432.

Hökfelt, T., R. Elde, O. Johansson, R. Luft, G. Nilsson, and A. Arimura (1976). Immunohistochemical evidence for separate populations of somatostatin-containing and substance P-containing primary afferent neurons in the rat, *Neuroscience* **1**:131–136.

Hökfelt, T., J. O. Kellerth, G. Nilsson, and B. Pernow (1975a). Substance P: localization in the central nervous system and in some primary sensory neurons, *Science* **190**:889–890.

Hökfelt, T., J. O. Kellerth, G. Nilsson, and B. Pernow (1975b). Experimental immunohistochemical studies on the localization and distribution of substance P in cat primary sensory neurones, *Brain Res.* **100**:234–252.

Hökfelt, T., B. Meyerson, G. Nilsson, B. Pernow, and C. Sachs (1976). Immunohistochemical evidence for substance P-containing nerve endings in the human cortex, *Brain Res.* **104**:181–186.

Hori, S. (1968). The presence of bradykinin-like polypeptide, kinin-releasing and destroying activity in brain, *Jpn. J. Physiol.* **18**:772–787.

Hughes, J., T. W. Smith, H. W. Kosterlitz, L. A. Fothergill, B. A. Morgan, and H. R. Morris (1975). Identification of two related pentapeptides from the brain with potent opiate agonist activity, *Nature (London)* **258**:577–579.

Hunt, C. C. and E. R. Perl (1960). Spinal mechanisms concerned with skeletal muscle, *Physiol. Rev.* **40**:538–579.

Inouye, A. and K. Kataoka (1962). Sub-cellular distribution of the substance P in the nervous tissues, *Nature (London)* **193**:585.

Jack, J. J. B., S. Miller, R. Porter, and S. J. Redman (1971). The time course of minimal excitatory post-synaptic potentials evoked in spinal motoneurones by group Ia afferent fibers, *J. Physiol. (London)* **215**:353–380.

Juan, H. and F. Lembeck (1974). Action of peptides and other algesic agents on paravascular pain receptors of the isolated perfused rabbit ear, *Naunyn-Schmiedebergs Arch. Pharmakol.* **283**:151–164.

Konishi, S. and M. Otsuka (1974a). Excitatory action of hypothalamic substance P on spinal motoneurones of newborn rats, *Nature (London)* **252**:734–735.

Konishi, S. and M. Otsuka (1974b). The effects of substance P and other peptides on spinal neurons of the frog, *Brain Res.* **65**:397–410.

Kosterlitz, H. W. and J. Hughes (1975). Some thoughts on the significance of enkephalin, the endogenous ligand, *Life Sci.* **17**:91–96.

Krnjević, K. (1976). Effects of substance P on central neurons in cats, in *Substance P*, von Euler, U. S. and B. Pernow, eds. Raven Press, New York, in press.

Krnjević, K. and M. E. Morris (1974). An excitatory action of substance P on cuneate neurones, *Can. J. Physiol. Pharmacol.* **52**:736–744.

Lambert, G. A. and W. J. Lang (1970). The effects of bradykinin and eledoisin injected into the cerebral ventricles of conscious rats, *Eur. J. Pharmacol.* **9**:383–386.

LaMotte, C., C. B. Pert, and S. H. Snyder (1976). Opiate receptor binding in primate spinal cord: distribution and changes after dorsal root section, *Brain Res.* **112**:407–412.

Leeman, S. E. and R. Hammerschlag (1967). Stimulation of salivary secretion by a factor extracted from hypothalamic tissue, *Endocrinology* **81**:803–810.

Lembeck, F. (1953). Zur Frage der zentralen Übertragung afferenter Impulse. III. Das Vorkommen und die Bedeutung der Substanz P in der dorsalen Wurzeln des Rückenmarks, *Arch. Exp. Pathol. Pharmakol.* **219**:197–213.

Lembeck, F. and K. Starke (1968). Substanz P und Speichelsekretion, *Naunyn-Schmiedebergs Arch. Pharmakol.* **259**:375–385.

Lembeck, F. and G. Zetler (1971). Substance P, pp. 29–71 in *International Encyclopedia of Pharmacology and Therapeutics,* Walker, J. M., ed. Pergamon Press, Oxford.

Meinardi, H. and L. C. Craig (1966). Studies on substance P, pp. 594–607 in *Hypotensive Peptides*, Erdos, E. G., N. Back, and F. Sicuteri, eds. Springer-Verlag, New York.

Melo, J. C. and F. G. Graeff (1975). Effect of intracerebroventricular bradykinin and related peptides on rabbit operant behavior, *J. Pharmacol. Exp. Ther.* **193**:1–10.

Mendell, L. M. (1966). Physiological properties of unmyelinated fiber projection to the spinal cord, *Exp. Neurol.* **16**:316–332.

Mroz, E. A., M. J. Brownstein, and S. E. Leeman (1976). Evidence for substance P in the habenulo-interpeduncular tract, *Brain Res.* **113**:597–599.

Otsuka, M. and S. Konishi (1976). Substance P and excitatory transmitters of primary sensory neurons, *Cold Spring Harbor Symp. Quant. Biol.* **40**:135–143.

Pearson, L., G. A. Lambert, and W. J. Lang (1969). Centrally mediated cardiovascular and EEG responses to bradykinin and eledoisin, *Eur. J. Pharmacol.* **8**:153–158.

Pela, I. R., C. Gardey-Lavassort, P. Lechat, and M. Rocha e Silva (1975). Brain kinins and fever induced by bacterial pyrogens in rabbits, *J. Pharm. Pharmacol.* **27**:793–794.

Phillis, J. W. (1976). Is β-(4-chlorophenyl)-GABA a specific antagonist of substance P on cerebral cortical neurons? *Experientia* **32**:593–594.

Phillis, J. W. and J. J. Limacher (1974a). Substance P excitation of cerebral cortical Betz cells, *Brain Res.* **69**:158–163.

Phillis, J. W. and J. J. Limacher (1974b). Excitation of cerebral cortical neurons by various polypeptides, *Exp. Neurol.* **43**:414–423.

Powell, D., S. E. Leeman, G. W. Tregear, H. D. Niall, and J. T. Potts (1973). Radioimmunoassay for substance P, *Nature (London) New Biol.* **241**:252–254.

Puil, E., K. Krnjević, and R. Werman (1976). Effects of Lioresal on cat motoneurons, *Fed. Proc.* **35**:307.

Rall, W., R. E. Burke, T. G. Smith, P. G. Nelson, and K. Frank (1967). Dendritic location of synapses and possible mechanisms for the monosynaptic EPSP in motoneurons, *J. Neurophysiol.* **30**:1169–1193.

Randić, M. and H. H. Yu (1976). Effects of 5-hydroxytryptamine and bradykinin in cat dorsal horn neurones activated by noxious stimuli, *Brain Res.* **11**:197–203.

Ryall, R. W. (1964). The subcellular distributions of acetylcholine, Substance P, 5-hydroxytryptamine, γ-aminobutyric acid and glutamic acid in brain homogenates, *J. Neurochem.* **11**:131–145.

Saito, K., S. Konishi, and M. Otsuka (1975). Antagonism between Lioresal and substance P in rat spinal cord, *Brain Res.* **97**:177–180.

Shaw, J. E. and P. W. Ramwell (1968). Release of a substance P polypeptide from the cerebral cortex, *Am. J. Physiol.* **215**:262–267.

Shikimi, T. and H. Iwata (1970). Pharmacological significance of peptidase and proteinase in the brain. II. Purification and properties of a bradykinin inactivating enzyme from rat brain, *Biochem. Pharmacol.* **19**:1399–1407.

Stern, P. and V. Dobrič (1957). Über die Wirkung der Substanz P in Zentralnervensystem, pp. 448–452 in *Psychotropic Drugs,* Garattini, S. and V. Ghetti, eds. Elsevier, Amsterdam.

Stern, P. and J. Hadzović (1973). Pharmacological analysis of central actions of synthetic substance P, *Arch. Int. Pharmacodyn. Ther.* **202**:259–262.

Stewart, J. M., C. J. Getto, K. Neldner, E. B. Reeve, W. A. Krivoy, and E. Zimmerman (1976). Substance P and analgesia, *Nature (London)* **262**:784–785.

Studer, R. O., A. Trzeciak, and W. Lergier (1973). Isolierung und Aminosäuresequenz von Substanz P aus Pferdedarm, *Helv. Chim. Acta* **56**:860–866.

Takahashi, T., S. Konishi, D. Powell, S. E. Leeman, and M. Otsuka (1974). Identification of the motoneuron-depolarizing peptide in bovine dorsal root as hypothalamic substance P, *Brain Res.* **73**:59–69.

Takahashi, T. and M. Otsuka (1975). Regional distribution of substance P in the spinal cord and nerve roots of the cat and the effect of dorsal root section, *Brain Res.* **87**:1–11.

Tregear, G. W., H. D. Niall, J. T. Potts, S. E. Leeman, and M. M. Chang (1971). Synthesis of substance P, *Nature (London) New Biol.* **232**:87–89.

Vogler, K., W. Haefely, A. Hürlimann, R. O. Studer, W. Lergier, R. Strässle, and K. H. Berneis (1963). A new purification procedure and biological properties of substance P, *Ann. N. Y. Acad. Sci.* **104**:378–389.

von Euler, U. S. (1936). Preparation of substance P, *Scand. Arch. Physiol.* **73**:142–144.

von Euler, U. S. and J. H. Gaddum (1931). An unidentified depressor substance in certain tissue extracts, *J. Physiol. (London)* **72**:74–87.

von Euler, U. S. and F. Lishajko (1961). Presence of substance P in subcellular particles of peripheral nerves, pp. 109–112 in *Proceedings of the Scientific Society of Bosnia and Herzegovia,* Vol. 1, *Symposium on Substance P*, Sarajevo.

Walker, R. J., J. A. Kemp, H. Yajima, K. Kitagawa, and G. N. Woodruff (1976). The action of substance P on mesencephalic reticular and substantia nigral neurones of the rat, *Experientia* **32**:214–215.

Yajima, H. and K. Kitagawa (1973). Studies on peptides. XXXIV. Conventional synthesis of the undecapeptide amide corresponding to the entire amino acid sequence of bovine substance P, *Chem. Pharmacol. Bull.* **21**:682–683.

Zetler, G. (1961). Zwei neue pharmakologisch aktive polypeptide in einem Substanz P-haltigen Hirinextrakt, *Naunyn-Schmiedebergs Arch. Exp. Pathol. Pharmakol.* **242**:330–352.

Zetler, G. (1970a). Biologically active peptides (Substance P), pp. 135–148 in *Handbook of Neurochemistry*, Vol. IV, *Control Mechanisms in the Nervous System*, Lajtha, A., ed. Plenum Press, New York.

Zetler, G. (1970b). Distribution of peptidergic neurons in mammalian brain, pp. 287–295 in *Aspects of Neuroendocrinology. V. International Symposium on Neurosecretion*, Bargman, W. and B. Scharrer, eds. Springer-Verlag, Berlin.

Zuber, H. (1966). Purification of substance P, pp. 584–593 in *Hypotensive Peptides*, Erdos, E. G., N. Back, and F. Sicuteri, eds. Springer-Verlag, New York.

TRH, LHRH, and Somatostatin: Distribution and Physiological Action in Neural Tissue

L. P. Renaud

Montreal General Hospital, Montreal, Quebec

This decade has witnessed considerable progress in our understanding of hypothalamic regulation of the pituitary-endocrine axis. It appears reasonably certain that the brain-pituitary link is mediated by peptide "releasing factors" liberated into the pituitary portal vessels from nerve endings of specialized hypothalamic neurosecretory neurons (cf. Harris, 1955). The structural characterization of three of these peptide messengers, i.e., TRH (thyrotropin-releasing hormone), LH-RH (luteinizing hormone-releasing hormone), and GH-RIH (SRIF or somatostatin), has opened up substantial avenues for investigation of their mode of action at the pituitary level. Coincident with the development of specific radioimmunoassays for these peptides has been the rather surprising discovery of their localization in both the median eminence and in other areas of the CNS, and certain extraneural tissues. A wealth of data suggest that these peptides also influence both animal behavior and neural excitability. In this presentation, I shall endeavor to review highlights of the experimental material that support a neural function for each of these three peptides, and to outline some of the histological and physiological studies that have attempted identification of these "peptidergic" neural elements.

Thyrotropin-Releasing Hormone

The first peptide to be structurally characterized (Figure 1) (Nair, Barrett, Bowers, and Schally, 1970; Burgus, Dunn, Desiderio, Ward, Vale, and Guillemin, 1970) is involved in the release of both TSH (thyrotropin-secreting hormone) and prolactin (Vale and Rivier,

RELEASING-HORMONE STRUCTURES

TRH — PYRO-GLU-HIS-PRO-NH$_2$

GNRH — PYRO-GLU-HIS-TRYP-SER-TYR-GLY-LEU-ARG-PRO-GLY-NH$_2$

GHIH — H-ALA-GLY-CYS-LYS-ASN-PHE-PHE-TRP-LYS
         THR-PHE-THR-SER-CYS-OH

FIGURE 1. Structural formulae for thyrotropin-releasing hormone (TRH), gonadotropin-releasing hormone or luteinizing hormone-releasing hormone (GNRH), and somatostatin (growth hormone-inhibiting hormone, GHIH).

1975). Although TRH (and the other releasing factors) is generally considered to be released directly into the portal circulation from median eminence nerve terminals, there is evidence that TRH may also be released into the cerebrospinal fluid and then transported to the anterior pituitary via the hypophysial portal vessels (Oliver, Ben-Jonathan, Mical, and Porter, 1975). Although initial localization studies using bioassay techniques have described a rather restricted TRH distribution, mainly in the median eminence, dorsomedial hypothalamic nucleus, and preoptic area (Krulich, Quijada, Hefco, and Sundberg, 1974), specific and sensitive radioimmunoassays have localized TRH throughout the CNS (Table 1). Within the hypothalamus, TRH is concentrated mainly in the median eminence, the anterior part of the ventromedial nucleus, the periventricular region, and the arcuate and dorsomedial nuclei (Brownstein, Palkovits, Saavedra, Bassiri, and Utiger, 1974). This distribution, however, only reflects about one-third of brain TRH content, with most TRH being found in extrahypothalamic regions, notably in the preoptic area and septal region, thalamus, amygdala, and brain stem (Winokur and Utiger, 1974; Jackson and Reichlin, 1974; Oliver, Eskay, Ben-Jonathan, and Porter, 1974).

An investigation of the source of this hypothalamic and extrahypothalamic TRH has led to interesting observations. Brownstein and his colleagues (Brownstein, Utiger, Palkovits, and Kizer, 1975*b*) have shown that hypothalamic deafferentation drastically reduces the hypothalamic TRH content without having a significant effect on extrahypothalamic TRH (Table 1). Thus it would appear that extrahypothalamic TRH does not arise from mediobasal hypothalamic TRH-producing neurons. Conversely, much of the mediobasal hypothalamic TRH is probably synthesized elsewhere and transported to the hypothalamic mediobasal area. Median eminence TRH presumably is produced by neurosecretory neurons located anterior to the median eminence, because stimulation in the anterior hypothalamic area can evoke an elevation of plasma TSH levels (Martin and Reichlin, 1972). In favor of the argument of multiple sites of TRH production are the observations of in vitro TRH biosynthesis in both hypothalamic and extrahypothalamic brain fragments (Mitnick and Reichlin, 1971; McKelvy, 1974; Grimm-Jørgensen and McKelvy, 1974); although this

TABLE 1. *Distribution of TRH in the CNS*

	Immunoreactive TRH in rat brain[a]		
Brain area	Area weight (mg)	TRH content (ng)	% of total TRH
Hypothalamus	32.6 ± 1.5	4.1 ± 0.2	31.2 ± 2.3
Forebrain	399.0 ± 8.9	3.5 ± 0.3	25.6 ± 2.1
Brainstem	185.0 ± 5.5	2.1 ± 0.1	16.9 ± 1.8
Posterior diencephalon	213.3 ± 8.7	1.9 ± 0.2	13.8 ± 1.7
Posterior cortex	622.8 ± 11.5	1.3 ± 0.1	10.6 ± 0.7
Cerebellum	244.0 ± 5.1	0.26 ± 0.03	2.1 ± 0.3

Brain TRH (pg/mg tissue wet weight) distribution in different vertebrates[b]

Species	Brain stem	Cerebellum	Olfactory lobe	Cerebral cortex	Hypothalamus
Rat	4–5	1–3	5–8	1–3	240–300
Snake	129–359	85–186	750–764	264–381	393–731
Frog	40–85	368–724	220–444	71–150	1,520–3,620

Brain TRH (ng/g of tissue) in rat brain: effects of hypothalamic deafferentation[c]

Area	Sham operated	Deafferentated
Hypothalamus	489 ± 59	117 ± 21[d]
Preoptic area	108 ± 16	95 ± 16
Septum	85 ± 29	85 ± 14
Amygdala	23 ± 3	31 ± 5
Caudate	21 ± 5	19 ± 4
Medulla	19 ± 3	16 ± 2
Pons	15 ± 3	9 ± 2
Cerebellum	2 ± 0.2	3 ± 1

[a] Adapted from Winokur and Utiger (1974).
[b] Adapted from Jackson and Reichlin (1974).
[c] Adapted from Brownstein et al. (1975b).
[d] Significantly different $P < 0.001$.

has been observed in forebrain fragments, it does not appear to occur in cerebral cortex (Mitnick and Reichlin, 1971).

TRH enjoys a wide phylogenetic distribution in both hypothalamic and extrahypothalamic brain areas of mammals, reptiles, amphibians, fish (Jackson and Reichlin, 1974), and gastropods (Grimm-Jørgensen, McKelvy, and Jackson, 1975). TRH is found in the brain of many poikilotherms (Table 1); however, synthetic TRH is *not* capable of stimulating release of TSH in these animals (Vandesande and Aspeslagh, 1974). Although TRH is present in the CNS of the axolotl, it does not regulate metamorphosis (a process usually controlled by the thyroid axis) in this Mexican salamander (Taurog, Oliver, Eskay, Porter, and McKenzie, 1974). Evidently, TRH represents an ancient molecule whose function is by no means restricted to the regulation of TSH secretion. This has prompted the suggestion that TRH may act as a neural modulator or possibly as a neural transmitter agent within the CNS (Jackson and Reichlin, 1974; Wilbur, Montoya, Plotnikoff, White, Genrich, Renaud, and Martin, 1976).

As might be expected, brain TRH appears localized to neural elements. With the indirect immunofluoroescent technique, TRH-containing nerve terminals are observed in both the medial part of the external layer of the median eminence, the dorsomedial hypothalamic nucleus and perifornical area of the hypothalamus, and in extrahypothalamic regions, such as nucleus accumbens, the lateral septal nucleus, and several motor nuclei of the brain stem and spinal cord (Hökfelt, Fuxe, Johansson, Jeffcoate, and White, 1975b,c). Differential

TABLE 2. *Regional distribution of [³H]TRH binding in rat brain*[a]

	High-affinity binding		Low-affinity binding	
Region (n)	K_D (nM)	No. of sites (fmol per mg protein)	K_D (μM)	No. of sites (pmol per mg protein)
Cerebral cortex (7)	47 ± 5	110 ± 13	5 ± 1	30 ± 2
Hypothalamus (2)	52	190	9	46
Hippocampus (1)	36	150	3	39
Midbrain (1)	32	100	6	34
Corpus Striatum (1)	38	60	7	35
Pons-medulla oblongata (1)	27	40	2	7
Cerebellum (2)	ND	ND	0.9	7

[a] Adapted from Burt and Snyder (1975). ND, none detected.

subcellular fractionation studies in hypothalamic tissue indicate that TRH is located in the synaptosomal fraction (Barnea, Ben-Jonathan, Colston, Johnston, and Porter, 1975), similar to the subcellular localization of other known neurotransmitters (Whittaker, 1969). Burt and Snyder (1975) have demonstrated high-affinity TRH binding sites in brain, with an approximate correspondence between the dissocation constant of the binding site and the endogenous levels of TRH in brain (Table 2).

There have now been numerous behavioral studies that indicate psychotrophic actions of TRH, further support for a direct action of TRH in the CNS (Prange, Nemeroff, Lipton, Breese, and Wilson, 1976; Wilbur et al., 1976); these effects appear to be independent of the pituitary-thyroid axis. What is still uncertain is the mechanism of action of TRH in the brain; suggestions from available data indicate some form of interaction with endogenous neurotransmitter agents, e.g., monoamines (Green and Grahame-Smith, 1974; Keller, Bartholini, and Pletscher, 1974) or acetylcholine (Yarbrough, 1976).

In an attempt to determine whether it does influence neuronal excitability directly, TRH has been applied to central neurons by microiontophoresis (Dyer and Dyball, 1974; Steiner, 1975; Renaud and Martin, 1975a,b; Renaud, Martin, and Brazeau, 1975, 1976). Preliminary in vitro experiments that measured the release of tritiated TRH (Renaud and Martin, 1975b) demonstrated that TRH could be ejected as a cation from aqueous 5 to 10 mM solutions in the physiological pH range. For certain sensitive cells, TRH appears to reduce glutamate-evoked or spontaneous spike discharge activity (e.g., Figure 2); on the other hand, discharges evoked by acetylcholine appear to be enhanced (cf. Yarbrough, 1976). TRH-sensitive neurons appear to be located at various levels of the neural axis, although the proportionate numbers of TRH-sensitive cells declines in extrahypothalamic regions (Table 3). It is curious that TRH at relatively low iontophoretic currents can also influence the activity of neurons in the cerebellar cortex, an area containing little or no TRH by radioimmunoassay (Brownstein et al., 1974), or TRH high-affinity receptor binding sites (Table 2).

A large number of structural analogues of TRH have been synthesized and tested for activity in a variety of biological systems. In general, the in vivo TSH- and prolactin-releasing potency of these analogues is correlated with their ability to compete with TRH for binding to pituitary cells (Grant, Vale, and Guillemin, 1973; Vale and Rivier, 1975). However, TRH receptors in brain and in pituitary appear to be different.

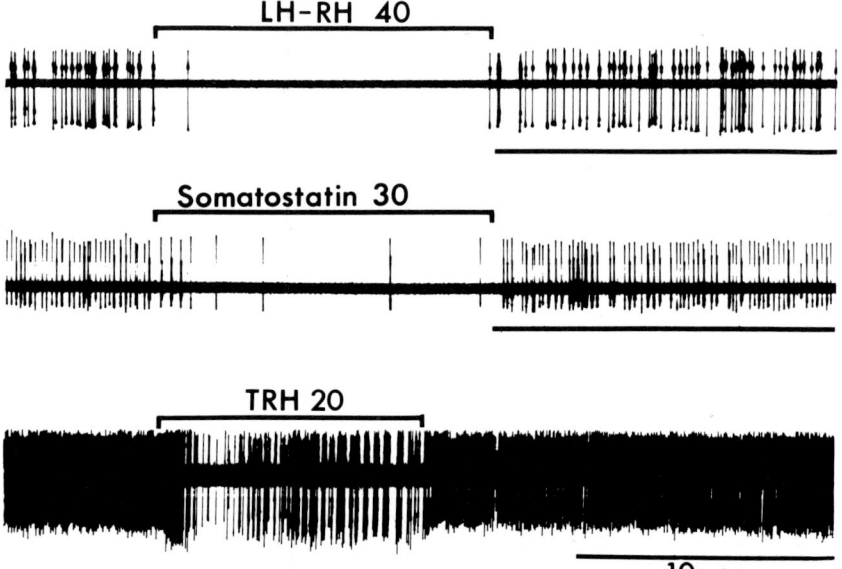

FIGURE 2. Representative oscillograph traces to indicate the depressant effects of microiontophoretic application of luteinizing hormone-releasing hormone (LH-RH), cyclic somatostatin, and TRH on the frequency of spike discharges recorded from three separate neurons. The cell in the top trace was located in the ventromedial nucleus, the cell in the middle trace was recorded from parietal cortex, and the cell in the lower trace was recorded from the cerebellar cortex of pentobarbital anesthesized Sprague-Dawley rats. The numbers above each bar indicate the microiontophoretic current applied in nanoamperes. The time calibration (10 sec) is represented by the horizontal bar below each trace. From Wilbur et al. (1976).

The behavioral activities of a series of TRH analogues do not correlate well with their relative hypophysiotrophic potencies; in general, adenohypophyseal tissue is more discriminating than brain tissue (cf. Prange, Breese, Jahnke, Martin, Cooper, Cott, Wilson, Alltop, Lipton, Bissette, Nemeroff, and Loosen, 1975b). Burt and Snyder (1975) have also noted some similar discrepancies in the ability of certain TRH analogues to compete with TRH for binding to high-affinity binding sites in membrane preparations of brain and pituitary tissue. There is general agreement that the 3-methyl-His-TRH analogue, which has approximately 10-fold the potency in TSH release as native TRH, is also more potent in the nervous system (Prange et al., 1975b; Burt and Snyder, 1975). Preliminary iontophoretic studies with this analogue (Figure 3)

TABLE 3. Survey of central peptide-sensitive neurons[a]

Peptide	Site	No. tested	No. responsive
TRH	Cuneate nucleus	43	12 (28%)
	Cerebellar cortex	66	28 (42%)
	Cerebral cortex	36	17 (47%)
	Hypothalamus (HVM)	50	30 (60%)
LH-RH	Cerebellar cortex	17	13 (76%)
	Hypothalamus (HVM)	16	13 (81%)
Somatostatin	Cerebellar cortex	9 (L)	5 (55%)
		9 (C)	5 (55%)
	Cerebral cortex	13 (L)	11 (84%)
		15 (C)	12 (80%)
	Hypothalamus (HVM)	14 (C)	11 (78%)
		12 (L)	10 (83%)

[a] Somatostatin was tested in both the linear (L) and cyclized (C) form. Responsive neurons demonstrated a decrease in excitability within 10 sec of peptide application by microiontophoresis. HVM refers to hypothalamic ventromedial nucleus. Adapted from Renaud, Martin, and Brazeau (1975).

offer a further indication of its enhanced potency over native TRH. Whether the structure-activity relationships will remain generally similar for pituitary and brain tissue remains to be determined; it is possible that brain TRH receptors exhibit significant differences in their structural preferences.

Luteinizing Hormone-Releasing Hormone

The decapeptide luteinizing hormone-releasing hormone (LH-RH) (Figure 1) was the second hypothalamic peptide to receive structural characterization (Amoss, Burgus, Blackwell, Vale, Fellows, and Guillemin, 1971; Schally, Arimura, Baba, Nair, Matsuo, Redding, Debeljuk, and White, 1971). This, therefore, was the long-sought hypothalamic factor described by McCann and his colleagues to have LH-releasing activity (McCann, Taleisnik, and Friedman, 1960). The development of sensitive radioimmunoassays for LH-RH has yielded information not only on total LH-RH content in brain, reported to be about 2 to 5 ng in the rat (Araki, Toran-Allerand, Ferin, and Vande Wiele, 1975; Jonas, Burger, Comming, Findlay, and Kretser, 1975), but also on its distribution. Tissue sections of various brain regions indicate that LH-RH is localized mainly to the hypothalamus (Palkovits, Arimura, Brownstein, Schally, and Saavedra, 1974; Brownstein, Palkovits, Saavedra, and Kizer, 1976) and circumventricular organs

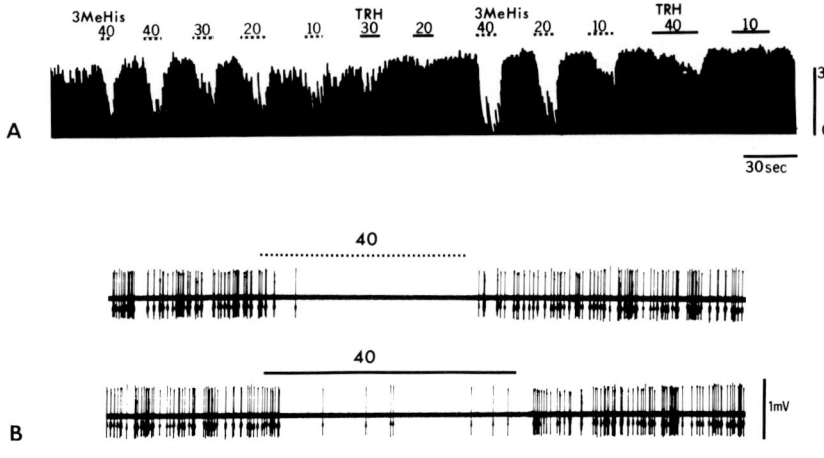

FIGURE 3. (A) Polygraph frequency traces of the spike discharge activity of a cerebellar cortical neuron and its response to iontophoretic TRH and the TRH analogue 3-methyl-His TRH. Note that the TRH analogue evokes a greater decrease in firing frequency than the TRH itself. The vertical bar on the right represents 30 spikes/sec. (B) Action of LH-RH (upper trace) and an LH-RH analogue (lower trace: Des-His^2, D-Ala^6, Pro^9, ethylamide LH-RH) on the spike discharge frequency of a hypothalamic ventromedial nucleus neuron. Note the similarity in the depressant effects of the native compound and the LH-RH analogue, despite the fact that the analogue is more potent in terms of pituitary LH release. The numbers above each horizontal bar indicate the current (in nanoamperes) used to release each substance. From Renaud, Martin, and Brazeau (1976).

(Kizer, Palkovits, and Brownstein, 1976; Brownstein, Palkovits, and Kizer, 1976). Little LH-RH had been located elsewhere in the nervous system.

Within the hypothalamus, high concentrations of LH-RH are found notably within the median eminence and arcuate nucleus (Palkovits et al., 1974), whereas lesser amounts can be detected in the preoptic and anterior hypothalamic area (Kalra, 1976; Wheaton, Krulich, and McCann, 1976). In female rats, brain tissue LH-RH levels vary with the stage of the estrus cycle; the fact that brain LH-RH can also be altered by castration and estrogen treatment suggests that gonadal steroids are in some way involved in the control of hypothalamic LH-RH (Araki, Ferin, Zimmerman, and Vande Wiele, 1975; Kalra, 1976; Kobayashi, Lu, and Yen, 1976). LH-RH biosynthesis in hypothalamic tissue is also in part governed by levels of gonadal steroids (Moguilevsky, Enero, and

Szwarcfarb, 1974), as are the levels of hypothalamic LH-RH peptidases (Griffiths, Hooper, Jeffcoate, and Holland, 1975), enzymes possibly involved in any central functions of LH-RH.

Where, specifically, is brain LH-RH distributed? Cytochemical studies have confirmed the presence of LH-RH in a network of nerve fibers and terminals in the external layer of the median eminence, and in the organum vasculosum of the lamina terminalis (Hökfelt, Fuxe, Goldstein, Johansson, Park, Fraser, and Jeffcoate, 1974; Kordon, Kerdelhue, Pattou, and Jutisz, 1974; Zimmerman, Hsu, Ferin, and Kozlowski, 1974; Baker, Dermody, and Reel, 1975; Sétáló, Vigh, Schally, Arimura, and Flerkó, 1975b). Neuronal localization is confirmed by subcellular fractionation studies that strongly support the presence of LH-RH in nerve terminals (Pelletier, Labrie, Puviani, Arimura, and Schally, 1974; Ramirez, Gautron, Epelbaum, Pattou, Zamura, and Kordon, 1975), where LH-RH appears to be associated with a specific population of dense granules (Goldsmith and Ganong, 1975; Taber and Karavolas, 1975; Naik, 1975a).

Although some conflicts have arisen regarding the origin of these LH-RH nerve fibers, there are several clues to suggest that they may originate from neuronal perikarya located at more rostral levels. (1) There is a pronounced drop in mediobasal hypothalamic LH-RH levels after anterior hypothalamic deafferentation (Brownstein, Arimura, Schally, Palkovits, and Kizer, 1976; but cf. Silverman, 1976) in association with a rise in preoptic LH-RH levels (Kalra, 1976). (2) LH-RH nerve fibers in the mediobasal hypothalamus are diminished in number after anterior hypothalamic deafferentation (Sétáló et al., 1976). (3) Neuronal perikarya containing immunoreactive LH-RH have been reported scattered throughout the medial preoptic and suprachiasmatic region (Barry, DuBois, and Carette, 1974; Sétáló et al., 1976); other authors have described LH-RH neuronal perikarya in the arcuate and ventromedial nuclei of different species (Zimmerman et al., 1974; Leonardelli and Dubois, 1974; Naik, 1975b; Zimmerman, 1976). In accordance with these findings, one can visualize at least two parts to the LH-RH peptidergic system, i.e., the preoptic tuberoinfundibular pathway, which originates from cells in the preoptic region, and a second network localized to the mediobasal hypothalamic region. Presumably the interplay between these two systems governs both the tonic and cyclic release of LH from adenohypophysis during the female ovulatory cycle.

A substantial body of evidence based on behavioral studies indicates that LH-RH might have some independent role in the brain aside from its ability to regulate function in the pituitary-gonad axis. Subcutaneous administration of less than 500 ng of LH-RH to ovariectomized and/or hypophysectomized and adrenalectomized female rats primed with estrogen will elicit the lordotic posturing associated with mating behavior, and will also accelerate ejaculation in the castrated testosterone-treated male rat (Moss and McCann, 1973, 1975; Pfaff, 1973; Moss, 1975; Moss, McCann, and Dudley, 1975b). The time course of this response is curious, with a maximal behavioral pattern being observed only 6 to 8 h after injection. Evidently these results suggest a direct effect of LH-RH on the nervous system. A similar proposition has been advanced to explain the unusually early return of sexual potency in some human hypogonadal males treated with LH-RH (Mortimer, McNeilly, Fisher, Murray, and Besser, 1974). What is puzzling about this effect is the mechanism. In plasma, LH-RH is reported to have a half-life of only a few minutes (Jonas et al., 1975; Saito, Musa, Oshima, Yamamota, and Funato, 1975). Furthermore, Dupont and his colleagues (Dupont, Labrie, Pelletier, Puviani, Coy, Coy, and Schally, 1974) have not detected LH-RH in the CNS after systemic administration, thereby indicating the presence of a blood-brain barrier for this decapeptide. Evidently, how systemically administered LH-RH reaches central neurons is not yet resolved. The fact that such a minute quantity elicits behavioral responses argues for a physiological mechanism. It is also relevant that direct administration of 50 ng of LH-RH into the medial preoptic area or arcuate-ventromedial area of the hypothalamus initiates lordotic behavior, whereas similar injections into lateral hypothalamus or cerebral cortex are not effective (Foreman and Moss, 1975).

Further characterization of LH-RH action at cellular levels has been derived from microiontophoretic experiments. LH-RH can be ejected from aqueous solutions (Kelly and Moss, 1976) and, although the absolute numbers of LH-RH-sensitive neurons varies from study to study, different investigators have reported enhancement or depression of spontaneous or chemically evoked unit activity from neurons in the preoptic and mediobasal hypothalamic areas and elsewhere (Dyer and Dyball, 1974; Kawakami and Sakuma, 1974, 1976; Renaud et al., 1975, 1976; Kelly and Moss, 1976; Moss, 1976; Moss, Kelly, and Dudley, 1976). In some instances, the cellular responses have been gradual; in others, responses were quite brisk, with relatively low iontophoretic currents (e.g., Figures 2 and 3).

Preliminary microiontophoretic studies have been performed using LH-RH analogues to ascertain whether central neurons can discriminate between these analogues and the native LH-RH molecules (Moss, 1976; Renaud et al., 1976). Based on spike discharge frequency it would appear that some central LH-RH-sensitive cells do not manifest the potency range of LH-RH analogues, as determined by their ability to evoke pituitary LH release (Figure 3); in other instances, the responses compare favorably (cf. Moss, 1976). The available data do not permit further discussion on the presence or characterization of LH-RH receptor sites in brain, or differences between these receptor sites and LH-RH receptor sites in the adenohypophysis (cf. Labrie, Borgeat, Ferland, Lemay, Dupont, Lemaire, Pelletier, Barden, Drouin, De Lean, Belanger, and Jolicoeur, 1975).

Somatostatin (SRIF, GH-RIH)

Recognition that the hypothalamus contained a factor that depressed adenohypophyseal GH secretion has led to the structural characterization of the tetradecapeptide somatostatin (Brazeau, Vale, Burgus, Ling, Butcher, Rivier, and Guillemin, 1973). To the delight of neuroscientists and endocrinologists alike, the development of a specific radioimmunoassay for somatostatin (e.g., Arimura, Sato, Coy, and Schally, 1975) has permitted identification of somatostatin's presence in both central and peripheral neural tissues and in such extraneural tissues as the gut and pancreas (Hökfelt, Effendić, Hellerström, Johansson, Luft, and Arimura, 1975a). In the nervous system, somatostatin can be found in many areas, but is localized in highest concentration within the hypothalamus, where substantial amounts are found predominantly within the median eminence, arcuate, ventromedial and ventral premammillary nuclei, and the periventricular region (Brownstein, Arimura, Sato, Schally, and Kizer, 1975a). Earlier studies with bioassay could not demonstrate such high levels of somatostatin within the ventromedial nucleus (Vale, Rivier, Palkovits, Saavedra, and Brownstein, 1974; Vale, Brazeau, Rivier, Brown, Ross, Rivier, Burgus, Ling, and Guillemin, 1975), possibly owing to the presence of both somatostatin and a growth hormone-releasing factor in this nucleus. A more recent investigation of somatostatin content in various parts of individual hypothalamic nuclei has demonstrated the uniform distribution of somatostatin within the ventromedial nucleus, but has also confirmed that somatostatin levels here are not as high as in the arcuate nucleus or the median eminence (Palkovits, Brownstein, Arimura, Sato, Schally, and Kizer, 1976).

Immunohistochemical studies have visualized somatostatin-containing nerve fibers in mediobasal hypothalamus, notably in the arcuate and ventromedial nuclei and external zone of the median eminence, as well as in the preoptic area (Dubois, Barry, and Leonardelli, 1974; Dubois and Kolodziejczyk, 1975; Hökfelt, Effendić, Johansson, Luft, and Arimura, 1974; Hökfelt et al., 1975a; Sétáló, Vigh, Schally, Arimura, and Flerkó, 1975a). Neuronal perikarya immunoreactive for somatostatin have been described recently in the hypothalamus (Dubois and Kolodziejczyk, 1975) and spinal cord (Hökfelt, Elde, Johansson, Luft, Nilsson, and Arimura, 1976). These observations indicate the presence of peptidergic neural pathways for somatostatin, in addition to those already described earlier for TRH and LH-RH. In the hypothalamus, much of the local somatostatin content probably arises from local neural elements; the presence of neuronal perikarya immunoreactive for somatostatin in extrahypothalamic areas, such as the amygdala (Hökfelt, personal communication), supports the existence of independent "somatostatinergic" pathways.

Recent studies in our laboratories have concentrated on the development of a specific immunoassay for somatostatin and on its subcellular distribution (Tsang, Tan, Brazeau, Lal, Renaud, and Martin, 1975; Epelbaum, Brazeau, Tsang, Brawer, and Martin, 1977). Somatostatin

TABLE 4. Regional distribution of SRIF in brain[a]

Brain region	No. of exp	Wet weight (mg)	pg SRIF/ fragment	pg SRIF/ mg wet weight
Total MBH	7	16.7 ± 0.8[b]	22,239 ± 2,160	1,397 ± 208
ME[c]	7	1.4 ± 0.2	17,656 ± 1,036	15,470 ± 2,421
Remaining Hypothalamus[d]	7	13.9 ± 1.4	3,837 ± 604	266 ± 45
APO	7	13.3 ± 0.5	4,414 ± 387	338 ± 37
CMA	7	30.5 ± 1.2	8,212 ± 574	272 ± 23
BLA	7	34.1 ± 1.9	12,214 ± 1,472	351 ± 23
CX	7	42.0 ± 4.4	3,750 ± 404	93 ± 16
Spinal cord	7	34.0 ± 3.2	3,696 ± 508	114 ± 18
Pineal gland	7	2.3 ± 0.3	250	

[a] Adapted from Epelbaum et al. (1977).
[b] Mean ± SE.
[c] Median eminence (ME).
[d] Hypothalamus excluding medial basal hypothalamus (MBH). Abbreviations: APO, preoptic area; CMA, corticomedial amygdala; BLA, basolateral amygdala; CX, cortex.

TABLE 5. *Subcellular distribution of SRIF in different brain regions*[a]

	Protein (μg/mg equivalent)	LDH (μM NADH$_2$/h/ equivalent)	SRIF (pg/equivalent)		
			MBH	APO	Amygdala
H	88.53 ± 6.92[b] (7)[c]	115.00 ± 10.00 (4)[c]	15,331 ± 1,574 (7)[c]	5,276 ± 724 (6)[c]	12,076 ± 2,607 (5)[c]
S	62.62 ± 10.44	97.35 ± 10.55	14,815 ± 2,013	4,528 ± 452	10,943 ± 807
P	18.44 ± 0.85	12.70 ± 1.52	2,588 ± 883	1,370 ± 474	2,324 ± 680
S$_2$	22.53 ± 4.75	50.16 ± 7.61	1,362 ± 698	499 ± 112	686 ± 194
P$_2$	39.28 ± 5.75	40.35 ± 9.70	15,401 ± 1,787	6,200 ± 1,138	9,755 ± 1,812

[a] Adapted from Epelbaum et al. (1977).
[b] Mean ± SE.
[c] Numbers in parentheses indicate separate experiments.

is localized mostly within the synaptosomal fraction in mediobasal hypothalamus, medial preoptic area, and extrahypothalamic regions, such as the amygdala and cerebral cortex (Table 4). Over 80% of the hormone present in the homogenate from mediobasal hypothalamus, preoptic area, and amygdala is concentrated in the crude mitochondrial fraction (P$_2$), and 60 to 70% is concentrated in the synaptosomal band of the sucrose purification gradient (Table 5), suggesting that most brain somatostatin is in fact concentrated in nerve terminals. It is appropriate, therefore, that Pelletier and his colleagues (Pelletier, Labrie, Arimura, and Schally, 1974) have confirmed neuronal localization of somatostatin at the electron microscope level within secretory granules of median eminence nerve endings. We have also demonstrated that somatostatin can modify calcium uptake and calcium release from synaptosomal preparations (Tsang et al., 1975). The latter may reflect a role for somatostatin in neural transmission, but does not distinguish between a pre- and postsynaptic site of action.

Several laboratories have reported behavioral changes with systemic or intraventricular somatostatin injections (Plotnikoff, Kastin, and Schally, 1974; Brown and Vale, 1975; Cohn, 1975; Prange, Breese, Jahnke, Cooper, Cott, Wilson, Lipton, and Plotnikoff, 1975a; Rezak, Havlicek, Hughes, and Friesen, 1975). Applied by microiontophoresis, somatostatin appears to exert a potent depressant action on the activity of central neurons (Figure 2) (Renaud et al., 1975, 1976). If, as these studies suggest, somatostatin does exert some role in neural function, the specific nature of this role and its mechanism are far from clear. Its presence in nerve cells and nerve terminals in the mediobasal hypothalamus and the amygdala, two structures known to exert control over GH secretion from adenohypophysis (Martin, Kontor, and Mead, 1973), may indicate some role in a central feedback loop for GH

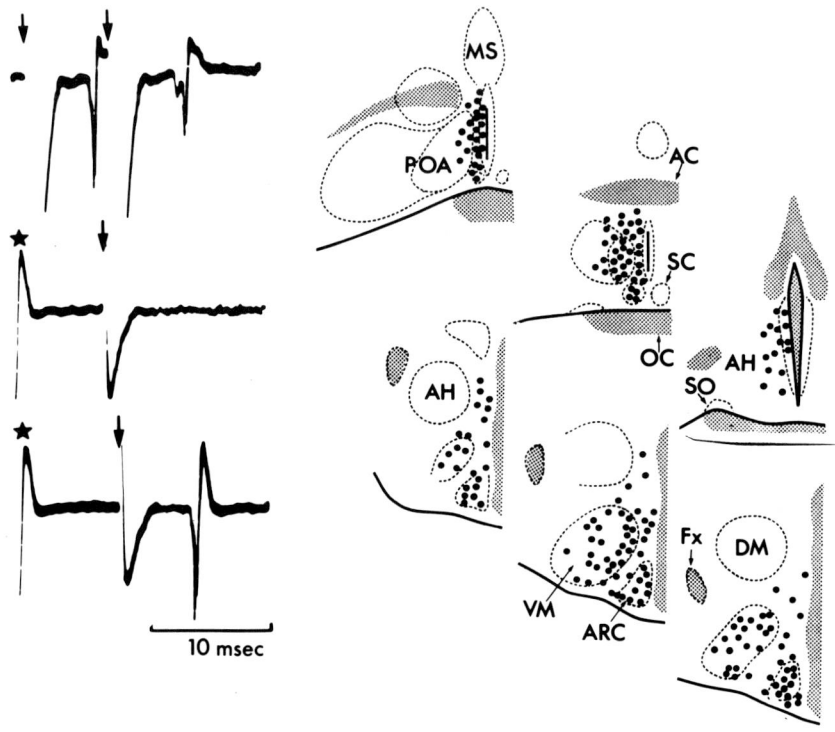

FIGURE 4. Tuberoinfundibular neurons. On the left, three representative oscilloscope traces display the characteristic antidromic response of a tuberoinfundibular neuron after median eminence stimulation (at the arrowheads). The upper trace displays constant latency responses at high frequency; the lower traces illustrate collision at the appropriate intervals between a spontaneous action potential (represented by a star) and the antidromic spike. On the right, the approximate locations of medial basal hypothalamic and preoptic tuberoinfundibular neurons are indicated by black dots. All cells displayed antidromic invasions after median eminence stimulation. Abbreviations: AC, anterior commissure; AH, anterior hypothalamic area; ARC, arcuate nucleus; DM, dorsomedial hypothalamic nucleus; Fx, fornix; MS, medial septum; OC, optic chiasm; POA, preoptic area; SC, suprachiasmatic nucleus; SO, supraoptic nucleus; VM, ventromedial nucleus.

secretion. One might speculate that somatostatin-containing primary afferent neurons in the spinal cord are engaged in specific sensory modality perceptions.

Tuberoinfundibular Neurons: Electrophysiological Studies

A study of the neural distribution, subcellular and immunocytochemical localization, and presumed functional role of hypothalamic-releasing factors would be incomplete without some consideration of the electrophysiology of the neurons that are presumed to be associated with neurosecretion of these particular peptides. The following is a brief review of certain electrophysiological features of hypothalamic tuberoinfundibular cells. The electrophysiological definition of a "tuberoinfundibular neuron" refers to a neuron located in the basal forebrain that exhibits antidromic invasion after stimulation is applied to the surface of the median eminence (Figure 4). This pattern of response implies axon termination in the median eminence. One must assume that these neurons belong to the hypothalamic parvicellular neuronal system that has been described by morphologists to project to the portal vessel capillaries in the median eminence (Szentágothai, Flerkó, Mess, and Halász, 1968). By analogy with neural events associated with secretion of hormones in the supraoptic and paraventricular neurohypophyseal system (Dyball and Koizumi, 1969; Dyball, 1971; Wakerley and Lincoln, 1973; Arnauld, Dufy, and Vincent, 1975; Dreifuss, Tribollet, and Baertschi, 1976), one also assumes that neurosecretion in the tuberoinfundibular system (i.e., the peptidergic neurosecretory cells responsible for elaboration of the release or release-inhibiting factors) is also associated with activity in this neural network.

Based on the criteria defined above for antidromic identification, neuronal perikarya which are considered to represent tuberoinfundibular cells have been identified in two main areas (Figure 4): (1) in the mediobasal hypothalamus, with cells located in the arcuate, ventromedial, dorsomedial, and dorsal premammillary nuclei and periventricular region (Makara, Harris, and Spyer, 1972; Sawaki and Yagi, 1973; Harris and Sanghera, 1974; Moss, Kelly, and Riskind, 1975; Renaud, 1976a,c); and (2) in the suprachiasmatic, periventricular, and medial preoptic areas and adjacent anterior hypothalamic regions (Makara et al., 1972; Renaud, 1976b). There are two points worthy of note: first, some of these cells are suitably situated to conform to the Halász definition of the hypophysiotrophic area (Halász, 1969) and the preoptic-tuberoinfundibular pathway; second, their overall distribution is compatible with the localization of neuronal perikarya that demonstrate immunocytochemical localization of hypothalamic peptides that we considered earlier. Electrophysiological studies have also indicated the presence of axon collaterals within the tuberoinfundibular system (Harris and Sanghera, 1974; Yagi and Sawaki, 1974; Renaud, 1975, 1976a,c; Sawaki and Yagi, 1976). In summary (Figure 5), terminal branching in the tuberoinfundibular pathway is suggested by the occasional observation of antidromic invasion at two discrete latencies. The presence of recurrent postsynaptic inhibitory patterns after median

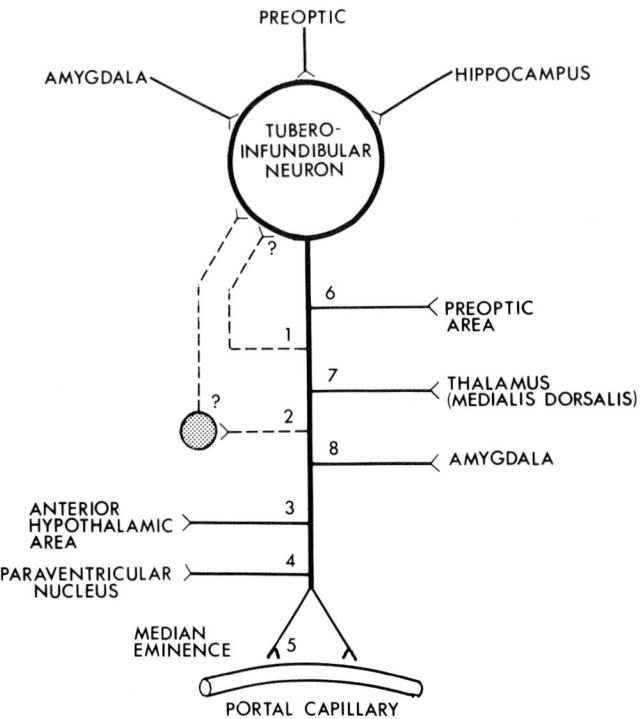

FIGURE 5. Schematic illustration of the tuberoinfundibular system, based on electrophysiological observations. The solid vertical line represents the main axon, which terminates on the median eminence portal capillary plexus. Intrahypothalamic axon collaterals (1 through 5) and extrahypothalamic collaterals (6 through 8) are illustrated as off-shoots of the main axon. Afferent fibers to the tuberoinfundibular neuronal system include those from amygdala, preoptic area, and hippocampus, and are illustrated schematically at the top of the figure. Adapted from Renaud, Martin, and Brazeau (1976).

eminence stimulation is further evidence for local axon collaterals in the hypothalamus; antidromic activation of tuberoinfundibular cells both from the median eminence and from other hypothalamic sites (anterior hypothalamic area and paraventricular nuclei), and from extrahypothalamic regions (preoptic area, amygdala, and medialis dorsalis nucleus of the thalamus), indicate extensive axon aborization in the tuberoinfundibular system. Collaterals and branching have also been observed in the axons of cells immunoreactive with antisera to LH-RH (Barry et al., 1974).

Electrophysiology has facilitated study of the afferent connections in the tuberoinfundibular system. Evidence acquired to date indicates that amygdalofugal fibers appear to innervate specifically those tuberoinfundibular cells located within the ventromedial nucleus, but not elsewhere in the mediobasal hypothalamus or the preoptic area (Renaud, 1976b,c). Stimulation of the hippocampus influences the excitability of tuberoinfundibular cells located in more medial parts of the mediobasal hypothalamus (Renaud, 1976b), whereas preoptic-

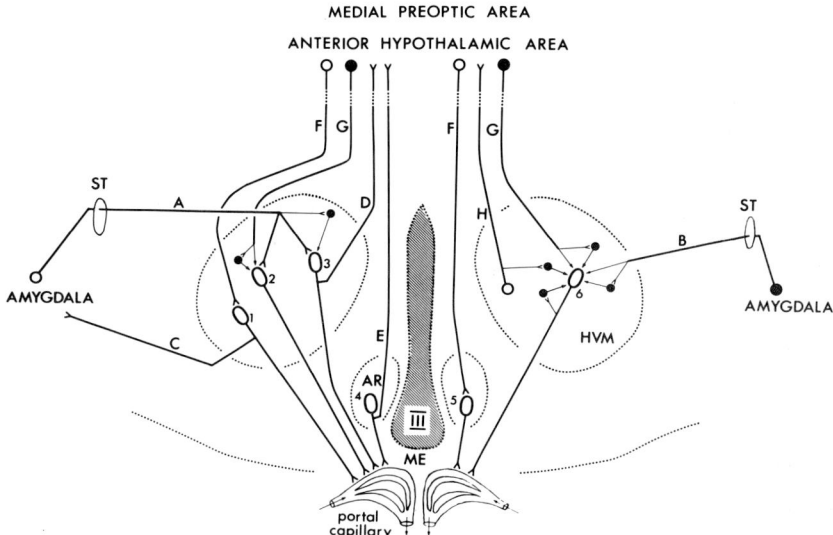

FIGURE 6. Schematic coronal section through the medial basal hypothalamus outlining the relative positions of the ventromedial (HVM) and arcuate (AR) nuclei. The figure illustrates postulated connections between tuberoinfundibular neurons (1 through 6) connected directly to the median eminence (ME) portal capillary plexus, the amygdala, and medial preoptic and anterior hypothalamic areas. Principal connections are depicted by heavy continuous lines. Tuberoinfundibular neurons in each VM (1 through 3,6) receive connections from both amygdala and more rostral regions, whereas arcuate tuberoinfundibular neurons (4,5) are mostly connected only with rostral areas. Extrahypothalamic afferents presumed to mediate excitatory connections originate from open circles (A,F); extrahypothalamic inhibitory connections are shown to originate from filled circles (B,G), and may be mediated either directly or through afferent collateral pathways to local inhibitory interneurons (identified as small filled circles). The fine continuous lines indicate intranuclear recurrent or afferent collateral inhibitory pathways. Note that axons of some tuberoinfundibular neurons (1,3,4) bifurcate and send fibers to the amygdala (C) and medial preoptic area (D,E). Adapted from Renaud (1977).

anterior hypothalamic stimulation sites alter activity of tuberoinfundibular cells located throughout the mediobasal hypothalamus (Renaud, 1976b, 1977). Thus it has been possible to provide at least part of the neural circuitry through which these extrahypothalamic areas may modify the activity of hypothalamic tuberoinfundibular neurons (Figure 6).

Despite the abundance of neuroendocrine data implicating monoamines in hypothalamic regulation of adenohypophysis, little is known about the neuropharmacology of tuberoinfundibular cells. Recently, Moss and his colleagues have demonstrated that microiontophoretic application of both norepinephrine and dopamine, as well as hypothalamic peptides, can modify the activity of arcuate nucleus tuberoinfundibular cells (Moss et al., 1975a, 1976). Recurrent inhibition in the tuberoinfundibular system appears to be picrotoxin-sensitive (Yagi and Sawaki, 1974; Sawaki and Yagi, 1976), thereby suggesting that gamma-aminobutyric acid may be a neural transmitter in the recurrent inhibitory pathway.

CONCLUSIONS

In this presentation, only the highlights of a rapidly expanding field of interest in peptide actions on neural tissue have been presented. The data overwhelmingly favor a role for TRH, LH-RH, and somatostatin (to mention but three of the hypothalamic peptides) in neural behavior. Their localization in neuronal perikarya, fibers, and terminals outside of the median eminence, and the presence of axon collaterals in the tuberoinfundibular system, suggest that these peptides may be liberated at central synaptic sites (Renaud, 1975), either alone or in association with other neurotransmitter substances (cf. Mroz, Brownstein, and Leeman, 1976). Their ability to induce changes in behavior and neuronal excitability increases the possibility that these agents may serve as some form of neural modulator and possibly even as neurotransmitters themselves. Further details are required on the nature and specificity of high-affinity receptor binding sites in the brain, and on structure-function relationships at central receptor sites, in addition to studies on the mechanisms of action. The electrophysiological observations are interesting, but still cannot be precisely correlated with immunohistochemical data. There is little doubt that the current multidisciplinary emphasis being devoted to peptide research will indeed answer many of the questions posed today in this promising area.

ACKNOWLEDGMENTS

The Medical Research Council of Canada provided financial support for the work conducted in our laboratories.

REFERENCES

Amoss, M., R. Burgus, R. Blackwell, W. Vale, R. Fellows, and R. Guillemin (1971). Purification, amino-acid composition and N-terminus of hypothalamic luteinizing-hormone releasing factor (LRF) of ovine origin, *Biochem. Biophys. Res. Commun.* **44:**205–210.

Araki, S., M. Ferin, E. A. Zimmerman, and R. L. Vande Wiele (1975a). Ovarian modulation of immunoreactive gonadotropin–releasing hormone (Gn-RH) in the rat brain: evidence for a differential effect on the anterior and midhypothalamus, *Endocrinology* **96:**644–650.

Araki, S., C. D. Toran-Allerand, M. Ferin, and R. L. Vande Wiele (1975b). Immunoreactive gonadotropin-releasing hormone (Gn-RH) during maturation in the rat: ontogeny of regional hypothalamic differences, *Endocrinology* **97:**693–697.

Arimura, A., H. Sato, D. H. Coy, and A. V. Schally (1975). Radioimmunoassay for GH-release inhibiting hormone, *Proc. Soc. Exp. Biol. Med.* **148:**784–792.

Arnauld, E., B. Dufy, and J-D. Vincent (1975). Hypothalamic supraoptic neurones: rates and patterns of action potential firing during water deprivation in the unanaesthetized monkey, *Brain Res.* **100:**315–325.

Baker, B. L., W. C. Dermody, and J. R. Reel (1975). Distribution of gonadotropin-releasing hormone in the rat brain as observed with immunocytochemistry, *Endocrinology* **97:**125–135.

Barnea, A., N. Ben-Jonathan, C. Colston, J. M. Johnston, and J. C. Porter (1975). Differential sub-cellular compartmentalization of thyrotropin releasing-hormone (TRH) and gonadotropin releasing hormone (LRH) in hypothalamic tissue, *Proc. Natl. Acad. Sci. U.S.A.* **72:**3153–3157.

Barry, J., M. P. Dubois, and B. Carette (1974). Immunofluorescence study of the preoptico-infundibular LRF neurosecretory pathway in the normal, castrated or testosterone-treated male guinea pig, *Endocrinology* **95:**1416–1423.

Brazeau, P., W. Vale, R. Burgus, N. Ling, M. Butcher, J. Rivier, and R. Guillemin (1973). Hypothalamic polypeptide that inhibits secretion of immunoreactive pituitary growth hormone, *Science* **179:**77–79.

Brown, M. and W. Vale (1975). Central nervous system effects of hypothalamic peptides, *Endocrinology* **96:**1333–1336.

Brownstein, M., A. Arimura, H. Sato, A. V. Schally, and J. S. Kizer (1975a). The regional distribution of somatostatin in the rat brain, *Endocrinology* **96:**1456–1461.

Brownstein, M., A. Arimura, A. V. Schally, M. Palkovits, and J. S. Kizer (1976). The effect of surgical isolation of the hypothalamus on its luteinizing hormone-releasing hormone content, *Endocrinology* **98:**662–665.

Brownstein, M. J., M. Palkovits, and J. S. Kizer (1976). On the origin of luteinizing hormone-releasing hormone (LH-RH) in the supraoptic crest, *Life Sci.* **17**:679–682.

Brownstein, M. J., M. Palkovits, J. M. Saavedra, R. M. Bassiri, and R. D. Utiger (1974). Thyrotropin-releasing hormone in specific nuclei of rat brain, *Science* **185**:267–269.

Brownstein, M. J., M. Palkovits, J. M. Saavedra, and J. S. Kizer (1976). Distribution of hypothalamic hormones and neurotransmitters within the diencephalon, pp. 1–23 in *Frontiers in Neuroendocrinology*, Martini, L. and W. F. Ganong, eds. Raven Press, New York.

Brownstein, M. J., R. D. Utiger, M. Palkovits, and J. S. Kizer (1975*b*). Effect of hypothalamic deafferentation on thyrotropin-releasing hormone levels in rat brain, *Proc. Natl. Acad. Sci. U.S.A.* **72**:4177–4179.

Burgus, R., T. F. Dunn, D. Desiderio, D. N. Ward, W. Vale, and R. Guillemin (1970). Characterization of ovine hypothalamic hypophysiotropic TSH-releasing factor, *Nature (London)* **226**:321–325.

Burt, D. R. and S. H. Snyder (1975). Thyrotropin releasing hormone (TRH)—apparent receptor binding in rat-brain membranes, *Brain Res.* **93**:309–328.

Cohn, M. L. (1975). Cyclic AMP, thyrotropin releasing factor and somatostatin: key factors in the regulation of the duration of narcosis, pp. 485–500 in *Molecular Mechanisms of Anesthesia*, Fink, B. R., ed. Raven Press, New York.

Dreifuss, J. S., E. Tribollet, and A. J. Baertschi (1976). Excitation of supraoptic neurones by vaginal distention in lactating rats; correlation with neurohypophyseal hormone release, *Brain Res.* **113**:600–605.

Dubois, M. P., J. Barry, and J. Leonardelli (1974). Mise en evidence par immunofluorescence et repartition de la somatostatine (SRIF) dans l'eminence mediane des vertebrés, mammifères, oiseaux, amphibians et poissons, *C. R. Acad. Sci.* **272**:1899–1902.

Dubois, M. P. and E. Kolodziejczyk (1975). Centres hypothalamiques du rat sécrétant la somatostatine: répartition des péricaryons en 2 systèmes magno et parvocellulaires (étude immunocytologique), *C.R. Acad. Sci.* **281**:1737–1740.

Dupont, A., F. Labrie, G. Pelletier, R. Puviani, D. H. Coy, E. J. Coy, and A. V. Schally (1974). Organ distribution of radioactivity and disappearance of radioactivity from plasma after administration of (^{3}H) luteinizing hormone-releasing hormone to mice and rats, *Neuroendocrinology* **16**:65–73.

Dyball, R. E. J. (1971). Oxytocin and ADH secretion in relation to electrical activity on antidromically identified supraoptic and paraventricular units, *J. Physiol.* **214**:245–256.

Dyball, R. E. J. and K. Koizumi (1969). Electrical activity in the supraoptic and paraventricular nuclei associated with neurohypophyseal hormone release, *J. Physiol.* **201**:711–722.

Dyer, R. G. and R. E. J. Dyball (1974). Evidence for a direct effect of LRF and TRF on single unit-activity in rostral hypothalamus, *Nature (London)* **252**:486–488.

Epelbaum, J., P. Brazeau, D. Tsang, J. Brawer, and J. B. Martin (1977). Subcellular distribution of radioimmunoassayable somatostatin in rat brain, *Brain Res.*, in press.

Foreman, M. M. and R. L. Moss (1975). Enhancement of lordotic behavior by intrahypothalamic infusion of luteinizing hormone-releasing hormone, *Abstr. Annu. Meet. Soc. Neurosci.*, 5th, New York, p. 435.

Goldsmith, P. C. and W. F. Ganong (1975). Ultrastructural localization of luteinizing hormone releasing hormone in the median eminence of the rat, *Brain Res.* **97**:181–193.

Grant, G., W. Vale, and R. Guillemin (1973). Characteristics of the pituitary receptor for thyrotropin releasing factor, *Endocrinology* **92**:1629–1633.

Green, A. R. and D. G. Grahame-Smith (1974). TRH potentiates behavioral changes following increased brain 5-hydroxytryptamine accumulation in rats, *Nature (London)* **251**:524–526.

Griffiths, E. C., K. C. Hooper, S. L. Jeffcoate, and D. T. Holland (1975). The effect of gonadectomy and gonadal steroids on the activity of hypothalamic peptidases inactivating luteinizing hormone-releasing hormone (LH-RH), *Brain Res.* **88**:384–388.

Grimm-Jørgensen, Y. and J. F. McKelvy (1974). Biosynthesis of thyrotropin releasing factor by newt (*Triturus Viridescens*) brain in vitro. Isolation and characterization of thyrotropin releasing factor, *J. Neurochem.* **23**:471–478.

Grimm-Jørgensen, Y., J. F. McKelvy, and I. M. D. Jackson (1975). Immunoreactive thyrotrophin releasing factor in gastropod circumesophageal ganglia, *Nature (London)* **254**:620.

Halász, B. (1969). The endocrine effects of isolation of the hypothalamus from the rest of the brain, pp. 307–342 in *Frontiers in Neuroendocrinology*, Ganong, W. F. and L. Martini, eds. Oxford University Press, London.

Harris, G. W. (1955). *Neural Control of Pituitary Gland*. Edward Arnold, London.

Harris, M. C. and M. Sanghera (1974). Projection of medial basal hypothalamic neurones to the preoptic anterior hypothalamic areas and the paraventricular nucleus in the rat, *Brain Res.* **81**:401–411.

Hökfelt, T., S. Effendić, C. Hellerström, O. Johansson, R. Luft, and A. Arimura (1975). Cellular localization of somatostatin in endocrine-like cells and neurons of the rat with special references to A_1-cells of the pancreatic islets and to the hypothalamus, *Acta Endocrinol.* **80** (Suppl. 200): 1–40.

Hökfelt, T., S. Effendić, O. Johansson, B. Luft, and A. Arimura (1974). Immunohistochemical localization of somatostatin (growth-hormone release-inhibiting factor) in guinea-pig brain, *Brain Res.* **80**:165–169.

Hökfelt, T., R. Elde, O. Johansson, R. Luft, G. Nilsson, and A. Arimura (1976). Immunohistochemical evidence for separate populations of somatostatin-containing and substance P-containing primary afferent neurons in the rat, *Neuroscience* **1**:131–136.

Hökfelt, T., K. Fuxe, M. Goldstein, O. Johansson, D. Park, H. Fraser, and S. L. Jeffcoate (1974*b*). Immunofluorescence mapping of central monoamine and releasing hormone (LRH) systems, pp. 381–392 in *Anatomical Neuroendocrinology*, Stumpf, W. E. and L. D. Grant, eds. S. Karger, Basel.

Hökfelt, T., K. Fuxe, O. Johansson, S. Jeffocate, and N. White (1975*b*). Distribution of thyrotropin-releasing hormone (TRH) in the central nervous system as revealed with immunohistochemistry, *Eur. J. Pharmacol.* **34**:389–392.

Hökfelt, T., K. Fuxe, O. Johansson, S. L. Jeffcoate, and N. White (1975c). Thyrotropin releasing hormone (TRH)-containing nerve terminals in certain brain stem nuclei and in the spinal cord, *Neurosci. Lett.* **1**:133–139.

Jackson, I. M. D. and S. Reichlin (1974). Thyrotropin-releasing hormone (TRH)—distribution in hypothalamic and extrahypothalamic brain-tissues of mammalian and submammalian chordates, *Endocrinology* **95**:854–862.

Jonas, H. A., H. G. Burger, I. A. Comming, F. K. Findlay, and D. M. Kretser (1975). Radioimmunoassay for luteinizing hormone releasing hormone (LHRH): its application to the measurement of LHRH in ovine and human plasma, *Endocrinology* **96**:384–393.

Kalra, S. P. (1976). Tissue levels of luteinizing hormone-releasing hormone in the preoptic area and hypothalamus, and serum concentrations of gonadotropins following anterior hypothalamic deafferentation and estrogen treatment in the female rat, *Endocrinology* **99**:101–107.

Kawakami, M. and Y. Sakuma (1974). Responses of hypothalamic neurons to the microiontophoresis of LH-RH, LH and FSH under various levels of circulating ovarian hormones, *Neuroendocrinology* **15**:290–307.

Kawakami, M. and Y. Sakuma (1976). Electrophysiological evidences for possible participation of periventricular neurons in anterior pituitary regulation, *Brain Res.* **101**:79–94.

Keller, H. H., G. Bartholini, and A. Pletscher (1974). Enhancement of cerebral noradrenaline turnover by thyrotropin-releasing-hormone, *Nature (London)* **248**:528–529.

Kelly, M. J. and R. M. Moss (1976). Quantitative evaluation and determination of the biological potency of iontophoretically applied luteinizing hormone releasing hormone (LRH), *Neuropharmacology* **15**:325–328.

Kizer, J. S., M. Palkovits, and M. J. Brownstein (1976). Releasing factors in the circumventricular organs of the rat brain, *Endocrinology* **98**:311–317.

Kobayashi, R. M., K. H. Lu, and S. S. C. Yen (1976). Effects of ovariectomy and estrogen on regional concentrations of hypothalamic LRF and pituitary LH secretion in the rat, *Abstr. Annu. Meet. Soc. Neurosci.*, 6th, Toronto, p. 674.

Kordon, C., B. Kerdelhue, E. Pattou, and M. Jutisz (1974). Immunocytochemical localization of LH-RH in axons and nerve terminals of the rat median eminence, *Proc. Soc. Exp. Biol. Med.* **147**:122–127.

Krulich, L., M. Quijada, E. Hefco, and D. K. Sundberg (1974). Localization of thyrotropin-releasing factor (TRF) in the hypothalamus of the rat, *Endocinrology* **95**:9–17.

Labrie, F., B. Borgeat, L. Ferland, A. Lemay, A. Dupont, S. Lemaire, G. Pelletier, N. Barden, J. Drouin, A. De Lean, A. Belanger, and P. Jolicoeur (1975). Mechanism of action of hypothalamic hypophysiotropic hormones, pp. 109–129 in *Hypothalamic Hormones: Chemistry, Physiology, Pharmacology and Clinical Uses*, Motta, M., P. G. Crossignani, and L. Martini, eds. Academic Press, New York.

Leonardelli, J. and M. P. Dubois (1974). Commandes aminergique et cholinergique des cellules hypothalamiques élaboratrices de LH-RH chez le cobaye, *Ann. Endocrinol.* **35**:639–645.

Makara, G. B., M. C. Harris, and K. M. Spyer (1972). Identification and distribution of tuberoinfundibular neurones, *Brain Res.* **40**:283–290.

Martin, J. B., J. Kontor, and P. Mead (1973). Plasma GH responses to hypothalamic hippocampal and amygdaloid electrical stimulation: effects of variation of stimulation parameters and treatment with α-methyl-paratyrosine (α-MT), *Endocrinology* **92**:1354–1361.

Martin, J. B. and S. Reichlin (1972). Plasma thyrotropin (TSH) response to hypothalamic electrical stimulation and to injection of synthetic thyrotropin releasing hormone (TRH), *Endocrinology* **90**:1079–1089.

McCann, S. M., S. Taleisnik, and H. M. Friedman (1960). LH-releasing activity in hypothalamic extracts, *Proc. Soc. Exp. Biol. Med.* **104**:432–434.

McKelvy, J. F. (1974). Biochemical neuroendocrinology. I. Biosynthesis of thyrotropin releasing hormone (TRH) by organ cultures of mammalian hypothalamus, *Brain Res.* **65**:489–502.

Mitnick, M. and S. Reichlin (1971). Thyrotropin-releasing hormone: biosynthesis by rat hypothalamic fragments in vitro, *Science* **172**:1241–1242.

Moguilevsky, J. A., M. A. Enero, and B. Szwarcfarb (1974). Luteinizing hormone-releasing hormone—biosynthesis by rat hypothalamus *in vitro*. Influence of castration, *Proc. Soc. Exp. Biol. Med.* **147**:434–437.

Mortimer, C. H., A. S. McNeilly, T. A. Fisher, M. A. F. Murray, and G. M. Besser (1974). Gonadotrophin-releasing hormone therapy in hypogonadal males with hypothalamic or pituitary dysfunction, *Br. Med. J.* **4**:617–621.

Moss, R. L. (1975). Relationship between the central regulation of gonadotropin and mating behavior in female rats, pp. 55–76 in *Reproductive Behavior*, Montagna, W. and W. A. Sadler, eds. Plenum Press, New York.

Moss, R. L. (1976). Role of hypophysiotropic neurohormones in mediating neural and behavioral events, *Fed. Proc.*, in press.

Moss, R. L., M. J. Kelly, and C. A. Dudley (1976). Effect of peptide hormones on extracellular electrical activities of preoptic-hypothalamic neurons, *Abstr. Annu. Meet. Soc. Neurosci.*, 6th, Toronto, p. 652.

Moss, R. L., M. Kelly, and P. Riskind (1975a). Tuberoinfundibular neurons: dopaminergic and norepinephrinergic sensitivity, *Brain Res.* **89**:265–277.

Moss, R. L. and S. M. McCann (1973). Induction of mating behavior in rats by luteinizing hormone-releasing factor, *Science* **181**:177–179.

Moss, R. L. and S. M. McCann (1975). Action of luteinizing hormone-releasing faction (LRF) in the initiation of lordosis behavior in the estrone primed ovariectomized female rat, *Neuroendocrinology* **17**:309–318.

Moss, R. L., S. M. McCann, and C. A. Dudley (1975b). Releasing hormones and sexual behavior, *Prog. Brain Res.* **42**:37–46.

Mroz, E. A., M. J. Brownstein, and S. E. Leeman (1976). Evidence for substance P in the habenulo-interpenduncular tract, *Brain Res.* **113**:597–599.

Naik, D. V. (1975a). Immuno-electron microscopic localization of luteinizing hormone-releasing hormone in the arcuate nuclei and median eminence of the rat, *Cell Tissue Res.* **157**:437–455.

Naik, D. V. (1975b). Immunoreactive LH-RH neurons in the hypothalamus identified by light and fluorescent microscopy, *Cell Tissue Res.* **157**:423–436.

Nair, R. M. G., J. F. Barrett, C. Y. Bowers, and A. V. Schally (1970). Structure of porcine thyrotropin releasing hormone, *Biochemistry* **9**:1103–1106.

Oliver, C., N. Ben-Jonathan, R. S. Mical, and J. C. Porter (1975). Transport of thyrotropin-releasing hormone from cerebrospinal fluid to hypophyseal portal blood and the release of thyrotropin, *Endocrinology* **97**:1138–1143.

Oliver, C., R. L. Eskay, N. Ben-Jonathan, and J. C. Porter (1974). Distribution and concentration of TRH in the rat brain, *Endocrinology* **96:**540–546.

Palkovits, M., A. Arimura, M. Brownstein, A. V. Schally, and J. M. Saavedra (1974). Luteinizing hormone-releasing hormone (LH-RH) content of the hypothalamic nuclei in rat, *Endocrinology* **95:**554–558.

Palkovits, M., M. J. Brownstein, A. Arimura, H. Sato, A. V. Schally, and J. S. Kizer (1976). Somatostatin content of the hypothalamic ventromedial and arcuate nuclei and the circumventricular organs in the rat, *Brain Res.* **109:**430–434.

Pelletier, G., F. Labrie, A. Arimura, and A. V. Schally (1974). Electron microscopic immunohistochemical localization of growth hormone-release inhibiting hormone (somatostatin) in the rat median eminence, *Am. J. Anat.* **140:**445–450.

Pelletier, G., F. Labrie, R. Puviani, A. Arimura, and A. V. Schally (1974). Immunohistochemical localization of luteinizing hormone-releasing hormone in rat median-eminence, *Endocrinology* **95:**314–317.

Pfaff, D. W. (1973). Luteinizing hormone-releasing factor potentiates lordosis behavior in hypophysectomized ovariectomized female rats, *Science* **182:**1148–1149.

Plotnikoff, N. P., A. J. Kastin, and A. V. Schally (1974). Growth hormone release inhibiting hormone:neuropharmacological studies, *Pharmacol. Biochem. Behav.* **2:**693–696.

Prange, A. J., Jr., G. R. Breese, G. D. Jahnke, B. R. Cooper, J. M. Cott, I. C. Wilson, M. A. Lipton, and N. P. Plotnikoff (1975a). Parameters of alteration of pentobarbital response by hypothalamic polypeptides, *Neuropsychobiology* **1:**121–131.

Prange, A. J., Jr., G. R. Breese, G. D. Jahnke, B. R. Martin, B. R. Cooper, J. M. Cott, I. C. Wilson, L. B. Alltop, M. A. Lipton, G. Bissette, C. B. Nemeroff, and P. T. Loosen (1975b). Modification of pentobarbital effects by natural and synthetic polypeptides: dissociation of brain and pituitary effects, *Life Sci.* **16:**1907–1914.

Prange, A. J., Jr., C. B. Nemeroff, M. A. Lipton, G. R. Breese, and I. C. Wilson (1976). Peptides in the central nervous system, in *Handbook of Psychopharmacology*, Iverson, L. L., S. D. Iverson, and S. H. Snyder, eds. Plenum Press, New York.

Ramirez, V. D., J. P. Gautron, J. Epelbaum, E. Pattou, A. Zamura, and C. Kordon (1975). Distribution of LH-RH in subcellular fractions of the basomedial hypothalamus, *Mol. Cell. Endocrinol.* **3:**339–350.

Renaud, L. P. (1975). Electrophysiological evidence to suggest that hypothalamic releasing (inhibiting) peptides may be liberated from nerve terminals in the CNS, *Abstr. Annu. Meet. Soc. Neurosci.*, 5th, New York, p. 441.

Renaud, L. P. (1976a). Tuberoinfundibular neurons in the basomedial hypothalamus of the rat: electrophysiological evidence for axon collaterals to hypothalamic and extrahypothalamic areas, *Brain Res.* **105:**59–72.

Renaud, L. P. (1976b). Tuberoinfundibular neurons: electrophysiological studies on afferent and efferent connections, *Physiologist* **19:**338.

Renaud, L. P. (1976c). Influence of amygdala stimulation on the activity of identified tuberoinfundibular neurones in the rat hypothalamus, *J. Physiol.* **260:**237–252.

Renaud, L. P. (1977). Influence of medial preoptic-anterior hypothalamic area stimulation on the excitability of mediobasal hypothalamic neurones in the rat, *J. Physiol.* **264:**541–564.

Renaud, L. P. and J. B. Martin (1975a). Thyrotropin releasing hormone (TRH)—depressant action on central neuronal activity, *Brain Res.* **86:** 150–154.

Renaud, L. P. and J. B. Martin (1975b). Microiontophoresis of thyrotropin-releasing hormone (TRH). Effects on the activity of central neurons, pp. 354–356 in *Anatomical Neuroendocrinology*, Stumpf, W. E. and L. D. Grant, eds. S. Karger, Basel.

Renaud, L. P., J. B. Martin, and P. Brazeau (1975). Depressant action of TRH, LH-RH and somatostatin on activity of central neurons, *Nature (London)* **255:**233–235.

Renaud, L. P., J. B. Martin, and P. Brazeau (1976). Hypothalamic releasing factors: physiological evidence for a regulatory action on central neurons and pathways for their distribution in brain, *Pharmacol. Biochem. Behav.* **5:** Suppl. 1, 171–178.

Rezak, M., V. Havlicek, K. R. Hughes, and H. Friesen (1975). Central action of somatostatin: role of hippocampus, *Abstr. Annu. Meet. Soc. Neurosci.*, 5th, New York, p. 394.

Saito, S., K. Musa, I. Oshima, S. Yamamoto, and T. Funato (1975). Radio-immunoassay for luteinizing hormone in plasma, *Endocrinol. Jpn.* **22:** 247–293.

Sawaki, Y. and K. Yagi (1973). Electrophysiological identification of cell bodies of the tuberoinfundibular neurones in the rat, *J. Physiol.* **230:**75–85.

Sawaki, Y. and K. Yagi (1976). Inhibiton and facilitation of antidromically identified tuberoinfundibular neurones following stimulation of the median eminence in the rat, *J. Physiol.***260:**447–460.

Schally, A. V., A. Arimura, Y. Baba, R. M. G. Nair, J. Matsuo, T. W. Redding, L. Debeljuk, and W. F. White (1971). Isolation and properties of FSH and LH-releasing hormone, *Biochem. Biophys. Res. Commun.* **43:**393–399.

Sétáló, G., S. Vigh, A. V. Schally, A. Arimura, and B. Flerkó (1975a). GH-RIH containing elements in the rat hypothalamus, *Brain Res.* **90:**352–356.

Sétáló, G., S. Vigh, A. V. Schally, A. Arimura, and B. Flerkó (1975b). LH-RH containing neural elements in the rat hypothalamus, *Endocrinology* **96:**135–142.

Sétáló, G., S. Vigh, A. V. Schally, A. Arimura, and B. Flerkó (1976). Immuno-histological study of the origin of LH-RH containing nerve fibers of the rat hypothalamus, *Brain Res.* **103:**597–602.

Silverman, A. J. (1976). Distribution of luteinizing hormone-releasing hormone (LHRH) in the guinea pig brain, *Endocrinology* **99:**30–41.

Steiner, F. A. (1975). Electrophysiological mapping of brain sites sensitive to corticosteroids, ACTH and hypothalamic releasing hormones, pp. 270–275 in *Anatomical Neuroendocrinology*, Stumpf, W. E. and L. G. Grant, eds. S. Karger, Basel.

Szentágothai, J., B. Flerkó, B. Mess, and B. Halász (1968). *Hypothalamic Control of the Anterior Pituitary.* Akademiai Kiado, Budapest.

Taber, C. A. and H. J. Karavolas (1975). Subcellular localization of LH releasing activity in the rat hypothalamus, *Endocrinology* **96:**446–452.

Taurog, A., C. Oliver, R. L. Eskay, J. C. Porter, and J. M. McKenzie (1974). The role of TRH in the neoteny of the Mexican axolotl, *Gen. Comp. Endocrinol.* **24**:267–279.

Tsang, D., A. T. Tan, P. Brazeau, S. Lal, L. P. Renaud, and J. B. Martin (1975). Subcellular distribution of somatostatin in extrahypothalamic brain tissue, *Abstr. Annu. Meet. Soc. Neurosci.*, 5th, New York, p. 450.

Vale, W., P. Brazeau, C. Rivier, M. Brown, B. Ross, J. Rivier, R. Burgus, N. Long, and R. Guillemin (1975). Somatostatin, *Recent Prog. Hor. Res.* **31**:365–397.

Vale, W. and C. Rivier (1975). Hypothalamic hypophysiotropic hormones, pp. 195–238 in *Handbook of Psychopharmacology*, Vol. 5, Iversen, L., S. D. Iversen, and S. H. Snyder, eds. Plenum Press, New York.

Vale, W., C. Rivier, M. Palkovits, J. M. Saavedra, and M. Brownstein (1974). Ubiquitous brain distribution of inhibitors of adenohypophyseal secretion, *Endocrinology* **94**:A 128.

Vandesande, F. and M. R. Aspeslagh (1974). Failure of thyrotropin releasing hormone to increase ^{125}I uptake by the thyroid of Rana temporaria, *Gen. Comp. Endocrinol.* **23**:355–356.

Wakerley, J. B. and D. W. Lincoln (1973). The milk ejection reflex of the rat: a 20- to 40-fold acceleration in the firing of paraventricular neurones during oxytocin release, *J. Endocrinol.* **57**:477–493.

Wheaton, J. E., L. Krulich, and S. M. McCann (1976). Localization of luteinizing hormone-releasing hormone in the preoptic area and hypothalamus of the rat using radioimmunoassay, *Endocrinology* **97**:30–38.

Whittaker, V. P. (1969). The synaptosome, pp. 327–364 in *Handbook of Neurochemistry*, Vol. 2, Lajtha, A., ed. Plenum Press, New York.

Wilbur, J. F., E. Montoya, N. Plotnikoff, W. F. White, R. Genrich, L. Renaud, and J. B. Martin (1976). Gonadotropin-releasing hormone and thyrotropin-releasing hormone: distribution and effects in the central nervous system, *Recent Prog. Hor. Res.*, **32**:117–153.

Winokur, A. and R. D. Utiger (1974). Thyrotropin-releasing hormone — regional distribution in rat brain, *Science* **185**:265–267.

Yagi, K. and Y. Sawaki (1974). Recurrent inhibition and facilitation: demonstration in the tuberoinfundibular system and effects of strychnine and picrotoxin, *Brain Res.* **84**:155–159.

Yarbrough, G. G. (1976). TRH potentiates excitatory actions of acetylcholine on cerebral cortical neurones, *Nature (London)* **263**:523–524.

Zimmerman, E. A. (1976). Localization of hypothalamic hormones by immunocytochemical techniques, pp. 29–62 in *Frontiers in Neuroendocrinology*, Vol. 4, Martini, L. and W. F. Ganong, eds. Raven Press, New York.

Zimmerman, E. A., K. C. Hsu, M. Ferin, and G. P. Kozlowski (1974). Localization of gonadotropin-releasing hormone (GH-RH) in the hypothalamus of the mouse by immunoperoxidase technique, *Endocrinology* **95**:1–8.

ENKEPHALINS, ENDORPHINS, AND OPIATE RECEPTORS

Hans W. Kosterlitz, John Hughes, John A. H. Lord, and Angela A. Waterfield

University of Aberdeen, Aberdeen, Scotland

INTRODUCTION

About a year ago, the first paper (Hughes, Smith, Kosterlitz, Fothergill, Morgan, and Morris, 1975b) was published giving the structures of the two pentapeptides that are present in the CNS and interact with opiate receptors. One of the peptides is H-Tyr-Gly-Gly-Phe-Leu-OH or leucine-enkephalin. The other peptide, methionine-enkephalin, has the sequence H-Tyr-Gly-Gly-Phe-Met-OH, which, as was pointed out in the paper, is identical with sequence 61–65 of ovine β-lipotropin (Figure 1), first isolated and sequenced by Li, Barnafi, Chrétien, and Chung (1965). This sequence is present also in the β-lipotropins of porcine, bovine, camel, or human origin (Gráf, Barát, Cseh, and Sajgó, 1971; Pankov and Iudaev, 1972; Li and Chung, 1976a,b). No analogue of β-lipotropin has yet been discovered in which methionine^{65} is replaced by leucine.

It is of interest to recall at this point the anticipatory statement C. H. Li made in 1968: "It should not be surprising that the hormone (β-lipotropin) may have other unexpected activities when subjected to extensive biological examination." One of the most important findings that followed the discovery of the presence of the methionine-enkephalin sequence in β-lipotropin was the opiate-like behavior shown by the fragments of lipotropin commencing at Tyr^{61} and having different lengths of amino acid residues. The presence of five amino acids appears to be essential, because the tetrapeptides, LPH$_{61-64}$ and LPH$_{62-65}$, are almost inactive (Morgan, Smith, Waterfield, Hughes, and Kosterlitz, 1976; Hambrook, Morgan, Rance, and

H-Glu-Leu-Thr-Gly-Glu-Arg-Leu-Glu-Gln-Ala-
                5   10

Arg-Gly-Pro-Glu-Ala-Gln-Ala-Glu-Ser-Ala-
              15   20

Ala-Ala-Arg-Ala-Glu-Leu-Glu-Tyr-Gly-Leu-
              25   30

Val-Ala-Glu-Ala-Glu-Ala-Ala-Glu-Lys-Lys-
              35   40

Asp-Ser-Gly-Pro-Tyr-Lys-Met-Glu-His-Phe-
              45   50

Arg-Trp-Gly-Ser-Pro-Pro-Lys-Asp-Lys-Arg-
              55   60

Tyr-Gly-Gly-Phe-Met-Thr-Ser-Glu-Lys-Ser-
              65   70

Gln-Thr-Pro-Leu-Val-Thr-Leu-Phe-Lys-Asn-
              75   80

Ala-Ile-Ile-Lys-Asn-Ala-His-Lys-Lys-Gly-Gln-OH
              85   90

FIGURE 1. Amino acid sequence of ovine β-lipotropin. From Li and Chung (1976a).

Smith, 1976). On the other hand, LPH_{61-68}, LPH_{61-69}, LPH_{61-76} (α-endorphin), LPH_{61-77} (γ-endorphin), LPH_{61-87} (C'-fragment), LPH_{61-89}, and LPH_{61-91} (C-fragment or β-endorphin) all have considerable affinity to the binding sites of the opiate receptors and are active in the guinea pig ileum and mouse vas deferens (Bradbury, Smyth, Snell, Birdsall, and Hulme, 1976; Guillemin, Ling, and Burgus, 1976; Cox, Goldstein, and Li, 1976; Lazarus, Ling, and Guillemin, 1976; Lord, Waterfield, Hughes, and Kosterlitz, 1976; Ling, Burgus, and Guillemin, 1976; Waterfield, Smokcum, Hughes, Kosterlitz, and Henderson, 1977).

Lipotropin$_{61-91}$ (C-fragment or β-endorphin) is particularly interesting in that it has a very potent antinociceptive action after injection into the cerebral ventricles or into the brain substance dorsal to the periaqueductal grey of the mesencephalon (Feldberg and Smyth, 1976; Loh, Tseng, Wei, and Li, 1976; Pert, 1976); it is also active after intravenous injection (Tseng, Loh, and Li, 1976). One of the reasons for this good antinociceptive effect is the resistance of β-endorphin to enzymatic inactivation (Pert, Bowie, Fong, and Chang, 1976).

In the guinea pig ileum and the mouse vas deferens, β-endorphin has a slower onset and offset of action than either of the two enkephalins. The fast onset of action and the rapid inactivation of the enkephalins appear to make them good candidates for a possible role of inhibitory neurotransmitters or neuromodulators. At the same time, these characteristics make it much more difficult to examine their putative physiological roles. To show that they have pharmacological actions in the whole animal, they have to be applied by iontophoresis close to neurons in the brain or spinal cord when they will depress the firing rates of these neurons, some of which have been shown to belong to the nociceptive pathways (Hill, Pepper, and Mitchell, 1976). This effect is rapid both in onset and offset, and in most cells is reversed by naloxone (e.g., Bradley, Briggs, Gayton, and Lambert, 1976; Davies and Dray, 1976; Zieglgänsberger, Fry, Herz, Moroder, and Wünsch, 1976; Duggan, Hall, and Headley, 1976). The enkephalins have only a small and transient antinociceptive effect, even after injection into the cerebral ventricles. This is probably due to their rapid enzymatic inactivation, because the D-alanine^2 analogue of methionine-enkephalin, which is enzyme resistant, is a good antinociceptive agent (Pert et al., 1976).

From this survey of the chemical and biological properties of the enkephalins and endorphins, it seems necessary to conclude that we are dealing with a series of compounds that have one characteristic in common, namely, that they interact with the opiate receptors. There are, however, considerable quantitative and probably qualitative differences between the members of the series, apparently incompatible with the assumption of a single receptor.

In two of the major systems of neurotransmission it has been established that there is more than one type of receptor for the released transmitter mediating different physiological functions. In the cholinergic system, acetylcholine interacts with both the muscarinic and nicotinic receptors, which can be differentiated by the specific antagonists atropine and (+)-tubocurarine or hexamethonium. In the catecholaminergic system, the situation is more complex: noradrenaline can interact with α_1- and α_2-receptors and also with β_1- and β_2-receptors, which are again distinguished by specific antagonists. Adrenaline has most, if not all, the actions of noradrenaline, but it is not a major neurotransmitter; furthermore, it is present mainly in an endocrine organ, the medulla of the adrenal gland. A third member of the catecholaminergic system is dopamine, which is differentiated from noradrenaline by a specific antagonist and several other characteristics.

What is the evidence for the presence of more than one opiate receptor and more than one endogenous opioid agonist subserving different physiological functions? Portoghese (1965) discussed the possibility that opiates might have more than one binding mode. His method for detecting similarities or differences in molecular binding modes compared the variation of activity in two or more different series of compounds when identical changes of the N-substituent were made. A parallel change in activity is suggestive of similar binding modes, whereas a nonparallel relationship is indicative of dissimilar interactions. Two years later, Martin (1967) introduced the concept of receptor dualism. The basis of this hypothesis was the observation by Houde and Wallenstein (1956) that, in man, the interaction between morphine and nalorphine is biphasic, because low doses of nalorphine antagonize the analgesic action of morphine, whereas higher doses increase analgesia. The receptor dualism hypothesis proposes that nalorphine interacts as an antagonist with the morphine receptor, but as an agonist with a receptor different from the morphine receptor. Martin and his colleagues examined this concept by studying the effects of various opioid drugs on the behavior and reflex activity of the chronic spinal dog, and thus distinguished between three types of receptors: morphine is the prototype agonist for the μ-receptor, ketocyclazocine is the prototype agonist for the κ-receptor, and N-allylnorcyclazocine is the prototype agonist for the σ-receptor (Martin, Eades, Thompson, Huppler, and Gilbert, 1976; Gilbert and Martin, 1976).

Parallel Assays of Enkephalins and Endorphins

Receptors with different properties present in a mixed receptor population are readily differentiated when antagonists are used that are specific for the different receptors. If such specific antagonists are not available, the agonist activities are assayed simultaneously in several systems. If the rank order of potency varies in the different assays, the assay tissues may be assumed to have identical receptors. If, on the other hand, there is no correlation of the rank order of potency in the different bioassays, the receptor populations are not identical (Chang and Gaddum, 1933).

Two of the assay systems that have been used in our analyses are based on pharmacological responses, namely the contractions of the guinea pig ileum or its myenteric plexus-longitudinal muscle prepara-

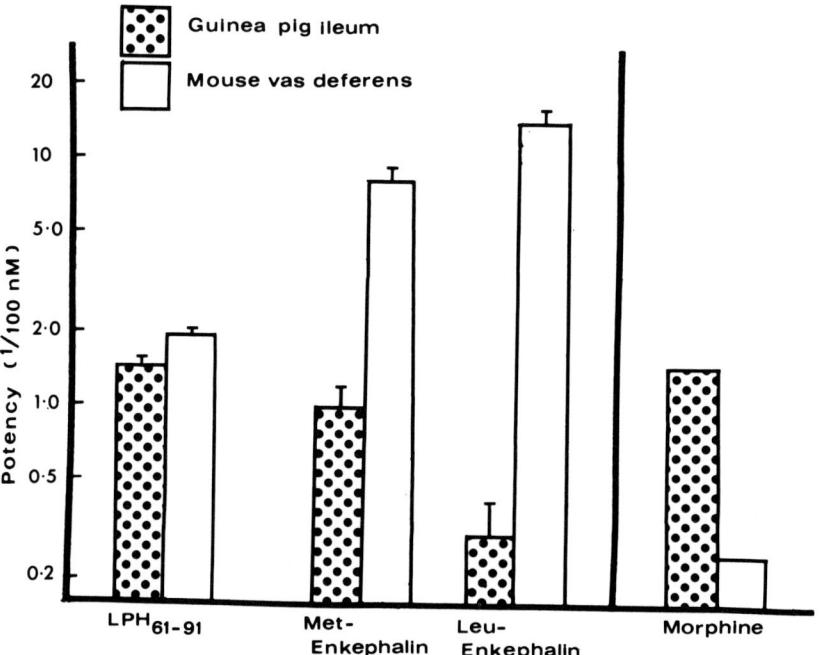

FIGURE 2. The potencies of natural porcine β-endorphin, synthetic methionine-enkephalin, leucine-enkephalin, and morphine in the guinea pig ileum and mouse vas deferens. Potencies are given on the ordinate as the reciprocals of the ID_{50} values expressed in units of 100 nM.

tion (Kosterlitz and Watt, 1968) and the mouse vas deferens (Hughes, Kosterlitz, and Leslie, 1975a). The other two systems depend on the inhibition of the binding of two different ligands in brain homogenates, namely [^{3}H]naloxone (1 nM) and [^{3}H]leucine-enkephalin (0.86 nM). To reduce enzymatic inactivation to its minimum, the incubation was carried out at 0°C for 150 min (Lord et al., 1976).

When LPH_{61-91} (C-fragment or β-endorphin), methionine-enkephalin, leucine-enkephalin, and morphine are assayed in the guinea pig ileum and mouse vas deferens and their potencies are plotted as the reciprocals of the ID_{50} values, it is found that natural LPH_{61-91} is equipotent in the two preparations (Figure 2). LPH_{61-65} (methionine-enkephalin) is more potent than LPH_{61-91} in the mouse vas deferens, whereas in the guinea pig ileum, it is less active. These differences in potency become even more pronounced when methionine is replaced by leucine, the resulting leucine-enkephalin being about 50 times more potent in the vas deferens than in the guinea pig ileum. In contrast, the alkaloid morphine is about six times more potent in the guinea pig ileum than in the mouse vas deferens.

Because LPH_{61-91} may well be the parent substance of shorter peptides and, particularly, of methionine-enkephalin, it is of interest that it is about equiactive not only in the guinea pig ileum (ID_{50} of the natural porcine peptide is 75 ± 6.0 nM, n = 4, and of the synthetic ovine peptide 85 ± 6.6 nM, n = 4) and mouse vas deferens (53 ± 4.0 nM, n = 4, and 70 ± 5.8 nM, n = 4, respectively), but also in its ability to inhibit [^{3}H]leucine-enkephalin binding (ID_{50} of the synthetic ovine peptide is 1.51 ± 0.19 nM, n = 3) and [^{3}H]naloxone binding (2.23 ± 0.16 nM, n = 3). For this reason, it was decided to compare the relative potencies of peptides, morphine, and naloxone in the four assay systems and relate the results to β-endorphin as a standard of reference (Table 1). As far as inhibition of [^{3}H]leucine-enkephalin binding is concerned, β-endorphin is the most potent of the peptides, followed by D-alanine^2-methionine-enkephalin, methionine-enkephalin itself, and leucine-enkephalin; the methionine-enkephalin analogues N-CH$_3$-Tyr-Gly-Gly-Phe-Met amide and LPH_{61-76} (α-endorphin) are weak inhibitors. Morphine and naloxone are least effective, the inhibition by morphine sometimes not exceeding 30 to 40%. By far the most potent inhibitors of [^{3}H]naloxone binding are naloxone and β-endorphin, followed by the N-CH$_3$-Tyr-Gly-Gly-Phe-Met amide, methionine-enkephalin, its D-alanine^2 analogue, N-CH$_3$-Tyr^1-methionine-enkephalin, morphine, leucine-enkephalin, and finally α-endorphin. β-Endorphin is about 16 times more potent than morphine as an inhibitor of [³H]naloxone binding, a value that agrees well with the factor of 10 found for the natural porcine peptide under different experimental conditions by Bradbury et al. (1976); naloxone is 1.3 times more potent than β-endorphin in our experiments, and it was 1.4 times more potent in the experiments of Bradbury et al. (1976).

To allow for the variation in the absolute values, the ratios of inhibition of [³H]leucine-enkephalin binding to inhibition of [³H]naloxone binding were calculated and compared to the ratio for β-endor-

TABLE 1. *The relative potencies (β-endorphin equals 1) of opioid peptides, morphine, and naloxone to inhibit saturable binding of [³H]leucine-enkephalin and [³H]naloxone in homogenates of guinea pig brain and to depress the electrically induced contractions of the mouse vas deferens and guinea pig ileum*[a]

Compound	Inhibition of binding of:		Ratio of leucine-enkephalin/ naloxone	Inhibition of contractions of:		Ratio of mouse vas deferens/ guinea pig ileum
	[³H]leucine-enkephalin	[³H]naloxone		mouse vas deferens	guinea pig ileum	
β-Endorphin (LPH$_{61-91}$)	1	1	1	1	1	1
α-Endorphin (LPH$_{61-76}$)	0.036 (4)	0.016 (3)	2.2	2.4 (6)	0.38 (7)	6.3
Methionine-enkephalin (LPH$_{61-65}$)	0.64 (17)	0.19 (9)	3.4	5.5 (16)	0.88 (31)	6.2
N-CH$_3$-Tyr^1-methionine-enkephalin	0.20 (4)	0.072 (3)	3.6	1.3 (5)	1.3 (6)	1.0
N-CH$_3$-Tyr^1-methionine-enkephalin amide	0.068 (3)	0.27 (3)	0.25	1.8 (4)	3.3 (5)	0.56
D-Ala^2-methionine-enkephalin	0.76 (3)	0.11 (3)	6.9	31 (7)	5.3 (8)	5.9
Leucine-enkephalin	0.43 (18)	0.038 (5)	11	9.0 (9)*	0.34 (13)	26
Morphine	0.002 (3)	0.062 (4)	0.03	0.14 (7)*	1.2 (6)*	0.12
Naloxone	0.030 (3)	1.3 (3)	0.02	—	—	—

[a] The ID$_{50}$ value of synthetic ovine β-endorphin for inhibition of [³H]leucine-enkephalin binding at 0°C in the absence of Na$^+$ was 1.51 ± 0.19 nM (3), and of [³H]naloxone binding, 2.23 ± 0.16 nM (3). The relative potencies of the other compounds were the ratio of the ID$_{50}$ value of β-endorphin to the ID$_{50}$ value of the compound under test; the number of observations are given in parentheses. In view of the considerable variation between preparations, methionine-enkephalin or leucine-enkephalin was used as internal standard except for the values indicated by asterisks. The ID$_{50}$ value of methionine-enkephalin was 12.8 ± 1.2 nM (16) in the mouse vas deferens, and 96.2 ± 8.7 nM (31) in the guinea pig ileum; the ID$_{50}$ values of leucine-enkephalin were 7.8 ± 0.8 nM (8) and 463 ± 59 nM (10), respectively. The mean ID$_{50}$ values of β-endorphin were 69.8 ± 5.8 nM (4) in the mouse vas deferens and 85.0 ± 6.6 nM (4) in the guinea pig ileum, adjusted to the mean ID$_{50}$ values of leucine-enkephalin, which served as internal standard.

phin as a standard of reference (Table 1). It was found that α-endorphin, and methionine-enkephalin and its N-CH$_3$-tyrosine[1] analogue inhibit [^{3}H]leucine-enkephalin binding more than [^{3}H]naloxone binding. This pattern of activity is particularly marked with leucine-enkephalin and D-alanine[2]-methionine-enkephalin. In contrast, N-CH$_3$-Tyr-Gly-Gly-Phe-Met amide and, particularly, morphine and naloxone, inhibit [^{3}H]naloxone binding better than [^{3}H]leucine-enkephalin binding.

In summary, we have found that opioid peptides and opiate alkaloids show considerable variations in their affinity to the opiate receptors identified by [^{3}H]leucine-enkephalin and [^{3}H]naloxone binding. These observations lead to the question of whether or not there are physiological correlates to these differences. We tested this possibility, in the first instance, in the two in vitro preparations, the mouse vas deferens and the guinea pig ileum.

In the mouse vas deferens, all peptides tested are more potent than β-endorphin, particularly D-alanine[2]-methionine-enkephalin, leucine-enkephalin, and methionine-enkephalin (Table 1). Even α-endorphin, which is a weak agonist both in binding tests and in the guinea pig ileum, is in the mouse vas deferens somewhat more potent than β-endorphin. The two N-CH$_3$-tyrosine[1] analogues of methionine-enkephalin are about equipotent with β-endorphin. Morphine is the only compound tested in this series that is weaker than β-endorphin. A very different pattern has been found in the guinea pig ileum. About equiactive with β-endorphin are methionine-enkephalin, its N-CH$_3$-tyrosine[1] analogue, and morphine. More potent are the D-alanine[2]-analogue of methionine-enkephalin and, particularly, N-CH$_3$-Tyr-Gly-Gly-Phe-Met amide; less potent are α-endorphin and leucine-enkephalin.

The ratios of activity in the mouse vas deferens to activity in the guinea pig ileum were calculated and again compared to β-endorphin as the standard of reference (Table 1). In general, the pattern was similar to that found for the ratios of activity in inhibiting [^{3}H]leucine-enkephalin binding to activity in inhibiting [^{3}H]naloxone binding, although the absolute values of the ratios differed between the two groups. For instance, leucine-enkephalin and D-alanine[2]-methionine-enkephalin, which inhibit [^{3}H]leucine-enkephalin binding much better than [^{3}H]naloxone binding, are also much more potent in the mouse vas deferens than in the guinea pig ileum. At the other end of the spectrum, N-CH$_3$-Tyr-Gly-Gly-Phe-Met amide and morphine inhibit

[³H]naloxone binding better than [³H]leucine-enkephalin binding, and are more active in the guinea pig ileum than in the mouse vas deferens.

These findings are not compatible with the view that the receptor populations in the homogenate of guinea pig brain, in the guinea pig ileum, and in the mouse vas deferens are homogeneous and identical. At first sight, this appears to be surprising, because there is such good correlation between the analgesic activity of many narcotic analgesics with their activities in the guinea pig ileum and mouse vas deferens, and their ability to inhibit [³H]naloxone binding in rat brain homogenates (Kosterlitz and Waterfield, 1975; Hughes et al., 1975a; Creese and Snyder, 1975). The first discrepancy in this relationship was found for certain benzomorphans, which are unusual in that they do not substitute for morphine in the morphine-dependent monkey, although they have strong antinociceptive activity reversible by naloxone. In the two in vitro bioassay preparations, too, these benzomorphans have unusual pharmacological effects (Hutchinson, Kosterlitz, Leslie, Waterfield, and Terenius, 1975). First, their relative agonist potencies in the mouse vas deferens are only 25% of those in the guinea pig ileum when related to normorphine as a standard of reference. Second, these benzomorphans require, in both assay preparations, three to six times more naloxone (pA_2 of 7.9 to 8.05) for the antagonism of their agonist actions than is needed for the antagonism of the classical analgesics, e.g., morphine or normorphine (pA_2 of 8.5 to 8.7). These findings suggest that both preparations contain receptors other than those with which the classical analgesics interact. In the chronic spinal dog, Martin and his colleagues (Martin et al., 1976; Gilbert and Martin, 1976) showed that two members of this group, ketocyclazocine and ethylketocyclazocine, had effects different from those of morphine, and they suggested that these compounds interacted with κ-receptors rather than with the typical morphine or μ-receptors. From our experiments it would appear that both the guinea pig ileum and the mouse vas deferens have μ- and κ-receptors. Because the mouse vas deferens is less sensitive to these unusual benzomorphans, it may be assumed that in the mouse vas deferens the proportion of κ-receptors to μ-receptors is smaller than in the guinea pig ileum.

As far as methionine-enkephalin and leucine-enkephalin are concerned, naloxone antagonizes these peptides as readily as normorphine does (K_e of about 2.5 nM corresponding to pA_2 of 8.6) in the guinea pig

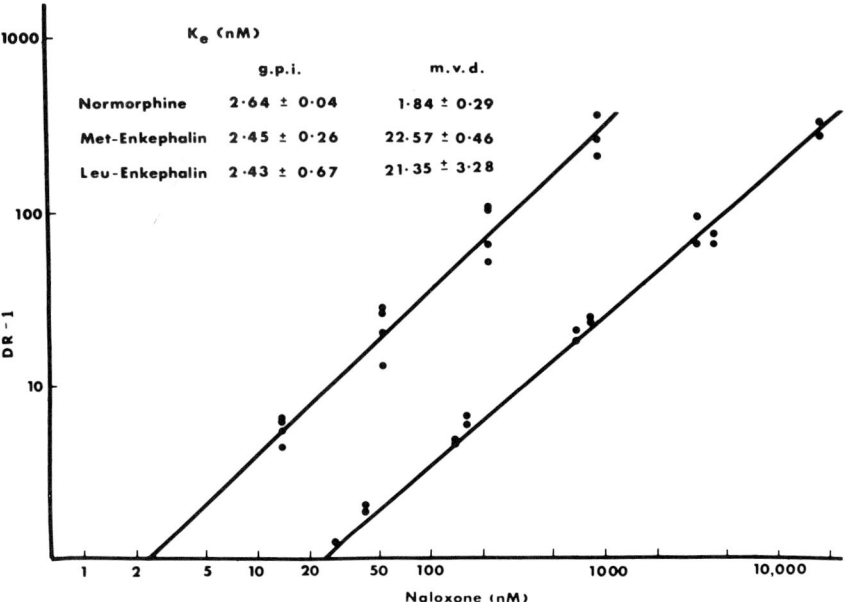

FIGURE 3. The determination of the dissociation equilibrium constant K_e, or its negative logarithm pA_2, of naloxone. The agonists are normorphine, methionine-enkephalin, and leucine-enkephalin. The regression lines are for methionine-enkephalin, on the left in the guinea pig ileum and on the right in the mouse vas deferens.

ileum (Figure 3). On the other hand, in the mouse vas deferens, naloxone is much less effective as an antagonist against the peptides (K_e of about 22 nM corresponding to pA_2 of 7.65) than against normorphine (K_e of about 1.8 nM corresponding to pA_2 of 8.75). Similar results have been obtained for all opioid peptides thus far investigated (unpublished observations). Following a line of argument similar to that used for the differentiation between μ- and κ-receptors in our assay systems, we are led to the conclusion that the opioid peptides act on populations of receptors that are different in the mouse vas deferens from those in the guinea pig ileum. In the latter tissue, the peptides seem to interact mainly with μ-receptors, whereas in the mouse vas deferens they probably act on ∂-receptors (Lord et al., 1976). Because high affinity to the [^{3}H]leucine-enkephalin binding sites in homogenates of guinea pig brain is associated with high pharmacological activity in the mouse vas deferens (Table 1), it is possible that the ∂-receptor is associated with high affinity to leucine-enkephalin.

The question arises now of whether or not it is possible to correlate the different receptors with different physiological functions. The only functional property of the enkephalins and endorphins that has so far been subjected to some analysis is their antinociceptive effect. Of the compounds given in Table 1, results have been published for methionine-enkephalin by several laboratories who have agreed that it is a weak antinociceptive agent even after administration into the cerebral ventricles or the central periaqueductal grey. However, replacement of glycine² by D-alanine, which makes the compound resistant to enzymatic degradation, converts methionine-enkephalin to a potent antinociceptive agent (Pert, 1976; Pert et al., 1976). Similarly, introduction of N-CH$_3$ at the N-terminal tyrosine, and an amide group at the C-terminal methionine makes methionine-enkephalin less readily inactivated by peptidases, and the resulting N-CH$_3$-Tyr-Gly-Gly-Phe-Met amide has an antinociceptive action after injection into the third ventricle of cats (Feldberg and Smyth, 1977). β-Endorphin is a very potent antinociceptive agent, and α-endorphin is a relatively weak one (Feldberg and Smyth, 1976; Pert, 1976). If we consider the abilities of these compounds and of morphine to inhibit [³H]leucine-enkephalin binding and [³H]naloxone binding, we find that the pattern of these compounds is quite heterogeneous: β-endorphin is the most potent inhibitor, acting equally well on [³H]leucine-enkephalin and [³H]naloxone; N-CH$_3$-Tyr-Gly-Gly-Phe-Met amide is four times more potent as an inhibitor of naloxone binding than of leucine-enkephalin binding; in contrast, Tyr-D-Ala-Gly-Phe-Met is seven times more potent as an inhibitor of leucine-enkephalin than of naloxone binding; finally, morphine is 30 times more potent as an inhibitor of naloxone than of leucine-enkephalin binding. A similar lack of correlation exists between antinociceptive action of the peptides and their relative potency in the two bioassay preparations, particularly the mouse vas deferens. It would follow, therefore, that antinociceptive action is not closely correlated with the degree of interaction of a peptide with μ-receptors or ∂-receptors. There are two main possible explanations for these observations: either all receptors, i.e., μ-, ∂-, and κ-receptors, can mediate antinociception, or all compounds act to varying degrees on one common receptor mediating antinociception.

CONCLUSIONS

The possible physiological functions of the endorphins and enkephalins have not yet been elucidated. There are similarities in principle, but important differences in detail between the actions of morphine and those of the peptides, as for instance, antinociception (e.g., Pert, 1976), effects on the extrapyramidal motor system (e.g., Bloom, Segal, Ling, and Guillemin, 1976; Jacquet and Marks, 1976) and possibly on the release of pituitary hormones and, finally, tolerance and dependence (e.g., Wei and Loh, 1976). Detailed examination in vivo is made difficult by the rapid destruction of the naturally occurring pentapeptides. Therefore, a direct comparison of the stable long-chain peptides with the pentapeptides is not possible in vivo, unless iontophoretic application is used. When the pentapeptides are made resistant to enzymatic inactivation by blocking the N- and C-termini or by introduction of an unnatural amino acid, the experiments reported in this paper show that their relative affinities to the various binding sites or receptors are changed.

One of the most interesting findings of the present investigation is that β-endorphin inhibits equally well [^{3}H]leucine-enkephalin and [^{3}H]naloxone binding and is also equipotent in the guinea pig ileum and mouse vas deferens. This observation may be interpreted as indicating that β-endorphin, which is possibly a precursor of other opioid peptides, interacts equally well with several or perhaps all opiate receptors. The shorter peptide, methionine-enkephalin, is in several aspects different from its putative parent substance in that it has greater affinity to the binding site of [^{3}H]leucine-enkephalin than to that of [^{3}H]naloxone, that it is more potent in the mouse vas deferens than in the guinea pig ileum and, finally, that it is readily inactivated by peptidases. Thus, it would appear that methionine-enkephalin is designed for a more specialized function than is β-endorphin; furthermore, the short duration of action of methionine-enkephalin makes it particularly suitable for transmitting or modulating neuronal impulses, whereas β-endorphin could fulfil the function of a neurohumoral agent of prolonged action.

It is interesting to note how readily small changes in the molecule change the characteristics of methionine-enkephalin. The replacement of glycine^2 by D-alanine not only prevents degradation by peptidases, but also shifts the relative affinity in favor of the [^{3}H]leucine-enkephalin binding site, whereas for N-CH$_3$-Tyr-Gly-Gly-Phe-Met amide there is an increase in the relative affinity to the [^{3}H]naloxone binding site.

These changes in relative affinity are paralleled by changes in the relative activity in the two bioassay preparations, a relative increase in potency in the mouse vas deferens occurring concomitantly with a relative increase in affinity to the [³H]leucine-enkephalin binding site. There is, however, so far no explanation for the sometimes large changes in absolute activity. For instance, in the mouse vas deferens the D-alanine² analogue of methionine-enkephalin is over 30 times more potent than β-endorphin, although the affinity to the binding site of [³H]leucine-enkephalin is slightly less than that of β-endorphin. Furthermore, N-CH₃-Tyr-Gly-Gly-Phe-Met amide is somewhat more active than β-endorphin in both bioassay preparations, but its affinity to the binding site of [³H]naloxone is only 27%, and its affinity to the binding site of [³H]leucine-enkephalin is only 7%, of that of β-endorphin. Similar discrepancies between inhibition of [³H]naloxone binding and pharmacological activity in bioassay preparations have been noted with some narcotic analgesics, for instance, fentanyl and ethylketocyclazocine (Kosterlitz and Leslie, unpublished observations).

If it is permissible to assume that the endorphins and the enkephalins have physiological functions of a neuronal and endocrine character, then it follows that the opioid peptidergic systems are of considerable complexity. There are several agonists that seem to be matched by the presence of multiple receptors. These circumstances are similar to those found in the catecholamine system, but whereas in the latter the action of the transmitter is terminated by its reuptake in the nerve terminals, in the opioid peptidergic system inactivation of the rapidly acting pentapeptides appears to be by enzymatic degradation similar to that of acetylcholine. It is tempting to compare the neuroendocrine element of the catecholamine system, adrenaline, with the member of the peptidergic system, which may also have a neuroendocrine function, β-endorphin. Adrenaline is present in high concentration in the adrenal medulla, and large accumulations of β-endorphin and α-endorphins are found in the intermediate and anterior lobes of the pituitary gland (Ling et al., 1976). Adrenaline is essential for the fight or flight reaction. β-Endorphin may be of importance in similar situations: could the often-reported lack of pain perception on the battle field or the reduced pain experienced during childbirth be explained on this basis? Because morphine specifically reduces the levels of luteinizing hormone and testosterone in the serum of rats (Cicero, Wilcox, Bell, and Meyer, 1976), could it be possible that the longer-chain endorphins of the pituitary play some role in the control of sexual functions? However, the other components of the two systems, noradrenaline and dopamine on the one hand,

and methionine-enkephalin and leucine-enkephalin on the other, are present in lower concentrations in widely spread areas of the central and autonomic nervous systems (Simantov and Snyder, 1976; Smith, Hughes, Kosterlitz, and Sosa, 1976). This would be compatible with the role of neuromodulator or neurotransmitter suggested for the enkephalins. Future experimental work will decide whether or not these speculations are justified.

ACKNOWLEDGMENTS

This research was supported by grants from the U.K. Medical Research Council, the U.S. National Institute on Drug Abuse (DA 00662), and the U.S. Committee on Problems of Drug Dependence. Grateful acknowledgment is made of the following gifts: [^{3}H]leucine-enkephalin (Radiochemical Centre), [^{3}H]naloxone (National Institute on Drug Abuse), natural porcine C-fragment or β-endorphin, and N-CH$_3$-Tyr^1-methionine-enkephalin amide (Drs. H. F. Bradbury and D. G. Smyth), synthetic ovine β-endorphin (Dr. C. H. Li), synthetic α-endorphin (Dr. R. Guillemin), methionine-enkephalin, leucine-enkephalin, D-alanine^2-methionine-enkephalin, and N-CH$_3$-Tyr^1-methionine-enkephalin (Dr. B. A. Morgan; Reckitt and Colman), naloxone (Endo Laboratories), and normorphine (Dr. E. L. May).

REFERENCES

Bloom, F., D. Segal, N. Ling, and R. Guillemin (1976). Endorphins: profound behavioral effects in rats suggest new etiological factors in mental illness, *Science* **194**:630–632.

Bradbury, A. F., D. G. Smyth, C. R. Snell, N. J. M. Birdsall, and E. C. Hulme (1976). C fragment of lipotropin has a high affinity for brain opiate receptors, *Nature (London)* **260**:793–795.

Bradley, P. B., E. Briggs, R. J. Gayton, and L. A. Lambert (1976). Effects of microiontophoretically applied methionine-enkephalin on single neurones in rat brain stem, *Nature (London)* **261**:425–426.

Chang, H. C. and J. H. Gaddum (1933). Choline esters in tissue extracts, *J. Physiol. (London)* **79**:255–285.

Cicero, T. J., C. E. Wilcox, R. D. Bell, and E. R. Meyer (1976). Acute reductions in serum testosterone levels by narcotics in the male rat; stereospecificity blockade by naloxone and tolerance, *J. Pharmacol. Exp. Ther.* **198**:340–346.

Cox, B. M., A. Goldstein, and C. H. Li (1976). Opioid activity of a peptide, β-lipotropin-(61–91), derived from β-lipotropin, *Proc. Natl. Acad. Sci. U.S.A.* **73**:1821–1823.

Creese, I. and S. H. Snyder (1975). Receptor binding and pharmacological activity of opiates in the guinea-pig intestine, *J. Pharmacol. Exp. Ther.* **194**:205–219.

Davies, J. and A. Dray (1976). Effects of enkephalin and morphine on Renshaw cells in feline spinal cord, *Nature (London)* **262**:603–604.

Duggan, A. W., J. G. Hall, and P. M. Headley (1976). Morphine, enkephalin and the substantia gelatinosa, *Nature (London)* **264**:456–458.

Feldberg, W. and D. G. Smyth (1976). The C-fragment of lipotropin—a potent analgesic, *J. Physiol. (London)* **260**:30–31P.

Feldberg, W. and D. G. Smyth (1977). Analgesia produced in cats by the C-fragment of lipotropin and by a synthetic pentapeptide, *J. Physiol. (London)* **265**:25–27P.

Gilbert, P. E. and W. R. Martin (1976). The effect of morphine- and nalorphine-like drugs in the nondependent, morphine-dependent and cyclazocine-dependent chronic spinal dog, *J. Pharmacol. Exp. Ther.* **198**:66–82.

Gráf, L., E. Barát, G. Cseh and M. Sajgó (1971). Amino acid sequence of porcine β-lipotropic hormone, *Biochim. Biophys. Acta* **229**:276–278.

Guillemin, R., N. Ling, and R. Burgus (1976). Endorphines, peptides d'origine hypothalamique et neurohypophysaire à activité morphinomimétique. Isolement et structure moléculaire d'α-endorphine, *C.R. Acad. Sci.* **274**:783–785.

Hambrook, J. M., B. A. Morgan, M. J. Rance, and C. F. C. Smith (1976). Mode of deactivation of the enkephalins by rat and human plasma and rat brain homogenates, *Nature (London)* **262**:782–783.

Hill, R. G., C. M. Pepper, and J. F. Mitchell (1976). Depression of nociceptive and other neurones in the brain by iontophoretically applied met-enkephalin, *Nature (London)* **262**:604–606.

Houde, R. W. and S. L. Wallenstein (1956). Clinical studies of morphine-nalorphine combinations, *Fed. Proc.* **15**:440–441.

Hughes, J., H. W. Kosterlitz, and F. M. Leslie (1975a). Effect of morphine on adrenergic transmission in the mouse vas deferens. Assessment of agonist and antagonist potencies of narcotic analgesics, *Br. J. Pharmacol.* **53**:371–381.

Hughes, J., T. W. Smith, H. W. Kosterlitz, L. A. Fothergill, B. A. Morgan, and H. R. Morris (1975b). Identification of two related pentapeptides from the brain with potent opiate agonist activity, *Nature (London)* **258**:577–579.

Hutchinson, M., H. W. Kosterlitz, F. M. Leslie, A. A. Waterfield, and L. Terenius (1975). Assessment in the guinea-pig ileum and mouse vas deferens of benzomorphans which have strong antinociceptive activity but do not substitute for morphine in the dependent monkey, *Br. J. Pharmacol.* **55**:541–546.

Jacquet, Y. F. and N. Marks (1976). The C-fragment of β-lipotropin: an endogenous neuroleptic or antipsychotogen? *Science* **194**:632–635.

Kosterlitz, H. W. and A. A. Waterfield (1975). In vitro models in the study of structure-activity relationships of narcotic analgesics, *Annu. Rev. Pharmacol.* **15**:29–47.

Kosterlitz, H. W. and A. J. Watt (1968). Kinetic parameters of narcotic agonists and antagonists, with particular reference to N-allylnoroxymorphone (naloxone), *Br. J. Pharmacol.* **33**:266–276.

Lazarus, L. H., N. Ling, and R. Guillemin (1976). β-Lipotropin as a prohormone for the morphinomimetic peptides, endorphins and enkephalins, *Proc. Natl. Acad. Sci. U.S.A.* **73**:2156–2159.

Li, C. H. (1968). β-Lipotropin, a new pituitary hormone, *Arch. Biol. Med. Exp.* **5**:55–61.

Li, C. H., L. Barnafi, M. Chrétien, and D. Chung (1965). Isolation and amino-acid sequence of β-LPH from sheep pituitary glands, *Nature (London)* **208**:1093–1094.

Li, C. H. and D. Chung (1976*a*). Isolation and structure of an untriakontapeptide with opiate activity from camel pituitary gland, *Proc. Natl. Acad. Sci. U.S.A.* **73**:1145–1148.

Li, C. H. and D. Chung (1976*b*). Primary structure of human β-lipotropin, *Nature (London)* **260**:622–624.

Ling, N., R. Burgus, and R. Guillemin (1976). Isolation, primary structure, and synthesis of α-endorphin and γ-endorphin, two peptides of hypothalamic-hypophysial origin with morphinomimetic activity, *Proc. Natl. Acad. Sci. U.S.A.* **73**:3942–3946.

Loh, H. H., L. F. Tseng, E. Wei, and C. H. Li (1976). β-Endorphin is a potent analgesic agent, *Proc. Natl. Acad. Sci. U.S.A.* **73**:2895–2898.

Lord, J. A. H., A. A. Waterfield, J. Hughes, and H. W. Kosterlitz (1976). Multiple opiate receptors, pp. 275–280 in *Opiates and Endogenous Opioid Peptides*, Kosterlitz, H. W., ed. North-Holland Publishing Co., Amsterdam.

Martin, W. R. (1967). Opioid antagonists, *Pharmacol. Rev.* **19**:463–521.

Martin, W. R., C. G. Eades, J. A. Thompson, R. E. Huppler, and P. E. Gilbert (1976). The effects of morphine- and nalorphine-like drugs in the nondependent and morphine-dependent chronic spinal dog, *J. Pharmacol. Exp. Ther.* **197**:517–532.

Morgan, B. A., C. F. C. Smith, A. A. Waterfield, J. Hughes, and H. W. Kosterlitz (1976). Structure-activity relationships of methionine-enkephalin, *J. Pharm. Pharmacol.* **28**:660–661.

Pankov, Iu. A. and N. A. Iudaev (1972). Polnaia posledovatel'nost'aminokislotnykh ostatkov v molekule svinogo beta-lipotropina, *Biokhimiya* **37**:994–1004.

Pert, A. (1976). Behavioral pharmacology of D-alanine^2-methionine-enkephalin amide and other long-lasting opiate peptides, pp. 8–94 in *Opiates and Endogenous Opioid Peptides*, Kosterlitz, H. W., ed. North-Holland Publishing Co., Amsterdam.

Pert, C. B., D. L. Bowie, B. T. W. Fong, and J.-K. Chang (1976). Synthetic analogues of met-enkephalin which resist enzymatic destruction, pp. 79–86 in *Opiates and Endogenous Opioid Peptides*, Kosterlitz, H. W., ed. North-Holland Publishing Co., Amsterdam.

Portoghese, P. S. (1965). A new concept on the mode of interaction of narcotic analgesics with receptors, *J. Med. Chem.* **8**:609–616.

Simantov, R. and S. H. Snyder (1976). Brain-pituitary opiate mechanisms: pituitary opiate receptor binding, radioimmunoassays for methionine enkephalin and leucine enkephalin, and [^{3}H]enkephalin interactions with the opiate receptor, pp. 41–48 in *Opiates and Endogenous Opioid Peptides*, Kosterlitz, H. W., ed. North-Holland Publishing Co., Amsterdam.

Smith, T. W., J. Hughes, H. W. Kosterlitz, and R. P. Sosa (1976). Enkephalins: isolation, distribution and function, pp. 57–62 in *Opiates and Endogenous Opioid Peptides*, Kosterlitz, H. W., ed. North-Holland Publishing Co., Amsterdam.

Tseng, L.-F., H. H. Loh, and C. H. Li (1976). β-Endorphin as a potent analgesic by intravenous injection, *Nature (London)* **263**:239–240.

Waterfield, A. A., R. W. J. Smokcum, J. Hughes, H. W. Kosterlitz, and G. Henderson (1977). *In vitro* pharmacology of the opioid peptides, enkephalins and endorphins, *Eur. J. Pharmacol.*, in press.

Wei, E. and H. Loh (1976). Chronic, intracerebral infusion of morphine and peptides with osmotic minipumps, and the development of physical dependence, pp. 303–310 in *Opiates and Endogenous Opioid Peptides*, Kosterlitz, H. W., ed. North-Holland Publishing Co., Amsterdam.

Zieglgänsberger, W., J. P. Fry, A. Herz, L. Moroder, and E. Wünsch (1976). Enkephalin-induced inhibition of cortical neurones and the lack of this effect in morphine tolerant/dependent rats, *Brain Res.* **115**:160–164.

Angiotensin-Sensitive Sites in the Brain Ventricular System

M. Ian Phillips, D. Felix, W. E. Hoffman, and D. Ganten

University of Iowa, University of Zürich, and University of Heidelberg

The classical view that hypothalamic hormones have singular functions has had to be changed because it has become clear that these peptide hormones not only have multiple effects, but are also broadly distributed throughout the brain and body. For example, somatostatin, which was originally considered to be a growth hormone-release inhibitor, is a tetradecapeptide that also inhibits insulin, glucagon, and gastrin release. Furthermore, somatostatin is found not only in the hypothalamus, but also in the stomach and pancreas (Hökfelt, Efendic, Hellerström, Johansson, Luft, and Arimura, 1975). Similarly, substance P is found in neural tissue and in the gut, and certain peptides associated initially only with the gut, such as gastrin and vasoactive intestinal peptide (VIP), have recently been found in the brain (Pearse, 1976).

It has now been shown that the octapeptide angiotensin II, once thought of as a vasoconstrictor, has a large number of properties and a wide distribution that includes the brain, as well as many other tissues (Ganten, Hutchinson, Schelling, Ganten, and Fischer, 1976a). This augmented view of its function has emerged as a result of the discovery of iso-renin-angiotensin systems in brain (Ganten, Minnich, Granger, Hayduk, Brecht, Barbeau, Boucher, and Genest, 1971; Fischer-Ferrario, Nahmod, Goldstein and Finkielman, 1971), salivary glands, gonads, and other tissues (Ganten, Schelling, Vecsei, and Ganten, 1976b). These iso-renins are distinguished from kidney renin by virtue of their independent action on extrarenal tissues where the naturally

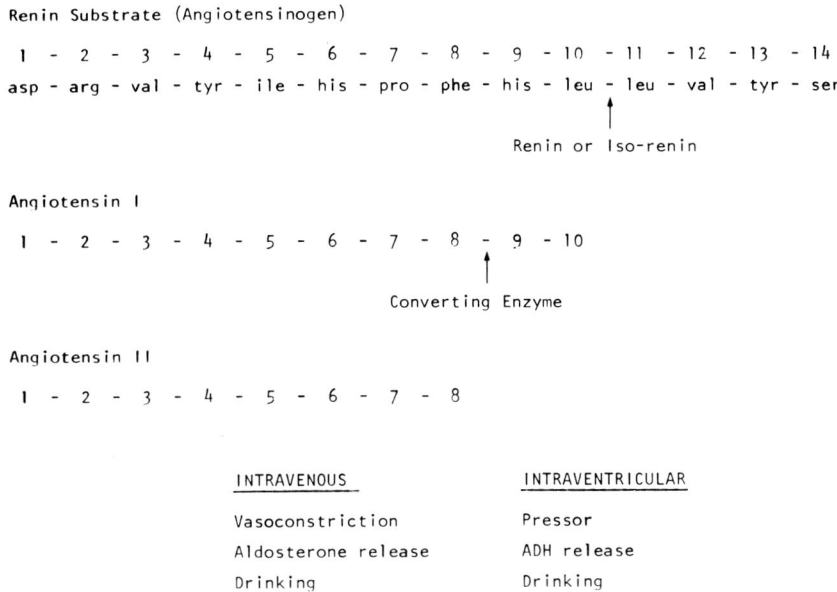

FIGURE 1. The amino acid sequences of the renin-angiotensin system and the changes that occur in the formation of angiotensin II. The latter is responsible for the effects listed when given intravenously or intraventricularly.

occurring renin substrate (angiotensinogen) is present. Iso-renins are characterized by their ability to hydrolyze the substrate between the 10 and 11 leucyl-leucyl bond to form angiotensin I (Figure 1). The iso-renin is a specific enzyme and does not degrade angiotensin I. Iso-renin (or angiotensinogenase) concentration is not dependent on the presence of renin from the kidney, since similar levels are maintained even after nephrectomy. Concentrations in the brain (about 20 ng of angiotensin I/mg of protein per hour) are 30 to 40 times higher than plasma levels (Ganten, Schelling, Hoffman, Phillips, and Ganten, 1977). All the components of a renin-angiotensin system are present in the brain. In addition to iso-renin, these components include the substrate (angiotensinogen) angiotensin I-converting enzyme and angiotensinase (Ganten et al., 1976a; Yang and Neff, 1972). Furthermore, angiotensin receptors have been demonstrated in brain tissue (Nicoll and Barker, 1971; Sakai, Marks, George, and Koestner, 1974; Phillips and Felix, 1976). In this paper, we will focus on the physiological action of angiotensin II and the current search for its receptors in the brain, as a possible model peptide.

Why Peptides?

One may ask why peptides should have so many functional roles and be so widely distributed. First of all, peptides are short chains of amino acids. Longer chains of 12 to 14 or more amino acids are considered to be polypeptides and longer chains still are designated as macropeptides or proteins. Because the peptide structure is small, it is easily formed and quickly inactivated by enzyme action. The sequence of amino acids in the peptide offers a number of possible permutations; for example, in the case of angiotensin a large number of analogues can be produced which compete with the angiotensin II molecule for receptor occupancy. The peptides developed early in evolution, and their wide distribution in the body may be traced ontogenetically back to their presence in the primordial cells in the embryo (Pearse, 1976). Of broad interest to neuroscientists is the fact that many peptides produce profound effects on behavior. Behavior is basically a physiological mechanism developed to maintain physiological homeostasis. Simple examples are hunger or thirst, or the movement of an animal from one temperature to another to maintain its body temperature. More subtle changes are involved in learning and memory, but one can view these as physiological mechanisms selected early in evolution as necessary sophistications for sustaining physiological balance over long periods of time. Peptides are involved in these behavioral mechanisms, as well as in the classical physiological mechanisms. De Wied and his colleagues (De Wied, 1976) have shown that ACTH, a polypeptide of 39 amino acids, has an effect on learning in, for example, a conditioned avoidance situation. Furthermore, they have demonstrated that the active components of the polypeptide are the amino acid sequences between 4 and 7 (De Wied, 1976). Fewer amino acids have no effect, whereas more amino acids produce no increase in the effect. ACTH is released in response to stress and provides physiological protection against inflammation. The behavioral counterpart of this response appears to consist of increasing attentiveness during stress, and ACTH has continued to play a role in this development. Another peptide that has been investigated is the nonadecapeptide vasopressin (ADH). This hormone not only plays a role in water balance, but, as De Wied has shown, is also involved in memory. The connection between water balance and memory is not hard to speculate upon and it should be emphasized that ADH is released by stress, too. Angiotensin is also involved in water balance. It is associated with increased hypertension during states of hypovolemia (Severs and Daniels-Severs, 1973). On the basis of deductive reasoning, Fitzsimons (1972) has proposed that angiotensin is also a thirst hormone, and Epstein, Fitzsimons, and Rolls (1970) have demonstrated that angiotensin infusions will produce drinking behavior. Whether angiotensin has more subtle effects on learning and memory remains to be investigated. Because angiotensin injections into the brain release both ACTH (Reid and Day, 1977) and ADH (Mouw, Bonjour, Malvin and Vander, 1971), angiotensin may act indirectly; this effect may be the most significant, because this peptide may potentially control the release of other peptides.

Search for Receptors

It has been shown that angiotensin II(AII)-induced drinking occurs after both intravenous (i.v.) injections and injections into various brain areas (Booth, 1968; Epstein et al., 1970). Severs, Summy-Long, Daniels-Severs, and Connor (1971) have further shown that AII injected into the brain in relatively small quantities elevates blood pressure and induces drinking behavior. Since this discovery, it has been demonstrated that renin injected directly into the ventricles of the brain elicits drinking (Reid and Ramsay, 1975). Angiotensin I (AI) also stimulates drinking, but it is ineffective when SQ 20881 is present (Cooling and Day, 1974). SQ 20881 is a nonapeptide that inhibits the conversion of AI to AII. AII effectively elicits drinking behavior, but can be inhibited by a specific competitor analogue, such as Sar-1-Ala-8-AII (Swanson, Marshall, Needleman, and Sharpe, 1973), or by AII antibodies (Epstein, Fitzsimons, and Johnson, 1973). Thus, the active peptide for these drinking and blood pressure effects is the octapeptide AII. The actual site of injection in the brain, however, has proved to be less important than it was first thought to be. If, when the cannula is placed in the brain, it penetrates the ventricles, and AII is injected through it, some AII usually escapes into the ventricular system (Johnson and Epstein, 1975). For this reason, attention is currently focused upon the ventricular system in the search for AII receptor sites. The actual receptors are the starting points for entry into the complex brain circuits that control thirst, blood pressure, and ADH release. By defining these receptors, we should eventually be able to study these neural circuits for such physiological mechanisms in as precise a way as the sensory systems are now being studied.

Peripheral and Central Effects

Since AII occurs endogenously (because release of renin by the kidney affects levels of angiotensin in the plasma), it may be asked whether the effects of injecting angiotensin into the brain merely mimic the action of angiotensin produced peripherally.

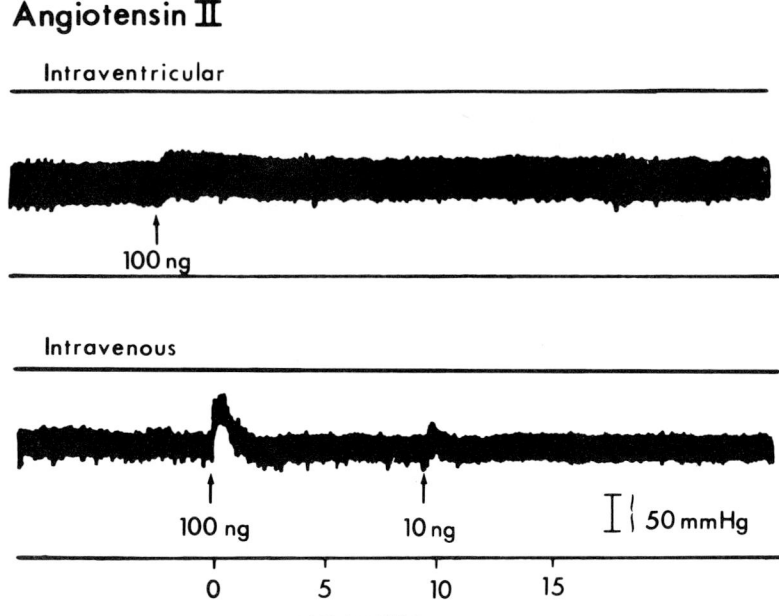

FIGURE 2. Blood pressure responses to AII by two different routes of administration.

Responses to intraventricular (IVT) AII may be characterized differently from responses to AII given intravenously. First, the blood pressure response to AII i.v. is fast (occurring within 10 sec), and short; on the other hand, the response to IVT AII occurs more slowly (30 sec) and lasts much longer (10 to 15 min) (Figure 2). Second, one can increase the blood pressure response by increasing the dose of AII i.v., but the pressor response to the IVT angiotensin levels off above 500 ng, and no further increase in the pressor response is seen (Figure 3). This implies that, in the ventricles, angiotensin has a threshold effect on the pressor response. The quick response to AII after i.v. injection is due to its effect on local receptors in the walls of blood vessels (Page and McCubbin, 1968), whereas the slower response to AII IVT is presumably due to the time it takes for the AII injected into the lateral ventricles to reach appropriate receptor sites. Third, AII IVT has no effect on kidney function, whereas AII i.v. causes a decrease in GFR, plasma flow, and Na^+ excretion (Weet, Hoffman, and Phillips, 1977).

ADH release by AII i.v. is a matter of controversy. Bonjour and

Malvin (1970) reported a release of ADH after i.v. AII, but Share and his colleagues (Shade and Share, 1975) were not able to confirm this. In our laboratory, we have not found convincing evidence for the release of ADH by AII given peripherally. AII IVT, however, consistently produces an ADH release response (Keil, Summy-Long, and Severs, 1975). We have calculated that the amount of ADH released by an injection of 50 ng of AII is 2 to 3 mU, which is actually sufficient to produce a pressor response (Hoffman and Phillips, 1977).

Drinking behavior is more easily and more reliably obtained by injections of AII into the ventricles than by infusion or injection of AII i.v. (Epstein et al., 1970). It has been pointed out by Abraham, Baker, Blaine, Denton, and McKinley (1975), however, that the concentration of AII injected IVT is relatively enormous. They have based their

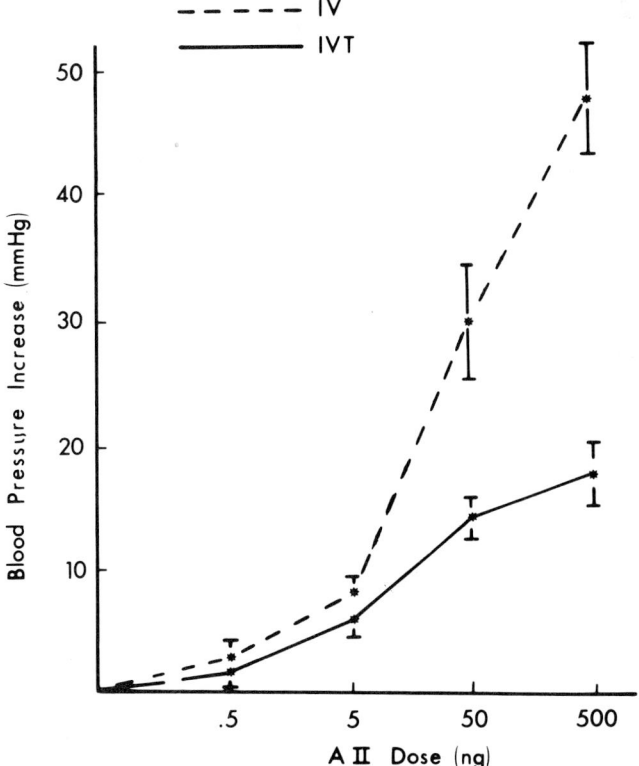

FIGURE 3. Relationship between blood pressure responses and dose of AII given by two different routes of administration.

calculations on an effective IVT dose of 0.1 ng in 0.5 µliters, as reported by Simpson and Routtenberg (1973), which would be equivalent to 20,000 ng per 100 ml, whereas drinking (at least in sheep) occurs when the blood concentration levels reach 100 ng per 100 ml. The 0.5 µliters of AII, however, is injected into a certain volume of CSF, and an unknown amount of the AII travels up the sides of the cannula. In addition, CSF is a dynamic medium and moves the concentrated solution away from the injection site, and, in so doing, may also move the dose away from the receptive area. We have found that an injection of 50 pg in 1 µliter of AII is sufficient to produce drinking and a blood pressure response if the cannula is aimed at the anterior part of the third ventricle. Although this is still a high dose, the important point is that, within the ventricles, there are different sensitivities to AII, and until we can calculate the amount of AII that reaches the receptors we shall not be able to say whether the doses are physiological or not (see Figure 10).

In summary, there are differences between the IVT and i.v. routes of injection of AII, which means that the peripheral effects of angiotensin are not responsible for all the effects seen by central angiotensin injections.

Voyage Through the Ventricles

Since the focus of attention is on ventricular sites of action, we shall briefly consider some of the anatomical features of the ventricular system. Let us imagine a voyage in the ventricles. Starting from the choroid plexus of one of the lateral ventricles where CSF is largely produced (Davson, 1970), we would see the ventricle walls covered with undulating cilia (Figure 4). The CSF would be shunted backwards and forwards with each heartbeat, but the overall direction would be toward the third ventricle. We would enter the third ventricle via the foramen of Monroe and there, where the choroid plexi of both lateral ventricles meet, we would see above us the subfornical organ pendulously hanging from the roof of the third ventricle (Figure 4B). A striking feature of this organ is that it is devoid of the mass of cilia so characteristic of the ventricle walls. One would see three zones in the subfornical organ, a partially ciliated anterior zone, a sparsely ciliated central zone, and a posterior zone containing large bulbous cells and occasional clumps of cilia (Phillips, Balhorn, Leavitt, and Hoffman, 1974a) (Figure 4C). If we then journeyed down the face of the anterior third ventricle, moving over the hump caused by the anterior commissure, we would see the apex of the organum vasculosum of the lamina terminalis (OV). This apex would stand out as another region that has no cilia or very few cilia. As we travel down the OV toward the base of the third ventricle we find that the cells are flat (Figure 4D) and have frequent strands of axon-like structures sweeping across the surface, disappearing down between the clefts of the cells. At the base of the OV, we would be in the optic recess, where it is quite possible that the flow of CSF is slower than in other parts of the ventricular system due to the narrowing of the recess. On the floor of the ventricle above the optic chiasm are clumps of cilia, and these give way to the oligociliated floor of the median eminence (ME), which is usually dotted with numerous small vesicles on the surface (Figure 4E). Rising above the ME, one again encounters the ciliated wall of the ventricle. Here, CSF may enter or exit through gap junctions within the wall (see Figure 5). Further caudal, the ME descends into the infundibular recess (IR). Travelling upward to the dorsal third ventricle, we again meet the choroid plexus as it terminates at the pineal recess. Below the dorsal third ventricle is the subcommissural organ, which guards the entrance to the cerebral aqueduct. The subcommissural organ has rounded, rather than flattened cells, but these too have few cilia—usually only a single cilium for each cell (Figure 4F). After the narrow cerebral aqueduct, one enters the cavernous fourth ventricle, with walls carpeted with cilia (Figure 4G), and little change is seen until one arrives at the very end of the fourth ventricle beneath the tent-like cover of the isolated choroid plexus. There we find the bare surface of the area postrema (Figure 4H), positioned at the dividing point for CSF to flow down into the spinal cord through the spinal canal, or up to the arachnoid villae via the cisterna magna. Of these areas, the area postrema, the subfornical organ, and the anterior third ventricle are regions that have been proposed as mediators of the angiotensin effects. These areas are circumventricular organs (CVO) that are known to have an imperfect blood-brain barrier. In addition to these areas, a location within the cerebral aqueduct, the subnucleus medialis, has also been proposed as a site of AII receptors.

Area Postrema

The evidence for the area postrema being involved in AII pressor action comes from the fact that intravertebral injections of angiotensin are more effective in producing a pressor response than are i.v. injections (Dickinson and Thomas, 1959). When the area postrema is

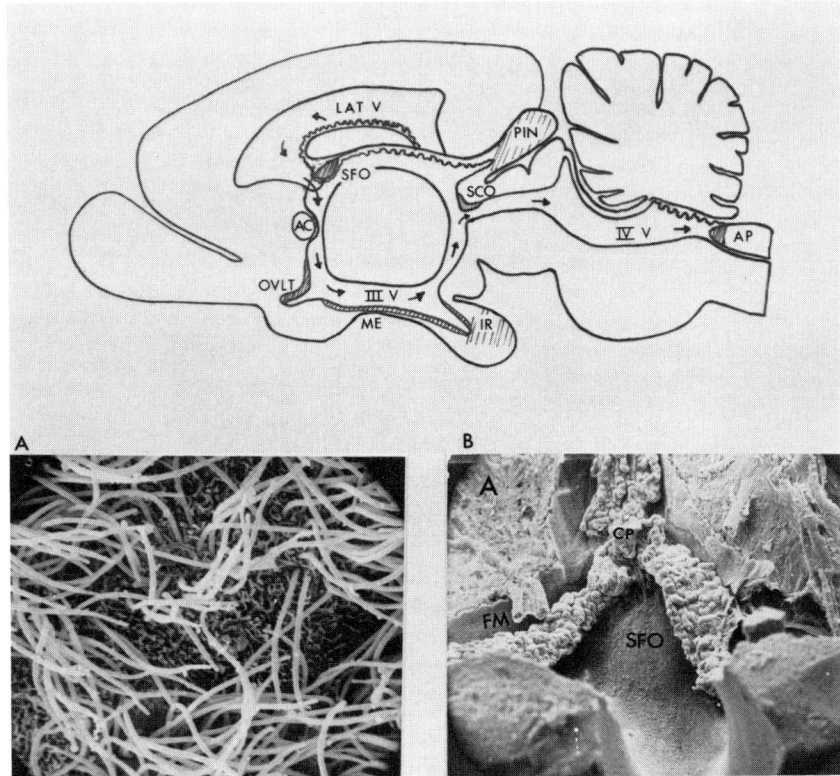

FIGURE 4. The ventricular system in the brain of the rat showing the circumventricular organs. Abbreviations: AC, anterior commissure; OVLT, organum vasculosum of the lamina terminalis; ME, median eminence; III V, third ventricle; IR, infundibular recess and hypophysis; SCO, subcommisural organ; PIN, pineal gland; IV V, fourth ventricle; AP, area postrema; Lat V, lateral ventricle; SFO, subfornical organ. The arrows indicate the route that was followed as described in the text. (A) Scanning electron microscope (SEM) photomicrograph of ciliated wall of lateral ventricle ($\times 4,500$). (B) The subfornical organ and choroid plexus (CP) in the third ventricle just beyond the foramen of Monroe (FM) ($\times 67$). (C) High-power view of surface of the subfornical organ ($\times 220$). (D) The OVLT ($\times 560$). (E) The surface of the ME, which is often covered in numerous microvilli and a few cilia ($\times 4,230$). (F) Subcommisural organ showing columnar ependymal cells ($\times 1,980$). (G) Ciliated wall of cerebral aqueduct ($\times 4,500$). (H) Area postrema ($\times 2,050$).

ablated, the response to vertebral artery infusion of angiotensin is entirely abolished (Joy and Lowe, 1970). Microinjection of AII into the area postrema causes systemic pressor responses (Ueda, 1968). The response to i.v. angiotensin II is reduced after area postrema ablation

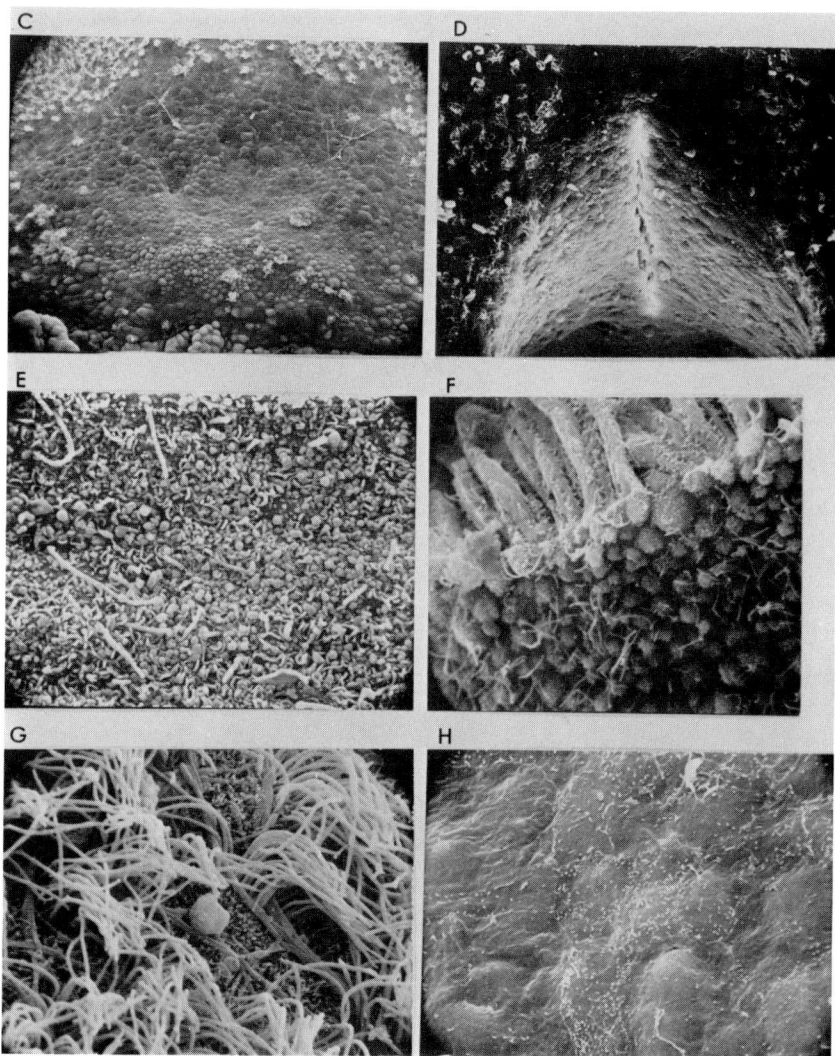

(Scroop, Katic, Joy, and Lowe, 1971). Analysis of the evidence reveals that two issues are involved. (1) The evidence strongly indicates that angiotensin has its effect on the area postrema when injected via the vertebral artery (Sweet and Brody, 1970). (2) The evidence is weak that the area postrema might be responsive on the ventricular side. When AII was injected intraventricularly directly above the area postrema in rats, we were not able to obtain pressor effects (Phillips and

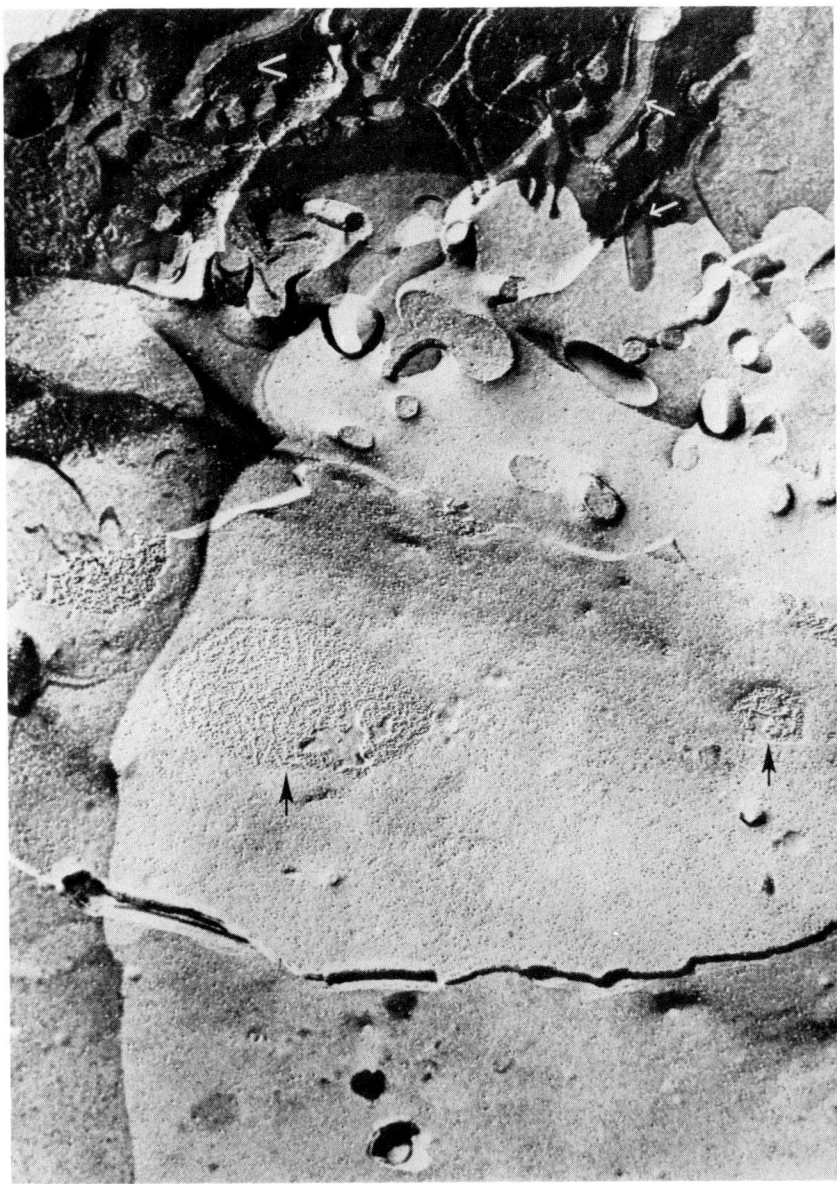

FIGURE 5. Freeze fracture of a ciliated ependymal cell showing gap junctions (black arrows) in the cell wall and cilia (white arrows) in the ventricle (V). Deshmukh, Larsen, and Phillips, unpublished observations (×75,000).

Hoffman, 1977); nor were Ferrario, Gildenberg, and McCubbin (1972) able to obtain effects in their experiments with dogs. The only evidence for AII getting to the area postrema by the ventricular route is from the microinjection studies performed by Ueda. Microinjections, however, penetrate the surface of the area postrema and deliver the angiotensin to the same area that the blood-borne angiotensin could reach. We therefore conclude that although the area postrema is probably a site of action of AII from the blood side, particularly the intravertebral route, it is not a receptor site on the ventricular side. The fact that ablation of the area postrema does not entirely abolish the effects of AII i.v. means that the area postrema cannot be the only site of action for blood pressure in the brain.

Subnucleus Medialis

The subnucleus medialis or the nucleus mesencephalicus profundus of the cat has been proposed as a site for AII receptors by Deuben and Buckley (1970). This nucleus lies close to the cerebral aqueduct, which is a ciliated region in the rat. Because most of the ciliated regions contain gap junctions through which the CSF can flow, it is quite probable that AII in the ventricular system could reach this nucleus. Deuben and Buckley showed that lesioning the area abolishes the pressor effect to IVT AII in the cat. In the rat, however, our data suggest that the subnucleus medialis does not appear to be essential for mediating the AII IVT pressor response. These data are obtained by using the plugging technique in which a cream plug is injected into the ventricles (Hertz, Albus, Matys, Schubert, and Toschenachi, 1970). The procedure we use is as follows: rats are implanted with two cannulae, one in the area that is to be plugged, and another through which angiotensin is to be administered. After recovery from the operation, the rats are tested first with AII to make sure that the cannula is effective. At least 1 h later, a microplug of 1 to 2 μliters of cold cream (Nivea) is injected through the other cannula. Within 0.5 h of the plugging, the rat is again tested with the peptide. Following the test, black india ink in the same volume is injected through the same cannula as in the test injection. The rat is immediately killed by overdose with Nembutal, and the brain is carefully removed and frozen. The frozen brain is then cut sagittally on a freezing microtome to reveal the third ventricle. The sections are photographed. In this short time between plugging and testing there is no apparent development of hydrocephalus. The plug itself produces no behavioral or physiological effects that we can detect. One can see the areas reached by the peptide from the distribution of the dye, and because the plug is white, the results come out in an uncompromising black and white (Figure 6). After plugging the entire cerebral aqueduct, we were still able to produce blood pressure and drinking responses to AII injected into the third ventricle or the lateral ventricle. Therefore, we conclude that in the rat the receptive sites are more anterior than the cerebral aqueduct.

Subfornical Organ

In his review of thirst in 1972, Fitzsimons made the suggestion that the subfornical organ might be a likely candidate as a dipsogenic

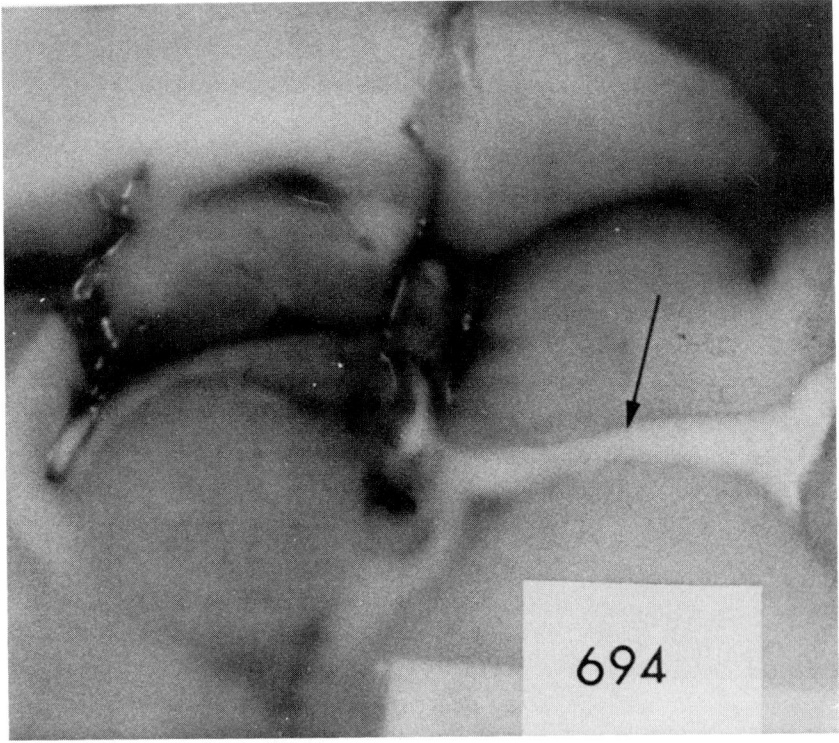

FIGURE 6. Example of histology of rat brain ventricle (sagittal section) in which the cerebral aqueduct has been filled by a cream plug shortly before testing. Blood pressure and drinking responses were still obtained from animals plugged in this way by injections of AII in the third ventricle.

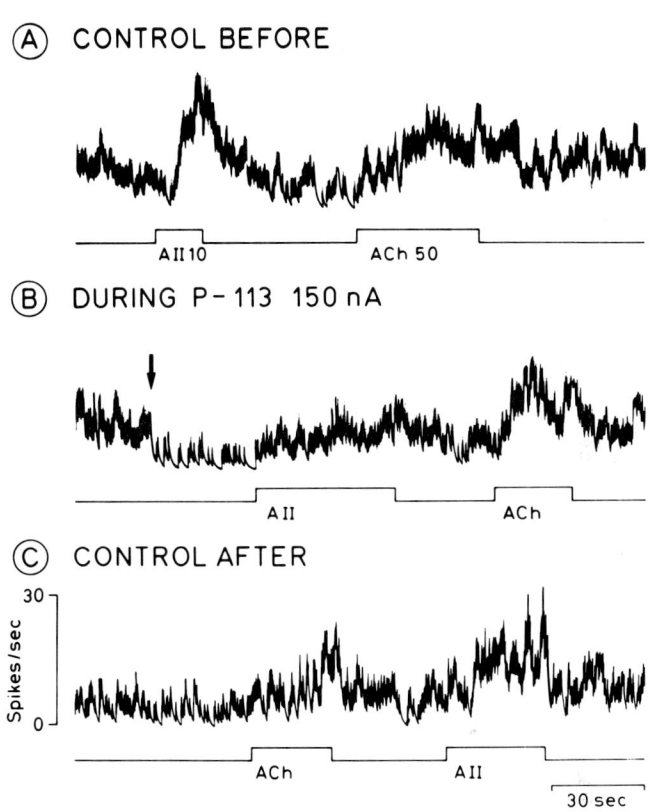

FIGURE 7. The effect of microiontophoretic application of AII and ACh on subfornical organ neurons in the cat. P 113 equals saralasin, a competitive angiotensin antagonist.

receptor for angiotensin II. Evidence to support this hypothesis came from studies by Simpson and Routtenberg (1973) in which they injected angiotensin into the preoptic area and found that, after ablation of the subfornical organ, the response was abolished or very much diminished. We initially supported this result when we injected AII directly into the ventricles and found that the effect on drinking behavior was abolished by subfornical organ lesion (Phillips, Leavitt, and Hoffman, 1974b). Due to the unique location of the subfornical organ in a very narrow part of the ventricles, we found that our lesions could block passage of CSF from the lateral to the third ventricle. This led us to reinterpret our results as due to ventricular obstruction of the AII injected into the lateral

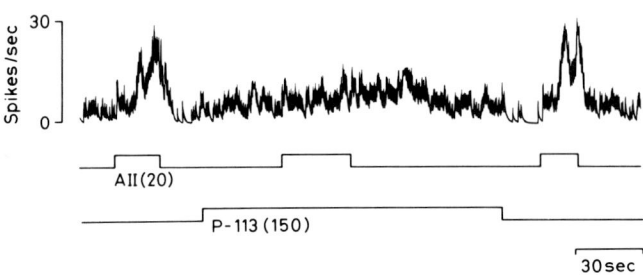

FIGURE 8. The effect of AII on a cell (or cells) that responded only to angiotensin and the effect on this response by P 113 ejection.

ventricle, and made us realize that there must be other sites within the ventricular system beyond the level of the subfornical organ that were also receptive to AII for the dipsogenic response (Buggy, Fisher, Hoffman, Johnson, and Phillips, 1975; Hoffman and Phillips, 1976b). Nevertheless, Simpson (1975) showed that i.v. injections of AII are less effective after lesioning of the subfornical organ.

Further, microiontophoretic studies on the subfornical organ indicate that neurons specifically sensitive for AII exist in the subfornical organ (Felix and Akert, 1974; Phillips and Felix, 1976; Felix, 1976). These studies were carried out on cats in which the subfornical organ was visualized by careful removal of one hemisphere in an unanesthetized preparation. A five-barrelled micropipette entered the subfornical organ from the ventricular surface side and penetrated into the neural elements below. In total, microinjections of AII excited 116 out of 161 neurons recorded in the subfornical organ, and there was a dose-response relationship. In addition, i.v. injections of AII excited neurons in this area (Felix and Akert, 1974). The neurons were not responsive to bradykinin, a nonapeptide (Arg-Pro-Pro-Gly-Phe-Ser-Pro-Phe-Arg) or eledoisin and physalaemin, which are both undecapeptides. Some of the same neurons were responsive to acetylcholine, but we could differentiate between those cells that were specifically responsive to AII and those cells that responded to both AII and acetylcholine (Figures 7 and 8). The cells that were specifically responsive to AII not only responded to low-current injection levels, but were also blocked in their response by low injection levels of a competitive antagonist for AII, Sar-1-Ala-8-angiotensin (P 113). Acetylcholine-stimulated neurons were not affected by P 113. Control injections of saline vehicle had no effect. In cortex and hippocampus (CA1), AII was not notably excitatory.

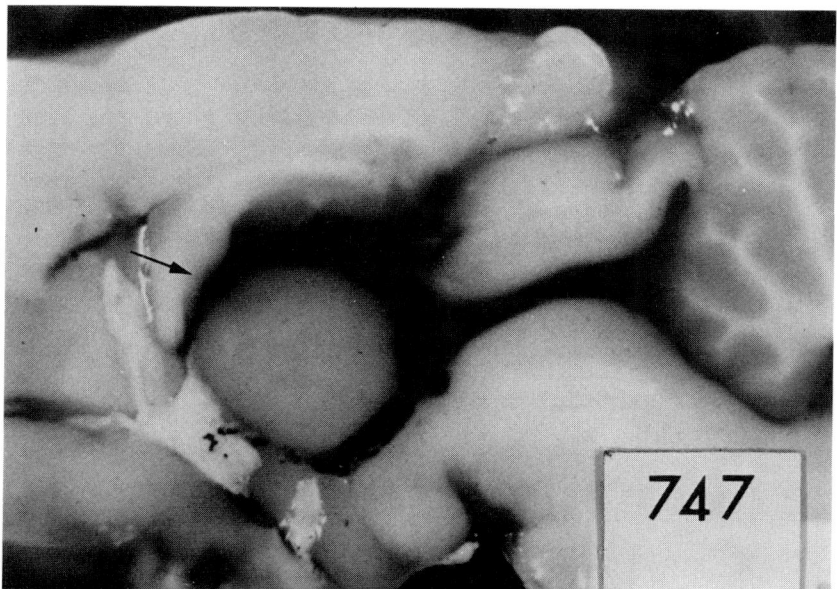

FIGURE 9. The histology of a rat brain that did not respond to angiotensin after the anterior third ventricle was plugged. Note that black dye had reached the surface of the SFO (black arrow).

Thus, there is evidence for AII receptive neurons within the subfornical organ (SFO). Felix and Akert (1974) also showed that direct application of angiotensin to the surface of the SFO could excite neurons. However, because the micropipettes punctured the surface, the angiotensin was reaching sites that could also be reached by systemic injection. Simpson (1975) has shown that small amounts of angiotensin are effective when injected directly into the subfornical organ, whereas an injection of angiotensin into the ventricles requires a higher dose. This may be explained if the subfornical organ, like the area postrema, has receptive elements on the systemic side, but not on the ventricular side. Again, evidence from our plugging studies convinces us that this is the case. Plugging the third ventricle prevented AII IVT from producing dipsogenic or pressor responses, even though the dye clearly indicates that the AII could reach the surface of the SFO (Figure 9). This result has been repeated in experiments with five rats. Also, we could not excite neurons in the SFO of rats by IVT AII when the electrode tip was lowered into SFO tissue from the dorsal side, leaving the ventricular surface intact (Phillips, et al., 1974b).

In summary, we propose that the subfornical organ, although not a unique dipsogenic receptor for AII in the brain, is a receptor site that is available to blood-borne AII, but not to ventricular AII.

Anterior Ventral Third Ventricle

There are three lines of evidence pointing to the importance of the arterior third ventricle region as a receptor site for AII. First, from our plugging studies, the anterior ventral third ventricle—which would contain the OV and ME—appeared to be essential for both the pressor and dipsogenic effects of AII IVT in rats (Phillips and Hoffman, 1977; Hoffman and Phillips, 1976a). In addition, Andersson, Leksell, and Lishajko (1975) have shown that, in goats, lesions of the anterior surface of the third ventricle result in hypodipsia or adipsia. Johnson and Buggy (1976) have demonstrated similar effects on thirst in rats after making small electrolytic lesions in the region of the OV. We have used a Halasz knife and approached the OV between the olfactory bulbs. By this route, the knife enters the lamina terminalis only and does not affect preoptic tissue. After OVLT cutting, we find that rats (n = 5) are unresponsive to IVT AII (Phillips and Hoffman, 1977). Third, we find that when small (33-gauge) cannulae are lowered into the narrow anterior third recess, we can produce blood pressure and drinking responses to less than 50 pg of AII. This is a lower dose than that administered at any other ventricular site (Figure 10).

Thus, based on plugging, lesioning, and injection data, we currently favor the view that the anterior third ventricle is a receptor site for AII for blood pressure and drinking effects. Whether this site is on the ventricular surface or on the brain side of the ventricular wall remains a question. To answer this question, we need to know about the permeability of the CVOs to peptides in the CSF.

Blood-Brain Barrier and Angiotensin

After an i.v. injection of horseradish peroxidase (HRP) and subsequent histochemical reactions with 3-3'diaminobenzidine, the brown reaction product can be seen in the fenestrated capillaries and in the perivascular space of the area postrema, ME, and OV (Weindl and Joynt, 1972). However, the reaction product does not reach the CSF of the ventricle because passage is prevented by the tight junctions of the ependyma cells (Brightman and Reese, 1969). Conversely, HRP injected into the ventricles does not cross these apical tight junctions and enter

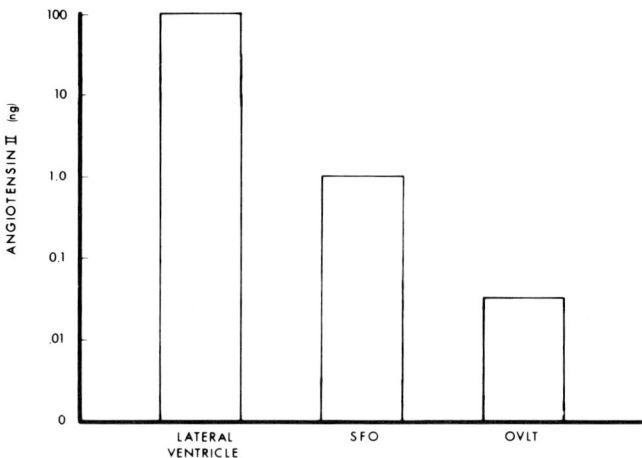

FIGURE 10. Comparative sensitivities of different sites within the ventricles to AII. Note the scale is logarithmic. Abbreviations: SFO, subfornical organ. OVLT, organum vasculosum.

the brain at these CVOs. HRP in the ventricles can cross through the gap junctions in the third ventricle wall of ciliated ependyma, but the technique demonstrates clearly that tight junctions in the CVOs are impervious to HRP. This indicates that AII could reach perivascular sites when given i.v., but probably would not reach the same sites when given IVT. It may be argued that because the molecular weight of HRP is 45,000 and that of AII is only 1,000, the octapeptide can travel where the enzyme cannot. However, the molecular diameter is probably the more important factor for penetration between cells, and the HRP molecule is only 5 nm in diameter. The size of the AII molecule has not been published to our knowledge, and its structure is apparently controversial (Printz, Némethy, and Bleich, 1972). Even when markers of much smaller molecular weight are injected IVT, such as [^{3}H]arginine (molecular weight 175) or [^{3}H]phenylalanine (molecular weight 166), the OV and ME were not penetrated (Weindl and Joynt, 1972). Similar studies on choroid plexus (Hashimoto and Hama, 1968) indicate that HRP can escape from the vasculature through the endothelial fenestrations, but is blocked from entering the ventricle by the tight junctions. Reese and Brightman (1968) also showed that HRP injected into the ventricles did not gain access to peripheral circulation. All these experimental results lead us to conclude that AII does not normally get into the ventricles from intravenous injection, although it has limited access to the brain in the regions of the CVOs where the blood-brain barrier is imperfect. Furthermore, AII in the ventricles cannot pass directly into these same sites. It might be possible for AII IVT to get to other brain areas by diffusing from the CSF through gap junctions in ciliated ependyma (Figure 5), but the HRP data indicate that it would not arrive at the same sites as the i.v. AII.

Autoradiographic Studies

Two studies using autoradiographic techniques have shown the presence of radioactivity after injections of labeled angiotensin i.v. (Volicer and Loew, 1971; Johnson, 1975). Radioactivity was seen in the CSF, the choroid plexus, the lateral ventricle, and the subfornical organ. Preliminary data from Johnson showed that a 250-ng injection of tritiated AII infused for 10 min produced detectable amounts of labeled substance in the CSF 4 min after injection. Ganten et al. (1976a), using a polyacrylamide gel, found that the radioactivity in the CSF was attached to nonimmunoreactive AII fragment. Infusion of unlabeled AII i.v. did not lead to an increase of immunoreactive AII in CSF perfusate, and they concluded that neither native AII nor ^{3}H-labeled AII penetrates into the CSF from the vascular side. There was, however, a dose difference of several orders of magnitude between the studies. Ganten et al. used 120 ng/kg/min. Johnson used 2 μg of AII and Volicer and Loew used even higher doses. It is possible that at such high doses, which would cause extreme hypertension, there would be sufficient capillary pressure to mechanically expel plasma containing angiotensin through the choroid plexus or even by disruption of the ependymal tight junctions. This is a hypothesis that could be tested and would also explain the reports of intraventricular antagonism of angiotensin by P 113.

Interaction Between P 113 and AII

All the possible combinations of blockade of angiotensin by P 113 by different routes have been investigated. In a ratio of 5:1, P 113 inhibits AII drinking and blood pressure responses when both are given IVT or when both are administered i.v. (Cooling and Day, 1974; Epstein et al., 1973). What is intriguing in terms of the blood-brain barrier is that an injection of P 113 IVT can block the effects of AII given i.v. (Cooling and Day, 1974; Johnson and Schwob, 1975). As proposed above, the levels of AII used in these studies would produce very high blood pressures and could force an opening of the blood-brain barrier. P 113 i.v. can also block the effects of AII IVT (Hoffman and Phillips, 1976b). This would mean that both the peptide and the antagonist are probably acting on the same site. The question is, where is this site? Because we have already argued that the CSF ependyma barriers would exclude P 113 from the site that AII could reach by systemic injection, we are forced to review our own interpretation of the P 113 effects. Thus, in our experiment it was only the high dose of P 113 injected i.v. (72 μg) that caused a block of AII IVT pressor and dipsogenic effects, and the effect was partial. We suggested that a fraction of P 113 could pass into the CSF and, thus, with a larger dose, a bigger fraction gained entry to the ventricles. We now have evidence that this dose of P 113 was causing an increase in blood pressure. We find that a bolus injection of 25 to 50 or more μg of P 113 i.v. is agonistic, causing a blood pressure increase of +30 mm Hg (Phillips, Mann, Dietz, Hoffman, and Ganten, 1977). The response is identical in topography to that produced by a high dose of AII i.v. in a bolus injection. Therefore, the results with P 113 might be due to high blood pressures that result from the AII or P 113 injections breaking down the brain CSF barrier. When angiotensin was coupled with HRP or cytochrome c and injected into mice at pressor doses lower than those used above, vesicles containing the reaction product were seen in the choroid plexus and the extracellular space surrounding blood vessels. At these dose levels, however, the reaction product did not empty into the ventricular compartment (Richardson and Beaulnes, 1971). More studies of this kind need to be done using rats and high doses of angiotensin to resolve the possibility that high pressure may force P 113 or AII into the ventricles.

Local Ischemia Hypothesis

When it was discovered that injections of angiotensin given intravertebrally cause a greater blood pressure effect than those given via the i.v. route, Dickinson and Thomas (1959) hypothesized that the effect was due to local ischemia of the vasomotor centers. This stimulated some ingenious experiments by Gildenberg (1969), who ligated the basilar artery during infusions of the intravertebral artery and located the effect of angiotensin at the level of the area postrema, thus excluding the vasomotor centers. Recently, the same type of explanation for angiotensin dipsogenic effects has been applied, namely, that AII IVT causes local vasoconstriction in "thirst centers." Nicolaidis and Fitzsimons (1975) reported that an infusion of papaverine before an injection of AII IVT prevented the drinking response to the peptide, whereas the drinking response to carbachol IVT persisted. The authors interpreted this to mean that because papaverine has a powerful vasodilator effect, it had prevented angiotensin from causing vasoconstriction in a dipsogenic receptive area. The second piece of evidence was that prostaglandin E, also presumed to be a vasodilator, caused a blockade of the angiotensin response. This latter result has received support from Kenny and Epstein (1975), who showed that prostaglandin E attenuated AII IVT drinking. Phillips, Phipps, and Hoffman (1976) have shown that the prostaglandin inhibitor meclofenamate given before AII IVT leads to prolonged and increased drinking in response to AII. A possible interpretation of these results is that central angiotensin stimulates the synthesis of prostaglandins that counteract the angiotensin dipsogenic effect. This was an appealing explanation for the cessation of drinking that occurs in rats infused with AII IVT. However, the story is a little more complicated than it first appeared. Rats that respond to AII by drinking isotonic saline persist in drinking large amounts of saline during a continuous 1-h infusion of AII. Rats that prefer water drink only in the first 15 min of a 1-h infusion of AII IVT. Thus, if the hypothesis were true, one would have to postulate separate mechanisms for saline drinking and for water drinking in response to AII. Leksell (1976) has shown that prostaglandin E IVT in the goat actually produces drinking. We have not been able to support the finding of Nicolaidis and Fitzsimons on the effects of papaverine. We surrounded a bolus injection of AII (50 ng of IVT) with a bolus of papaverine before and an infusion after the injection. The papaverine was given at 90 μg in 3 μliters before AII, and 30 μg/μliter was infused after AII for 5 min. We were unable to inhibit angiotensin effects on either blood pressure or drinking (n = 6) by this procedure. Although there may be procedural details, such as the doses given, that could explain the conflict between results, it would still have to be proved that papaverine and prostaglandin E are vasodilators on cerebral vasculature in order for the ischemia hypothesis to be valid.

Surface Receptor Hypothesis

AII might also act from the ventricles by diffusion, by microiontophoretic action, or by receptors on the ependymal surface that are connected to subependymal neurons. Diffusion would be through the ciliated ependymal wall and, from there, eventually a small quantity might reach and activate receptive neurons. The plug and dye studies (Hoffman and Phillips, 1976a, b; Phillips and Hoffman, 1977) show, however, that when access to the anterior third ventricle is plugged, there is no response to AII, even though use of the dye indicates that AII could diffuse through the walls of the third ventricle above the plug. A microiontophoretic effect was proposed by Weindl in another context (Weindl and Joynt, 1972), but this effect could be used as a possible explanation of the mechanism for AII in the ventricles. This concept proposes that substances that diffuse through the gap junctions of ciliated ependyma can activate periventricular neurons microiontophoretically. The axons of such neurons could reach the effective neurons in the circuitry for blood pressure and drinking responses. Again, the dye injection data rule this possibility out for drinking and blood pressure; however, we have not tested ADH release under plugging conditions. We have attempted to block the release of ADH by simultaneous IVT injections of haloperidol, 6-hydroxydopamine, and P 113 (Hoffman and Phillips, 1977). Only P 113 was effective in stopping

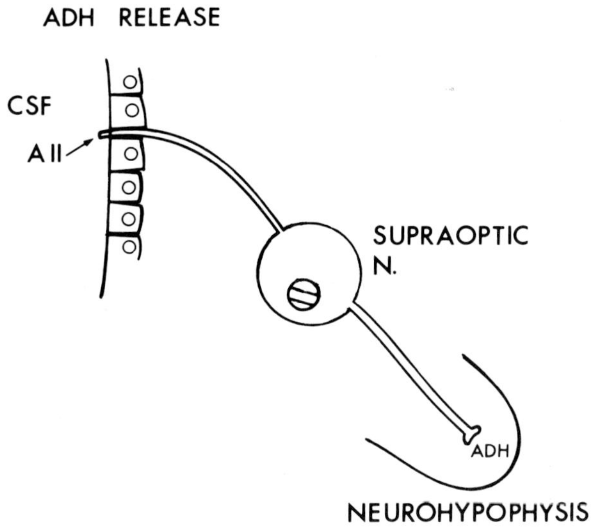

FIGURE 11. Possible explanation for the release of vasopressin (ADH) by intraventricular AII. The peptide may stimulate hypothetical dendrites of ADH-containing magnocells or diffuse through the intracellular space to microiontophoretically excite the cell, causing ADH release.

the release of ADH. This suggested to us that perhaps AII directly stimulates cells involved in the release of vasopressin either through stimulating dendrites, which reach the ventricles, or by a microiontophoretic action as described above (Figure 11). Nicoll and Barker (1971) showed that angiotensin stimulated supraoptic neurons when applied microiontophoretically. Intravenous injections of angiotensin, however, did not stimulate these cells, indicating that angiotensin had to reach the surface of the neurons. Recently, we (Knowles and Phillips, unpublished observations) have found that injections of AII into the third ventricle stimulate supraoptic neurons. Thus, electrophysiological evidence appears to support the possibility that AII acts microiontophoretically after it diffuses from the ventricles, as far as vasopressin is concerned.

The third possibility is that there are surface receptors that can be activated by AII IVT. This would explain why the plug over the surface prevents elicitation of blood pressure and dipsogenic responses. It also implies that small quantities of AII applied to the surface would be effective. We have lowered 33-gauge cannulae into the optic recess and tested the threshold doses of AII and found these to be below 50 pg in 1 μliter. At 50 pg, a 5-mm Hg increase in blood pressure and 2- to 5-ml dipsogenic responses were recorded in six rats. The histology showed the cannulae to be in the lower third ventricle about 1 mm above the optic recess and, therefore, the dose injected was diluted in CSF. Nicolaidis and Fitzsimons (1975) also found that injection of AII into the ventral anterior third ventricle produced greater responses than an equivalent injection in the area of the subfornical organ. The exact nature of such putative surface receptors is not known. Our scanning electron microscopy (SEM) shows numerous supraependymal structures crossing the surface of the OV, ME, and other parts of the ventricles. We have removed the ependymal surface from the OV region by the use of thin, dry glass. The ependymal tissue was then fixed in glyoxylic acid, dried, and treated with formaldehyde vapor for fluorescence microscopy. By using this method, we have seen beaded varicosities containing catecholamines that are very similar in size and shape to the structures seen in SEM (Figure 12; Phillips, Brody, and Azzam, unpublished observations). Lorez and Richards (1973) found numerous serotonin-containing structures on the ependymal surface of the ventricles, but in the area where we found catecholamine-containing varicosities, their data showed an absence of 5-HT-fluorescence. Thus, it appears that catecholamine-containing fibers traverse the surface of

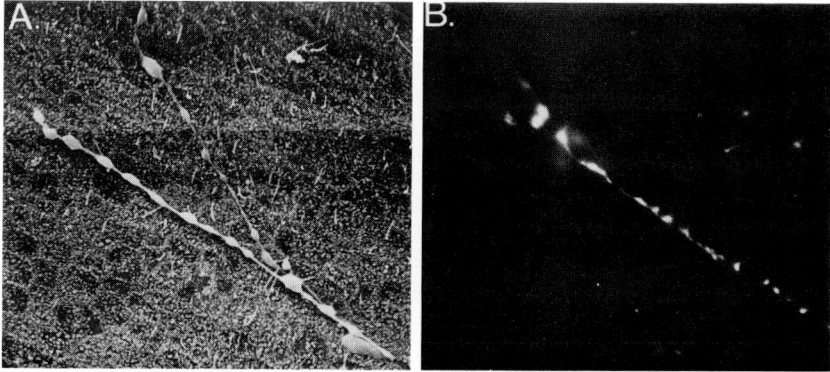

FIGURE 12. Similar appearance of supraependymal structures in the anterior third ventricle region. (A) Supraependymal structures viewed by scanning electron microscopy (×1,350). (B) Different tissue viewed by fluorescence microscopy for catecholamines (×1,100). Phillips and Brody, unpublished observations.

the OV and ME. From SEM studies, we know that these fibers descend beneath the surface into the neuronal and perivascular regions. The possibility exists that these fibers could be stimulated by AII, because in the periphery, AII has been shown to stimulate noradrenaline release and to inhibit noradrenaline uptake (Palaic and Khairallah, 1967).

The Brain Iso-Renin-Angiotensin System

If endogenous sytemic angiotensin or angiotensin injected i.v. does not reach the ventricles and angiotensin injected IVT does not leak out of the ventricles, then one must ask what physiological role receptors in the ventricles would have. We consider an IVT AII injection as a probe that unlocks a physiological mechanism for which the normal key is the endogenous brain angiotensin.

The evidence for brain angiotensin has been steadily mounting since the discovery of iso-renin and angiotensin in the brain (Ganten et al., 1971; Fischer-Ferrario et al., 1971). This evidence includes the following: (1) Addition of renin to the CSF produces the effects seen with angiotensin, thereby demonstrating the presence of angiotensinogen and converting enzyme (Reid and Ramsay, 1975). (2) Hoffman, Schelling, Phillips, and Ganten (1977) have found that in nephrectomized rats, injections of renin substrate extracted from either dog plasma or rat plasma, or made synthetically (tetradecapeptide), are followed by drinking behavior. This gives strong evidence for the

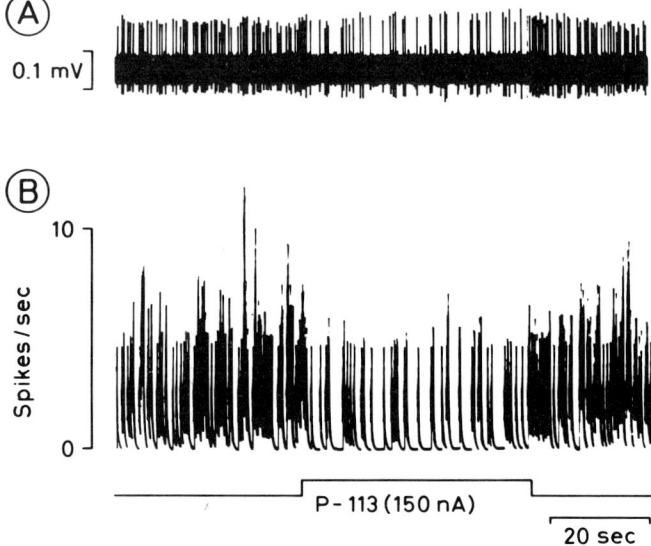

FIGURE 13. Slowing of spontaneous firing rate of SFO neurons by ejection of saralasin (P 113).

presence of iso-renin in the absence of kidney renin being available to act physiologically on these substrates in the ventricles. (3) Injections of angiotensin antagonist into the ventricles reduces blood pressure in spontaneously hypertensive rats. This was first demonstrated in the Smirk strain by Hutchinson, Schelling, and Ganten (1975) and Ganten, Hutchinson, and Schelling (1975), where high levels of angiotensin in the CSF were also assayed. Phillips, Phipps, Hoffman, and Leavitt (1975) independently demonstrated similar effects in SH rats of the Okamoto strain when the blood pressure was measured by the tail-cuff method. Sweet, Columbo, and Gaul (1976) and Schoelkens (1976) have also reported blood pressure decreases in the Okamoto strain after injection of angiotensin analogues. Their data differ in the age at which they saw the effect. Sweet et al. saw the effect in old rats, whereas Schoelkens saw the effect in young rats. In the case of Phillips et al. (1975) the rats were older (more than 3 months old). Recently, with H. Mann we have repeated the effect with P 113 in spontaneously hypertensive rats of the stroke-prone strain. In addition to this evidence, Finkielman, Fischer-Ferrario, Diaz, Goldstein, and Nahmod (1972) have found higher levels of AII in the CSF of essential hypertensive patients. All these data suggest that endogenous angiotensin has a pathophysiological role in contributing to hypertension, and the studies themselves are evidence for the presence of endogenously produced angiotensin. (4) In the microiontophoretic studies, we noted a slowing of cellular activity when P 113 was applied alone in the subfornical organ (Figure 13). This is suggestive of endogenous angiotensin maintaining higher rates of activity. (5) Fuxe, Ganten, Hökfelt, and Bolme (1976), by using the indirect method, report showing angiotensin or angiotensin-like immunofluorescent compounds in the brain. The highest levels of fluorescent angiotensin are associated with the ME, the medulla, the spinal cord, and the hypothalamus. These levels persisted in the absence of peripheral renin produced by nephrectomy. The fluorescence so far has been located in axons and only to a limited extent in cell bodies. It is too soon to say yet whether this represents the limit of sensitivity of the fluorescence technique or the true distribution of endogenous angiotensin. (6) In brain assays of iso-renin, the levels of the enzyme are higher than in plasma, and present after nephrectomy (Ganten et al., 1976a, b).

CONCLUSIONS

We have presented the case that, in the brain, there are two types of receptor sites for angiotensin: one that is available to angiotensin in the blood and the other that is available to endogenously formed angiotensin (Figure 14). The emphasis has been on a ventricular site for the latter, but the broad distribution of angiotensin-like immunoreactivity indicates that the ventricular sites are not exclusive, but only technically convenient to study. With further mapping of the brain by immunochemical techniques it will be possible to apply neurophysiological study to other brain sites. Indeed, the evidence so far implies that angiotensin is formed intracellularly (Ganten et al., 1976a) and is concentrated in nerve terminals (Fuxe et al., 1976), and its presence in CSF may be incidental.

In seeking a unifying principle for the bewildering number of actions of angiotensin and other peptides on the brain, we are drawn to the conclusion that there is peptidergic action on the membranes of neurons, possibly postsynaptic, and it is the neurons that are different by virtue of their connections to the brain circuitry mediating blood pressure, water balance, etc. It is surprising how physically close such neurons are, and we have had only limited success so far in separating, for example, the pressor response from the drinking response to AII.

The peptidergic action of angiotensin on the membrane may lie in an

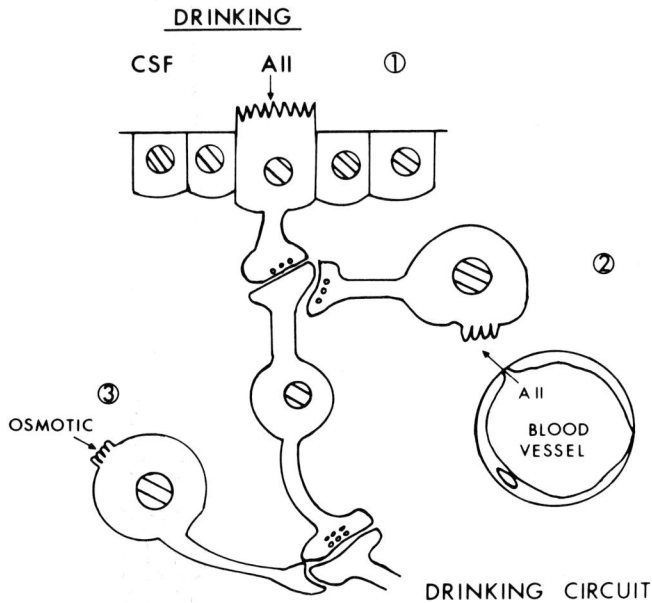

FIGURE 14. Schematic diagram of possible receptor cells for angiotensin central effects, e.g., thirst. (1) A receptor cell with the receptive surface on the ventricular wall for which some of our evidence suggests a distribution in the anterior third ventricle. This may not be the exclusive site, but one which is available to test procedures. (2) A receptor cell found in circumventricular organs where the blood-brain barrier is insufficient to keep out AII in the blood. Both types of receptors could have a common neural output to a circuit that controls drinking behavior. (3) A cell in brain tissue receptive to osmotic changes that also stimulates the drinking circuit. The presence of such a receptor has been disputed by Andersson.

effect on Na^+-K^+-ATPase. Evidence for this comes from experiments by Andersson (1977), who has shown a profound dependence of angiotensin on Na^+ levels in CSF. Low Na^+ levels or inhibition of Na^+-K^+-ATPase blocks the effects of AII on thirst and ADH release.

In the next few years, we should see the resolution of the questions currently asked about angiotensin. Is its action on the brain of peripheral or endogenous origin? Is there a way to trigger the release of endogenous angiotensin? Is angiotensin a neural transmitter for certain cells? All these questions equally apply to other peptides and, given the rapid progress in research on angiotensin, it may serve as a model for the action of peptides on neural function.

ACKNOWLEDGMENT

We thank Judy Phipps for technical assistance in some of these experiments. The work was supported by National Science Foundation grant BNS 75-16346, National Institute of Mental Health Research Scientist Development Award II 3K02-MH70983-0151, and a Humboldt Foundation grant to M.I.P.

REFERENCES

Abraham, S. F., R. M. Baker, E. H. Blaine, D. A. Denton, and M. J. McKinley (1975). Water drinking induced in sheep by angiotensin—a physiological or pharmacological effect? *J. Comp. Physiol. Psychol.* **88**:503–518.

Andersson, B. (1977). Central sodium-angiotensin interaction, in *Central Actions of Angiotensin*, Buckley, J. P. and C. Ferrario, eds. Pergamon Press, New York, in press.

Andersson, B., G. Leksell, and F. Lishajko (1975). Perturbations in fluid balance induced by medially placed forebrain lesions, *Brain Res.* **19**:261–275.

Bonjour, J. P. and R. L. Malvin (1970). Plasma concentrations of ADH in conscious and anesthetized dogs, *Am. J. Physiol.* **218**:1128–1132.

Booth, D. (1968). Mechanism of action of norepinephrine in eliciting an eating response on injection into the rat hypothalamus, *J. Pharmacol. Exp. Ther.* **160**:336–348.

Brightman, M. W. and T. S. Reese (1969). Junctions between intimately opposed cell membranes in the vertebrate brain, *J. Cell Biol.* **40**:648–677.

Buggy, J., A. E. Fisher, W. E. Hoffman, A. K. Johnson, and M. I. Phillips (1975). Ventricular obstruction: effect of drinking induced by intracranial angiotensin, *Science* **190**:72–74.

Cooling, M. J. and M. D. Day (1974). Inhibition of renin-angiotensin induced drinking in the cat by enzyme inhibitors and by analogue antagonists of angiotensin II, *Clin. Exp. Pharmacol. Physiol.* **1**:389–396.

Davson, H. (1970). *Physiology of the Cerebrospinal Fluid.* J. A. Churchill, London.

Deuben, R. R. and J. P. Buckley (1970). Identification of a central site of action of angiotensin II, *J. Pharmacol. Exp. Ther.* **170**:139–146.

De Wied, D. (1976). Hormonal influence on motivation, learning, and memory processes, *Hosp. Pract.* **11**:123–131.

Dickinson, C. J. and A. D. Thomas (1959). Vertebral and internal carotid arteries in relation to hypertension and cerebrovascular disease, *Lancet* **2**:46–48.

Epstein, A. N., J. T. Fitzsimons, and A. K. Johnson (1973). Peptide antagonists of the renin-angiotensin system and the elucidation of the receptors for angiotensin-induced drinking, *J. Physiol. (London)* **238**:34P–35P.

Epstein, A. N., J. T. Fitzsimons, and B. Rolls (1970). Drinking induced by injection of angiotensin into the brain of the rat, *J. Physiol. (London)* **210**:457–474.

Felix, D. (1976). Peptide and acetylcholine action on neurones of the cat subfornical organ, *Naunyn-Schmiedebergs Arch. Pharmacol.* **292**:15–20.

Felix, D. and K. Akert (1974). The effect of angiotensin II on neurones of the cat subfornical organ, *Brain Res.* **76**:350–353.
Ferrario, C. M., P. L. Gildenberg, and J. W. McCubbin (1972). Cardiovascular effects of angiotensin mediated by the central nervous system, *Circ. Res.* **30**:257–262.
Finkielman, S., C. Fischer-Ferrario, A. Diaz, D. J. Goldstein, and V. E. Nahmod (1972). A pressor substance in the cerebrospinal fluid of normotensive and hypertensive patients, *Proc. Natl. Acad. Sci. U.S.A.* **69**:3341–3344.
Fischer-Ferrario, C., V. E. Nahmod, D. J. Goldstein, and S. Finkielman (1971). Angiotensin and renin in rat and dog brain, *J. Exp. Med.* **133**:353–361.
Fitzsimons, J. T. (1972). Thirst, *Physiol. Rev.* **52(2)**:468–559.
Fuxe, K., D. Ganten, T. M. Hökfelt, and P. Bolme (1976). Immunohistochemical evidence for the existence of angiotensin II-containing nerve terminals in the brain and spinal cord in the rat, *Neurosci. Lett.* **2**:229–234.
Ganten, D., J. Hutchinson, and P. Schelling (1975). The intrinsic brain iso-renin angiotensin system: its possible role in central mechanisms of blood pressure regulation, *Clin. Sci. Mol. Med.* **48**:265s–268s.
Ganten, D., J. S. Hutchinson, P. Schelling, U. Ganten, and H. Fischer (1976a). The iso-renin angiotensin systems in extrarenal tissue, *Clin. Exp. Pharmacol. Physiol.* **3**:103–126.
Ganten, D., J. E. Minnich, P. Granger, K. Hayduk, H. M. Brecht, A. Barbeau, R. Boucher, and J. Genest (1971). Angiotensin-forming enzyme in brain tissue, *Science* **173**:64–65.
Ganten, D., P. Schelling, W. E. Hoffman, M. I. Phillips, and U. Ganten (1977). The measurement of extrarenal iso-renins, in *Proceedings on Symposium for Methodology of the Renin Angiotensin System,* Krause, H., ed., in press.
Ganten, D., P. Schelling, P. Vecsei, and U. Ganten (1976b). Iso-renin of extrarenal origin, *Am. J. Med.* **60**:760–772.
Gildenberg, P. L. (1969). Localization of a site of angiotensin vasopressor activity in the brain, *Physiologist* **12**:235.
Hashimoto, P. H. and K. Hama (1968). An electron microscope study on protein uptake into brain regions devoid of the blood-brain barrier, *Med. J. Osaka Univ.* **18**:331–346.
Hertz, A., K. Albus, J. Matys, P. Schubert, and H. J. Toschenachi (1970). On the central sites for the antinociceptive action of morphine and fentanyl, *Neuropharmacology* **9**:539–551.
Hoffman, W. E. and M. I. Phillips (1976a). The effect of SFO lesions and ventricular blockade on drinking induced by angiotensin II, *Brain Res.* **108**:59–73.
Hoffman, W. E. and M. I. Phillips (1976b). Evidence for Sar^1-Ala^8-angiotensin II crossing the blood cerebrospinal fluid barrier to antagonize central effects of angiotensin II, *Brain Res.* **109**:541–552.
Hoffman, W. E. and M. I. Phillips (1977). The role of ADH in the pressor response to intra-ventricular angiotensin II, in *Central Actions of Angiotensin,* Buckley, J. P. and C. Ferrario, eds. Pergamon Press, New York, in press.
Hoffman, W. E., P. Schelling, M. I. Phillips, and D. Ganten (1976). Evidence for local angiotensin formation in brain of nephrectomized rats, *Neurosci. Lett.,* **3**:299–303.

Hoffman, W. E., P. G. Schmid, M. I. Phillips, J. Falcon, and J. F. Weet (1977). Release of pressor amounts of antidiuretic hormone by intraventricular injections of angiotensin II and carbachol, *Neuropharmacology*, in press.
Hökfelt, T., S. Efendic, C. Hellerström, O. Johansson, R. Luft, and A. Arimura (1975). Cellular localization of somatostatin in endocrine-like cells and neurons of the rat with special reference to the A_1-cells of pancreatic islets and the hypothalamus, *Acta Endocrinol.* **80**(Suppl. 200):1–41.
Hutchinson, J. S., P. Schelling, and D. Ganten (1975). Effect of centrally administered AII and P113 on blood pressure in conscious rats, *Pflügers Arch. Europ. J. Physiol.* **355**:R 28.
Johnson, A. K. (1975). The role of the cerebral ventricular system in angiotensin induced thirst, pp. 117–122 in *Control Mechanisms of Drinking,* Peters, G., J. T. Fitzsimons, and L. Peters-Haefeli, eds. Springer-Verlag, Heidelberg.
Johnson, A. K. and J. Buggy (1976). Angiotensin (AII) and intracellular dehydration induced drinking: mediation by tissue surrounding anteroventral third ventricle (AV3V), *Fed. Proc.* 814 (Abstr.).
Johnson, A. K. and A. N. Epstein (1975). The cerebral ventricles as the avenue for the dipsogenic action of intracranial angiotensin, *Brain Res.* **86**:399–418.
Johnson, A. K. and J. E. Schwob (1975). Cephalic angiotensin II receptor mediating drinking to systemic angiotensin II, *Pharmacol. Biochem. Behav.* **3**:1076–1084.
Joy, M. D. and R. D. Lowe (1970). Evidence that the area postrema mediates the central cardiovascular response to angiotensin II, *Nature (London)* **228**:1303–1304.
Keil, L. C., J. Summy-Long, and W. B. Severs (1975). Release of vasopressin by angiotensin II, *Endocrinology* **96**:1063–1064.
Kenney, N. J. and A. N. Epstein (1975). The antidipsogenic action of prostaglandin E_1 (PGE_1), *Neuroscience* **1**:469.
Leksell, L. G. (1976). Influence of prostaglandin E_1 on cerebral mechanisms involved in the control of fluid balance, *Acta Physiol. Scand.* **96**:1–9.
Lorez, H. P. and J. G. Richards (1973). Distribution of indolealkylamine nerve terminals in the ventricles of the rat brain, *Z. Zellforsch. Mikrosk. Anat.* **144**:511–522.
Mouw, D., J. P. Bonjour, R. L. Malvin and A. Vander (1971). Central action of angiotensin in stimulating ADH release, *Am. J. Physiol.* **220**:239–242.
Nicolaidis, S. M. and J. T. Fitzsimons (1975). La dependance de la prise d'eau induite par l'angiotensine II envers la fonction vasomotrice cerebrale locale chez le Rat, *C. R. Acad. Sci. (Paris)* **281**:D 1417–1420.
Nicoll, R. A. and J. L. Barker (1971). Excitation of supraoptic neurosecretory cells by angiotensin II, *Nature (London) New Biol.* **233**:172–173.
Page, I. H. and J. W. McCubbin (1968). Renal Hypertension. Yearbook Medical Publishers, Inc., Chicago.
Palaic, D. and P. Khairallah (1967). Effect of angiotensin on uptake and release of norepinephrine by brain, *Biochem. Pharmacol.* **16**:2291–2298.
Pearse, A. G. E. (1976). Peptides in the brain and intestine, *Nature (London)* **262**:92–94.
Phillips, M. I., L. Balhorn, M. Leavitt, and W. Hoffman (1974a). Scanning electron microscope study of the rat subfornical organ, *Brain Res.* **80**:95–110.

Phillips, M. I. and D. Felix (1976). Specific angiotensin II receptive neurons in the cat subfornical organ, *Brain Res.* **109**:531–540.

Phillips, M. I. and W. E. Hoffman (1976). Regional study of cerebral ventricle sensitive sites to angiotensin II, *Brain Res.* **110**:313–330.

Phillips, M. I. and W. E. Hoffman (1977). Sensitive sites in the ventricular system for blood pressure and drinking responses to angiotensin, in *Central Actions of Angiotensin*, Buckley, J. P. and C. Ferrario, eds. Pergamon Press, New York, in press.

Phillips, M. I., M. Leavitt, and W. E. Hoffman (1974b). Experiments on angiotensin II and the subfornical organ in the control of thirst, *Fed. Proc.* **33**:563.

Phillips, M. I., H. Mann, R. Dietz, W. E. Hoffman, and D. Ganten (1977). Effect of intraventricular and intravenous administration of saralasin in renal and spontaneous hypertensive rats, *Fed. Proc.* **36**:810.

Phillips, M. I., J. Phipps, and W. E. Hoffman (1976). Central interaction of prostaglandins and angiotensin II on drinking blood pressure and ADH release, *Abstr. Annu. Meet. Soc.* Neurosci., 6th, Toronto, p. 307.

Phillips, M. I., J. Phipps, W. E. Hoffman, and M. Leavitt (1975). Reduction of blood pressure by intracranial injection of angiotensin blocker (P113) in spontaneously hypertensive rats (SHR), *Physiologist* **18**(3):350.

Printz, M. P., G. Némethy, and P. Bleich (1972). Proposed models for angiotensin II in aqueous solution and conclusions about receptor topography, *Nature (London) New Biol.* **237**:135–140.

Reese, T. S. and M. W. Brightman (1968). Similarity in structure and permeability to peroxidase of epithelia overlying fenestrated cerebral capillaries, *Anat. Rec.* **160**:414.

Reid, I. A. and R. Day (1977). Interactions and properties of some components of the renin-angiotensin system in brain, in *Central Actions of Angiotensin*, Buckley, J. P. and C. Ferrario, eds. Pergamon Press, New York, in press.

Reid, I. A. and D. J. Ramsay, (1975). The effects of intracerebroventricular administration of renin on drinking and blood pressure, *Endocrinology* **97**(3):536–542.

Richardson, J. B. and A. Beaulnes (1971). The cellular site of action of angiotensin, *J. Cell Biol.* **51**:419–432.

Sakai, K. K., B. H. Marks, J. George, and A. Koestner (1974). Specific angiotensin II receptors in the organ culture canine supraoptic nucleus cells, *Life Sci.* **14**:1337–1344.

Schoelkens, B. A. (1976). Central hypotensive action of an angiotensin II-antagonist in conscious rats with experimental hypertension, *IRCS Med. Sci.* **4**:320.

Scroop, G. C., F. Katic, M. D. Joy, and R. D. Lowe (1971). Importance of central vasomotor effects in angiotensin-induced hypertension, *Br. Med. J.* **1**:324–326.

Severs, W. B. and A. E. Daniels-Severs (1973). Effects of angiotensin on the central nervous system, *Pharmacol. Rev.* **25**:415–449.

Severs, W. B., J. Summy-Long, A. E. Daniels-Severs, and J. D. Connor (1971). Influence of adrenergic blocking drugs on central angiotensin effects, *Pharmacology (Basel)* **5**:205–214.

Simpson, J. B. (1975). Subfornical organ involvement in angiotensin-induced drinking, pp. 123–126 in *Control Mechanisms of Drinking*, Peters, G., J. T. Fitzsimons, and L. Peters-Haefeli, eds. Springer-Verlag, Heidelberg.
Simpson, B. and A. Routtenberg (1973). Subfornical organ: site of drinking elicitation by angiotensin II, *Science* **181:**1172–1174.
Shade, R. E. and L. Share (1975). Vasopressin release during nonhypotensive hemorrhage and angiotensin II infusion, *Am. J. Physiol.* **228:**149–154.
Swanson, L. W., G. R. Marshall, P. Needleman, and L. G. Sharpe (1973). Characterization of central angiotensin II receptor involved in the elicitation of drinking in the rat, *Brain Res.* **49:**441–446.
Sweet, C. S. and M. J. Brody (1970). Central inhibition of reflex vasodilatation by angiotensin and reduced renal pressure, *Am. J. Physiol.* **219:**1751–1758.
Sweet, C. S., J. C. Columbo, and S. K. Gaul (1976). Comparative antihypertensive effects of inhibitors of the renin-angiotensin system by central and peripheral administration in the malignant and spontaneously hypertensive rat, *Fed. Proc.* **35:**1056 (Abstr.).
Ueda, H. (1968). Renin-angiotensin system and central nervous system, *Proc. Eur. Congr. Cardiol.* **5:**249–251.
Volicer, L. and C. G. Loew (1971). Penetration of angiotensin II into the brain, *Neuropharmacology* **10:**631–636.
Weet, J. F., W. E. Hoffman, and M. I. Phillips (1976). Effect of intraventricular angiotensin II injections on renal function, *Physiologist* **19:**408.
Weindl, A. and R. J. Joynt (1972). The median eminence as a circumventricular organ, pp. 280–297 in *Brain Endocrine Interaction. Median Eminence: Structure and Function,* Knigge, K. M., D. E. Scott and A. Weindl, eds. S. Karger, Basel.
Yang, H. Y. T. and N. H. Neff (1972). Distribution and properties of angiotensin converting enzyme of rat brain, *J. Neurochem.* **19:**2443–2450.

Peptides as Neurohormones

Jeffery L. Barker and Thomas G. Smith, Jr.

National Institute of Neurological and Communicative Disorders and Stroke, Bethesda, Maryland

INTRODUCTION

The advent of immunohistochemical and more refined biochemical techniques has established the presence of peptides and indicated their distribution in the nervous system (Ganten, Minnich, Granger, Hayduk, Brecht, Barbeau, Boucher, and Genest, 1971; Ganten, Hutchinson, Schelling, Ganten, and Fischer, 1976; Brownstein, Palkovits, Saavedra, Bassiri, and Utiger, 1974; Hökfelt, Kellerth, Nilsson, and Pernow, 1975; Hughes, Smith, Kosterlitz, Fothergill, Morgan, and Morris, 1975). One early hypothesis that emerged regarding possible functional roles of peptides in the nervous system attempted to account for peptide effects simply in terms of the traditional concept of a neurotransmitter that mediates rapid cell-to-cell events at specialized "synaptic" junctions between contiguous nerve cells (Nicoll and Barker, 1971a; Konishi and Otsuka, 1974; Phillis and Limacher, 1974; Dyer and Dyball, 1974; Renaud, Martin, and Brazeau, 1975; Saito, Konishi, and Otsuka, 1975; Frederickson and Norris, 1976; La Motte, Pert, and Snyder, 1976; Brown, 1976). Another early notion suggested that some peptides might act in more of a "neuromodulatory" manner distinct from a conventional transmitter role (Henry, Krnjević, and Morris, 1975). Still another possibility—unspecified at the time—was suggested by the observation that angiotensin, a peptide derived from a circulating precursor, specifically excited supraoptic neurosecretory cells in the hypothalamus (Nicoll and Barker, 1971b). However, the preparations and physiological techniques initially employed permitted little more than preliminary and incomplete data to define functional roles for peptides in the nervous system (for review, see Barker, 1976, 1977a).

To begin to define the roles of peptides in neuronal function it will be necessary to satisfy certain criteria analogous to those used to identify neurotransmitter molecules as mediators of particular synaptic transmissions (Werman, 1966). These criteria include: (1) the demonstration of the in vivo synthesis and release of peptides by nerve or other cells; (2) the demonstration of physical avenues of communication between peptidergic cells and their target neuronal cells; (3) the demonstration of effects by a peptide on the target neurons that are identical to the physiology of the peptidergic pathway; and (4) similar actions of antagonists both on the physiological effects of the peptidergic pathway and on the pharmacological effects of the peptide. Satisfying such criteria in the CNS is difficult. An alternative approach to this problem is to use preparations of neuronal tissue that do not have the same complex geometry and inherent difficulties as the CNS, but that might provide insight into the physiological roles of peptides in the nervous system. We have used one such preparation—an invertebrate nervous system—to examine the effects of peptides on neuronal membrane properties. Invertebrate nervous systems have become increasingly useful as models of the vertebrate nervous system to study basic neurobiological questions at the single cell and defined circuit level (see Kandel, 1976). The preparations have the advantage of containing large, easily identifiable nerve cells that permit long-term study with intracellular recordings of the cell's electrophysiological properties. In this article we will discuss recent observations obtained in the invertebrates, which indicate that some peptides can act on nerve cells in a manner quite unlike the classical effects of neurotransmitters.

Excitatory Peptide Effects

The principal observation is that vasopressin, oxytocin, and related peptides, which are synthesized in the vertebrate hypothalamus, cause a long-lasting increase in the excitability of several identified neurons found in the land snail *Otala lactea* and in the marine mollusc *Aplysia californica* (Barker and Gainer, 1974; Barker, Ifshin, and Gainer, 1975). This effect is illustrated in Figure 1. In part, the increase in excitability is reflected in an increase in the number and frequency of action potentials evoked by a standard intracellular injection of depolarizing current or by an increase in the average frequency of spontaneously occurring action potentials. The two cells excited by lysine-vasopressin (LVP) have similar physiological and biochemical properties. Both synthesize low-molecular-weight proteins (Gainer, 1972*a*, *b*; Strumwasser, 1973; Gainer and Barker, 1974; Loh, Barker, and Gainer, 1976; Strumwasser

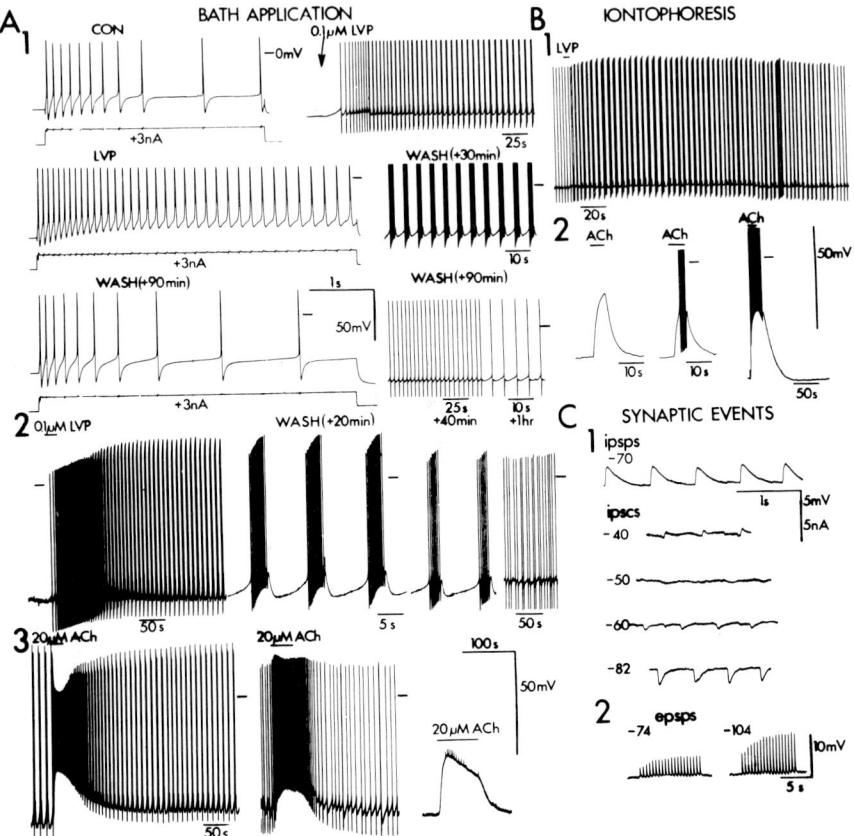

FIGURE 1. Phenomenology of vasopressin effect compared to synaptic events. (A1) Intracellular recording from cell 11 in *Otala*. The cell is inactive but can generate action potentials upon injection of 3 nA of depolarizing current recorded on current trace below voltage trace (CON). A 3-min bath application of 0.1 μM vasopressin (LVP), at arrow, excites cell and induces bursting pacemaker potential activity. Depolarizing current injection causes higher-frequency, sustained action potential activity. Bursting pacemaker activity still present after washing (WASH [+30 min]) for 30 min in peptide-free medium. After 90 min (WASH[+90 min]), excitability approaches control level although cell still generates beating pacemaker activity. Original resting potential: −50 mV. (A2) Experiment is similar to that in (A1), showing a 30-sec bath application of peptide inducing long-lasting bursting pacemaker activity in an inactive cell (LVP). Beating pacemaker activity is still present after 1 h of wash (+1 h). (A3) 30- and 50-sec bath applications of 20 μM ACh to the peptide-sensitive cell rapidly and intensely excite the cell for a period that only briefly outlasts the application of ACh. Rightmost trace:longer application of ACh is associated with a decay in depolarizing response (desensitization). Resting potential:−70 mV. (B1) A

and Wilson, 1976) and both generate endogenous pacemaker potentials (Carpenter and Gunn, 1970; Carpenter, 1973, Gainer, 1972b; Strumwasser, 1973; Barker and Gainer, 1975a). In addition, the electrical properties and biochemistry of the cell present in *Otala* appear to vary with the general state of activity of the snail (Gainer, 1972a, b; Barker and Gainer, 1975b; Loh et al., 1976). When the snail is dormant, the cell is either electrically silent, generates randomly occurring action potentials, or exhibits a beating pattern of pacemaker activity and does not synthesize low-molecular-weight proteins; on the other hand, when the snail is active, the cell typically generates bursting pacemaker potential (BPP) activity and synthesizes low-molecular-weight proteins. BPP activity is characterized by slow oscillations of membrane potential coupled to trains or "bursts" of action potentials. The excitatory effect of LVP is also associated with a long-lasting transformation of the membrane properties of the cell so that it now generates BPP activity (Figure 1). In those cells already generating BPP activity, such as the peptide-sensitive cell found in an active *Otala* snail or the analogous cell in *Aplysia*, the peptide enhances this activity, increasing the amplitude of the pacemaker potential and the number of action potentials produced during the depolarized phase of the pacemaker potential. The induction of pacemaker activity has not been observed after application of either acetylcholine (ACh) or serotonin, two putative neurotransmitters that excite the peptide-sensitive cell (Barker, 1975). The time course of excitation produced by either bath application or iontophoresis of ACh onto the peptide-sensitive cell is very much shorter, when compared to the duration of the peptide response, and relaxes upon termination of ACh application (Figure 1). Exactly why the time course of the peptide effect is so prolonged relative to that of the conventional transmitters is not clear. Presumably, both types of molecules diffuse away from the sites of action at similar rates so that the prolonged time course of LVP

5-sec iontophoresis from a micropipette with 1 mM LVP solution induces bursting pacemaker activity that lasts several minutes. (B2) Iontophoresis from a micropipette with 0.5 M ACh solution briefly depolarizes and excites a peptide-sensitive cell. Resting potentials: −75 mV, −60 mV, and −70 mV. (C1) Spontaneous inhibitory synaptic potentials and currents recorded in L_3 (*Aplysia*). The amplitude and polarity of the currents are linearly dependent on voltage and are absent at the potential where the electrochemical driving force underlying the event (−50 mV) is zero. (C2) Evoked excitatory synaptic potentials recorded in crayfish muscle, showing facilitation of postsynaptic potentials. In this and subsequent figures, zero membrane potential is indicated by an "−0 mV," as in A1 CON or by a bar near the spikes of a voltage trace, as in A1 LVP.

reflects either prolonged binding or brief binding with long-term changes.

Another significant difference between ACh and LVP is the threshold concentration required to elicit an observable effect. The threshold is approximately micromolar for ACh and nanomolar for LVP. In addition, the ACh response can be elicited over the entire range of realizable membrane potentials and is associated with an increase in membrane conductance (Barker, 1975). Because the magnitude of the conductance change is essentially independent of membrane potential and because a potential change, per se, cannot evoke the conductance change, such conductances are, by definition, voltage-independent conductances (Barker, 1975). By relating the amplitude of the ACh voltage response to the membrane potential, a membrane potential can be extrapolated for which there would be no voltage response. This potential reveals the sum of the ionic driving forces involved in the response and is less negative than the resting potential. Moreover, the ACh response is due to activation of ACh receptor-coupled conductances whose net driving force is at a membrane level less negative than the threshold for action potential generation. Hence, an ACh response can lead to the excitation of action potentials.

Spontaneously occurring synaptic potentials reveal similar properties: brevity and voltage-independent conductances (Figure 1C). The synaptic events that are illustrated have a driving force more negative than the threshold for action potential generation and excitation. Hence, they inhibit excitation. Two other aspects of synaptic physiology common to a number of forms of synaptic transmission include "desensitization," that is, attenuation of the postsynaptic response in the continued presence of the transmitter (Figure 1A3), and frequency-dependent facilitation of the amplitude of the synaptic response (Figure 1C2). Neither of these aspects has been studied with reference to peptide actions.

Some preliminary work has been carried out in an attempt to extract from the snail nervous system a peptide factor with actions similar to vasopressin (Ifshin, Gainer, and Barker, 1975). Crude extracts of the nervous system revealed a low-molecular-weight substance whose activity was abolished with pronase (Ifshin et al., 1975). Subsequent research by Mayeri and collaborators have localized an active substance influencing a cluster of neurosecretory cells, the so-called bag cells, in the *Aplysia* abdominal ganglion (Mayeri and Simon, 1975). Peptide extracts of the bag cells yield material that produces effects similar to

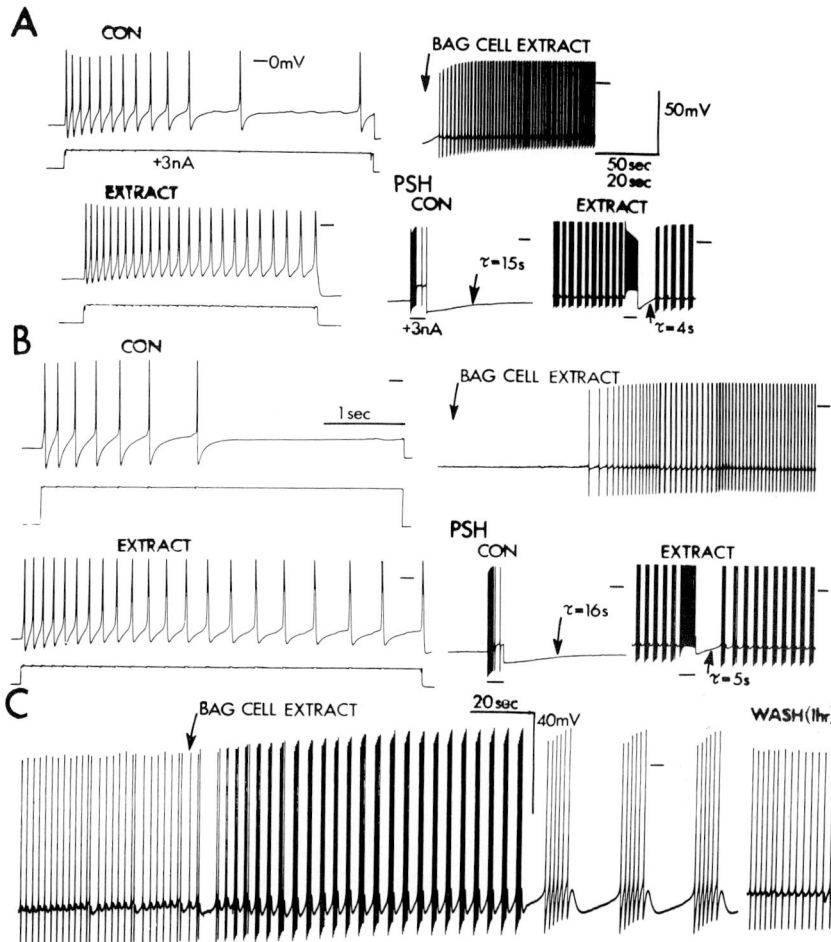

FIGURE 2. Effect of bag cell extract (from *Aplysia*) on membrane potential activity and membrane excitability of cell 11 of *Otala*. (A and B) Two examples of increased membrane excitability induced by extract on electrically silent cell 11 from dormant snails. Excitability, assessed by injection of 3 nA depolarizing currents, produces more spikes and a higher rate of spike activity after extract (EXTRACT) than in control (CON). Decay of post-stimulus hyperpolarization is shortened from a time constant of 15 to 16 sec in control (PSH:CON) to 4 to 5 sec in the presence of extract (PSH:EXTRACT) (right-hand traces). Resting potentials: −48 mV in (A), −46 mV in (B). (C) A 1-min application of bag cell extract produces bursting pacemaker activity that outlasts application. Recovery to control after 1 h (WASH [1 h]) (right-hand trace).

vasopressin on the peptide-sensitive snail cell (Figure 2). Further characterization of the factor is necessary to determine its structure and relationship to the active vertebrate peptides.

The initial observations of the long time course and pacemaker character of the peptide and bag cell extract excitation were useful in providing phenomenology of reliable quality, obtained under well-controlled experimental conditions. To examine the biophysical mechanisms underlying these excitatory actions, we have used the electrophysiological technique of voltage clamping, a method that permits control of the membrane potential and allows examination of the currents underlying the membrane's conductances, including those that are voltage- and time-dependent. For these measurements, two microelectrodes are placed in the cell body: one electrode is used to record the membrane potential of the cell, while the other is used to pass the current required to control the membrane potential. These microelectrodes are connected to a closed-loop electronic system in a negative feedback configuration. In this way the cell's membrane potential can be "clamped" to a given holding potential and thence commanded in a step-wise fashion to any desired potential. The current flowing across the membrane is monitored with an operational amplifier, which holds the extracellular space at a virtual ground potential.

Clamping the cell's membrane to the resting potential in the case of electrically silent cells (about −50 mV) or to −50 mV in cells spontaneously generating a low-amplitude beating pattern of pacemaker activity requires little, if any, observable net current (Figure 3). No net current flow is observed if the cell is properly clamped to its resting potential, becasue the algebraic sum of all currents flowing across a membrane with such resting potential is zero. Cells generating beating pacemaker activity do not have stable resting potentials and, therefore, clamping the membrane to a potential that approximates the "average" potential of the cell about halfway between the excursions of the beating pacemaker potential reveals an inwardly directed current of small magnitude (as in Figure 3). Presumably, this inward current is the force necessary to keep the membrane depolarized enough to attain threshold for action potential generation. Clamping the membrane potential of the same cell to the same potential after addition of the peptide, when the cell is generating BPP activity, now shows the gradual development of considerably more inwardly directed current (Figure 3). (The gradual development of this inward-going current is mainly due to the decay of an outwardly directed K^+ current, which was activated by the cell's

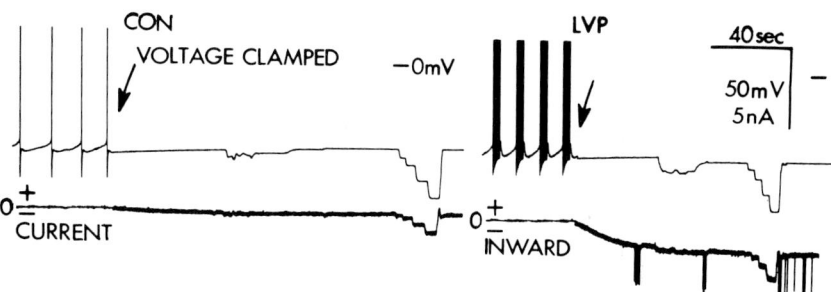

FIGURE 3. LVP induces persistent inward holding current. Voltage traces are above current traces. Under control conditions (CON), the unclamped membrane potential behavior of a cell is characterized by beating pacemaker activity. Voltage clamp of membrane to potential approximating a "resting" potential (−50 mV; at arrow) reveals just detectable, net inward membrane current. Hyperpolarizing step commands, near end of trace, show direct relationship between voltage and current. Addition of LVP induces bursting pacemaker activity ("LVP" before arrow), and when the cell's potential is clamped to −50 mV (at arrow), a gradually developing net inward current results. Current responses to hyperpolarizing steps show a slight increase in membrane conductance. Downward deflections on current trace in LVP are fast-spike currents resulting from action potentials in unclamped and remote axon regions of cell.

membrane just before clamping and is superimposed on a steady inward current. This will be discussed below.) The presence of considerable inwardly directed current over a wide membrane potential range produces a depolarizing bias that insures sustained depolarization of the membrane into a region of potential where the fast voltage-dependent conductances underlying action potentials and the slow voltage-dependent conductances underlying pacemaker potentials can be activated. At present, we do not have consistent evidence to indicate the ionic basis of the apparently voltage-independent conductance underlying the steady inward current. It may reflect inactivation of a hyperpolarizing (K^+) conductance or activation of a depolarizing (Na^+/Ca^{2+}) conductance or both. Furthermore, no clear and consistent changes in the leakage conductance of the cell have been observed. The "leakage" conductance is, by definition, the conductance derived from the slope of the linear current-voltage relationship found at large, negative membrane potentials. The leakage conductance, therefore, is voltage independent. A small increase in this slope can be seen in Figure 3, where slightly more inward current is evoked during the hyperpolarizing command steps in the presence of the peptide, whereas no change in

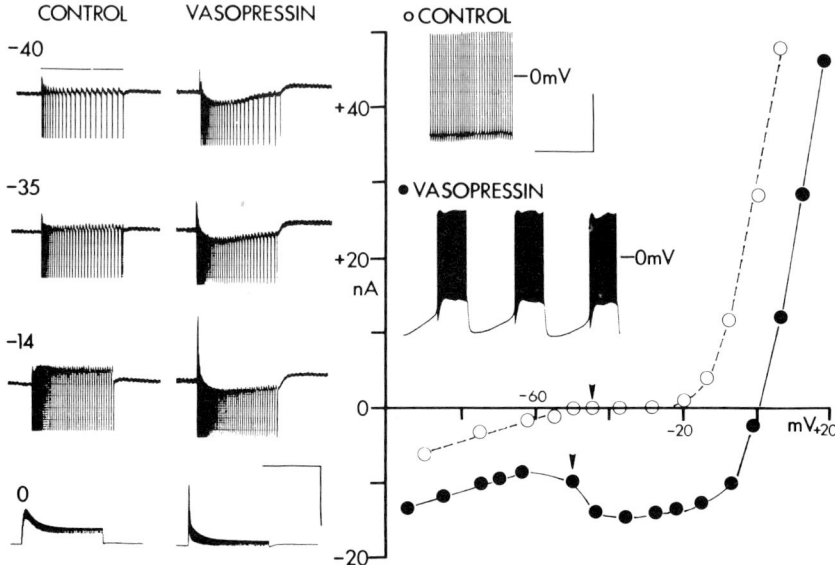

FIGURE 4. Vasopressin alters steady-state, voltage-clamp, current voltage (I-V) curve. Recordings are from peptide-sensitive cell from the snail before (CONTROL) and after the bath application of 1 μM vasopressin (VASOPRESSIN). Membrane potential activity is illustrated in insets of I-V plot on right. Control trace shows beating pacemaker activity. Vasopressin induces bursting pacemaker activity. Zero membrane potential: "0 mV." Left: Membrane of cell voltage, clamped and 5-sec voltage steps imposed (during time indicated by bar above current trace marked "−40"). Currents are shown at different depolarizing voltage steps (to membrane potentials indicated by numbers above traces) under control conditions and in presence of vasopressin. Rapid downward current events represent action potential currents. Presence of slow inward current that decreases during the command is apparent in the vasopressin-treated membrane. Right: I-V curve derived from quasi-steady-state currents using most negative or least positive current evoked after 1 sec during command. Current axis (nA), voltage axis (mV). Cell's membrane held at −45 mV in control and −50 mV in vasopressin (downward arrows). Calibrations: Left, 10 nA (upper three traces) and 40 nA (lowermost traces), 5 sec; right (inset), 50 mV, 20s. From Barker and Smith (1976).

the slope is evident over the same potential range in the experiment illustrated in Figure 4. Whatever the precise mechanisms, the presence of a depolarizing bias allows continued activation of the conductances underlying pacemaker and action potentials, which would not otherwise be activated if the membrane were to remain hyperpolarized relative to threshold for their activation.

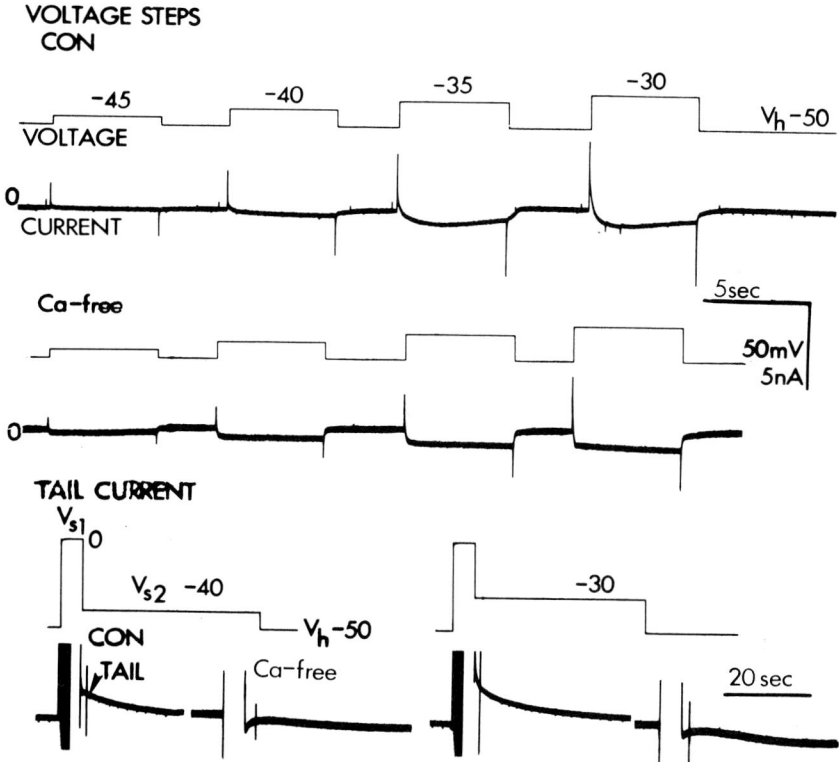

FIGURE 5. Effect of Ca^{2+} on pacemaker currents. Recordings are from R_{15} in *Aplysia* voltage clamped to -50 mV (V_h) under control conditions (10 mM Ca^{2+}, 50 mM Mg^{2+}) and after washing for 30 min in Ca^{2+}-free medium (60 mM Mg^{2+}). Amplitude of pacemaker potential increases from 12 mV in control to 30 mV in Ca^{2+}-free medium (not illustrated). VOLTAGE STEPS. Time-dependent decrease in steady inward current in control (CON) observed at commands to -35 mV and -30 mV is absent in nominally Ca^{2+}-free solution (Ca free). TAIL CURRENT. Outward tail current evoked by double-step voltage commands to 0 mV(V_{s1}) and then to -40 mV or -30 mV(V_{s2}) from holding potential (V_h) of -50 mV is markedly diminished in Ca^{2+}-free solution.

In addition to enhanced excitability, another effect of the peptide is an activation of pacemaker conductances underlying the BPP activity. Such activity cannot be induced by depolarizing the membrane of a cell not spontaneously generating BPPs, as can be seen in the control traces in Figures 1 and 2. The two pacemaker conductances, with relatively slow kinetics, have been identified and are activated at membrane potentials within millivolts of threshold for activation of the fast

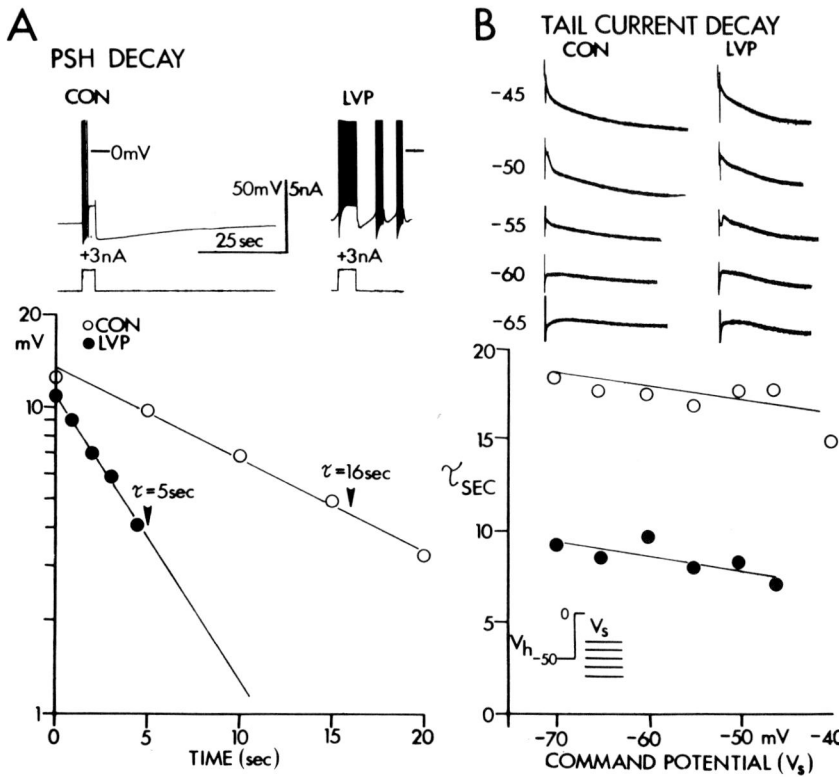

FIGURE 6. LVP shortens K⁺ pacemaker conductance decay. (A) Recording are from initially inactive cell in *Otala*. Under unclamped conditions, injection of 3 nA depolarizing current is followed by post-stimulus hyperpolarization (PSH) that decays with a time constant of 16 sec (CON). Addition of LVP induces bursting pacemaker activity. Now 3 nA depolarizing current injection is followed by PSH of approximately the same amplitude, but shorter time course (LVP) (time constant equals 5 sec). Resting potential: −50 mV. (B) Decay of outward tail current evoked by double-step voltage commands from holding potential (V_h) of −50 mV first to 0 mV for 5 sec and then to various other potentials under control conditions and in LVP. Tail currents observed during 2nd step potentials (indicated by numbers at left of traces) displayed above their time constants of decay. Decay is two-phased and voltage-dependent. The late, slow phase is 16 to 18 sec in control and 6 to 9 sec in LVP (right), approximating the membrane potential decay rates (left) of PSH in the two conditions.

conductances underlying action potentials (Smith, Barker, and Gainer, 1975; Figure 4). One conductance is evidenced by the presence of a persistent inward current, often seen at potentials subthreshold to the spike conductances (Wilson and Wachtel, 1974; Gola, 1974; Smith et al.,

1975; Eckert and Lux, 1976). In *Otala* and *Aplysia*, the amplitude of the inward current is directly dependent on extracellular Na^+ concentration (Smith et al., 1975) and inversely dependent on extra-cellular Ca^{2+} concentration (unpublished observations, Figure 5), and hence is a Na^+ conductance. The other conductance is activated at more depolarized potentials and is reflected in the appearance of slowly decaying, outwardly directed tail currents following step commands to more depolarized levels (Junge and Stephens, 1973; Smith et al., 1975; Figures 5, 6). These tail currents extrapolate to a reversal potential that varies with extracellular K^+ concentration (unpublished observations). Thus, the outwardly directed pacemaker current is presumably due to a K^+ conductance, which is slow to activate and slow to inactivate. Because the magnitudes of Na^+ and K^+ pacemaker conductances, once they are activated by the peptide, are a function of membrane potential, such conductances, by definition, are voltage dependent.

The time-dependent decrease in the amplitude of the inward-going current in normal solutions might be due either to inactivation of the Na^+ pacemaker conductance and/or to activation of the outward K^+ pacemaker conductance. That the latter may be sufficient to account for the observation is suggested by the lack of a decay in the inward current after bathing in solutions nominally free of Ca^{2+} and the virtual absence of slowly decaying, outward tail current under these conditions (Figure 5). Thus, the pacemaker K^+ conductance appears to be activated, at least partly, by Ca^{2+} ions, as reflected by the loss of slow outward currents under nominally Ca^{2+}-free conditions.

Peptide regulation of the pacemaker conductances alters the steady-state current-voltage curve of the cell so that net current flow across the membrane remains inward at potentials more depolarized than in control. This effectively shifts the steady-state current-voltage curve in a depolarizing direction. In those cells already generating low-amplitude BPP activity under control conditions, and already showing a steady-state current-voltage (I–V) curve with an N-shaped characteristic, the peptide enhances both the BPP activity and the region of negative slope, indicating that more voltage-dependent net Na^+ current is developed in its presence.

The enhanced activation of the K^+ pacemaker conductance by the peptide appears to have a threshold at potentials hyperpolarized relative to control (unpublished observations) and the decay of the conductance is faster, as evidenced by the shorter time constant of decay of the tail currents (Figure 6). More rapid inactivation of this K^+ conductance

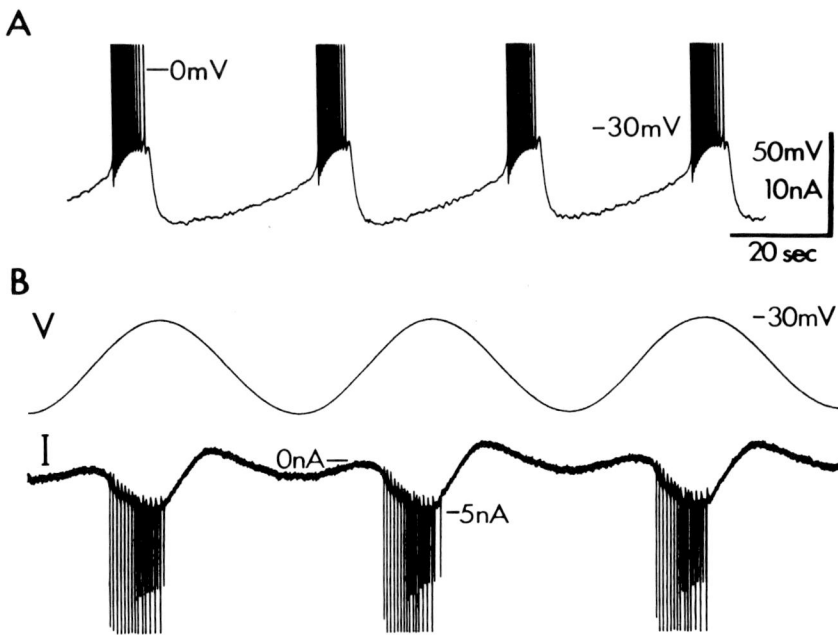

FIGURE 7. Dynamics of net membrane currents during simulated bursting pacemaker activity in *Otala*. (A) Recordings were made with CsCl microelectrodes from cell bathed in LVP and 10 mM Sr^{2+}. Under unclamped conditions, pacemaker potential amplitude is about 40 mV, oscillating between −34 mV and −74 mV. (B) After voltage clamping, a sinusoidal 50 mV command oscillating between −30 mV and −80 mV is imposed on the membrane (V) and the resulting net membrane current is recorded (I). At the beginning of the traces, voltage is −80 mV and net current is −2 nA. As membrane is depolarized, net current gradually becomes less negative until potential is about −40 mV, when net current becomes more negative, reaching −5 nA at peak of artificial pacemaker potential. While at peak of waveform net current is rapidly reversed, momentarily becoming positive during the hyperpolarizing phase of oscillation. Current decays monophasically as potential is polarized to −80 mV.

would effectively lead to a more rapid depolarization of the membrane potential after its activation. Activation of the conductance can be achieved under current clamp conditions by injecting depolarizing current, after which the membrane hyperpolarizes beyond the resting potential and then slowly repolarizes back to control potential. The time constant of this repolarization is about 16 sec in control and 5 sec in the same cell after addition of the peptide. These rates approximate the decay times of the K^+ pacemaker conductance under the two conditions, when measured with the voltage clamp. A more rapid inactivation of this conductance would act to shorten the period of pacemaker potential.

The progress and polarity of the membrane currents underlying the pacemaker potential can be observed under voltage clamp by imposing a sine-wave command that simulates, in an imperfect manner, the course of the pacemaker potential (Figure 7). During this simulated pacemaker potential activity several time- and voltage-dependent changes in the magnitude and polarity of the total membrane current are evident. As the membrane is depolarized from its initially hyperpolarized level at the beginning of the trace, net membrane current, which is inward (negative or depolarizing), gradually approaches and becomes zero about midway during the depolarizing phase of the simulated pacemaker waveform. The direction of the change in the current, that is, the current's time derivative, $\dot{I}$, is positive. Because the membrane potential change is also positive, that is, its time derivative, $\dot{V}$, is positive, then the *slope* conductance, dI/dV, during this phase is also positive. Further depolarization, however, leads to progressively *more* net inward membrane current until the peak depolarization of voltage waveform, at which potential net membrane current becomes progressively less negative. Thus, both during the late phase of the depolarizing, positive-going voltage change ($\dot{V} > 0$), and during the early phase of the hyperpolarizing, negative-going change ($\dot{V} < 0$), the corresponding current changes are of opposite sign: that is, when $\dot{V} > 0, \dot{I} < 0$, and when $\dot{V} < 0, \dot{I} > 0$. These results indicate that during these phases, the slope conductance is negative. Furthermore, these negative slope conductances probably correspond to the negative slope conductance region of the N-shaped I-V curve (Figure 4). The static, steady-state I-V curve provides no conclusive information as to whether its negative slope region is associated with the depolarizing or hyperpolarizing phases of the BPP. Figure 7 illustrates that the negative slope, as well as the negative I, is mainly related to the depolarizing phase of the BPP.

Subsequently, the polarity of the current is reversed, becoming outward (positive or hyperpolarizing). Eventually, the net outward current thus evoked decays monophasically ($\dot{I} < 0$) during the hyperpolarizing phase of the simulated pacemaker waveform, with a time constant that approximates the depolarization rate of the unclamped membrane during the interburst interval. Moreover, during this late, hyperpolarizing phase the slope conductance again becomes positive. To summarize the events associated with polarization of the membrane through a potential range, as would occur during spontaneously generated pacemaker potentials, sufficient depolarization of the membrane from an initially hyperpolarized level activates a conductance causing inward current to dominate until further depolarization allows activation of another conductance that rapidly leads to outward current predominating. The former conductance is primarily Na^+ and provides the sustained depolarizing phase of the pacemaker potential, whereas the latter is a K^+ conductance that acts to hyperpolarize the membrane. Thus, under unclamped conditions, the membrane potential continually oscillates as the depolarizing Na^+ pacemaker conductance and then the hyperpolarizing K^+ pacemaker conductance are sequentially activated in an alternating manner. The periodicity of the pacemaker oscillations appears to be determined mainly by the inactivation kinetics of the hyperpolarizing K^+ conductance; the slower the inactivation, the more prolonged is the slow depolarization and the longer is the period of oscillation. Calcium appears to play an important but incompletely defined regulatory role in the generation of pacemaker potentials (Barker and Gainer, 1975b), probably due to its regulation of the Na^+ and K^+ pacemaker conductances (Figure 5).

Several other voltage-dependent conductances, besides the two pacemaker conductances, can be identified on the basis of their distinctive voltage dependencies and kinetics. They are (1) a conductance activated at about -50 mV with a rapid time constant of decay of about 100 msec, which is inactivated at more depolarized potentials (Connor and Stevens, 1971a), and (2) a conductance activated at about -20 mV, which inactivates with a time constant of about 0.5 to 0.9 sec, and is the so-called delayed rectifying conductance (Katz, 1966). Both of these are K^+ conductances and neither the amplitudes nor the inactivation kinetics of these two conductances are affected by the peptide (unpublished observations). Peptide effects on activation kinetics of these conductances have yet to be examined.

The functional significance of the first, rapidly inactivating conductance to BPP activity remains unclear. Activation of this conductance would only be predicated on prior hyperpolarization of the cell's membrane sufficient to remove its inactivation processes, and would presumably tend to prolong a previous hyperpolarization (Neher, 1971). Inactivation of the conductance would increase the relative membrane resistance near threshold for action potential generation (Stevens, 1969; Connor and Stevens, 1971b). The second K^+ conductance is involved in controlling repolarization of the membrane during an action potential.

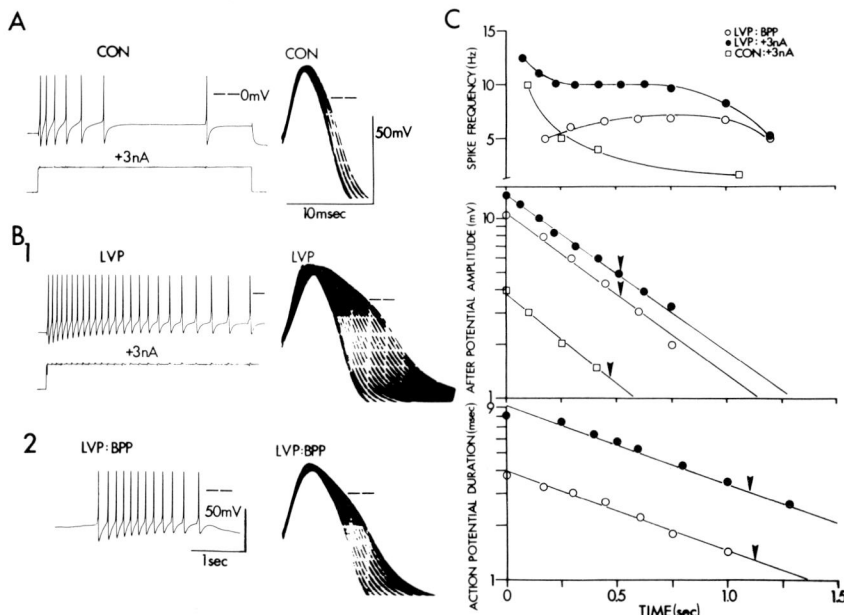

FIGURE 8. Action potential behavior in *Otala* during natural or stimulated train. Recordings from cell initially inactive (CON). (A) Injection of 3 nA depolarizing current initiates action potential train whose instantaneous frequency declines (C, top graph). After-potential amplitude declines during 3 nA stimulus with a time constant of about 0.5 sec (C, middle graph, arrowhead). Action potential duration increases during sustained depolarization (spike-triggered oscillographic traces in center), but quantitative analysis is not possible. (B1) Same depolarizing current stimulus to same cell after addition of LVP now generates action potential train whose instantaneous frequency is higher, and is maintained longer than in control (C, top graph). During stimulus, after-potential amplitude declines with time constant of about 0.5 sec (C, middle graph, arrowhead) and action potential duration increases with time constant of about 1.1 sec (C, bottom graph). Similar changes in instantaneous action potential frequency, and in kinetics of after-potential depression and of increase in action potential duration are present during a natural train of action potentials (B2 and C).

One of the important consequences of peptide regulation of pacemaker conductance activity is to produce a periodic depolarization of the cell sustained enough to cause a train of action potentials. During the train, action potential frequency remains relatively constant, while the amplitude of the after-potential progressively decreases and the duration of the action potential increases (Strumwasser, 1973; Figure 8). The time constant of change of the former event is about 0.5 sec, whereas that of the latter is about 1.1 sec. Similar kinetics for after-potential amplitude change are present under control conditions during a train evoked by injection of depolarizing current.

One might inquire as to why the action potentials are altered during an evoked or natural train. To gain insight into the membrane events surrounding these changes, we simulated a train of action potentials by using a repetitive series of brief voltage commands to 0 mV (Figure 9). The amplitudes of the currents evoked during such a repetitive sequence of commands decayed with a time constant that depended inversely on the frequency of the commands. The higher the frequency, the faster the decay rate and the greater the eventual decrease in amplitude relative to that of the first current evoked. That this phenomenon is due largely to a decay in a repetitively activated K^+ conductance is indicated by an observed depression of membrane conductance with little change in the equilibrium potential of the currents evoked at the end of a command train, relative to that at the start (unpublished observations). This conductance, with frequency-sensitive inactivation kinetics, appears to be identical to the delayed rectifying K^+ conductance activated at about -20 mV. Repolarization of action potentials is thus regulated by their frequency; the higher the frequency, the more rapidly and thoroughly depressed is the mechanism of repolarization. The sensitivity of inactivation kinetics to command frequency is unchanged by the peptide (Figure 9). The time constant of decay of the currents, evoked over a range of command frequencies similar to the natural frequencies of action potentials during BPP activity (3 to 8 Hz), approximates the time constant of change in after-potential amplitude observed during a BPP, suggesting that the two events are causally related. The progressive prolongation of action potentials during a BPP, which, like the depression in after-potential amplitude reflects a progressive inability of the membrane to repolarize during an action potential, is presumably also related to the frequency-sensitive decay of K^+ conductance. Thus, the membrane has a mechanism that complements the underlying pacemaker activity and produces a facilitated excitation during the depolarizing phases of the membrane potential oscillations.

What are the physiological consequences of pacemaking and the periodic generation of progressively longer action potentials? One possible consequence is the periodic, facilitated entry of Ca^{2+} into the cell body during the train of action potentials (Stinnakre and Tauc, 1973). If the train of action potentials is faithfully conducted along the axon of the cell and sequentially invades the axon terminal, there should be a periodic release of transmitter. If the axon terminal membrane also has a frequency-sensitive K^+ conductance associated with action potential repolarization, then there will be a progressive prolongation of each succeeding action potential invading the terminal. This would provide for a facilitated entry of Ca^{2+} and thereby produce a facilitated release of transmitter or neurosecretory product. Direct evidence for such a pulsatile, facilitated release is lacking because the terminals of the peptide-sensitive cell in *Aplysia* and *Otala* do not make synaptic

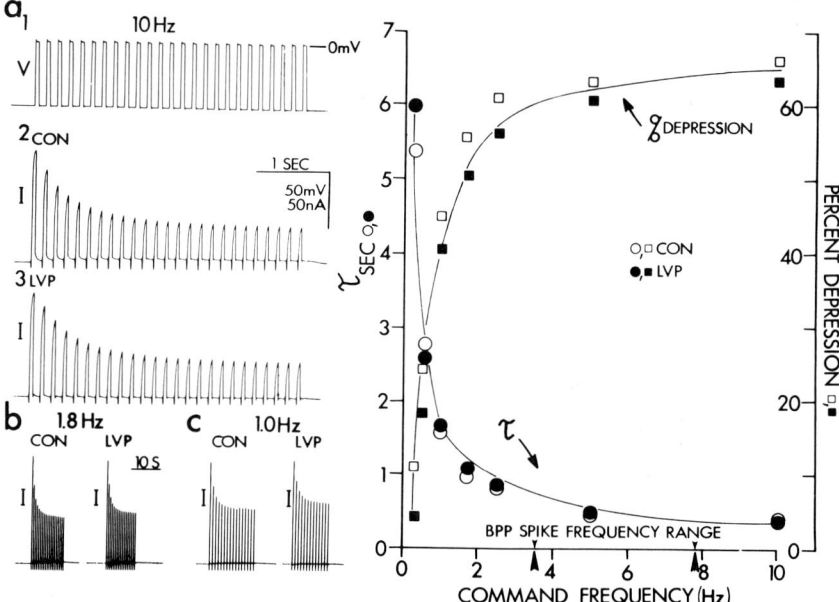

FIGURE 9. Frequency-sensitive inactivation of action potential ("delayed rectifier") K^+ conductance in *Otala*. Recordings are from a cell voltage clamped under control conditions or bathed in LVP. Action potential train is simulated by holding membrane at −50 mV and repetitively stepping to 0 mV using 50 msec commands (a1). With a repetition rate of 10 Hz, outward currents evoked during commands decline rapidly (time constant is approximately 0.5 sec) to less than 40% initial value with same kinetics in control (a2, CON) and in LVP (a3, LVP). At slower repetition rates, rate of decline and final depression is less (b,c). Time constant of decline and percent depression of outward current amplitude are plotted as a function of command frequency in graph on right. A hyperbolic relationship between the two parameters and frequency is evident. The higher the frequency, the faster and greater the decline in outward current. The range of natural action potential frequencies present during a bursting pacemaker potential are indicated by arrowheads on abscissa.

connections; therefore detailed examination of the output characteristics of the cell cannot be performed (Gainer, 1972a). However, another cell (L_{10}), which is presynaptic to the peptide sensitive cell (R_{15}) in *Aplysia*, does, on occasion, generate BPP activity (Frazier, Kandel, Kupfermann, Waziri, and Coggeshall, 1967). By recording from R_{15} one can observe the cholinergic excitatory postsynaptic events characteristic of presynaptic activity in L_{10} (Wachtel and Kandel, 1971; Figure 10). Voltage clamping R_{15} permits observation of the excitatory postsynaptic currents underlying the EPSPs. These currents are of constant amplitude and frequency when the presynaptic cell generates a constant frequency beating pacemaker potential type of activity (Figure 10B1: CON). When the presynaptic cell generates BPP activity, the excitatory synaptic currents are periodically present in R_{15} and are typically of progressively increasing amplitude and frequency (Figure 10B3). Integration, over time, of the output of the presynaptic cell, in terms of postsynaptic current under the two modes of presynaptic pacemaker activity, reveals a greater than 10-fold increase in output produced during BPP activity (Figure 10A). This is approximately threefold more than would have been expected had the same number and frequency of presynaptic action potentials present during a BPP led to postsynaptic currents of *constant* amplitude (Figure 10A: solid square). Thus, clustering of the presynaptic events at an intermittent, but fast, frequency has led to a facilitated, pulsatile release of transmitter. If postsynaptic events accurately reflect presynaptic activity, then this synaptic transmission and the changes in the postsynaptic events associated with the two modes of presynaptic pacemaker activity may be an adequate model of the output characteristics of other nerve cells whose membrane potential behavior changes from a beating pattern to BPP activity, as happens in cell 11 of *Otala* and R_{15} of *Aplysia* upon addition of the peptide. By inducing BPP activity, the peptide may provide for a facilitated, pulsatile release of transmitter or neurosecretory product.

A second consequence of the peptide's alteration in membrane properties is that the membrane attains considerably more nonlinear properties. In such cases, synaptic input to the membrane is therefore transformed in a much more nonlinear and amplified manner into output. If the nonspike membrane properties of the cell were close to linear, then synaptic input would be converted in a more or less arithmetic fashion into output. The presence of nonlinear membrane allows, for example, for an exponential conversion of input to output (Figure 10A) and, over

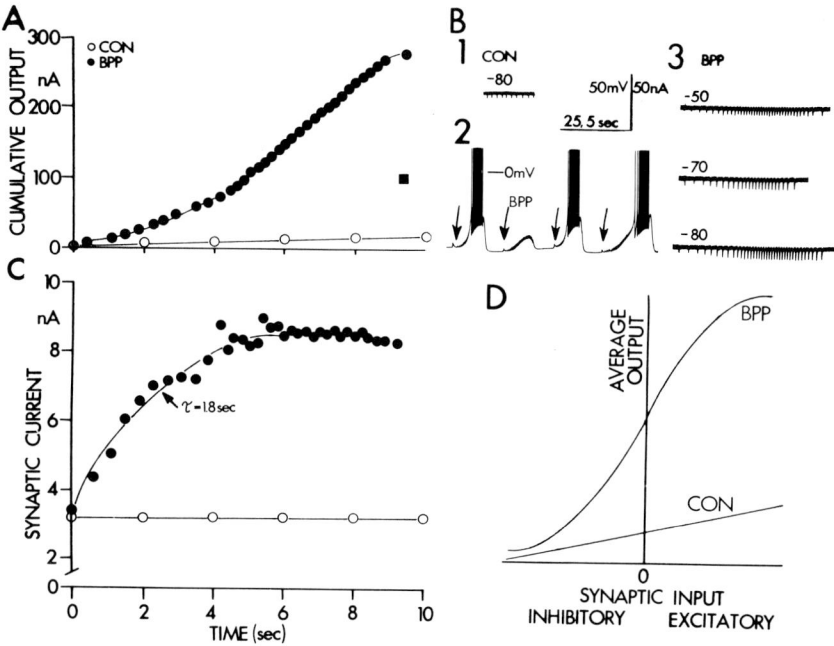

FIGURE 10. Physiological consequences of bursting pacemaker potential activity. Recordings are from R_{15}, which receives monosynaptic excitatory input from L_{10}. When L_{10} generates a beating pacemaker pattern of activity, unitary excitatory postsynaptic currents (EPSCs) are recorded in R_{15} voltage clamped at -80 mV (B1, CON). The constant-amplitude, constant-frequency EPSCs have been plotted in (C) and integrated over time in (A) as "cumulative output" of L_{10} (○). When L_{10} generates a bursting mode of pacemaker activity, a burst of excitatory postsynaptic potentials (B2, arrows) and EPSCs of increasing amplitude and frequency (B3) are recorded in R_{15}. Plotting the EPSC amplitude as a function of time (C) reveals a single exponential increase in EPSC amplitude (time constant equals 1.8 sec), which plateaus at 1.5 times the amplitude of EPSCs recorded when L_{10} generates beating pacemaker activity. Integrating the EPSC over time (A) shows 10-fold greater synaptic current accumulated during BPP activity. An approximately threefold increase in accumulated current would have been expected if each EPSC in the burst were of constant amplitude (■). Thus, the output of L_{10}, monitored by using EPSC amplitude in R_{15}, is facilitated during the physiological BPP activity. (D) Theoretical input-output relations of a cell with almost linear membrane properties (CON), generating beating pacemaker activity, compared to one with nonlinear membrane properties generating BPP activity (BPP). Average output of neurotransmitter or neurosecretory product is considerably increased in cell generating BPPs due to its facilitated pulsatile character, and the effect of synaptic input is much greater in BPP cell due to the nonlinear membrane.

the nonlinear range of membrane properties, synaptic input would have considerably more effect than it would with a linear membrane (Figure 10D).

One consequence of a facilitated Ca^{2+} entry at the level of the cell body may relate to the role of Ca^{2+} in cytoplasmic events. Ca^{2+} appears to play a role in synthesis and transport of low-molecular-weight proteins in R_{15} neurosecretory cells (Barker, 1977b). Although the details regarding the precise role of Ca^{2+} have yet to be formulated, a bathing medium nominally free of Ca^{2+} leads to a reduction in both the synthesis and transport of low-molecular-weight proteins. Thus, facilitated entry of Ca^{2+} into the cell body during BPP activity might play a role in the protein biochemistry of the cell.

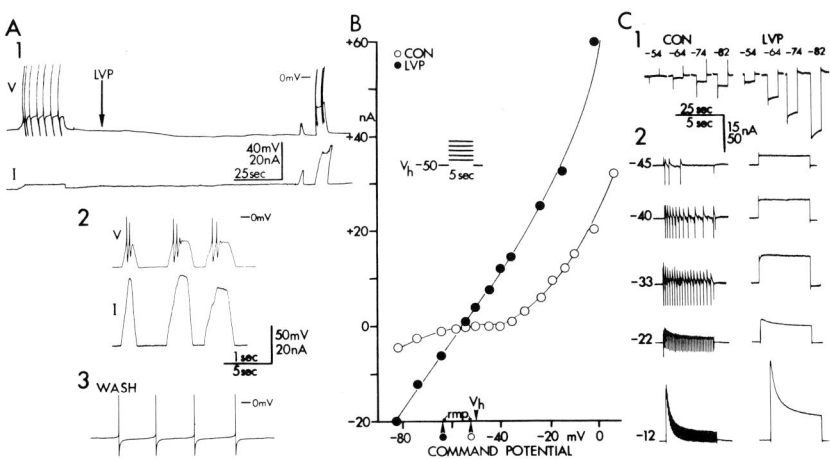

FIGURE 11. Inhibitory effects of LVP. Recordings are from unidentified cell adjacent to cell (cell 11) excited by LVP. (A1) Potential trace (V) above current trace (I). Cell is electrically inactive but generates repetitive series of action potentials upon injection of depolarizing current, as seen in the early part of the trace. Bath application of 0.1 μM LVP (arrow) hyperpolarizes membrane and much more current is required to generate action potentials: late part of trace. Traces were recorded on curvilinear pen recorder. (A2) Relatively fast, large depolarizing current pulses evoke small amplitude action potentials that rapidly accommodate. Rectilinear traces. (A3) Washing in peptide-free solution leads to recovery of spikes within minutes. (B) Steady-state I-V curves are derived from currents (C) observed at different potentials under voltage clamp in control solution and in LVP. A holding potential (V_h) of −50 mV and 5-sec commands were used to generate data. Membrane conductance considerably increased and I-V curve changed from nonlinear to mainly linear in LVP. Rmp: resting membrane potential. (C) Currents evoked during hyperpolarizing (1) and depolarizing commands (2). Note the absence of multiple action potential currents in LVP.

Inhibitory Peptide Effects

In addition to the enhanced excitability evoked by LVP, we have occasionally observed an inhibitory effect of vasopressin in *Otala* on an unidentified nerve cell that is located next to the cell (cell 11) excited by the peptide. An inhibitory effect has also been observed on cells in the left upper quadrant of the abdominal ganglion of *Aplysia* (unpublished observations), but the biophysical mechanisms underlying this effect have yet to be examined. The inhibitory effect of the peptide in *Otala* consists of a hyperpolarization of the membrane and is associated with a large increase in membrane conductance (Figure 11). These events rapidly reduce the excitability of the cell, effectively suppressing the generation of action potentials. Action potentials that can be elicited by

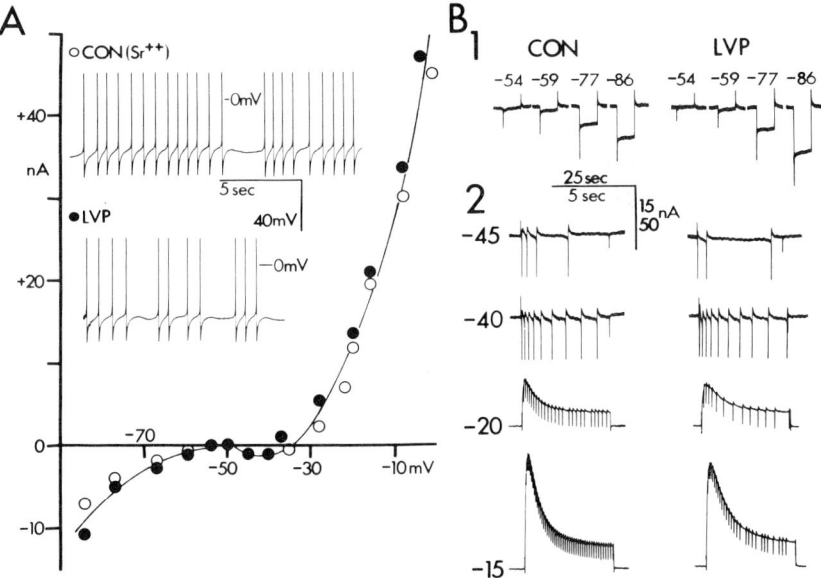

FIGURE 12. Absence of inhibitory peptide effect in the absence of Ca^{2+}. Recordings are from same cell as illustrated in Figure 11. Cell is now bathed in a solution nominally free of Ca^{2+} using equimolar Sr^{2+} as substituting divalent cation. Membrane potential behavior (insets in A) consists of spontaneous beating-(quasi) bursting pacemaker activity in both control and LVP. Little change is apparent after bath application of 0.1 μM LVP. I-V curve (A) derived from steady-state currents evoked by 5-sec hyperpolarizing and depolarizing commands from holding of −50 mV is similar with (●) and without (○) peptide in Sr^{2+}-containing solutions. (B) Currents were recorded during hyperpolarizing (1) and depolarizing commands (2). Notice presence of multiple action potential currents in LVP.

injection of depolarizing current are smaller in amplitude and rapidly accommodate (Figure 11A2). The steady-state current-voltage relations of the cell are likewise altered by the peptide over a wide range of membrane potential. Under control conditions, the current-voltage curve contains a nonlinear region, whereas, in the presence of the peptide, this region and the remainder of the curve become more linear. Thus, the peptide apparently has activated a voltage-independent conductance, which effectively shunts the voltage-dependent conductances, hyperpolarizes the membrane, and holds it below threshold for generating spikes. Although we have not determined the ionic basis of this increased conductance and hyperpolarization, the effects are probably due to an increased K^+ permeability. The change in the steady-state curve is the opposite of that induced by the peptide on the neighboring cell, where a nonlinear region was induced or enhanced. Examination of the steady-state currents evoked during various steps reveals the absence of multiple fast-spike currents in the presence of the peptide. The absence of these currents could reflect either insufficient depolarization of unclamped membrane, owing to the high conductance of the membrane, and/or a direct effect of the peptide on the conductance mechanisms underlying the fast-spike currents. All the inhibitory effects of the peptide are rapidly reversible, nonlinear membrane properties and full-amplitude action potentials being restored within minutes of washing away the peptide.

These effects of the peptide on the resting membrane properties are dependent on the presence of extracellular Ca^{2+}, because replacement of the medium with an equal concentration of Sr^{2+} abolished the inhibitory effects of the peptide on membrane properties (Figure 12). In Sr^{2+}, the cell shows a slight tendency to generate low-amplitude BPP activity. Full amplitude action potentials are also present under these conditions.

A closer examination of the currents underlying the action potentials, however, demonstrates a depressant effect of the peptide on the amplitude of the fast current that underlies the depolarizing phase of the action potential (Figure 13). Such an effect would complement the other actions of the peptide on this cell to reduce excitability. This inhibitory effect of the peptide is also dependent on extracellular Ca^{2+}. The depression of the rapid inward current cannot be entirely accounted for by the increase in leakage conductance induced by the peptide. If one assumes that leakage conductance is constant over a wide range of membrane potentials and that its contribution can be estimated by extending the slope of the I-V curve observed where leakage conductance dominates the membrane (at large, negative membrane potentials) to regions where other conductances dominate, then it is evident that only part of the decrease in inward current caused by the peptide observed in a Ca^{2+} medium relative to that seen in a Sr^{2+} medium is due to the increase in leakage conductance (Figure 13B). All of the apparent increase in outward current, however, is due to increased leakage.

Thus, the peptide suppresses excitation in this cell at several levels of

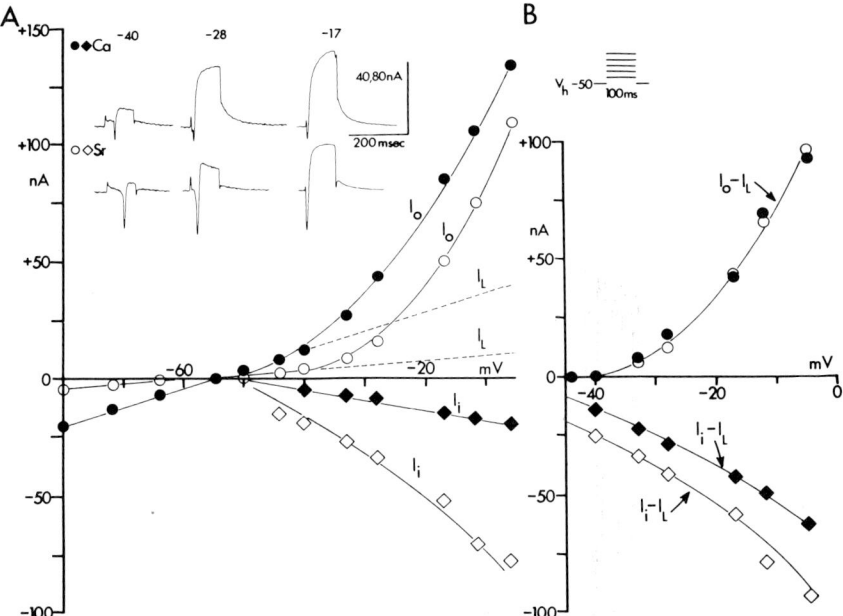

FIGURE 13. Selective depression of fast, inward spike currents by LVP in Ca^{2+}-containing solutions. Recordings are from same cell as illustrated in Figures 11 and 12 that was bathed in LVP solutions containing either 10 mM Ca^{2+} or 10 mM Sr^{2+}. Membrane voltage clamped to -50 mV and 100 msec hyper- and depolarizing commands imposed. Example of currents recorded for depolarizing commands to -40, -28, and -17 mV (insets of A) show rapidly activating and rapidly inactivating inward current succeeded by sustained outward current. Amplitudes of inward (I_i, diamond symbols) and outward currents (I_o, circles) are plotted as a function of command voltage. Slope of current-voltage relation is derived from hyperpolarizing commands (reflecting leakage conductance) extrapolated in a depolarizing direction to show underlying current due to leakage conductance (I_L). Considerably more inward, and somewhat less outward current is present in Sr^{2+} relative to that in Ca^{2+}. However, correcting for assumed contribution of I_L, by subtracing I_L at each potential from total I, shows that outward currents are identical (B). Only inward current is directly depressed in Ca^{2+} relative to that in Sr^{2+}.

excitability. It polarizes the membrane away from firing threshold and shunts incoming excitatory input, thereby effectively preventing excitatory synaptic potentials from producing sufficient voltage to evoke spikes. Furthermore, it acts on the cell's mechanism of excitation by specifically depressing the fast, voltage-dependent conductance that produces the spike's inward current. All of these inhibitory effects are dependent on the presence of extracellular Ca^{2+}, unlike the excitatory effects of the peptide on the neighboring cell (cell 11), which can be observed when Ca^{2+} is replaced by Sr^{2+} (unpublished observation). The physiological consequences of these effects are to prevent the cell from generating its own output and from responding to excitatory input. The combination of a high-conductance state of the membrane, coupled to a specific depression of the excitatory conductance involved in action potential generation, should markedly alter the input-output relations of the cell. Output should now be a less nonlinear function of input and have a low gain, whereas, in control, output was more nonlinearly related to input and operated at high gain.

CONCLUSIONS

Neurohormonal Communication

The evidence presented in this article demonstrates that specific peptides can markedly alter the excitability of nerve cells through multiple actions on voltage-dependent and voltage-independent conductances. The excitatory effect on identified molluscan neurons consists of a long-lasting depolarization and induction of pacemaker activity. The depolarization results from peptide regulation of voltage-independent conductances and insures that the membrane will be polarized into the potential region where the voltage-dependent Na^+ and K^+ pacemaker conductances are activated. The activity of these pacemaker conductances is also regulated by the peptide. The physiological consequences of these long-lasting events are to provide a facilitated, pulsatile output of transmitter or neruosecretory product and to make the input-output relations of the cell far more nonlinear. The inhibitory effects of the peptide render an unidentified cell almost completely inexcitable by hyperpolarizing the membrane and increasing a voltage-independent membrane conductance, and by specifically depressing a fast conductance underlying excitation. These inhibitory effects are rapidly reversible and dependent on extracellular Ca^{2+}, being absent in a Sr^{2+}-containing medium. The speed of recovery of the inhibitory effect contrasts with the slow recovery of the excitatory effect upon removal of the peptide. Moreover, whereas the inhibitory effect apparently has an obligating dependency on Ca^{2+}, the excitatory effect is affected by Ca^{2+}, but can occur in its absence.

All that has been discussed in this article is based on data obtained by a pharmacological approach, through application of peptides or peptide extracts to nerve cells. What is the physiology of the peptides that naturally exist in *Otala* and *Aplysia*? Peptide substances, which have qualitatively similar excitatory effects on the two cells excited by vasopressin, have been extracted from a specific cluster of neurosecretory cells (bag cells) in the abdominal ganglion of *Aplysia* (Mayeri and Simon, 1975; Figure 2). Electrical stimulation of the bag cells does not immediately lead to excitation, as would be expected if the bag cells were connected to other cells through synaptic junctions. Rather, there is a delay of seconds to minutes after stimulation before excitatory effects are evident (Mayeri and Simon, 1975). Furthermore, synapses between bag cells and other cells have not been observed; instead, bag cell processes appear to terminate in the connective tissue sheath surrounding the ganglion and its connectives. Thus, bag cell neurosecretory product is probably released into the hemolymph to diffuse both within the ganglion, as well as extra-ganglionically to induce egg laying (for review, see Arch, 1976). Although still incompletely defined, other effects of the bag cell neurosecretion on neuronal activity have been reported (Mayeri and Simon, 1975).

The evidence obtained, therefore, demonstrates that the physiology of the naturally occurring peptide does not resemble conventional chemical synaptic transmission, but rather, is analogous to the manner in which hormonal signals are conveyed over long distances by circulatory routes. (Neurohormonal communication is also unlike electrical synaptic transmission, which involves instantaneous transmission of electrical signals via low-resistance junctions between contiguous elements; for details see Bennett, 1966.) The differences and similarities between the two forms of communication in the nervous system are summarized in Table 1. Two important differences between synaptic transmission and neurohormonal communication appear to be in the distribution of the receptors and in the character of the receptor-coupled conductances that are activated in the postsynaptic or target cells. Synaptic transmission is localized, in that the postsynaptic receptors are most concentrated in the subsynaptic membrane, although extrasynaptic receptors are known to exist. In addition, synaptic

TABLE 1. *Synaptic transmission and neurohormonal communication*

Characteristic	Synaptic transmission	Neurohormonal communication
Avenue	Between contiguous cells in synaptic contact 200 Å synaptic cleft between adjacent pre- and postsynaptic neuronal membranes	Between remote cells without synaptic contact Extracellular space between one neuron and its target neurons
Distribution	Limited by axonal connections	Limited by appropriate receptors on target cells
Substance	Amino acid, catecholamine, ACh, peptide(?)	Peptide, ACh(?), catecholamine(?)
Release	Synaptic terminals Ca^{2+} dependent Facilitation Fatigue	Neurocirculatory terminals Ca^{2+} dependent
Effective concentration	Micromolar-millimolar	Nanomolar
Receptors	Subsynaptic localization Couple to one or more voltage-independent conductances Cooperativity Desensitization	Extrasynaptic localization Couple to one or more voltage-dependent and voltage-independent conductances
Actions	Rapid kinetics (msec-sec) Change in voltage-independent membrane properties Additive factor in input-output relations	Rapid and slow kinetics (sec-min-h) Change in voltage-independent and voltage-dependent membrane properties Additive and exponential factor in input-output relations
Function	Momentary regulation of single neuron excitability Simple and limited output	Sustained regulation of activity of multiple nerve cell aggregates Complex and concerted output

transmitters act on one or more voltage-independent conductances. By contrast, neurohormones activate receptors that are extrasynaptic, in that they bear no obvious anatomical relationship to other neuronal elements, and furthermore, they affect conductances that are voltage-independent and voltage-dependent. Synaptic events therefore regulate postsynaptic membrane properties in a more or less arithmetic manner. Under physiological conditions, temporal, spatial, cooperative, and kinetic characteristics of synaptic excitatory and inhibitory events determine the net synaptic current effective at any moment in regulating excitability. Pharmacological dissection of the synaptic input, allowing one or another species of synaptic transmission to be examined individually, shows that excitatory events increase, and inhibitory events decrease the postsynaptic cell's action potential frequency and number, and thus indirectly affect the output of a cell with linear membrane properties in a more or less direct manner. As measured either by nonspike changes in membrane potential or by spike frequency or number, output is therefore nearly a unitary power function of input. The function depends primarily on the linearity and time-variant properties of the extrasynaptic membrane of the postsynaptic cell over a wide range of membrane potential, especially near threshold for action potential generation. Because the voltage-dependent conductance mechanisms underlying spikes are not themselves directly affected by synaptic events, any power function in the input-output equation resulting from such nonlinearities is unchanged. Rather, the synaptic event acts as an additive factor in the input-output equation causing quantitative changes in the excitability of synaptically connected neuronal elements.

Neurohormonal regulation of excitability is a form of communication between one cell type and its diverse and distant target neurons. It is similar to hormonal regulation of peripheral, non-neural tissues. By way of analogy, neurohormonal communication may be likened to radio transmission and synaptic transmission may be likened to telephone messages. The former is broadcast widely without need of physical contact between sender and receiver, yet is only effective where there are properly "tuned receivers," called receptors. The latter is a private conversation mode of communication, dependent on "hard-wired" communication lines called axons and synapses. The avenue of neurohormonal communication is long distance relative to the several hundred angstroms at synapses. Although the invertebrate CNS is directly exposed to hemolymph in contrast to the vertebrate CNS, which is not except for the circumventricular organs, there are potentially two other avenues in which neurohormones or (hormones) could freely diffuse. They are the ventricular spaces, for diffusion over centimeters, and the extrasynaptic areas in the interstitium, for diffusion over micrometers. Specificity of communication is then predicated upon the appropriate receptor distribution. Some compensation for the effects of distance on effective concentration appears to have evolved, since neurohormones appear to be effective in nanomolar concentrations, which is at least three orders of magnitude more potent than neurotransmitters applied pharmacologically and six orders of magnitude more potent than transmitter concentration estimated to be physiologically present in synaptic clefts (Kuffler and Yoshikami, 1975). Long- and short-term changes in target cell excitability produced by neurohormones are accomplished through regulation of both receptor-coupled, voltage-independent, and voltage-dependent conductances underlying pacemaker and action potential activity. Such regulation means that neurohormones act as both additive and exponential factors in the input-output relations. The latter action significantly alters the transforming membrane upon which subsequent synaptic events may superimpose.

Although peptides have been proposed as neurohormones in this chapter, recent work suggests that conventional putative neurotransmitters (ACh and epinephrine) may also operate "hormonally" on particular cardiac tissues that are not innervated by neurons using these compounds as transmitters. For example, epinephrine has been shown to act on both voltage-dependent K^+ pacemaker conductance and voltage-independent conductances of Purkinje fibers (Tsien, 1974). In a similar fashion, ACh acts on resting and action potential conductances of auricular muscle (Giles and Noble, 1976).

Neurohormonal regulation of excitability represents a form of communication in the nervous system whereby one substance can alter the activity of a wide variety of target neurons. Teleologically, the nervous system may have elaborated such a mechanism, because one species of molecule can effectively and rapidly command and organize the long-lasting activity of a set of neurons whose concerted output would lead to an autonomic, endocrine, and/or motor behavior of survival value. Several examples of neurohormonal communication may have already been observed. For example, minute amounts of angiotensin injected into discrete areas of the CNS rapidly lead to an elevation of blood pressure, release of vasopressin, causing water retention, and drinking behavior (for recent articles, see Buckley, 1977). These events provide a concerted defense against circulatory volume deficits and are of survival value. Because a renin-angiotensin system has recently been found in the CNS (Ganten et al., 1976), we know that angiotensin derived from neuronal tissue may also operate as a neurohormone to regulate the required autonomic, endocrine, and motor activities. However, such neurohormonal regulation appears to operate *only* under conditions of exaggerated circulatory stress, e.g., hypovolemia and salt-and-water imbalance, since specific blockers of angiotensin receptors in the CNS are normally without effect and only disturb the response to the stress. Thus, angiotensin, acting as a neurohormone, may not be involved in the normal, daily maintenance of circulatory volume; only when severe deficit ensues is it released in the CNS to act neurohormonally.

Another example of neurohormonal communication may involve a species of peptide with analgesic activity. These peptides, when injected intracerebrally, can cause profound analgesia (Pert, Pert, Chang, and Fong, 1976), which is specifically reversed by coincident application of naloxone. The latter is an alkaloid with well-established properties as a specific antagonist to the variety of pharmacological effects of morphine. Naloxone does not alter pain perception in healthy humans (El-Sobky, Dostrovsky, and Wall, 1976), suggesting that these peptides with analgesic activity may not be released unless the pain is so severe as to be potentially incapacitating. An injury of such pain as to paralyze the organism would hardly be of survival value in a fight-or-flight situation. Thus, "opiate-like" peptides may be released primarily under pathological conditions where "physiological" analgesia is required, in order that the organism survive by making the appropriate motor response. Anecdotal evidence in support of this notion is based on the numerous observations of severely wounded animals or soldiers continuing to flee or fight.

Another example of neurohormonal communication may be reflected in the catatonia-like state produced by a peptide species whose structure overlaps that of the analgesic opiate-like peptide (Bloom, Segal, Ling, and Guillemin, 1976; Jacquet and Marks, 1976). Injection of this peptide into the periaqueductal gray region of the CNS produces long-lasting attenuation of motor activity without paralysis, per se, because the animal can be startled by auditory stimuli. Such a neurohormone might be operative especially in those species that do not use fight or flight as primary means of survival, but rather make themselves motionless either to avoid predators or to prey. Interestingly, the catatonia-producing peptide (β-endorphin) and a peptide hormone involved in the regulation of color (β-melanocyte-stimulating hormone) are both present in the sequence of a larger peptide hormone synthesized in the intermediate lobe of the pituitary (β-lipotropin). The latter thus appears to contain messages of survival value for both short-term motor, and long-term endocrine responses relating to camouflage. The brain is capable of synthesizing the endorphin sequences independent of the pituitary (Cheung and Goldstein, 1976). Presumably brain-derived endorphin mediates rapid attenuation of motor activity through central actions. Peripheral functions of intermediate-lobe endorphin have yet to be formulated.

Research on the physiological roles of peptides in neuronal function is just beginning. From the evidence obtained it appears that some peptides may belong to a neurohormonal class of chemically mediated communication in the nervous system that is operationally distinct from neurotransmitters and synaptic transmission. The potential importance of neurohormonal communication seems clear. It allows one substance to regulate the activity of functionally distinct neuronal elements, with complementary autonomic, endocrine, and motor outputs, in a manner analogous to peripheral hormonal regulation of distant and diverse non-neuronal target tissues. Presumably, neurohormones have been selected for and preserved by evolution because they constitute a relatively simple method of rapidly organizing the activity of a complex response of established physiological value. In this regard, neurohormones may be involved in the expression of basic drives and instincts (drinking, eating, mating, grooming, sleeping, aggression, nesting, hibernation, camouflage, imprinting, territoriality, societal instincts, and forms of communications, etc.). These speculative possibilities remain to be examined.

REFERENCES

Arch, S. (1976). Neuroendocrine regulation of egg laying in *Aplysia californica*, *Am. Zool.* **16**:167–175.

Barker, J. L. (1975). CNS depressants: effects on postsynaptic pharmacology, *Brain Res.* **92**:35–55.

Barker, J. L. (1976). Peptides: roles in neuronal excitability, *Physiol. Rev.* **56**:435–452.

Barker, J. L. (1977*a*). Physiological roles of peptides in the nervous system, pp. 295–343 in *Peptides in Neurobiology*, Gainer, H., ed. Plenum Press, New York.

Barker, J. L. (1977*b*). Peptide regulation of neuronal excitability: evidence for a neurohormonal role, in *Central Actions of Angiotensin*, Buckley, J. P. and C. Ferrario, eds. Pergamon Press, New York, in press.

Barker, J. L. and H. Gainer (1974). Peptide regulation of bursting pacemaker activity in a molluscan neurosecretory cell, *Science* **184**:1371–1373.

Barker, J. L. and H. Gainer (1975*a*). Studies on bursting pacemaker potential activity in molluscan neurons. I. Membrane properties and ionic contributions, *Brain Res.* **84**:461–477.

Barker, J. L. and H. Gainer (1975*b*). Studies on bursting pacemaker potential activity in molluscan neurons. II. Regulation by divalent cations, *Brain Res.* **84**:479–500.

Barker, J. L., M. Ifshin, and H. Gainer (1975). Studies on bursting pacemaker potential activity in molluscan neurons. III. Effects of hormones, *Brain Res.* **84**:501–513.

Barker, J. L. and T. G. Smith (1976). Peptide regulation of neuronal membrane properties, *Brain Res.* **103**:167–170.

Bennett, M. V. L. (1966). Physiology of electrotonic junctions, *Ann. N. Y. Acad. Sci.* **188**:242–269.

Bloom, F. E., D. Segal, N. Ling, and R. Guillemin (1976). Endorphins: profound behavioral effects suggest new etiological factors in mental illness, *Science* **194**:630–632.

Brown, B. E. (1976). Proctolin: a peptide transmitter candidate in insects, *Life Sci.* **17**:1241–1252.

Brownstein, M., M. Palkovits, J. M. Saavedra, R. M. Bassiri, and R. D. Utiger (1974). Thyrotropin releasing hormone in specific nuclei of the brain, *Science* **185**:267–269.

Buckley, J. P., and C. Ferrario, eds. (1977). *Central Actions of Angiotensin.* Pergamon Press, New York, in press.

Carpenter, D. O. (1973). Ionic mechanisms and models of endogenous discharge of *Aplysia* neurons, pp. 35–58 in *Neurobiology of Invertebrates, Mechanisms of Rhythm Regulation*, Salanki, J., ed. Akademiai Kiado, Budapest.

Carpenter, D. O. and R. Gunn (1970). The dependence of pacemaker discharge of *Aplysia* neurons upon Na$^+$ and Ca^{++}, *J. Cell. Physiol.* **75**:121–128.

Cheung, A. and A. Goldstein (1976). Failure of hypophysectomy to alter brain content of opioid peptides (endorphins), *Life Sci.* **19**:1005–1008.

Connor, J. A. and C. F. Stevens (1971*a*). Voltage clamp studies of a transient outward membrane current in gastropod neural somata, *J. Physiol. (London)* **213**:21–30.

Connor, J. A. and C. F. Stevens (1971*b*). Prediction of repetitive firing behavior from voltage clamp data on an isolated neurone soma, *J. Physiol. (London)* **213**:31–53.

Dyer, R. G. and R. E. J. Dyball (1974). Evidence for a direct effect of LRF and TRF on single unit activity in the rostral hypothalamus, *Nature (London)* **252**:486–488.

Eckert, R. and H. D. Lux (1976). A voltage-sensitive persistent calcium conductance in neuronal somata of *Helix, J. Physiol. (London)* **254**:129–151.

El-Sobky, A., J. O. Dostrovsky, and P. D. Wall (1976). Lack of effect of naloxone on pain perception in humans, *Nature (London)* **263**:783.

Frazier, W. T., E. R. Kandel, I. Kupfermann, R. Waziri, and R. E. Coggeshall (1967). Morphological and functional properties of identified neurons in the abdominal ganglion of *Aplysia californica, J. Neurophysiol.* **30**:1288–1351.

Frederickson, R. C. A. and F. H. Norris (1976). Enkephalin-induced depression of single neurons in brain areas with opiate receptors—antagonism by naloxone, *Science* **194**:440–442.

Gainer, H. (1972*a*). Effects of experimentally induced diapause on the electrophysiology and protein synthesis of identified molluscan neurons, *Brain Res.* **39**:387–402.

Gainer, H. (1972b). Electrophysiological behavior of an endogenously active neurosecretory cell, *Brain Res.* **39**:403–418.

Gainer, H. and J. L. Barker (1974). Synaptic regulation of specific protein synthesis in an identified neuron, *Brain Res.* **78**:314–319.

Ganten, D., J. S. Hutchinson, J. P. Schelling, U. Ganten, and H. Fischer (1976). The iso-renin angiotensin systems in extra-renal tissue, *Clin. Exp. Pharmacol. Physiol.* **2**:103–126.

Ganten, D., J. Minnich, P. Granger, K. Hayduk, H. M. Brecht, A. Barbeau, R. Boucher, and J. Genest (1971). Angiotensin-forming enzyme in brain tissue, *Science* **173**:64–65.

Giles, W. and S. J. Noble (1976). Changes in membrane currents in bullfrog atrium produced by acetylcholine, *J. Physiol. (London)* **261**:103–123.

Gola, M. (1974). Neurones à ondes-salves des molluscks, *Pflugers Arch. Eur. J. Physiol.* **352**:17–36.

Henry, J. L., K. Krnjević. and M. Morris (1975). Substance P and spinal neurons, *Can. J. Physiol. Pharmacol.* **53**:423–432.

Hökfelt, T., J. O. Kellerth, G. Nilsson, and B. Pernow (1975). Experimental immunohistochemical studies on the localization and distribution of substance P in cat primary sensory neurons, *Brain Res.* **100**:235–252.

Hughes, J., T. Smith, H. Kosterlitz, L. Fothergill, B. Morgan, and H. Morris (1975). Identification of two related pentapeptides from the brain with potent opiate agonist activity, *Nature (London)* **258**:577–579.

Ifshin, M., H. Gainer, and J. L. Barker (1975). Peptide factor extracted from molluscan ganglia that modulates bursting pacemaker activity, *Nature (London)* **254**:72–74.

Jacquet, Y. F. and N. Marks (1976). The C-fragment of β-lipotropin: an endogenous neuroleptic or antipsychotogen? *Science* **194**:632–635.

Junge, D. and C. L. Stephens (1973). Cyclic variation of potassium conductance in a burst generating neurone in Aplysia, *J. Physiol. (London)* **235**:155–173.

Kandel, E. R. (1976). *Cellular Basis of Behavior*. Freeman, San Francisco.

Katz, B. (1966). *Nerve, Muscle and Synapse*. McGraw-Hill, New York.

Konishi, S. and M. Otsuka (1974). The effects of substance P and other peptides on spinal neurons of the frog, *Brain Res.* **65**:397–410.

Kuffler, S. W. and D. Yoshikami (1975). The number of transmitter molecules in a quantum: an estimate from iontophoretic application of acetylcholine at the neuromuscular synapse, *J. Physiol. (London)* **251**:465–482.

La Motte, C., C. B. Pert, and S. H. Snyder (1976). Opiate receptor binding in primate spinal cord: distribution and changes after dorsal root section, *Brain Res.* **112**:407–412.

Loh, Y. P., J. L. Barker, and H. Gainer (1976). Neurosecretory cell protein metabolism correlated with diapause in the land snail, *Otala lactea, J. Neurochem.* **26**:25–30.

Mayeri, E. and S. Simon (1975). Modulation of synaptic transmission and burster neuron activity after release of a neurohormone in Aplysia, *Abstr. Annu. Meet. Soc. Neurosci.*, 5th, New York, p. 584.

Neher, E. (1971). Two fast transient current components during voltage clamp on snail neurons, *J. Gen. Physiol.* **58**:36–53.

Nicoll, R. A. and J. L. Barker (1971a). The pharmacology of recurrent inhibition in the supraoptic neurosecretory system, *Brain Res.* **35**:501–511.

Nicoll, R. A. and J. L. Barker (1971b). Excitation of supraoptic neurosecretory cells by angiotensin II, *Nature (London) New Biol.* **233**:172–174.

Pert, C. B., A. Pert, J. K. Chang, and B. T. W. Fong (1976). [D-Ala^2]-Met-enkephalinamide: a potent, long-lasting synthetic penta-peptide analgesic, *Science* **194**:330–332.

Phillis, J. W. and J. J. Limacher (1974). Excitation of cerebral cortical neurons by various polypeptides, *Exp. Neurol.* **53**:414–423.

Renaud, L. P., J. B. Martin, and P. Brazeau (1975). Depressant action of TRH, LHRH and somatostatin on activity of central neurons, *Nature (London)* **255**:233–235.

Saito, K., S. Konishi, and M. Otsuka (1975). Antagonism between Lioresal and substance P in rat spinal cord, *Brain Res.* **97**:177–180.

Smith, T. G., J. L. Barker, and H. Gainer (1975). Requirements for bursting pacemaker potential activity in molluscan neurons, *Nature (London)* **253**:450–452.

Stevens, C. F. (1969). Voltage clamp analysis of a repetitively firing neuron, pp. 76–84 in *Basic Mechanisms of the Epilepsies*. Jasper, H. H., A. A. Ward, and A. Pope, eds. Little, Brown and Co., Boston.

Stinnakre, J. and L. Tauc (1973). Calcium influx in active *Aplysia* neurons detected by injected aequorin, *Nature (London)* **242**:113–115.

Strumwasser, F. (1973). Neural and humoral factors in the temporal organization of behavior, *Physiologist* **16**:9–42.

Strumwasser, F. and D. L. Wilson (1976). Patterns of proteins synthesized in the R1S neuron of *Aplysia*, *J. Gen. Physiol.* **67**:691–702.

Tsien, R. W. (1974). Effects of epinephrine on the potassium pacemaker current of caridac Purkinje fibers, *J. Gen. Physiol.* **64**:293–305.

Wachtel, H. and E. R. Kandel (1971). Conversion of synaptic excitation to inhibition at a dual chemical synapse, *J. Neurophysiol.* **34**:56–68.

Werman, R. (1966). Criteria for identification of a central nervous system transmitter, *Comp. Biochem. Physiol.* **18**:745–766.

Wilson, W. A. and H. Wachtel (1974). Negative resistance characteristic essential for maintenance of slow oscillations in bursting neurons, *Science* **186**:932–934.

BIOCHEMICAL SEQUELAE OF SYNAPTIC ACTION

Chairman's Introduction

Floyd E. Bloom

The Salk Institute, La Jolla, California

Conventionally, neuronal activity is monitored by the detection of electrophysiological events or through estimates of neurotransmitter metabolism. In general, such appraisals require the assumption that the fundamental units of neuronal activity are the individual action potentials of single nerve cells, and that the "nth" observed action potential is physiologically and biochemically equivalent to any other.

This symposium dealt with experiments indicating that synaptic activity can, in fact, trigger multiple biochemical events whose duration clearly outlives individual action potentials. Some of these biochemical events, such as the synthesis of cyclic AMP or cyclic GMP and the activation of enzymes dependent on these cyclic nucleotides (see Kanof et al.), appear to mediate the effects of certain neurotransmitters. Other activity-related biochemical events are not yet attributable to a specific chemical intermediate. Events in this latter category have now been found to be capable of modulating the amount of transmitter released per impulse (and thus dependent on the interval between impulses; see Barondes et al.), and the extent to which the postsynaptic cell responds to a fixed amount of the released transmitter (thus, also interval dependent; see Kebabian et al.).

Taken together, these studies begin to sketch in the outlines of a dynamic continuum in which the transmitting and responding elements of a synaptic junction continually modify each other to achieve some sort of stabilized homeostasis. Clearly, the resolution of the processes responsible for this dynamic functional equilibrium will require the concerted efforts of many future symposiasts.

Modulation of Receptor Sensitivity in the Pineal: The Roles of Cyclic Nucleotides

John W. Kebabian, Martin Zatz, and Robert F. O'Dea

National Institute of Neurological and Communicative Disorders and Stroke, Bethesda, Maryland

INTRODUCTION

The pineal is a non-neural structure that is innervated by the postganglionic neurons of the sympathetic nervous system. The physical associations between the terminals of the postganglionic neurons and the parenchyma of the pineal do not demonstrate the specialized ultrastructural features that characterize the bona fide synapses between neurons in the central and the peripheral nervous systems (Wurtman, Axelrod, and Kelley, 1968; Bloom, Iversen, and Schmidt, 1970). Furthermore, the cells of the pineal are not electrically excitable and do not demonstrate the regenerative, self-propagating electrical phenomena that characterize neurons (Sakai and Marks, 1972). Thus, the pineal may appear to be an inappropriate object to discuss before the Society for Neuroscience in a symposium concerned with synaptic transmission. However, neurobiologists have repeatedly studied the pineal despite the fact that it is not a neural tissue. This historical fact does not justify the inclusion of the pineal in today's symposium.

The pineal can be easily studied because of its simple structure and function. This apparent simplicity of the pineal permits neurobiologists to use the gland as a model system in which it is possible to clarify a mechanism that may be related to the functioning of the brain. Subsequently, when the mechanism is well understood in this simple peripheral system, it is possible to attempt to demonstrate the same event in the brain. Thus, from the point of view of the present symposium, the pineal is presented as a model system in which it is possible to characterize events with a greater precision than is possible in the brain. Ultimately, it will be necessary to determine if similar mechanisms exist in the brain. Only such success will justify the study of the pineal, which is of minimal interest in its own right. A brief summary of the anatomy, biochemistry, and physiology of the pineal is presented to introduce this system.

Anatomy of the Pineal

The anatomy and biochemistry of the neurons innervating the pineal are well characterized. The pineal is innervated by the terminal arborization of the postganglionic sympathetic neurons. The somata of these neurons lie in the superior cervical ganglion and project to the pineal via the nervus cornarius. This anatomical organization permits the denervation of the pineal by bilateral superior cervical ganglionectomy. Similarly, it is possible to isolate the pineal and the postganglionic neurons from the rest of the nervous system with bilateral transection of the preganglionic axons in the cervical sympathetic chain. The neurotransmitter utilized by the postganglionic neurons is known to be norepinephrine. Thus, in studying the pineal, the extensive armamentarium of drugs known to influence the metabolism of catecholamines can be rationally utilized. Finally, because the pineal is outside the blood-brain barrier, drugs that are administered systemically will reach the pineal. The same is true of all target organs of the superior cervical ganglion.

Biosynthesis of Melatonin, the Pineal Hormone

Melatonin, 5 methoxy-N-acetyltryptamine, is a hormone synthesized in the pineal gland. In the past 18 years, since the discovery of this compound (Lerner, Case, Takahaski, Lee, and Mori, 1958), the enzymes responsible for the conversion of tryptophan to melatonin have been identified and characterized. Tryptophan is converted to 5 hydroxytryptophan by tryptophan hydroxylase (Lovenberg, Jequier, and Sjoderdsma, 1967); subsequently, this latter compound is converted to serotonin, 5 hydroxytryptamine, by L-aromatic amino acid decarboxylase (Snyder and Axelrod, 1964). Melatonin is formed from serotonin by successive N-acetylation and O-methylation by the enzymes serotonin N-acetyltransferase (Weissbach, Redfield, and Axelrod, 1960) and hydroxyindole-O-methyltransferase (Axelrod and

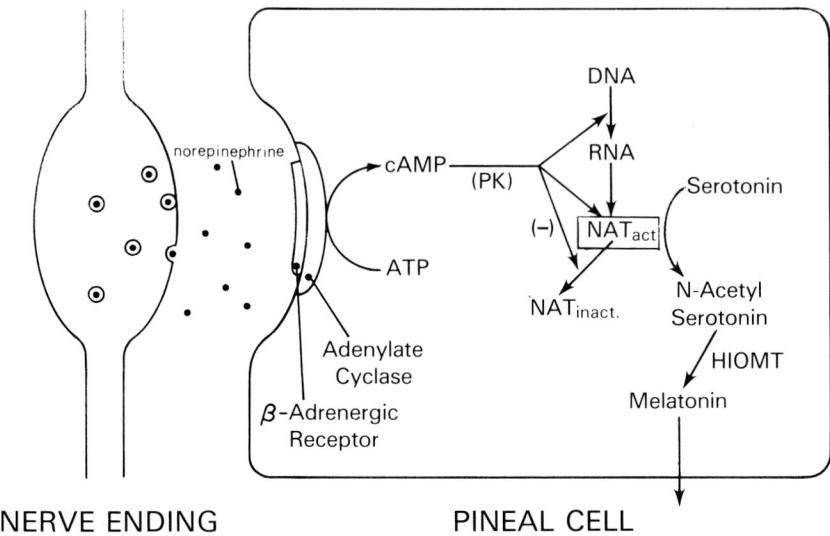

FIGURE 1. A simplified schematic diagram of the biochemical mechanisms regulating the synthesis of melatonin. Abbreviations: PK, cyclic AMP-dependent protein kinase; NAT_{act}, active serotonin N-acetyltransferase; NAT_{inact}, inactive serotonin N-acetyltransferase; HIOMT, hydroxyindole-O-methyltransferase.

Weissbach, 1961), respectively. The relatively simple, yet well-characterized, synthetic process for melatonin provides a unique experimental system in which the individual steps leading to the final physiological response of the gland can be monitored.

Mechanism of Action of Beta-Adrenergic Agonists in the Pineal

The intermediate steps between the stimulation of the beta-adrenergic receptor and the synthesis and release of melatonin have been identified (Figure 1). Beta-adrenergic stimulation causes a transient accumulation of cyclic AMP in the pineal (Deguchi and Axelrod, 1973). This is due to the stimulation of the beta-adrenergic receptor regulating adenylyl cyclase activity (Weiss and Costa, 1968a). Several hours after this rise in cyclic AMP, there is a gradual increase in the amount of N-acetyltransferase activity (Klein, Berg, and Weller, 1970; for a review, see Axelrod, 1974). This neurotransmitter-induced increase in N-acetyltransferase activity is blocked by beta-adrenergic antagonists. Several lines of evidence implicate cyclic AMP in the induction and maintenance of N-acetyltransferase activity. Thus, dibutyryl cyclic

AMP (but not cyclic AMP itself) causes a substantial increase in N-acetyltransferase activity (Klein and Weller, 1973). This effect of dibutyryl cyclic AMP bypasses the beta-adrenergic receptor and therefore is not affected by beta-adrenergic antagonists. Cholera toxin will also stimulate adenylyl cyclase activity by a mechanism independ-

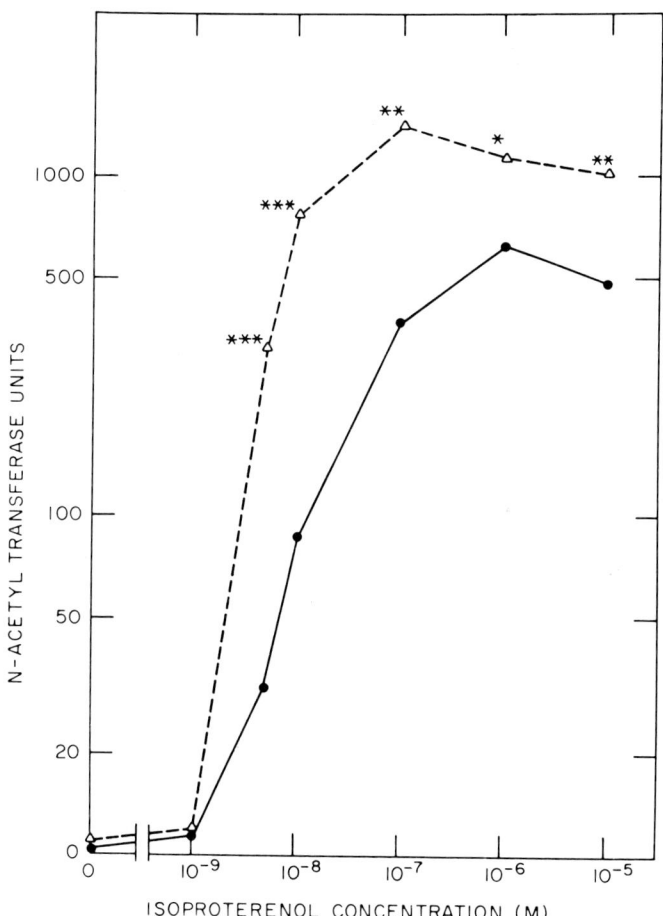

FIGURE 2. Diurnal change in sensitivity of rat pineal N-acetyltransferase to induction by L-isoproterenol in organ culture. Pineals obtained from animals killed at the end of the light period (△) or at the end of the dark period (●) were incubated in the presence of various concentrations of L-isoproterenol for 10 h. Glands were homogenized and assayed for N-acetyltransferase; units are pmol/gland per 10 min. Adapted from Romero and Axelrod (1974).

ent of the beta receptor. Such treatment will also induce
N-acetyltransferase activity (Minneman and Iversen, 1976a). Thus, the
cyclic AMP accumulation that occurs as a consequence of beta-
adrenergic stimulation, rather than occupancy of the beta-receptor per
se, induces the N-acetyltransferase activity.

Cyclic nucleotide-dependent protein kinase may be the intermediate
between the initial rise in cyclic AMP and the subsequent synthesis of
N-acetyltransferase (Figure 2). Cyclic nucleotide-dependent protein
kinase has been postulated to serve as the common mediator of the
diverse, tissue-specific effects of cyclic AMP. The specificity of the
response of a given tissue to cyclic AMP is envisioned to reside in the
ability of the enzyme to phosphorylate selected proteins within a given
tissue (Kuo and Greengard, 1969). The pineal is a rich source of the
cyclic AMP-dependent protein kinase; the enzyme from the bovine
pineal can phosphorylate nuclear proteins (Fontana and Lovenberg,
1971, 1973). Furthermore, isoproterenol stimulates the incorporation of
phosphate into a unique, nonhistone nuclear protein in the pineal
(Morrissey and Lovenberg, unpublished data). Because the increase in
N-acetyltransferase activity is sensitive to actinomycin D or cycloheximide, the synthesis of both RNA and protein can be invoked in
the induction and maintenance of this enzyme activity (Klein and Berg,
1970; Romero, Zatz, and Axelrod, 1975a). These observations suggest
that cyclic AMP-dependent protein phosphorylation may be the initial
step in the protein synthesis that causes the induction and maintenance
of N-acetyltransferase activity.

Continuous stimulation of the beta-adrenergic receptor is obligatory
to maintain the elevated N-acetyltransferase activity. During the night,
when the level of N-acetyltransferase activity is relatively high,
exposure of the rat to light causes a precipitous fall ($t_{1/2} < 5$ min) in the
enzyme activity (Deguchi and Axelrod, 1972). This loss of enzyme
activity results from the cessation of the sympathetic stimulation of the
pineal when the animal is exposed to light (see below). Pretreatment of
animals with the beta-adrenergic agonist L-isoproterenol prevents the
light-induced decrease in enzyme activity. Furthermore, the beta-
adrenergic antagonist propranolol mimics this effect of light. These
results demonstrate that continuous beta-adrenergic stimulation of the
pineal is required to maintain the elevated level of N-acetyltransferase
activity.

The beta-adrenergic receptor in the pineal is intimately involved in
regulating the rate of melatonin synthesis. Thus, N-acetyltransferase,

the neurotransmitter-induced enzyme, appears to be the pivotal synthetic enzyme in the metabolic pathway from serotonin to melatonin. When the enzyme activity increases, the content of pineal serotonin is diminished (Brownstein, Holz, and Axelrod, 1973a). At the same time, the content and the rate of synthesis of N-acetylserotonin and melatonin increase (Brownstein, Saavedra, and Axelrod, 1973b; Klein and Weller, 1973). These observations suggest that the beta-adrenergic receptor regulates cyclic AMP formation, which in turn induces the synthesis and maintenance of N-acetyltransferase activity, which ultimately regulates the rate of synthesis of melatonin.

Environmental Lighting and Physiological Activity in the Pineal

Environmental lighting can regulate the electrical activity in the postganglionic neurons innervating the pineal. Although in lower vertebrates, the parenchyma of the pineal possess photoreceptors, such structures are absent in mammalian pineals (Wurtman et al., 1968). However, the postganglionic sympathetic neurons are the final common pathway in a complex neuronal circuit by which environmental lighting can influence biochemical activity in the pineal. In view of the ability of exogenous norepinephrine to increase N-acetyltransferase activity in the pineal, it is not surprising that the endogenous norepinephrine within the sympathetic neurons can also induce enzyme activity. Thus, electrical stimulation of the preganglionic sympathetic fibers to the superior cervical ganglion will increase N-acetyltransferase activity (Volkman and Heller, 1971). During the night, when animals are in darkness, pineal N-acetyltransferase activity increases approximately 30-fold (Klein, Weller, and Moore, 1971). This increase in enzyme activity correlates with an enhanced electrical activity in the sympathetic neurons innervating the pineal of animals kept in the dark (Taylor and Wilson, 1970). Acute exposure of animals to light blocks this enhanced electrical activity and prevents the rise in N-acetyltransferase activity. Thus, the nocturnal rise in N-acetyltransferase activity can be attributed to the prolonged tonic stimulation of the gland by the norepinephrine released from the terminals of the sympathetic neurons innervating the pineal.

Sensitivity of the Pineal

The results of several studies indicate that the ability of the pineal to respond to beta-adrenergic stimulation is not a fixed, invariant parameter. Rather, the extent and the duration of the previous exposure of the pineal to agonists will influence the response of the pineal at a given moment. Prior stimulation will cause a subsequent diminution of the response, i.e., a state of relative "subsensitivity." The absence of stimulation produces a relatively enhanced response, i.e., a state of relative "supersensitivity." Such an alteration in the capacity of a tissue to respond to physiological stimulation is not unique to the pineal; indeed, such alterations are widespread and occur in a variety of tissues, including the mammalian brain. However, the clarity and precision that characterize our knowledge of the pineal gland are lacking from these other tissues, where the ultimate physiological response to physiological stimulation is either poorly defined or unknown.

The physiological stimulation of the pineal that accompanies the diurnal light-dark cycle can alter the sensitivity of the response of the pineal. Thus, the prolonged tonic sympathetic stimulation of the pineal gland that occurs during the night will decrease the capacity of the pineal to respond to beta-adrenergic stimulation. The biochemical basis for the physiological response of the pineal to sympathetic stimulation is well understood. Therefore, in examining the response of the pineal, more than the input and the final output of the gland can be measured. Many of the intermediate steps that participate in generating the final output of the tissue can be examined. One indicator of this change in the responsiveness of the pineal is the alteration in the induction of N-acetyltransferase activity (Romero and Axelrod, 1974). The decreased responsiveness is reflected as a diminution in the maximal response of the gland. In addition, the dose-response relationship between the concentration of agonist and the response is shifted to the right so that higher concentrations of drug are required to produce the measured response (Figure 2).

Cyclic AMP

Some of the mechanisms that regulate the response of the pineal to beta-adrenergic stimulation may involve the formation of cyclic AMP. Thus, the magnitude of the acute increase in cyclic AMP levels after beta-adrenergic stimulation varies during the light-dark cycle (Romero, Zatz, Kebabian, and Axelrod, 1975*b*). Injection of isoproterenol into animals after 12 h of exposure to darkness increases cyclic AMP levels in the pineal no more than twofold (Figure 3). Upon exposure to light and the cessation of the sympathetic stimulation of the pineal, the response to beta-adrenergic stimulation gradually increases. After 12 h of light, injection of isoproterenol increases cyclic AMP levels more than sixfold. When the animal is placed in darkness, the response to exogenous agonist is gradually decreased. This decrease in the capacity to accumulate cyclic AMP in response to beta-adrenergic stimulation parallels the loss of sensitivity that is reflected in the induction of N-acetyltransferase activity (see above). Thus, concomitant with the enhanced sympathetic stimulation that occurs at night, there is a reduction in the magnitude of the response to subsequent stimulation. In the absence of sympathetic stimulation (during exposure to light) there is a gradual recovery of sensitivity to beta-adrenergic stimulation.

Experimental procedures that diminish or enhance sympathetic stimulation of the pineal also alter the acute responses of cyclic AMP to

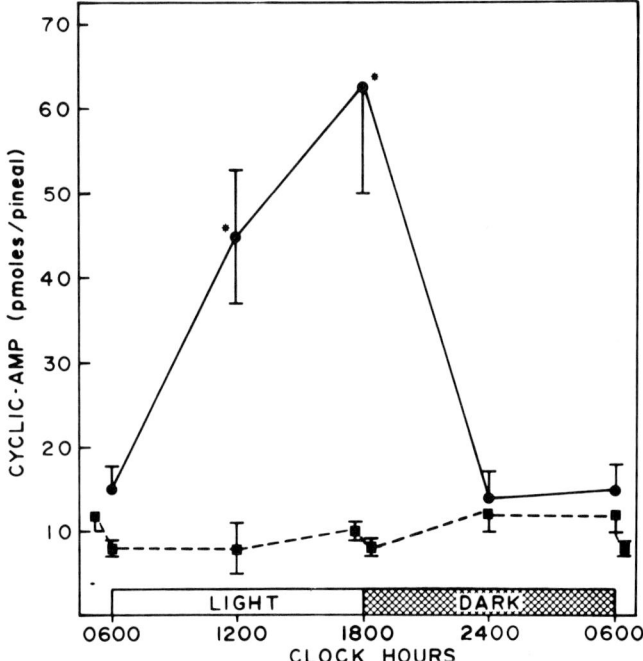

FIGURE 3. Diurnal variation in the accumulation of cyclic AMP after isoproterenol administration in the rat pineal gland. At the various times indicated, rats were injected with saline (■) or L-isoproterenol-bitartrate (●) (5 mg/kg) and pineal cyclic AMP levels were measured 10 min later. Results are means ± SEM. *$P < 0.05$ was compared with controls by Student's t test. Adapted from Romero et al. (1975b).

subsequent beta-adrenergic stimulation. Two hours after an injection of isoproterenol, the increase in cyclic AMP levels caused by a second identical dose of drug is reduced 85% in comparison with the response in untreated animals (Oleshansky and Neff, 1975a). Thus, a subsensitive response in terms of cyclic AMP accumulation can occur within several hours. Conversely, the response of cyclic AMP is enhanced after a period of diminished beta-adrenergic stimulation. After treatment with reserpine, which depletes the nerve terminals of norepinephrine, the response of cyclic AMP to acute stimulation is twice the control response (Deguchi and Axelrod, 1973). Similarly, denervation of the pineal causes a two- to fourfold increase in the response of the pineal (Strada and Weiss, 1974). A variation in the capacity of the pineal to accumulate cyclic AMP could reflect changes in its capacity either to synthesize or to degrade this cyclic nucleotide. Although changes in both adenylate cyclase and phosphodiesterase activities have been demonstrated, no single alteration in either of these enzyme activities can account for all of the variations in the capacity of the pineal to accumulate cyclic AMP or to regulate the activity of N-acetyl-transferase.

Adenylyl Cyclase

The adenylyl cyclase activity in homogenates of pineal gland is stimulated by catecholamines. A beta-adrenergic receptor is coupled to the enzyme and regulates its activity (Weiss and Costa, 1968a). Other hormones and putative neurotransmitters do not affect the enzyme activity. Thus, the hormone-sensitive adenylyl cylcase provides a marker for the beta-adrenergic receptor in the pineal. The recent development of high-affinity beta-adrenergic antagonists, which are radiolabeled to high specific activity, has permitted a direct investigation of the properties of the beta-adrenergic receptor (for a review, see Haber and Wrenn, 1976). We have used one such ligand, [^{3}H]dihydroalprenolol (Lefkowitz, Mukherjee, Coverstone, and Caron, 1974), to define binding sites in the pineal with properties similar to the beta-adrenergic receptor regulating adenylyl cyclase activity (Zatz, Kebabian, Romero, Lefkowitz, and Axelrod, 1976). The binding sites demonstrate high-affinity, stereospecific binding of a variety of compounds that parallels the biological potency of these compounds as agonists or antagonists of the beta-adrenergic receptor (Figure 4). The ability of several beta-adrenergic agonists to stimulate adenylyl cyclase activity in homogenates of pineal was measured (Table 1). The synthetic

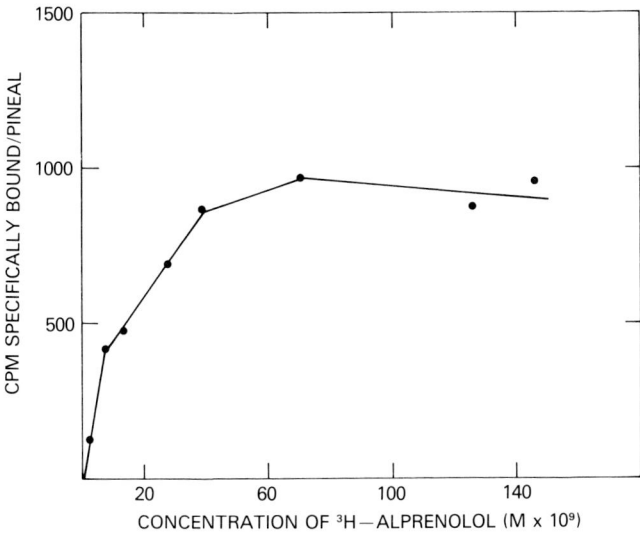

FIGURE 4. Effect of varying concentrations of L-[³H]alprenolol on the extent of L-[³H]alprenolol binding. Pineal homogenates were incubated with the indicated concentrations of L-[³H]alprenolol and were assayed for specifically bound radioactivity, the difference between total radioactivity bound and binding in the presence of 50×10^{-6} M D, L-propranolol. Adapted from Zatz et al. (1976).

TABLE 1. *Apparent affinity constants for beta-adrenergic agonists and antagonists*[a]

Compound	Affinity from binding assay (μM)	Affinity from adenylyl cyclase assay (μM)
Antagonists		
L-Alprenolol	0.022	0.017
D-Alprenolol	0.73	1.2
L-Propranolol	0.012	0.010
D-Propranolol	1.3	3.5
Agonists		
L-Isoproterenol	0.39	0.40
D-Isoproterenol	120.0	
L-Norepinephrine	5.3	3.0
D-Norepinephrine	1,200.0	
L-Epinephrine	9.3	8.0

[a] The effect of various concentrations of each compound on specific binding of L-[³H]dihydroalprenolol was determined. The concentration that inhibited specific binding by 50% was used to calculate the affinity of the specific binding site for the compound. The concentration of beta-adrenergic agonist that produced 50% of the maximal increase in adenylyl cyclase activity is listed. The affinity of the beta-adrenergic receptor regulating adenylyl cyclase for antagonists was calculated from the inhibition by various concentrations of drug of the stimulation of adenylyl cyclase activity by L-isoproterenol. Adapted from Zatz et al. (1976).

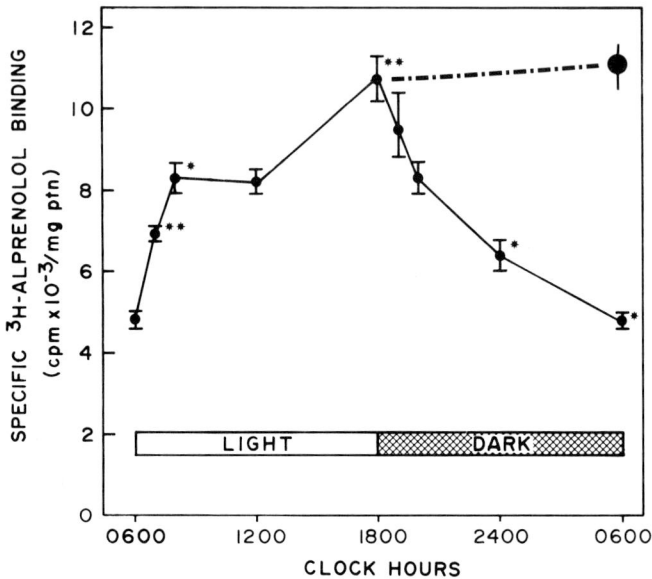

FIGURE 5. Diurnal variation in the number of specific beta-adrenergic binding sites in rat pineal gland. Each point is the average of multiple determinations made with each of two or three homogenates containing 7 to 10 pooled pineals. *$P < 0.05$; **$P < 0.01$ compared with immediately preceding time point. The broken line indicates the effect of exposure to an additional 12 h of light. Adapted from Romero et al. (1975b).

catecholamine L-isoproterenol is about 10-fold as potent an agonist as is the endogenous sympathetic neurotransmitter L-norepinephrine, which in turn is about twice as potent as L-epinephrine. Each catecholamine has the same intrinsic activity and causes the same maximal response of the enzyme. The D stereoisomers of these compounds are ineffective in stimulating adenylyl cyclase activity. Similarly, the compounds display the same relative affinity for the specific dihydroalprenolol binding sites (Table 1). Thus, L-isoproterenol is about 10-fold as potent as L-norepinephrine, which in turn is about twice as potent as epinephrine in competition with [^{3}H]dihydroalprenolol for the specific binding sites. Again, the D stereoisomers of these compounds have less affinity for these binding sites. The apparent affinities of the various beta-adrenergic agonists or antagonists were similar if determined by competition for specific binding sites or by stimulation of adenylyl cyclase activity. The properties of the specific binding sites and the beta-adrenergic receptor regulating adenylyl cyclase do not distinguish between these two entities.

Change in the properties of beta-adrenergic receptors may contribute to the changes in the sensitivity of the pineal. As was previously noted, the effectiveness of L-isoproterenol in stimulating the accumulation of cyclic AMP in the pineal increases during the day and decreases during the night. Similarly, the number of specific [^{3}H]dihydroalprenolol binding sites also exhibit a diurnal cycle that parallels the changes in the accumulation of cyclic AMP (Figure 5). Thus, the number of receptor sites increases almost twofold as the rat is exposed to light, reaching a maximal value at the end of the light period (Romero et al., 1975b). The number of specific binding sites then falls during the dark period, when sympathetic stimulation of the gland is enhanced. Exposure to light for an additional 12 h, replacing the dark period, is not accompanied by a further increase in the number of binding sites. In addition, such a treatment prevents the nocturnal fall in the number of specific binding sites.

Adenylyl cyclase activity in the pineal gland exhibits a small diurnal variation (Weiss, 1971). The effect of environmental lighting on adenylyl cyclase is seen clearly when pineals from animals kept in light overnight are compared with glands from animals exposed to the normal 12-h

TABLE 2. *Effect of environmental lighting and beta-adrenergic stimulation on adenylyl cyclase activity and specific binding of L-[^{3}H]dihydroalprenolol[a]*

Condition	Adenylate cyclase activity (pmol/mg protein per min)		K_a of L-Isoproterenol (μM)	Specific binding of L-[^{3}H]dihydroalprenolol (cpm/mg protein)	K_i of L-Isoproterenol (μM)
	No addition	L-Isoproterenol (100 μM)			
12 h in dark	23 ± 3	102 ± 2	0.2	6,500 ± 600	0.4
24 h in light	87 ± 10	225 ± 14	0.2	10,500 ± 600	0.6
24 h in light plus isoproterenol pretreatment	23 ± 1	52 ± 3	0.4	6,151 ± 500	0.7

[a] Aspects of the beta-adrenergic receptor-adenylyl cyclase complex are compared in pineals from animals exposed to darkness for 12 h, light for 24 h, or L-isoproterenol after exposure to continuous light for 24 h. Basal and maximally stimulated adenylyl cyclase activity, and the apparent affinity of the beta-adrenergic receptor regulating adenylyl cyclase for L-isoproterenol are presented, as are the number of specific L-[^{3}H]dihydroalprenolol binding sites and the calculated affinity of these binding sites for L-isoproterenol. Data from Kebabian et al. (1975).

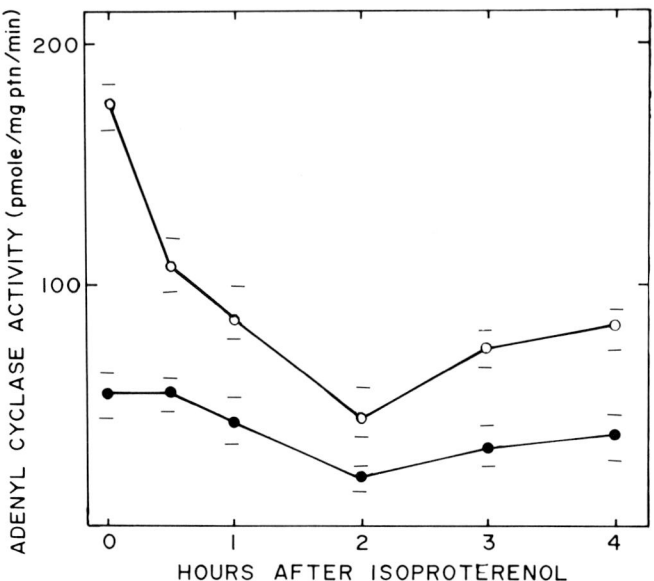

FIGURE 6. Time course of the L-isoproterenol-induced decrease in adenylyl cyclase activity in the rat pineal. Rats were kept in constant light for 27 h before injection of L-isoproterenol (5 mg/kg, subcutaneous) at 0 h. At the indicated times, groups of three rats were killed and the adenylyl cyclase activity was determined either in the absence (●) or in the presence (○) of 10 μM L-isoproterenol. The data represent the mean and range of three replicate samples, each assayed in duplicate. Adapted from Kebabian et al. (1975).

period of darkness when sympathetic stimulation of the gland is enhanced (Table 2). There is almost twice as much catecholamine-sensitive adenylyl cyclase activity in the homogenates of pineals from light-exposed animals. To test the hypothesis that the effect of darkness was related to the increase in beta-adrenergic stimulation during the night, we injected L-isoproterenol into light-exposed animals and subsequently measured specific binding sites and adenylyl cyclase activity in pineal homogenates (Figures 6 and 7) (Kebabian, Zatz, Romero, and Axelrod, 1975). Treatment with L-isoproterenol caused a fall in both the number of specific binding sites and in the amount of adenylyl cyclase activity. After 2 h of pharmacological beta-adrenergic stimulation, the number of specific binding sites and the amount of catecholamine-sensitive adenylyl cyclase were comparable to the values observed after 12 h of darkness. The changes in the number of available receptors and the amount of adenylyl cyclase may contribute to the changes in the maximal response of the pineal to beta-adrenergic stimulation. There is also, however, an apparent change in the potency of L-isoproterenol to induce N-acetyltransferase activity. We found no evidence for a consistent shift in the affinity of L-isoproterenol for the beta-adrenergic receptor that was studied either by [^{3}H]dihydroalprenolol binding or the catecholamine-sensitive adenylyl cyclase (Table 2).

Changes in potency of agonist are characteristic of denervation supersensitivity. Denervated glands have more adenylyl cyclase than pineals from sham-operated controls. However, we have been unable to demonstrate an increase in the number of [^{3}H]dihydroalprenolol binding sites in denervated glands. Thus, the mechanisms that effect a denervation supersensitivity, particularly the increased potency of L-isoproterenol, may affect intracellular sites rather than the beta-adrenergic receptor per se.

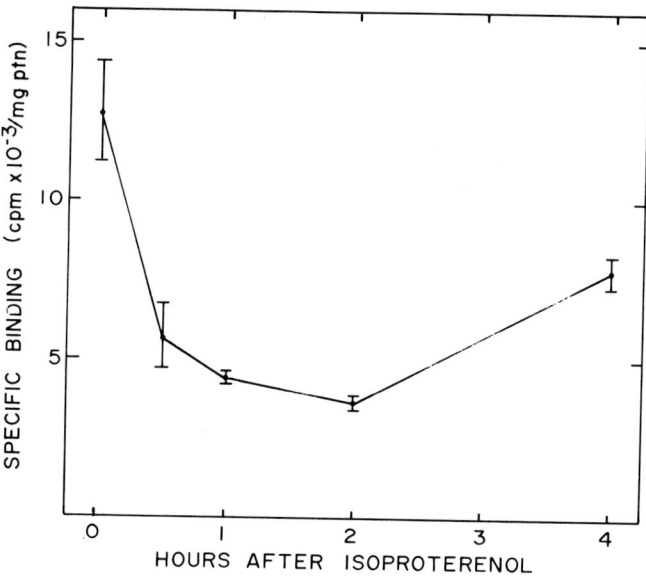

FIGURE 7. Time course of the L-isoproterenol-induced decrease in specific binding sites for L-[^{3}H]dihydroalprenolol. Rats were kept in constant light for 26 h before injection of L-isoproterenol (5 mg/kg) at 0 h. At the indicated times, groups of seven rats were killed and the specific binding of L-[^{3}H]alprenolol in the pineal homogenate was determined. The data represent the mean ± SEM of five replicate samples, each assayed in duplicate. Adapted from Kebabian et al. (1975).

Phosphodiesterase

The pineal gland contains substantial quantities of phosphodiesterase activity (Weiss and Costa, 1968b). Both the high K_m and the low K_m forms of the enzyme activity are present in this tissue (Oleshansky and Neff, 1975b). Phosphodiesterase activity may participate in the regulation of the level of cyclic AMP in the pineal gland. A trivial demonstration of this is the enhanced accumulation of cyclic AMP after beta-adrenergic stimulation in the presence of a phosphodiesterase inhibitor (Strada and Weiss, 1974). Similarly, alterations in the amount of endogenous phosphodiesterase activity may contribute to the development of supersensitive and subsensitive states in the pineal.

Stimulation of the beta-adrenergic receptor in the pineal gland can promote changes in phosphodiesterase activity. In vivo treatment with L-isoproterenol causes a transient 40 to 60% increase in phosphodiesterase, which is blocked by administration of L-propranolol or the protein synthesis inhibitor cycloheximide (Oleshansky and Neff, 1975b). The peak activity of this enzyme occurs at a time when a second injection of beta-adrenergic agonist produces a diminished response in pineal cyclic AMP (Oleshansky and Neff, 1975a). At the same time, adenylyl cyclase activity (measured under conditions that inhibit phosphodiesterase activity) is also diminished. A similar transient increase in phosphodiesterase activity has been shown to accompany a decline in cyclic AMP levels after irreversible activation of pineal adenylyl cyclase by cholera enterotoxin (Minneman and Iversen, 1976a).

The physiological regulation of phosphodiesterase has been studied in a diurnal lighting situation (Minneman and Iversen, 1976b). Phosphodiesterase activity in the rat pineal gland exhibits a diurnal rhythm for the hydrolysis of both cyclic AMP and cyclic GMP. Within 2 to 3 h after the onset of darkness, the enzyme activity reaches a maximal level 60 to 80% greater than that measured immediately before exposure to darkness. Throughout the remainder of the dark period, enzyme activity declines so that at the end of the night the level of enzyme activity is identical to that observed at the onset of darkness. This nocturnal rise in phosphodiesterase activity is prevented by prior treatment of the animals with L-propranolol or cycloheximide and is abolished by superior cervical ganglionectomy. These observations suggest that the transient increase in phosphodiesterase activity is caused by enhanced sympathetic stimulation. However, this transient alteration in phosphodiesterase activity cannot be invoked to explain the subsensitive state that has developed at the end of the period of dark exposure.

The rapid development of subsensitive responses in the pineal after beta-adrenergic stimulation probably is derived, in part, from the transient increase in cyclic nucleotide phosphodiesterase activity. The experiments discussed above clearly demonstrate a short-term enhancement of phosphodiesterase activity after acute beta-adrenergic stimulation. The existence of this phenomenon, however, does not exclude other factors as participants in the development of subsensitivity, nor does it adequately explain long-term changes in sensitivity observed either in the presence or in the absence of beta-adrenergic stimulation. As noted above, diurnal changes in the activity of phosphodiesterase cannot account for the diminished sensitivity at the end of the dark period because phosphodiesterase activity is the same at the beginning and the end of the night (Minneman and Iversen, 1976b). Furthermore, the development of supersensitivity in the pineal after denervation is not accompanied by any alteration in phosphodiesterase activity (Minneman and Iversen, 1976b). It is apparent, therefore, that changes in the activity of this enzyme contribute to the mechanism of rapid desensitization. However, the contribution of phosphodiesterase to long-term changes in sensitivity remains unclear.

Cyclic AMP-Dependent Protein Kinase

Cyclic nucleotide-dependent protein kinase has been proposed as a universal mechanism for the translation of changes in the intracellular concentrations of cyclic AMP into biochemical events (Kuo and Greengard, 1969). Because cyclic AMP has been implicated in the induction of N-acetyltransferase activity, the observation that the pineal gland is a rich source of cyclic AMP-dependent protein kinase activity would suggest that protein kinase may have a role in the induction and maintenance of N-acetyltransferase activity (Fontana and Lovenberg, 1971, 1973). The recent observation that dibutyryl cyclic AMP, which bypasses the receptor-adenylate cyclase complex, is more effective in inducing N-acetyltransferase activity in supersensitive glands than in subsensitive glands (Romero and Axelrod, 1975) prompted a search for the role of cyclic AMP-dependent protein kinase in the regulation of the sensitivity of the pineal gland to beta-adrenergic stimulation.

The activity of the cyclic AMP-dependent protein kinase varies under conditions that change the sensitivity of the response of the pineal to

TABLE 3. *Effect of L-isoproterenol and dibutyryl cyclic AMP in organ culture on protein kinase activity*[a]

Group[b]	Protein kinase activity (nmol of ^{32}P incorporated/ mg protein/10 min)			
	−cAMP		+cAMP	
	12 h dark	24 h light	12 h dark	24 h light
Control	2.1 ± 0.14 (7)	3.4 ± 0.10 (7)	6.4 ± 0.40 (7)	10.9 ± 0.67 (7)
Isoproterenol	2.6 ± 0.25 (7)	4.3 ± 0.33 (7)	5.7 ± 0.31 (7)	9.4 ± 0.67 (7)
Dibutyryl cAMP	6.9 ± 0.53 (6)	9.8 ± 0.55 (6)	7.8 ± 0.47 (6)	10.0 ± 0.62 (6)

[a] Pineal glands from rats exposed to 24 h of light or 12 h of darkness were placed in organ culture containing 10^{-7} M L-isoproterenol, 10^{-3} M dibutyryl cyclic AMP, or in control medium. After 20 min of incubation (L-isoproterenol) or 30 min of incubation (dibutyryl cyclic AMP), glands were homogenized in medium containing 500 mM NaCl and kinase activity was assayed in the presence and absence of 10^{-6} M cyclic AMP. Control glands did not differ between 20 and 30 min of incubation. Adapted from Zatz and O'Dea (1976).

[b] Statistical significance was as follows. (i) Control versus isoproterenol: light, −cAMP, $P < 0.05$, +cAMP, N.S.; dark, −cAMP, +cAMP, N.S. (ii) Dark versus light: −cAMP, $P < 0.001$, +cAMP, $P < 0.001$; after isoproterenol, −cAMP, $P < 0.01$, +cAMP, $P < 0.001$; after dbcAMP, −cAMP, $P < 0.01$, +cAMP, $P < 0.05$.

beta-adrenergic stimulation (Zatz and O'Dea, 1976). Supersensitive pineals have at least 60% more protein kinase activity, in both the presence and the absence of exogenous cyclic AMP, than do the subsensitive glands taken from rats at the end of the normal 12-h period in darkness (Table 3). Various compounds that promote the induction and maintenance of *N*-acetyltransferase activity were examined to determine their effect upon protein kinase activity in subsensitive and supersensitive pineals (Table 3). The effect of such treatments upon protein kinase activity in the absence of added cyclic nucleotide provides another indication of the relative sensitivity of the pineal, since cyclic AMP promotes the activation of this enzyme. Both isoproterenol and dibutyryl cyclic AMP increase the endogenous protein kinase activity in the absence of added cyclic AMP; a larger increase in enzyme activity occurs in the supersensitive glands than in the subsensitive glands. Furthermore, surgical or pharmacological treatments that, like light, reduce the sympathetic stimulation of the gland, also increase the cyclic AMP-dependent protein kinase activity (Table 4). Thus, either denervation or reserpine treatment markedly increases enzyme activity.

The mechanism responsible for the increase in protein kinase activity in supersensitive rat pineals is presently undefined. Kinetic analysis of the initial velocities of protein kinase activity as a function of varying concentrations of cyclic AMP, ATP, and histone (Zatz and O'Dea, 1976) have shown that the V_{max} in supersensitive preparations is consistently greater for each substrate examined, whereas no significant changes in the K_m for any substrate were noted when activities in light- and dark-exposed glands were compared. A greater concentration of the heat-stable kinase modulator (Appleman, Birnbaumer, and Torres, 1966; Walsh, Ashby, Gonzalez, Calkins, Fisher, and Krebs, 1971) in the subsensitive glands could produce differences in apparent V_{max}. However, additional experiments with heated and mixed preparations did not support this explanation. Furthermore, prior administration of cycloheximide did not block the increase in kinase observed in vivo after several hours of exposure to light, suggesting that this increase may not depend on new protein synthesis. More protein kinase activity appears to be present in the supernatant fraction of supersensitive glands, and the responsiveness of this enzyme to L-isoproterenol stimulation is enhanced under these conditions. These results suggest that protein phosphorylation may represent another physiological relevant control mechanism in the pineal. It is conceivable that the phosphorylation of one or more proteins may initiate the synthesis or maintain the N-acetyltransferase activity. Alterations in the capacity of the pineal to phosphorylate this hypothesized substrate protein could participate in the regulation of the physiological response to beta-adrenergic stimulation. It still remains to identify and to characterize the

TABLE 4. *Effects of denervation or reserpine on pineal protein kinase activity*[a]

Group	Protein kinase activity (nmol of ^{32}P incorporated/mg protein/10 min)	
	−cAMP	+cAMP
Sham operated	2.5 ± 0.1 (9)	7.3 ± 0.4 (9)
Denervated	4.2 ± 0.3 (9)[b]	13.9 ± 1.9 (9)[c]
Control	2.6 ± 0.2 (3)	9.0 ± 0.6 (3)
6 days reserpine	3.8 ± 0.2 (3)[d]	15.2 ± 0.7 (3)[c]
24 h reserpine	2.9 ± 0.2 (3)	12.7 ± 1.0 (3)[d]

[a] Rat pineals were denervated by bilateral superior cervical ganglionectomy 1 month before assay. Other rats were injected with reserpine (2.5 mg/kg, i.p.) once daily for 5 days or once (5 mg/kg, i.p.) 24 h before assay. All animals were killed at 0900 h after exposure to 12 h of darkness. Values shown are means ± SEM of determinations in three or nine separate experiments. Adapted from Zatz and O'Dea (1976).
[b] Significantly greater than control (or sham operated) with $P < 0.001$.
[c] Significantly greater than control (or sham operated) with $P < 0.01$.
[d] Significantly greater than control with $P < 0.05$, by Student's t test.

endogenous substrate protein (proteins?) for the cyclic AMP-dependent protein kinase in the pineal.

Cyclic GMP

This review has described a sequential series of regulatory components whose end point, the induction of N-acetyltransferase and the regulation of melatonin synthesis, can be related to the metabolism of cyclic AMP. The existence of bidirectional regulators in this system (e.g., inhibitors) has not been demonstrated. Recently, cyclic GMP and cyclic AMP were reported to have antagonistic regulatory influences in several biological systems, and it was proposed that cyclic GMP may function as an intracellular mediator whose effects oppose those mediated by cyclic AMP (Goldberg, Haddox, Nicol, Glass, Sanford, Kuehl, and Estensen, 1975). In an initial series of experiments, the addition of $10^{-3}M$ dibutyryl cyclic GMP had no effect on N-acetyltransferase induction in vitro under several assay conditions. In view of the recent reports that norepinephrine elevates cyclic GMP in vas deferens (Schultz, Hardman, Schultz, Baird, and Sutherland, 1973) and cerebellar tissue (Ferrendelli, Kinscherf, and Chang, 1975), the effect of adrenergic stimulation on pineal cyclic GMP was examined (O'Dea and Zatz, 1976) (Table 5). The neurotransmitter L-norepinephrine elevates pineal cyclic GMP five- to sevenfold. This response is dependent upon extracellular calcium and consists of two components: one that is stereospecific and inhibited by alpha-adrenergic antagonists, and another that is non-stereospecific and not blocked by

TABLE 5. Effects of agonists and antagonists on pineal cyclic GMP[a]

Agonist	Antagonist	cGMP (fmol/pineal)
None	None	139 ± 14 (23)
L-Isoproterenol (10^{-7})	None	440 ± 24 (23)
D-Isoproterenol (10^{-7})	None	452 ± 74 (6)
L-Isoproterenol (10^{-7})	L-Propranolol (10^{-7})	400 ± 18 (12)
D-Norepinephrine (10^{-5})	None	378 ± 38 (6)
L-Norepinephrine (10^{-5})	None	733 ± 61 (44)
L-Norepinephrine (10^{-5})	Phentolamine (2×10^{-5})	397 ± 70 (6)
L-Norepinephrine (10^{-5})	L-Propranolol (10^{-7})	869 ± 162 (12)

[a] Pineal glands were homogenized and cyclic GMP was assayed after 60 min of exposure to the various agents listed above. Antagonists were present in the culture medium, at the indicated molar concentrations, during a 15-min preincubation period before the addition of agonist, at the indicated molar concentrations, for the 60 min of incubation. Values are mean ± SEM for triplicate determinations in the indicated number of experiments.

alpha- or beta-adrenergic antagonists. This response of pineal cyclic GMP to catecholamines, unlike cyclic AMP, was not altered by prior exposure of rats to 24 h of light or 12 h of darkness. These data suggest that cyclic GMP is neither directly nor indirectly involved in the regulation of the metabolic events that follow stimulation of the postsynaptic beta-adrenergic receptor.

It appears likely that the mechanisms regulating the generation and actions of cyclic GMP in the pineal are distinct from those operative for cyclic AMP. Recently, we have shown that superior cervical ganglionectomy abolishes the stereospecific increase in cyclic GMP observed after L-norepinephrine, an effect quite different from that seen with regard to cyclic AMP. The presence of intact nerve terminals appears to be a prerequisite for the stereospecific generation of cyclic GMP. This last finding is especially interesting in that it is possible that the regulation of pineal cyclic GMP is intimately associated with the presynaptic process that modulates neurotransmitter uptake and release.

CONCLUSION

The relative anatomical and physiological simplicity of the pineal permits the detailed investigation of the biochemical mechanisms that participate in the modulation of the physiological response of this tissue. The stimulation of the gland, in addition to generating the overt response of the tissue, also reduces the capacity of the gland to respond to subsequent stimuli. Conversely, after the absence of stimulation, the maximal response of the tissue is expressed. No single biochemical alteration can account for the entire spectrum of phenomena that produce the states of relative supersensitivity and subsensitivity. Indeed, all the enzymatic mechanisms related to cyclic nucleotide metabolism (i.e., the specific binding sites, the adenylyl cyclase, phosphodiesterase, and cyclic AMP-dependent protein kinase) change so as to produce either a diminished or an augmented response. Although apparently similar phenomena occur in the CNS, the anatomical complexity of the brain does not permit as detailed an investigation as is possible in experiments using the pineal. Thus, the pineal gland serves as a useful model in which to investigate phenomena relevant to the brain. The extension of the results from the pineal to the brain will require substantially more work than has occurred to date. However, the pineal has helped to identify biological mechanisms that pertain to the brain.

REFERENCES

Appleman, M. M., L. Birnbaumer, and H. N. Torres (1966). Factors affecting the activity of muscle glycogen synthetase, *Arch. Biochem. Biophys.* **116:**39–43.

Axelrod, J. (1974). The pineal gland: a neurochemical transducer, *Science* **184:**1341–1348.

Axelrod, J. and H. Weissbach (1961). Purification and properties of hydroxyindole 0-methyltransferase, *J. Biol. Chem.* **236:**211–213.

Bloom, F. E., L. L. Iversen, and F. O. Schmidt (1970). Macromolecules in synaptic function, *Neurosci. Res. Program Bull.* **8:**313–439.

Brownstein, M., R. Holz, and J. Axelrod (1973a). The regulation of pineal serotonin by a *beta* adrenergic receptor, *J. Pharmacol. Exp. Ther.* **186:**109–113.

Brownstein, M., J. M. Saavedra, and J. Axelrod (1973b). Control of pineal N-acetylserotonin by a *beta* adrenergic receptor, *Mol. Pharmacol.* **9:**605–611.

Deguchi, T. and J. Axelrod (1972). Control of circadian change of serotonin N-acetyltransferase activity in the pineal organ by the β-adrenergic receptor, *Proc. Natl. Acad. Sci. U.S.A.* **69:**2547–2550.

Deguchi, T. and J. Axelrod (1973). Supersensitivity and subsensitivity of the β-adrenergic receptor in pineal gland regulated by catecholamine transmitter, *Proc. Natl. Acad. Sci. U.S.A.* **70:**2411–2414.

Ferrendelli, J. A., D. A. Kinscherf, and M. M. Chang (1975). Comparison of the effects of biogenic amines on cyclic GMP and cyclic AMP levels in mouse cerebellum, in vitro, *Brain Res.* **84:**63–73.

Fontana, J. A. and W. Lovenberg (1971). A cyclic AMP-dependent protein kinase of the bovine pineal gland, *Proc. Natl. Acad. Sci. U.S.A.* **68:**2787–2790.

Fontana, J. A. and W. Lovenberg (1973). Pineal protein kinase: effect of enzymatic phosphorylation on actinomycin D binding by, and template activity of, chromatin, *Proc. Natl. Acad. Sci. U.S.A.* **70:**755–758.

Goldberg, N. D., M. K. Haddox, S. E. Nicol, D. B. Glass, C. H. Sanford, F. A. Kuehl, and R. Estensen (1975). Biologic regulation through opposing influences of cyclic GMP and cyclic AMP: the ying yang hypothesis, pp. 307–330 in *Advances in Cyclic Nucleotide Research*, Vol. 5, Drummond, G. I., P. Greengard, and G. A. Robison, eds. Raven Press, New York.

Haber, E. and S. Wrenn (1976). Problems in identification of the beta-adrenergic receptor, *Physiol. Rev.* **56:**317–338.

Kebabian, J. W., M. Zatz, J. A. Romero, and J. Axelrod (1975). Rapid changes in rat pineal *beta*-adrenergic receptor: alterations in ^{3}H-(1)-alprenolol binding and adenylate cyclase, *Proc. Natl. Acad. Sci. U.S.A.* **72:**3735–3739.

Klein, D. C. and G. R. Berg (1970). Pineal gland: stimulation of melatonin production by norepinephrine involves cyclic AMP-mediated stimulation of N-acetyltransferase, pp. 241–263 in *Advances in Biochemical Psychopharmacology*, Vol. 3, Greengard, P. and E. Costa, eds. Raven Press, New York.

Klein, D. C., G. R. Berg, and J. Weller (1970). Melatonin synthesis: adenosine 3′,5′-monophosphate and norepinephrine stimulate N-acetyltransferase, *Science* **168:**979–980.

Klein, D. C. and J. L. Weller (1973). Adrenergic-adenosine 3',5'-monophosphate regulation of serotonin N-acetyltransferase activity and the temporal relationship of serotonin N-acetyltransferase activity to synthesis of ^{3}H-N-acetylserotonin and ^{3}H-melatonin in cultured rat pineal gland, *J. Pharmacol. Exp. Ther.* **186**:516–527.

Klein, D. C., J. L. Weller, and R. Y. Moore (1971). Melatonin metabolism: neural regulation of pineal serotonin N-acetyltransferase activity, *Proc. Natl. Acad. Sci. U.S.A.* **68**:3107–3110.

Kuo, J. F. and P. Greengard (1969). Cyclic nucleotide-dependent protein kinase. IV. Widespread occurrence of adenosine 3',5'-monophosphate-dependent protein kinase in various tissues and phyla of the animal kingdom, *Proc. Natl. Acad. Sci. U.S.A.* **64**:1349–1355.

Lefkowitz, R. J., C. Mukherjee, M. Coverstone, and M. G. Caron (1974). Stereospecific (^{3}H) (−)-alprenolol binding sites, β-adrenergic receptors and adenylate cyclase, *Biochem. Biophys. Res. Commun.* **60**:703–709.

Lerner, A. B., J. D. Case, Y. Takahaski, T. H. Lee, and W. Mori (1958). Isolation of melatonin, the pineal gland factor that lightens melanocytes, *J. Am. Chem. Soc.* **80**:2587.

Lovenberg, F. W., E. Jequier, and A. Sjoderdsma (1967). Tryptophan hydroxylation: measurement in pineal gland, brainstem, and carcinoid tumor, *Science* **155**:217–219.

Minneman, K. P. and L. L. Iversen (1976a). Cholera toxin induces pineal enzymes in culture, *Science* **192**:803–805.

Minneman, K. P. and L. L. Iversen (1976b). Diurnal rhythm in rat pineal cyclic nucleotide phosphodiesterase activity, *Nature (London)* **260**:59–61.

O'Dea, R. F. and M. Zatz (1976). Catecholamine-stimulated cyclic GMP accumulation in the rat pineal: apparent presynaptic site of action, *Proc. Natl. Acad. Sci. U.S.A.* **73**:3398–3402.

Oleshansky, M. A. and N. H. Neff (1975a). On the mechanism of tolerance to isoproterenol-induced accumulation of cyclic AMP in rat pineal in vivo, *Life Sci.* **17**:1429–1432.

Oleshansky, M. A. and N. H. Neff (1975b). Rat pineal adenosine cyclic 3',5'-monophosphate phosphodiesterase activity: modulation *in vivo* by a beta adrenergic receptor, *Mol. Pharmacol.* **11**:552–557.

Romero, J. A. and J. Axelrod (1974). Pineal β-adrenergic receptor: diurnal variation in sensitivity, *Science* **184**:1091–1092.

Romero, J. A. and J. Axelrod (1975). Regulation of sensitivity to *beta*-adrenergic stimulation in induction of pineal N-acetyltransferase, *Proc. Natl. Acad. Sci. U.S.A.* **72**:1661–1665.

Romero, J. A., M. Zatz, and J. Axelrod (1975a). *Beta*-adrenergic stimulation of pineal N-acetyltransferase: adenosine 3':5'-cyclic monophosphate stimulates both RNA and protein synthesis, *Proc. Natl. Acad. Sci. U.S.A.* **72**:2107–2111.

Romero, J. A., M. Zatz, J. W. Kebabian, and J. Axelrod (1975b). Circadian cycles in binding of ^{3}H-alprenolol to β-adrenergic receptor sites in rat pineal, *Nature (London)* **258**:435–436.

Sakai, K. K. and B. H. Marks (1972). Adrenergic effects on pineal cell membrane potential, *Life Sci.* **11**:285–291.

Schultz, G., J. G. Hardman, K., Schultz, C. E. Baird, and E. W. Sutherland

(1973). The importance of calcium ions for the regulation of guanosine 3':5'-cyclic monophosphate levels, *Proc. Natl. Acad. Sci. U.S.A.* **70**:3889–3893.

Snyder, S. H. and J. Axelrod (1964). A sensitive assay for 5-hydroxytryptophan decarboxylase, *Biochem. Pharmacol.* **13**:805–806.

Strada, S. J. and B. Weiss (1974). Increased response to catecholamines of the cyclic AMP system of rat pineal gland induced by decreased sympathetic activity, *Arch. Biochem. Biophys.* **160**:197–204.

Taylor, A. N. and R. W. Wilson (1970). Electrophysiological evidence for the action of light on the pineal gland in the rat, *Experientia* **26**:267–269.

Volkman, P. H. and A. Heller (1971). Pineal N-acetyltransferase activity: effect of sympathetic stimulation, *Science* **173**:839–840.

Walsh, D. A., C. D. Ashby, C. Gonzalez, D. Calkins, E. H. Fisher, and E. G. Krebs (1971). Purification and characterization of a protein inhibitor of adenosine 3',5'-monophosphate-dependent protein kinases, *J. Biol. Chem.* **246**:1977–1985.

Weiss, B. (1971). On the regulation of adenyl cyclase activity in rat pineal gland, *Ann. N.Y. Acad. Sci.* **185**:507–519.

Weiss, B. and E. Costa (1968*a*). Selective stimulation of adenyl cyclase of rat pineal gland by pharmacologically active catecholamines, *J. Pharmacol. Exp. Ther.* **161**:310–319.

Weiss, B. and E. Costa (1968*b*). Regional and subcellular distribution of adenyl cyclase and 3',5'-cyclic nucleotide phosphodiesterase in brain and pineal gland, *Biochem. Pharmacol.* **17**:2107–2116.

Weissbach, H., B. G. Redfield, and J. Axelrod (1960). Biosynthesis of melatonin: enzymatic conversion of serotonin to N-acetylserotonin, *Biochim. Biophys. Acta* **43**:352–353.

Wurtman, R. J., J. Axelrod, and D. Kelly (1968). *The Pineal*. Academic Press, New York.

Zatz, M., J. W. Kebabian, J. A. Romero, R. J. Lefkowitz, and J. Axelrod (1976). Pineal *beta* adrenergic receptor: correlation of binding of ^{3}H-L-alprenolol with stimulation of adenylate cyclase, *J. Pharmacol. Exp. Ther.* **196**:714–722.

Zatz, M. and R. F. O'Dea (1976). Regulation of protein kinase in rat pineal: increased V_{max} in supersensitive glands, *J. Cyclic Nucleotide Res.* **2**:427–439.

Cyclic Nucleotides and Phosphorylated Proteins in Neuronal Function

Philip Kanof, Tetsufumi Ueda, Isao Uno, and Paul Greengard

Yale University School of Medicine, New Haven, Connecticut

Neurotransmitter molecules, when released from the terminals of a presynaptic neuron, induce a change in the electrical properties of the membrane of the postsynaptic neuron by interacting with specific receptors located on the cell surface. The molecular nature of the events by which the binding of the neurotransmitter to its receptor is coupled with the alteration in the ionic properties of the nerve cell membrane remains poorly understood. However, there appear to be two general classes of mechanism by which this process can occur (Figure 1).

In one class (Figure 1A), the neurotransmitter receptor is thought to be coupled directly to an ionophore in such a manner that binding of the neurotransmitter to the receptor induces a conformational change in the ionophore, leading to a change in the permeability of the membrane to specific ions. One receptor that has been intensively studied by Changeux, Heilbronn, Karlin, Raftery, Reich, and their colleagues, and which appears to work in this manner, is the nicotinic cholinergic receptor.

A second general class of mechanisms (Figure 1B) by which a neurotransmitter could affect the electrical properties of postsynaptic neurons is through a process in which the binding of the neurotransmitter to its receptor on the outside of the cell membrane leads to the production of another molecule, a second messenger, on the inside of the cell. This second messenger could then initiate a sequence of biochemical reactions that would ultimately result in a change in the electrophysiological properties of the neuronal membrane. Such

A. "Receptor-Ionophore" Model

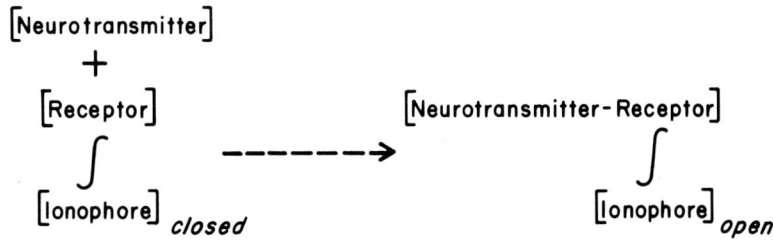

B. "Receptor – Second Messenger" Model

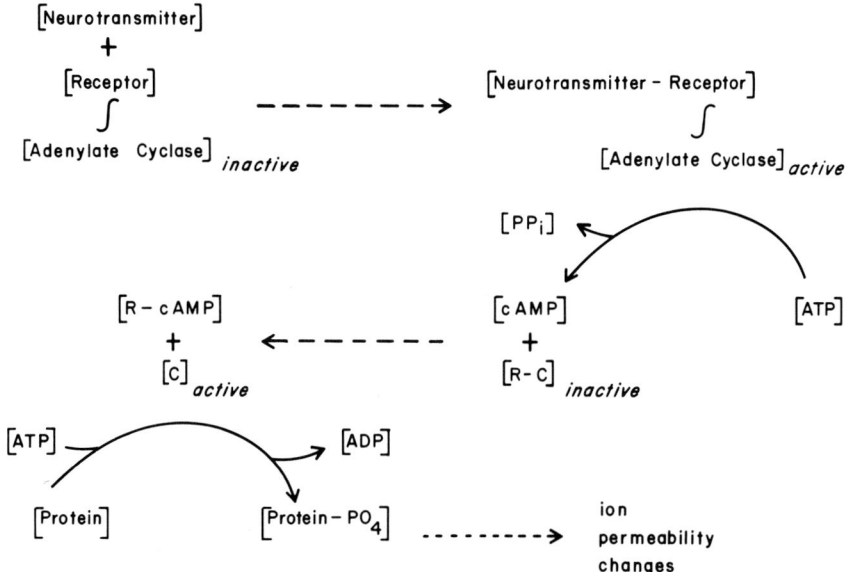

electrophysiological changes might be caused by a biochemical modification of a membrane protein involved in regulating the permeability of the membrane to specific ions.

Since the pioneering work of Earl Sutherland and his colleagues, great attention has been focused on possible roles for cyclic AMP as the intracellular second messenger for the action of many hormones on non-neuronal tissues (Robison, Butcher, and Sutherland, 1971). More recently, this interest in cyclic AMP has been extended to include its role as an intracellular mediator for the actions of certain neurotransmitters (Rall and Gilman, 1970; Drummond and Ma, 1973; Perkins, 1973; Von Hungen and Roberts, 1974; Bloom, 1975; Daly, 1975; Greengard, 1976; Nathanson, 1977). There is now considerable evidence that, at certain synapses, the effects on postsynaptic neurons of many putative neurotransmitters, including norepinephrine, dopamine, octopamine, serotonin, and histamine, are mediated by cyclic AMP. There is additional evidence that some of the effects of certain other

---

FIGURE 1. Schematic diagram illustrating two general classes of mechanisms by which binding of a neurotransmitter to its receptor can alter membrane permeability. Broken arrows denote non-enzymatic processes, i.e., processes that do not involve changes in the covalent structures of the reactants. Solid arrows denote enzymatic processes, i.e., processes that do involve changes in the covalent structures of the reactants. (1A) "Receptor-ionophore" model. The binding of the neurotransmitter to its receptor results in a conformational change in the receptor-ionophore complex, converting the ion channel from a closed to an open state. (1B) "Receptor-second messenger" model. The binding of the neurotransmitter to its receptor results in a conformational change in the receptor-adenylate cyclase complex, converting the catalytic component of adenylate cyclase from an inactive to an active state. The active adenylate cyclase catalyzes the conversion of ATP to cyclic AMP. Cyclic AMP then binds to an inactive protein kinase (RC), dissociating the holoenzyme into a free regulatory subunit-cyclic AMP complex (R-cAMP) and an active catalytic subunit (C). This active catalytic subunit catalyzes the protein kinase reaction, transferring a phosphate group from ATP to a protein acceptor. The phosphorylation of this protein results in the changes in ion permeability; the detailed molecular mechanism of this latter process is not yet understood. The receptor-second messenger model has, for illustrative purposes, been drawn for a receptor whose associated second messenger is cyclic AMP. However, in the most general case, the physiological effects subsequent to the binding of the neurotransmitter to its receptor may be mediated through other second messenger systems. Any such alternate second messenger system would have to include a generator of the second messenger (analogous to adenylate cyclase), the second messenger itself (analogous to cyclic AMP), an intracellular receptor for the second messenger (analogous to the regulatory subunit of the protein kinase), and a biochemical reaction catalyzed by the second messenger receptor (analogous to the protein kinase reaction).

TABLE 1. *Some criteria for the mediation by cyclic nucleotides of the postsynaptic effects of a neurotransmitter in the nervous system*[a]

A. Effect of stimulation of presynaptic neuronal pathways on cyclic nucleotide levels in intact tissue

1. Electrical stimulation of the neuronal pathway should increase tissue levels of the cyclic nucleotide in those regions of the nervous system innervated by that neuronal pathway.
2. This increase in cyclic nucleotide levels should be blocked by those agents that antagonize the postsynaptic physiological effects of electrical stimulation of the neuronal pathway.
3. This increase in cyclic nucleotide levels should be potentiated by phosphodiesterase inhibitors.
4. Cytochemical techniques should demonstrate that these various effects on cyclic nucleotide levels occur specifically in those postsynaptic cells which receive innervation from that neuronal pathway.

B. Effect of neurotransmitters on cyclic nucleotide levels in intact tissue

1. Exposure to the neurotransmitter should increase tissue levels of the cyclic nucleotide in those regions of the nervous system innervated by neurons containing that neurotransmitter.
2. This increase in cyclic nucleotide levels should be blocked by those agents that antagonize the postsynaptic physiological effects of the neurotransmitter.
3. This increase in cyclic nucleotide levels should be potentiated by phosphodiesterase inhibitors.
4. Cytochemical techniques should demonstrate that these various effects on cyclic nucleotide levels occur specifically in those postsynaptic cells that receive innervation from neurons containing the neurotransmitter.

C. Neurotransmitter-sensitive adenylate (or guanylate) cyclase

1. A neurotransmitter-sensitive adenylate (or guanylate) cyclase should be demonstrable in broken cell preparations from those regions of the nervous system innervated by neurons containing that neurotransmitter.
2. Activation by the neurotransmitter of this adenylate (or guanylate) cyclase should be blocked by pharmacological antagonists of the neurotransmitter receptor.
3. This neurotransmitter-sensitive adenylate (or guanylate) cyclase should have a subcellular distribution which parallels that of synaptic membranes.

D. Application of cyclic nucleotides

1. The cyclic nucleotide and its derivatives should mimic the electrophysiological effects (e.g., alteration of firing rate, change in membrane potential, change in membrane conductance, activation of an electrogenic pump) on the postsynaptic cell of stimulating the presynaptic neuronal pathway.
2. The cyclic nucleotide and its derivatives should mimic the electrophysiological effects on the postsynaptic cell of applying the putative neurotransmitter.
3. These effects of cyclic nucleotides should be potentiated by phosphodiesterase inhibitors.
4. These effects of cyclic nucleotides should not be blocked by pharmacological antagonists of the neurotransmitter receptor.

[a] Modified from Beam and Greengard (1976).

neurotransmitters, particularly those of acetylcholine on muscarinic cholinergic receptors, may be mediated by cyclic GMP.

One might anticipate that the synaptic potentials caused by activation of the two different classes of receptors shown in Figure 1 would have different characteristics. In the first case, where the binding of the neurotransmitter to the receptor induces a conformational change in an ionophore, the synaptic potential resulting from this one-step, non-enzymatic process characteristically has a very short latency and duration, on the order of several milliseconds. In contrast, the effects of cyclic nucleotides on the electrical properties of neuronal membranes appear to be mediated by means of a sequence of biochemical reactions, and the postsynaptic potential generated in this manner characteristically tends to have a much longer latency and duration, on the order of several hundred milliseconds to several seconds.

To be able to conclude that a certain neurotransmitter exerts its effects at a particular synapse by a mechanism involving cyclic

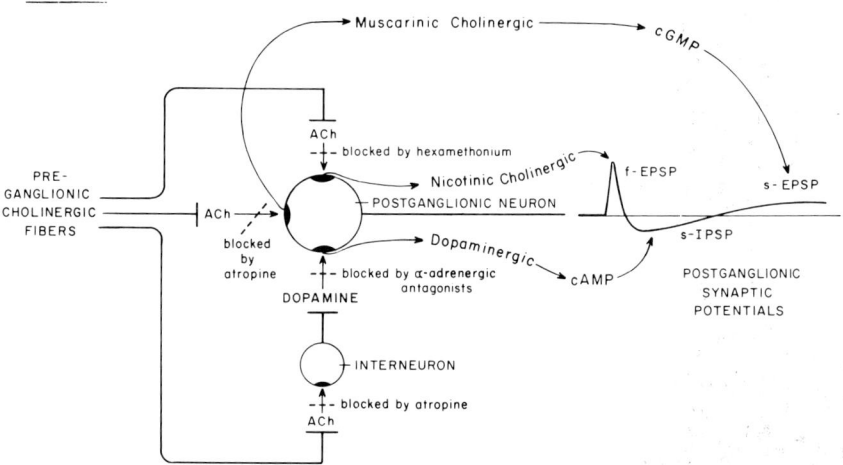

FIGURE 2. A schematic diagram of the principal synaptic connections in the mammalian superior cervical ganglion, and the postulated role of cyclic nucleotides in the genesis of the postganglionic synaptic potentials. The diagram shows the relationship between the various neuronal elements; the neurotransmitters released at the various synapses; the sensitivity of the synaptic receptors to different classes of specific antagonists; the electrical signs that accompany activation of the various postganglionic receptors after preganglionic stimulation; and the postulated involvement of cyclic nucleotides in the production of the electrophysiological responses. Abbreviations: ACh, acetylcholine; f-EPSP, fast excitatory postsynaptic potential; s-IPSP, slow inhibitory postsynaptic potential; s-EPSP, slow excitatory postsynaptic potential. Based on studies reviewed by Eccles and Libet (1961), Volle (1966), Libet (1970), Greengard and McAfee (1972), and Greengard and Kebabian (1974). Modified from Kalix et al. (1974).

nucleotides, certain criteria, presented in Table 1, must be met. In no single system where involvement of cyclic nucleotides in synaptic transmission is suspected have all of these criteria been met. However, there are two neuronal systems where many of these criteria have been fulfilled. These two systems are the vertebrate superior cervical ganglion and the Purkinje cells in the rat cerebellum.

The Superior Cervical Ganglion

A variety of anatomical, physiological, and pharmacological evidence supports the model for synaptic transmission in the vertebrate superior cervical ganglion presented in Figure 2. The principal neuronal cell in the superior cervical ganglion is the noradrenergic postganglionic cell that sends out its axon from the ganglion to innervate peripheral target tissues. The ganglion also contains dopaminergic interneurons called SIF cells (small intensely fluorescent cells), which synapse upon the postganglionic neurons. Both of these cell types receive preganglionic cholinergic innervation. When the preganglionic nerves to the superior cervical ganglion are electrically stimulated, the postganglionic potential recorded has three distinct phases. Each phase in this postganglionic potential is thought to be the consequence of a distinct mode of preganglionic cholinergic innervation.

In the principal pathway, acetylcholine released from preganglionic nerve terminals activates nicotinic cholinergic receptors located on the surface of the postganglionic neuron, and leads to the generation of a fast excitatory postsynaptic potential (f-EPSP). When a number of these f-EPSP's summate, an action potential is generated which is then propagated down the axon of the postganglionic cell. The generation of the f-EPSP does not appear to involve cyclic nucleotides; rather, it displays characteristics of the "receptor-ionophore" model described above. The f-EPSP is very rapid, with a duration of only a few milliseconds. Indeed, it would seem highly unlikely that the generation and termination of a postsynaptic potential over such a short time period could be the consequence of a series of biochemical reactions, such as those associated with cyclic nucleotide-mediated processes. In the second pathway of innervation, acetylcholine released from the nerve terminals of the preganglionic cholinergic fiber activates the dopaminergic interneuron, leading to the release of dopamine. This released dopamine activates a dopamine receptor on the postganglionic cell, which appears to be a dopamine-sensitive adenylate cyclase, and thereby leads to the generation of cyclic AMP intracellularly in the postganglionic cell. This cyclic AMP hyperpolarizes the postganglionic neuron, causing a slow inhibitory postsynaptic potential (s-IPSP). In the third pathway, acetylcholine released from the preganglionic nerve terminals activates a muscarinic cholinergic receptor located on the surface of the postganglionic cell, and leads to the generation of cyclic GMP intracellularly in the postganglionic cell. This cyclic GMP depolarizes the postganglionic neuron, causing a slow excitatory postsynaptic potential (s-EPSP). Thus, according to this model, cyclic AMP mediates dopaminergic transmission and leads to hyperpolarization of the postganglionic cell, whereas cyclic GMP mediates muscarinic cholinergic transmission leading to depolarization of the postganglionic cell. The net effect of these two types of slow membrane potential mediated by the cyclic nucleotides is to regulate the level of electrical excitability of the postganglionic cell and thereby to modulate nicotinic cholinergic transmission through the ganglion.

A number of the criteria listed in Table 1 for the mediation by cyclic nucleotides of the postsynaptic effects of a neurotransmitter have been fulfilled in the case of the slow postsynaptic potentials of the vertebrate superior cervical ganglion. The experimental evidence includes the following observations:

(1) Electrical stimulation of the preganglionic fibers leads to increased levels of cyclic AMP (McAfee, Schorderet, and Greengard, 1971) and cyclic GMP (Weight, Petzold, and Greengard, 1974) in the ganglion. The s-IPSP, as well as the increase in cyclic AMP levels, is blocked by pharmacological antagonists of alpha-adrenergic receptors, such as phentolamine (Kalix, McAfee, Schorderet, and Greengard, 1974); the s-EPSP, as well as the increase in cyclic GMP levels, is blocked by pharmacological antagonists of muscarinic receptors, such as atropine (Weight et al., 1974).

(2) Incubation of blocks of ganglionic tissue with dopamine causes an increase in cyclic AMP levels; this increase is blocked by phentolamine (Kebabian and Greengard, 1971). Incubation of blocks of ganglionic tissue with acetylcholine causes an increase in cyclic GMP levels; this increase is blocked by atropine (Kebabian, Steiner, and Greengard, 1975*b*). Cytochemical studies indicate that these increases in cyclic nucleotide levels are localized to the postsynaptic neuron (Kebabian, Bloom, Steiner, and Greengard, 1975*a*). In the experiment illustrated in Figure 3, slices of ganglion tissue were incubated either with dopamine or acetylcholine, and fluorescence micrographs were obtained after the

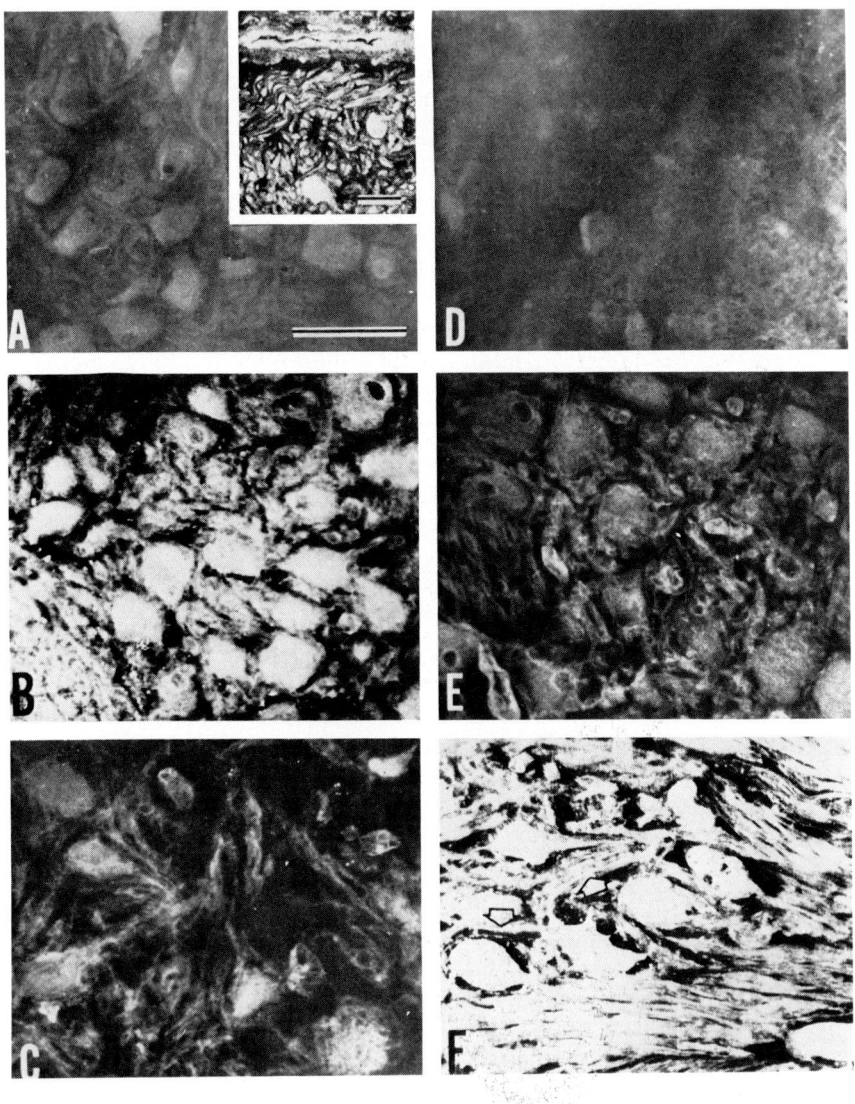

tissue was treated with fluorescein-labeled antibodies to cyclic AMP or cyclic GMP. In the control tissue slices, which were not exposed to neurotransmitter, negligible fluorescence staining of cyclic nucleotides in the ganglion was observed. When incubated in the presence of dopamine, the cell bodies of the postganglionic neurons demonstrated intense fluorescence when stained for cyclic AMP, but showed very little fluorescence staining for cyclic GMP. When slices were incubated in the presence of acetylcholine, the cell bodies, axons, and dendrites of the postganglionic cells demonstrated intense fluorescence when stained for cyclic GMP, but showed very little staining for cyclic AMP.

(3) In a cell-free homogenate of superior cervical ganglion, there is an adenylate cyclase activated by low concentrations of dopamine (Kebabian and Greengard, 1971).

(4) Electrophysiological results of applying either cyclic nucleotides, or agents that affect cyclic nucleotide metabolism, to the ganglion (Figure 4) further support a role for cyclic AMP as the mediator of the effects of dopamine on the s-IPSP, and a role for cyclic GMP as the mediator of the effects of acetylcholine on the s-EPSP (McAfee and Greengard, 1972). When a single supramaximal stimulus was applied to the preganglionic nerve and the postganglionic potential was recorded, the s-IPSP (but not the f-EPSP) was potentiated by theophylline, an inhibitor of phosphodiesterase, the enzyme that breaks down cyclic AMP. Exogenously applied dopamine, as was shown by Libet (1970), produced an inhibitory postsynaptic potential; the phosphodiesterase inhibitor theophylline increased the amplitude of this dopamine-induced hyperpolarization as well. Monobutyryl cyclic AMP, a lipid-soluble derivative of cyclic AMP, was able to mimic the hyperpolarization of the

FIGURE 3. Dark-field fluorescence micrographs illustrating the relative intensity of immunofluorescence staining either for cyclic AMP (A, B, C) or for cyclic GMP (D, E, F) in cryostat sections of bovine superior cervical ganglion. Tissue was incubated in Krebs-Ringer solution containing 1 mM SQ 20,006 (a phosphodiesterase inhibitor) as follows: (A, D) was incubated for 5 min with no other additions; (B, E) was incubated for 5 min with 100 μM dopamine; (C, F) was incubated for 2 min with 100 μM acetylcholine. All conditions used in the preparation of the photomicrographs (except inset in A) were identical, so that the relative brightness of the staining in the different figures (except inset in A) is directly comparable. The bar in A represents 100 μm and applies to all photomicrographs (except inset in A; bar in inset equals 100 μm). The inset in A illustrates the results of a 5-min incubation period with 100 μM norepinephrine plus 10 mM theophylline; positive staining is observed in two large neurons, the intima of a large vessel (above) and many small fusiform cells resembling fibroblasts. Taken from Kebabian et al. (1975a).

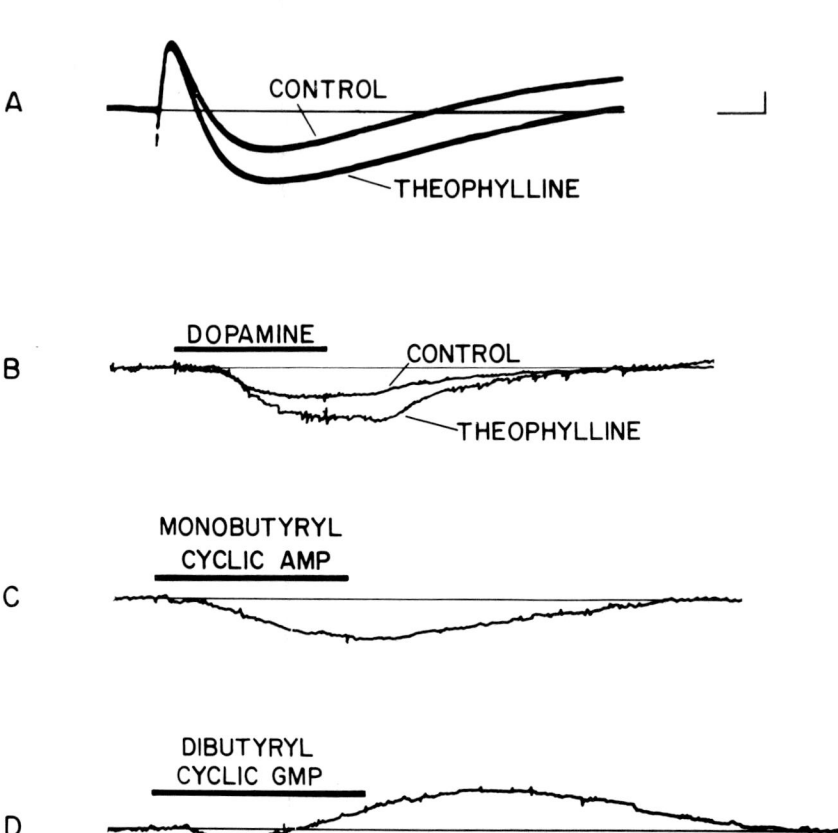

FIGURE 4. Effect of cyclic nucleotides, and of agents that affect cyclic AMP metabolism, on synaptic and resting membrane potentials recorded by means of the sucrose gap technique from postganglionic neurons of the superior cervical sympathetic ganglion of the rabbit. (A) Oscillographic traces of electrotonically conducted synaptic potentials elicited in response to a single supramaximum stimulus to the preganglionic nerve. Hexamethonium chloride (600 μM) was present to abolish propagated responses. Responses obtained in Locke solution and after 30 min of superfusion with Locke solution containing 1.5 mM theophylline are superimposed. (B) Resting membrane potential changes in response to a brief period of superfusion with dopamine. Responses to 50 μM dopamine before (control), and 30 min after, the start of superfusion with 2 mM theophylline are superimposed. (C, D) Changes in membrane potential in response to a brief period of superfusion with 2.5 mM monobutyryl cyclic AMP (C) or 25 μM dibutyryl cyclic GMP (D). The duration of superfusion with Locke solutions containing dopamine or cyclic nucleotides is indicated by the solid bars. All records are direct current recording, hyperpolarization downward. Calibration marks: (A) 1 sec, 800 μV; (B to D) 2 min, 400 μV. Modified from McAfee and Greengard (1972).

postsynaptic cell membrane produced by dopamine. Dibutyryl cyclic GMP, a lipid-soluble derivative of cyclic GMP, was able to mimic the depolarization of the postsynaptic cell membrane produced by acetylcholine acting at muscarinic receptors.

This combined body of biochemical, electrophysiological, and pharmacological evidence provides strong support for a role of cyclic nucleotides in the functioning of the superior cervical ganglion.

Noradrenergic Synapse Upon the Rat Cerebellar Purkinje Cell

The elegant studies conducted by Siggins, Hoffer, and Bloom on the noradrenergic innervation of Purkinje cells in the rat cerebellum provide strong evidence for the mediation by cyclic AMP of synaptic transmission in the CNS. Stimulation of the noradrenergic pathway arising from the locus coeruleus reduces the firing rate of cerebellar Purkinje cells (Hoffer, Siggins, Oliver, and Bloom, 1973). In this case, norepinephrine released from the presynaptic nerve terminals activates a beta-adrenergic receptor, which is coupled to an adenylate cyclase, on the postsynaptic cell.

Cytochemical techniques have demonstrated that the rise in cyclic AMP content of the cerebellum resulting either from stimulation of the locus coeruleus or from application of norepinephrine onto the cerebellar cortex occurs specifically in the Purkinje cells (Siggins, Battenberg, Hoffer, Bloom, and Steiner, 1973). The depression of cerebellar Purkinje cell firing due to stimulation of the locus coeruleus was potentiated by the phosphodiesterase inhibitor, theophylline (Siggins, Hoffer, and Bloom, 1971a). Iontophoresis of either norepinephrine or cyclic AMP onto the cerebellar Purkinje cell mimicked the depressant effect seen upon stimulation of the presynaptic noradrenergic pathway (Siggins et al., 1971a). Furthermore, it appears that norepinephrine and cyclic AMP exert their electrophysiological effects by a common mechanism (Siggins, Oliver, Hoffer, and Bloom, 1971b). Thus, by means of intracellular recording from Purkinje cells, it was shown that iontophoresis of either norepinephrine or cyclic AMP onto the cell resulted in an increase in the membrane resistance of the cell, suggesting that the ultimate biochemical event by which cyclic AMP mediates its depressant effect on Purkinje cell firing involves a decrease in the conductance of the cell membrane to certain specific ions. Interestingly, iontophoresed GABA also depressed the firing rate of cerebellar Purkinje cells; however, this inhibition, which is thought not

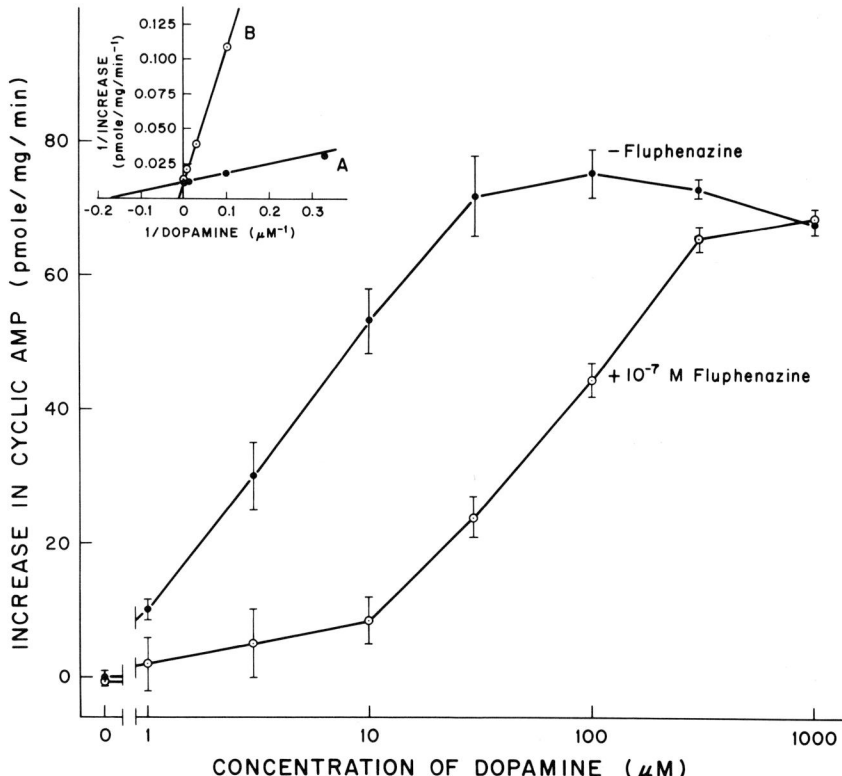

FIGURE 5. Effect of various concentrations of dopamine, in the absence (●) or presence (○) of 1×10^{-7} M fluphenazine, on adenylate cyclase activity in a particulate fraction of rat caudate nucleus rich in synaptic membranes. In the absence of added dopamine or fluphenazine, 48.1 pmol of cyclic AMP were formed per milligram wet weight of tissue per minute; in the presence of 0.1 μM fluphenazine, 47.9 pmol of cyclic AMP were formed. The increase in cyclic AMP above basal level (that is, the level in the absence of dopamine or fluphenazine) is plotted as a function of dopamine concentration. Inset: double-reciprocal plot of cyclic AMP increase as a function of dopamine concentration from 3 to 300 μM. (A) Control; (B) 1×10^{-7} M fluphenazine. Values represent the mean ± range of three replicate samples. Taken from Clement-Cormier et al. (1975).

to be mediated by cyclic nucleotides, is associated with a decrease, not an increase, in the membrane resistance.

Neurotransmitter-Sensitive Adenylate Cyclases in the Nervous System

The existence and properties of neurotransmitter-sensitive adenylate cyclases provide further support for a role of cyclic AMP in the mediation of synaptic transmission. Evidence has been obtained that the dopamine receptor in the caudate nucleus, the nucleus accumbens, and the olfactory tubercle may be the dopamine-binding portion of a dopamine-sensitive adenylate cyclase (Kebabian, Petzold, and Greengard, 1972; Clement-Cormier, Kebabian, Petzold, and Greengard, 1974; Miller, Horn, and Iversen, 1974; Makman, Mishra, and Brown, 1975; Clement-Cormier, Parrish, Petzold, Kebabian, and Greengard, 1975). As shown in Figure 5, low concentrations of dopamine stimulated the adenylate cyclase activity in a particulate fraction from rat caudate nucleus enriched in synaptic membranes; half-maximal stimulation of adenylate cyclase activity occurred with about 4 μM dopamine.

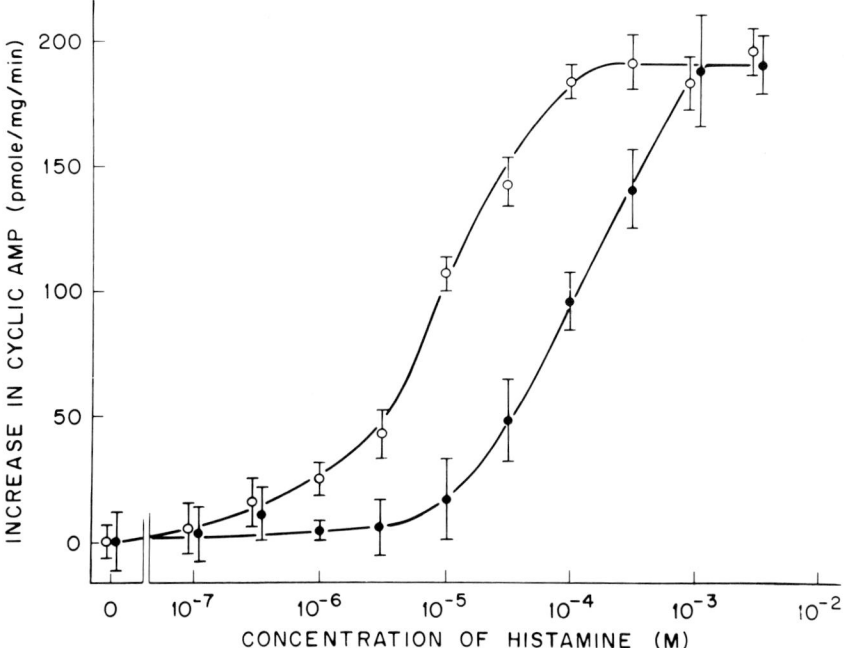

FIGURE 6. Effect of various concentrations of histamine, in the absence (○) or presence (●) of 10^{-5} M metiamide, on adenylate cyclase activity in homogenate of dorsal hippocampus from guinea pig brain. In the absence of added histamine or metiamide, 153 ± 4 pmol of cyclic AMP per minute per milligram protein were formed; in the presence of 10^{-5} M metiamide, 152 ± 10 pmol of cyclic AMP per minute per milligram protein were formed. The increase in cyclic AMP above basal level is plotted as a function of histamine concentration. Values represent the mean ± SEM of nine replicate samples in the absence, and three replicate samples in the presence, of histamine. Taken from Hegstrand et al. (1976).

Furthermore, very low concentrations of the antipsychotic drug fluphenazine, which is a potent antagonist of the physiological effects of dopamine at the dopamine receptor in the CNS, competitively inhibited the activation of this adenylate cyclase by dopamine. The inhibition constant (K_i) of the enzyme for fluphenazine was calculated to be 8×10^{-9}M. These and other studies suggest that the antipsychotic drugs may produce their Parkinsonian-like side effects by inhibiting the dopamine-sensitive adenylate cyclase in the caudate nucleus, and their therapeutic antipsychotic effects by inhibiting the dopamine-sensitive adenylate cyclase in cortical regions of the brain.

Recently, a possible role of cyclic AMP as a mediator for the effects of histamine in the CNS has also been investigated. From a number of different laboratories, there is now considerable biochemical evidence supporting the existence of histaminergic nerve pathways in the CNS (Garbarg, Barbin, Feger, and Schwartz, 1974; Barbin, Garbarg, Schwartz, and Storm-Mathisen, 1976), as well as electrophysiological evidence supporting the existence of histamine receptors in the brain through which neuronal excitability can be regulated (Haas, 1974; Haas and Bucher, 1975; Haas, Wolf, and Nussbaumer, 1975). A histamine-sensitive adenylate cyclase has been demonstrated in homogenates of several regions of guinea pig brain, including the hippocampus, neocortex, and corpus striatum (Hegstrand, Kanof, and Greengard, 1976). As shown in Figure 6, adenylate cyclase activity measured in a homogenate of guinea pig dorsal hippocampus was stimulated by low concentrations of histamine; half-maximal activation occurred with 8 μM histamine. Metiamide, which is a physiological antagonist of the effects of histamine on H_2 receptors, competitively inhibited the activation of this adenylate cyclase by histamine. The inhibition constant (K_i) of this enzyme for metiamide was calculated to be 0.87 μM, which is in excellent agreement with the K_i values for metiamide inhibition of the effects of histamine on H_2 receptors as calculated from measurements of physiological response using guinea pig atrium (0.92 μM) and rat uterus (0.75 μM) (Black, Durant, Emmett, and Ganellin, 1974). In contrast, mepyramine, a physiological antagonist of the effects of histamine on H_1 receptors, had no effect on the activation of this adenylate cyclase by histamine. These data suggest that the H_2 receptor in the CNS may be the histamine-binding portion of a histamine-sensitive adenylate cyclase.

The subcellular distribution of histamine-sensitive adenylate cyclase activity was studied (Kanof, Hegstrand, and Greengard, 1977), using

TABLE 2. *Distribution of histamine-sensitive adenylate cyclase activity in subcellular fractions of guinea pig cerebral cortex[a]*

Fraction	Protein (mg)	Total activity (pmol/min)		Specific activity (pmol/mg protein/min)	
		−Histamine	+Histamine (100 μM)	−Histamine	+Histamine (100 μM)
Primary subfractions					
Nuclear	18.0	972	1,458	54	81
Mitochondrial	42.4	3,434	7,208	81	170
Microsomal	22.9	893	1,649	39	72
Cell sap	25.5	ND[b]	ND	ND	ND
Starting material (homogenate)	142.2	6,826	13,509	48	95
Recovery (%)	77	78	76		
Mitochondrial subfractions					
M_1	29.8	4,857	8,612	163	289
$M_2 + M_3$	10.1	91	91	9	9
Starting material (mitochondrial)	42.4	3,434	7,208	81	170
Recovery (%)	94	144	121		
Subfractions of M_1 separated by sucrose density gradient centrifugation					
M_1 (0.8)	2.4	70	98	29	41
M_1 (1.0)	2.3	589	1,217	256	529
M_1 (1.2)	4.8	1,070	1,738	223	362
M_1 (1.4)	3.5	287	466	82	133
Pellet	0.7	40	57	57	82
Starting material	29.8	4,857	8,612	163	289
Recovery (%)	46	42	42		

[a] Taken from Kanof et al. (1977).
[b] ND, not detectable.

various subcellular fractions (DeRobertis, DeLores Arnaiz, and Alberici, 1967) prepared from guinea pig cerebral cortex (Table 2). Of the primary fractions, the highest total and specific activities of histamine-sensitive adenylate cyclase activity were present in the crude mitochondrial fraction, which contains most of the nerve endings. Enzyme activity was also found in the nuclear and microsomal fractions, but was not detectable in the cell sap. When the mitochondrial fraction was osmotically shocked and further fractionated, almost all of the histamine-sensitive adenylate cyclase activity appeared in the membranous M_1 subfraction. When this fraction was subjected to sucrose density gradient centrifugation, the bulk of the enzyme activity appeared in the M_1 (1.0) and the M_1 (1.2) subfractions, which are the fractions most highly enriched in synaptic membranes. The specific activity of this histamine-sensitive adenylate cyclase in the M_1 (1.0) subfraction was about fivefold greater than in the whole homogenate. These fractionation studies indicate that the subcellular distribution of this enzyme parallels the distribution of synaptic membrane fragments, and further support the possibility that the activation of this adenylate cyclase by histamine may be an early step in the sequence of biochemical events whereby histamine exerts certain of its physiological effects on neuronal elements.

Other neurotransmitter-sensitive adenylate cyclases have been found in neuronal tissue. Examples of such enzymes include a norepinephrine-sensitive adenylate cyclase in mammalian brain (Klainer, Chi, Freidberg, Rall, and Sutherland, 1962; Von Hungen and Roberts, 1973), and dopamine-sensitive, octopamine-sensitive, and serotonin-sensitive adenylate cyclases in invertebrate nervous tissue (Nathanson and Greengard, 1973; Nathanson and Greengard, 1974).

Protein Kinases, Endogenous Protein Kinase Substrates, and Protein Phosphatases in Mammalian Brain

In 1968, Dr. Edwin Krebs and his colleagues made the important discovery of a cyclic AMP-dependent protein kinase in skeletal muscle, and presented evidence that the effects of cyclic AMP in regulating glycogen breakdown in skeletal muscle were mediated through this cyclic AMP-dependent protein kinase (Walsh, Perkins, and Krebs, 1968). Subsequently, protein kinases were found in a wide variety of animal tissues (Kuo and Greengard, 1969), and the hypothesis was proposed that the diverse effects of cyclic AMP in various tissues might be mediated by regulating the activity of this family of enzymes. The appealing aspect of this protein kinase hypothesis was that it provided a mechanism by which one simple molecule, cyclic AMP, could achieve such a diversity of physiological and biochemical effects. According to this hypothesis, cyclic AMP need only regulate the activity of one class of enzymes, the protein kinases; the specificity of the action of cyclic AMP in the various tissues would then reside in the properties of the various protein kinases, and particularly in the properties of the substrate proteins for these protein kinases present in the different tissues.

There would appear to be at least three distinct functional roles for cyclic AMP and for protein phosphorylation mediated by cyclic AMP-dependent protein kinases in neuronal function (Figure 7). One role concerns the mediation of the postsynaptic potentials generated in response to certain neurotransmitters. According to our model, neurotransmitter released from presynaptic nerve terminals activates a neurotransmitter-sensitive adenylate cyclase present on the membrane of the postsynaptic cell, leading to the production of cyclic AMP in the immediate vicinity of the postsynaptic membrane. The newly formed cyclic AMP activates a cyclic AMP-dependent protein kinase present in the postsynaptic membrane, and this activated protein kinase catalyzes the phosphorylation of a substrate protein in the postsynaptic membrane, converting it from the non-phosphorylated state to the phosphorylated state. A key element in this model is the assumption that this substrate protein for the protein kinase can regulate the electrophysiological properties of the postsynaptic membrane. Thus, as a result of this protein becoming phosphorylated, the electrophysiological state of the postsynaptic membrane is altered. This alteration might be due to a change in passive ion conductance, or perhaps to a change in

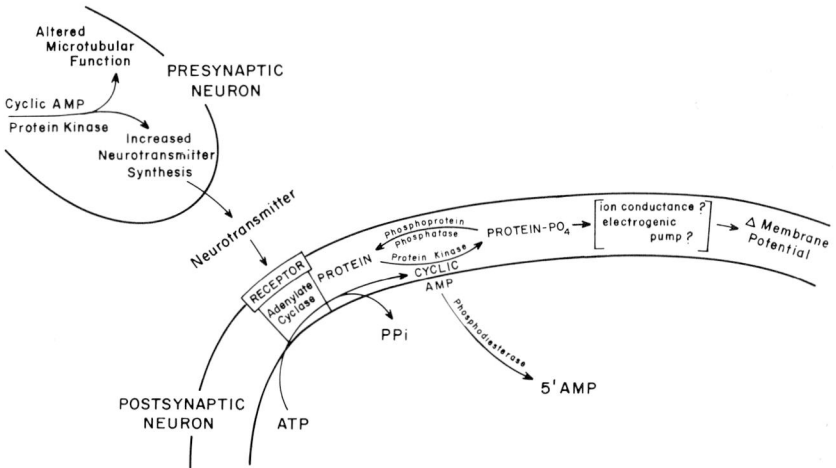

FIGURE 7. Some proposed roles for cyclic AMP and protein phosphorylation in neuronal function. (Microtubules are known to occur in dendrites, soma, and axons of neurons. Purely for convenience, regulation of microtubular function by cyclic AMP-dependent protein kinase is indicated as occurring in the presynaptic axon.) Taken from Greengard (1976).

the rate of an electrogenic pump; such an effect would lead to a change in membrane potential recognized as the classical postsynaptic potential. Because the postsynaptic potential is transient in nature, enzymatic machinery must exist for terminating this sequence of events. This enzymatic machinery includes a phosphodiesterase capable of hydrolyzing cyclic AMP to 5'-AMP, and a phosphoprotein phosphatase present in the postsynaptic membrane that dephosphorylates the substrate protein. As a result of the dephosphorylation of this permeability-controlling protein, the electrophysiological properties of the membrane return to their initial state, with the disappearance of the postsynaptic potential. Needless to say, this scheme is far from having been rigorously proven. We do not yet understand the molecular mechanism by which phosphorylation and dephosphorylation of a membrane protein might control membrane permeability. Moreover, although endogenous membrane-bound protein kinases, substrate proteins, and protein phosphatases have been found in synaptic membranes (see below), we have not yet proven the existence, or established the identity, of the phosphoprotein thought to be responsible for controlling membrane permeability.

In an attempt to understand more about the phosphoproteins that might be involved in the generation of the postsynaptic potential, as well as in other physiological effects of cyclic AMP in nervous tissue, a search was begun for endogenous protein substrates for the cyclic AMP-dependent protein kinase in nervous tissue (Johnson, Ueda, Maeno, and Greengard, 1972; Ueda, Maeno, and Greengard, 1973). In these studies, a synaptic membrane fraction from rat brain was incubated with [γ-^{32}P]ATP in the absence or presence of cyclic AMP for 15 sec. The protein kinase reaction was terminated by the addition of sodium dodecyl sulfate, which also solubilized the membrane proteins. The solubilized membrane proteins were then subjected to sodium dodecyl sulfate polyacrylamide gel electrophoresis and autoradiography in order to locate those proteins into which radioactive phosphate had been incorporated. It was observed that cyclic AMP markedly stimulated the phosphorylation, by an endogenous protein kinase, of two substrate proteins, designated Protein I and Protein II, present in these synaptic membrane fractions. In subsequent experiments (Figure 8), in which a different method of sodium dodecyl sulfate polyacrylamide gel electrophoresis was employed that allowed a higher resolution of proteins, it was found that Protein I could be separated into two distinct components, Protein Ia and Protein Ib (Krueger, Forn, and Greengard,

1975). As discussed below, Proteins Ia and Ib copurify and appear to be subunits of a single protein. It was found that the phosphorylation of Proteins I and II by the endogenous protein kinase was maximal within 5 sec, the earliest time that could be accurately studied (Ueda et al., 1973). Because the molecular events underlying synaptic transmission must be rapid, the rapid phosphorylation of these proteins is almost a prerequisite for serious consideration of the possibility that one or another of them might be involved in the generation of postsynaptic potentials.

Protein I appears to be present exclusively in nervous tissue; it has never been found in any non-neuronal tissue. Furthermore, Protein I appears to be present only in synaptic regions of the nervous system; subcellular distribution studies revealed it to be present in high concentrations in synaptic membranes and in synaptic vesicles, but not in any other subcellular fraction of nervous tissue. Protein I can be quantitatively extracted from synaptic membranes by treating the membranes with 0.1 M NH_4Cl. The ease of extraction indicates that Protein I is not an intrinsic membrane protein, and therefore not per se a transmembrane ion channel. However, the cyclic AMP-dependent phosphorylation and dephosphorylation of Protein I could be causally linked to the neurotransmitter-induced changes in the postsynaptic potential if Protein I were bound to an intrinsic, transmembrane protein. This intrinsic protein could be, for example, an ion channel, or an electrogenic pump. Then, according to this model, the functional activity of the intrinsic membrane protein could be altered by the neurotransmitter-induced cyclic AMP-dependent changes in the state of phosphorylation of Protein I, leading to the generation of the postsynaptic potential. Although this model has many attractive features, one should add that there is not yet any direct evidence that Protein I is the hypothetical phosphoprotein that mediates the effects of cyclic AMP on the postsynaptic potential.

In view of the potential importance of Protein I and Protein II in neuronal function, considerable efforts have recently been made to purify these proteins, and their associated kinases and phosphatases, from fractions rich in synaptic membranes. To have larger amounts of starting material, synaptic membranes from bovine brain rather than from rat brain were used for the purification of these proteins. Protein I has been purified to apparent homogeneity from bovine brain synaptic membranes (Ueda and Greengard, 1977). From approximately 2 kg of bovine brain, 600 μg of homogenous Protein I were obtained. This

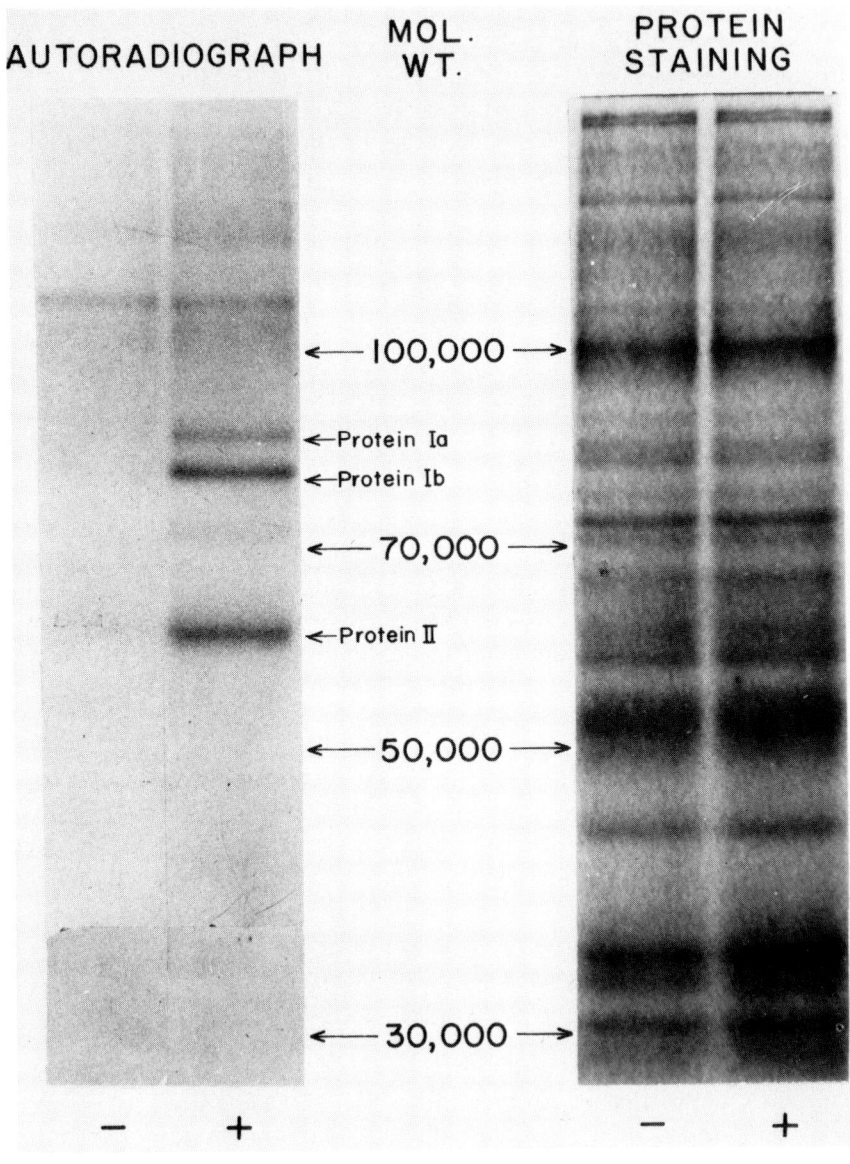

represents about a 5,000-fold purification calculated with respect to the crude synaptic membrane starting material.

The characteristics of this pure Protein I preparation have also been studied (Ueda and Greengard, 1977). In its native state, Protein I appears to exist as a mixture of a trimeric form, composed of Proteins Ia and Ib in a 1:2 molar ratio, and of the monomeric forms of the subunits. Proteins Ia and Ib have similar properties. The apparent molecular weights, on sodium dodecyl sulfate polyacrylamide gels, of Proteins Ia and Ib are 86,000 and 80,000, respectively. Both proteins are basic, with isoelectric points of 10.3 and 10.2, respectively. Each has a Stokes radius of about 60 Å, and each appears able to incorporate 1 mol of phosphate per mol of protein when subjected to phosphorylation by ATP and a protein kinase purified from synaptic membranes. The amino acid compositions of Proteins Ia and Ib are also similar. It is noteworthy that both proteins possess a high proline content (about 12%), and a high glycine content (about 11%). This high proline and glycine content is reminiscent of collagen. The amounts of these amino acids are not as high in Protein I as they are in collagen, but they are substantially higher than in many other proteins. Antibodies have been prepared to Protein I, and are being used to study the ultrastructural localization of Protein I in different regions of brain by immunocytochemical techniques (Ueda, Bloom, Battenberg, and Greengard, work in progress). These studies have verified the synaptic localization of Protein I in several regions of the brain.

Studies from several laboratories (Erlichman, Rosenfeld, and Rosen, 1974; Maeno, Reyes, Ueda, Rudolph, and Greengard, 1974) have shown that the catalytic subunit of certain types of protein kinase is capable of catalyzing the phosphorylation of the regulatory subunit of the protein kinase, a so-called "autophosphorylation" reaction. Protein II has now been purified to homogeneity and this protein appears to be identical to the regulatory subunit of the cyclic AMP-dependent protein kinase

FIGURE 8. Effect of cyclic AMP on endogenous protein phosphorylation in a synaptic membrane fraction from rat caudate nucleus. Subcellular fractions were prepared by the method of DeRobertis et al. (1967). Fraction M-1 (0.9), which was enriched in synaptic membranes, was incubated with 1 μM [γ-^{32}P]ATP for 15 sec at 30°C, in the absence (−) or presence (+) of 5 μM cyclic AMP. The reaction was terminated by the addition of sodium dodecyl sulfate, and an aliquot of the reaction product was then subjected to sodium dodecyl sulfate polyacrylamide gel electrophoresis, protein staining, and autoradiography. Left, phosphorylation of endogenous protein in the absence or presence of cyclic AMP; right, protein staining. Taken from Krueger et al. (1975).

present in the nerve cell membrane (Uno, Ueda, and Greengard, 1977b): the regulatory subunit of the brain membrane-derived protein kinase is phosphorylated by the catalytic subunit of this enzyme, and this autophosphorylated regulatory subunit migrates in the same position on a sodium dodecyl sulfate polyacrylamide gel as the exogenously phosphorylated Protein II; furthermore, both the regulatory subunit of the membrane-derived protein kinase and Protein II are able to bind ^{32}P-labeled 8-azido-cyclic AMP, a photoaffinity reagent that is highly specific for cyclic AMP-binding proteins (Pomerantz, Rudolph, Haley, and Greengard, 1975).

In bovine brain synaptic membranes, there appears to be only a single species of cyclic AMP-dependent protein kinase. This single enzyme catalyzes the phosphorylation of both Protein I and Protein II. In fact, each of these endogenous proteins is a much better substrate for this membrane-derived protein kinase than are the traditional protein kinase substrates, protamine and histone (Uno, Ueda, and Greengard, 1977a). As evidenced by the Michaelis constants, Proteins I and II each have about a 10-fold higher affinity for this protein kinase than do protamine, lysine-rich histone, or arginine-rich histone. Furthermore, the maximal reaction velocity at saturating substrate concentrations is about fivefold higher for Proteins I and II than it is for protamine and the two histones. Because the velocity of an enzyme reaction at low substrate concentrations is proportional to V_m/K_m, the rate of phosphorylation of Proteins I and II by this synaptic membrane-derived protein kinase, at low substrate concentrations, is about 50-fold greater than it is for protamine and the two histones.

The molecular properties of the protein kinase derived from brain membranes are very different from the properties of the cyclic AMP-dependent protein kinases purified to homogeneity from either brain cytosol or heart cytosol (Uno et al., 1977a). The molecular weights of the holoenzyme (177,000), regulatory subunit (55,000), and catalytic subunit (40,000) of the cyclic AMP-dependent protein kinases derived from brain and heart cytosol are identical to each other; however, these are different from the molecular weights of the holoenzyme (87,000), regulatory subunit (52,000), and catalytic subunit (40,000) of the protein kinase derived from brain membranes. In terms of quaternary structure, both of the cytosol protein kinases appear to exist as tetramers consisting of two regulatory subunits and two catalytic subunits (R_2C_2), whereas the brain membrane-derived kinase exists as a dimer of one regulatory subunit linked to one catalytic subunit (RC). In terms of their isoelectric points, the holoenzyme, regulatory subunit, and catalytic subunit of the two cytosol protein kinases are similar to one another, but are different from the holoenzyme and corresponding subunits of the brain membrane-derived enzyme. Similarly, the sedimentation coefficients of the two cytosol protein kinases are similar to one another, but are different from that of the membrane-derived enzyme. There are also antigenic differences between the cytosol and membrane-derived enzymes. The bovine heart cytosol protein kinase was purified to homogeneity, and antibodies to this enzyme were prepared. These antibodies cross-reacted with the bovine brain cytosol protein kinase, indicating that the two cytosol enzymes have certain antigenic similarities. However, these antibodies failed to cross-react with the membrane-derived protein kinase, indicating that this enzyme was antigenically very different from the two cytosol enzymes.

One other piece of evidence has been obtained which clearly illustrates the differences between membrane-derived and cytosol protein kinases (Uno et al., 1977a). Subunits from the bovine brain membrane-derived protein kinase, the bovine brain cytosol protein kinase, and the bovine heart cytosol protein kinase were isolated, and the ability of the regulatory subunits prepared from the three types of protein kinase to combine with, and thereby inhibit, the catalytic subunits of those three types of protein kinase was studied. As expected, the regulatory subunit was able to recombine with the catalytic subunit when the two subunits had been derived from the same source. Furthermore, the regulatory subunit of the heart cytosol protein kinase was able to combine with the catalytic subunit of the brain cytosol enzyme, and the regulatory subunit of the brain cytosol protein kinase was able to combine with the catalytic subunit of the heart cytosol enzyme. However, the regulatory subunit of the membrane-derived protein kinase could not inhibit the catalytic subunits of either of the cytosol kinases, nor could the catalytic subunit of the membrane-derived protein kinase be inhibited by the regulatory subunits of either of the cytosol kinases. A few years ago, it was found that the regulatory subunit of a cyclic AMP-dependent protein kinase prepared from bovine brain cytosol was capable of combining with, and thereby inhibiting, the catalytic subunit of a cyclic GMP-dependent protein kinase prepared from lobster muscle cytosol (Miyamoto, Petzold, Kuo, and Greengard, 1973). The fact that this interaction between regulatory and catalytic subunits occurred, although the subunits were from different tissues, different phyla, and different classes (with respect to cyclic nucleotide specificity) of protein kinase, suggested a low degree of specificity in the interaction of regulatory and catalytic subunits. Thus, the inability of the synaptic membrane-derived subunits to combine with the cytosol subunits is quite remarkable.

It is clear from the evidence presented above that the protein kinase prepared from synaptic membranes is very different from the protein kinase isolated from brain cytosol. Presumably, the highly specific properties of this membrane-derived kinase reflect a specific functional role for this enzyme in mediating the effects of cyclic AMP in membrane function. It will be interesting to see whether the properties of this protein kinase help in understanding more about the functional role of cyclic AMP at the synaptic membrane.

The protein phosphatases present in synaptic membranes that catalyze the dephosphorylation of Proteins I and II have also been studied (Uno et al., 1977b). When a Triton extract of a synaptic membrane fraction prepared from bovine brain was subjected to DEAE-cellulose column chromatography, two peaks of protein phosphatase activity were obtained. Both peaks catalyzed the dephosphorylation of protamine. One of these peaks catalyzed the dephosphorylation of Protein I but not of Protein II, whereas the other peak catalyzed the dephosphorylation of Protein II but not of Protein I. It is clear from these results that Protein I phosphatase is a different enzyme from Protein II phosphatase. Thus, this situation is in contrast to that of the membrane-derived protein kinase, where a single enzyme catalyzes the phosphorylation of both Protein I and Protein II. In earlier studies (Maeno and Greengard, 1972), it was found that the properties of synaptic membrane-derived protein phosphatase differed from those of protein phosphatases present in brain cytosol. As in the case of the protein kinases, it will be interesting to determine if the biochemical differences among the various phosphatases reflect different functional roles for phosphoproteins in neuronal physiology.

Cyclic AMP-Dependent Phosphorylation of Microtubular Protein

The physiological significance of microtubules in nerve cells is not yet well understood. However, there is evidence that their regulation may be important in axoplasmic transport and neurite outgrowth (Wuerker and Kirkpatrick, 1972). Early studies reported that cyclic AMP enhances the phosphorylation of tubulin (Goodman, Rasmussen, DiBella, and Guthrow, 1970), the major protein component of microtubules, suggesting the possibility that cyclic AMP-dependent protein phosphorylation might be able to affect microtubular function. Recently, in our laboratory (Sloboda, Rudolph, Rosenbaum, and Greengard, 1975), studies of endogenous protein phosphorylation were carried out on a preparation of microtubular protein that had been highly purified (Weisenberg, 1972; Borisy and Olmstead, 1972) by successive cycles of in vitro assembly and disassembly. In these studies, an aliquot of microtubular protein was incubated with [γ-^{32}P]ATP, with or without added cyclic AMP. The phosphorylation reaction was terminated by the addition of sodium dodecyl sulfate, and the proteins were subjected to sodium dodecyl sulfate polyacrylamide gel electrophoresis. As shown in Figure 9, the protein-staining pattern indicates that this preparation of

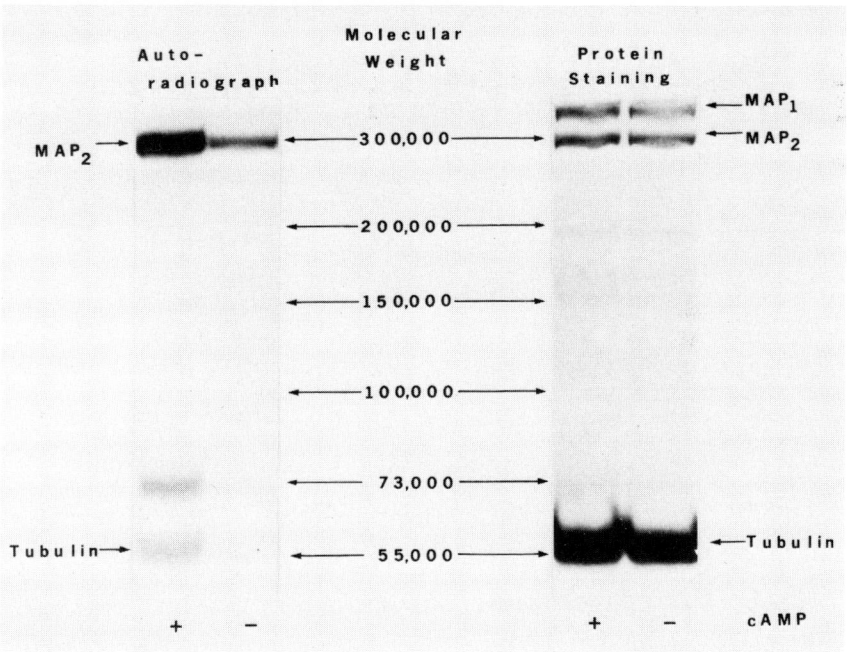

FIGURE 9. Effect of cyclic AMP on the endogenous phosphorylation of microtubule proteins. A 50 µg amount of three times assembled-disassembled microtubule protein was incubated with [γ-^{32}P]ATP for 30 sec at 30°C in the presence or absence of 10^{-5} M cyclic AMP. An aliquot of sodium dodecyl sulfate-solubilized protein was then subjected to polyacrylamide gel electrophoresis. The autoradiograph, showing ^{32}P incorporation, is on the left, and the protein-staining pattern is on the right. Taken from Sloboda et al. (1975).

purified microtubular protein contained not only tubulin, but also two high-molecular-weight proteins, designated microtubule-associated proteins 1 and 2, or MAP_1 and MAP_2. An autoradiograph of this gel revealed that cyclic AMP markedly stimulated the phosphorylation of one of these high molecular weight proteins, MAP_2, as well as of some other minor protein components of the microtubular preparation. The phosphorylation of MAP_2 was stoichiometric: in the absence of cyclic AMP, 1 mol of phosphate was incorporated per mol of MAP_2, whereas in the presence of cyclic AMP, 2 mol of phosphate were incorporated per mol of MAP_2. Studies are currently underway to determine whether the cyclic AMP-dependent phosphorylation of these microtubular proteins affects some parameter of microtubular function, such as the rate at which these microtubules transport material along their length, or the rate of assembly or disassembly of the microtubules.

Cyclic AMP-Dependent Protein Phosphorylation and Neurotransmitter Biosynthesis

Cyclic AMP-dependent protein phosphorylation seems to exert a regulatory role in the biosynthesis of certain neurotransmitters in presynaptic terminals. Tyrosine hydroxylase is the rate-limiting enzyme in catecholamine biosynthesis. This enzyme is activated in intact tissue by increased impulse flow along catecholaminergic nerve pathways

TABLE 3. *Activation of tyrosine hydroxylase by cyclic AMP and protein kinase*[a]

Additions to activation reaction mixture	Tyrosine hydroxylase activity (pmol DOPA/ mg protein/min)
None	7.5 ± 1.6
Cyclic AMP	7.1 ± 1.3
ATP + Mg^{2+}	13.4 ± 1.7
Cyclic AMP + ATP + Mg^{2+}	42.1 ± 4.6
Cyclic AMP + β-γ-methylene analogue of ATP + Mg^{2+}	7.5 ± 0.9
Protein kinase	7.7 ± 1.3
Protein kinase + ATP + Mg^{2+}	53.5 ± 7.1

[a] A 2-ml aliquot from a high-speed supernatant of rat hippocampi was applied to a Sephadex G-25 column. An aliquot (1.0 ml) from the void volume was added as enzyme to the activation reaction mixture. This activation reaction mixture was incubated at 37°C for 10 min in the absence or presence of 1 μM cyclic AMP, 0.1 mM Mg^{2+}, 2 μM ATP, or 2 μM β-γ-methylene analogue of ATP, and protein kinase (0.35 μg of protein), as indicated. The activation reaction was stopped by the addition of EDTA (final concentration, 0.2 mM); tyrosine was then added and tyrosine hydroxylase activity was determined. Modified from Morgenroth et al. (1975).

(Roth, Salzman, and Morgenroth, 1974). By what appears to be a similar mechanism, tyrosine hydroxylase is also activated by cyclic AMP both in slices (Goldstein, Anagnoste, and Shirron, 1973) and in high speed supernatants (Harris, Morgenroth, Roth, and Baldessarini, 1974) of rat brain. Recently, evidence has been obtained for the involvement of a protein kinase in the activation of tyrosine hydroxylase by cyclic AMP (Morgenroth, Hegstrand, Roth, and Greengard, 1975). In the experiment of Table 3, a high-speed supernatant of homogenized rat hippocampus was passed over a small Sephadex G-25 column in order to remove free ATP, cyclic AMP, metal ions, and other small molecules. The effluent in the void volume contained tyrosine hydroxylase activity, protein kinase activity, as well as many other soluble proteins. Aliquots of this preparation were preincubated in the absence or presence of various test substances known to be required for the protein kinase reaction, and then the tyrosine hydroxylase activity of the preparation was determined. In the presence of ATP and Mg^{2+}, cyclic AMP caused a threefold increase in tyrosine hydroxylase activity. However, when the ATP was replaced by the β-γ-methylene analogue of ATP, in which the terminal phosphate cannot be used for protein phosphorylation, no activation of tyrosine hydroxylase occurred. Exogenously added protein kinase also stimulated tyrosine hydroxylase activity, but only in the presence of ATP and Mg^{2+}, which are required for the protein kinase reaction. Other experiments showed that the activation of tyrosine hydroxylase by either cyclic AMP or exogenous protein kinase could be prevented by the addition to the preincubation mixture of any of several substances known (Miyamoto, Kuo, and Greengard, 1969; Walsh, Ashby, Gonzalez, Calkins, Fischer, and Krebs, 1971) to inhibit cyclic AMP-dependent protein kinase from mammalian brain.

There remain large gaps in our understanding of this process. The detailed mechanism of how protein kinase activates tyrosine hydroxylase has not yet been elucidated. It is possible that tyrosine hydroxylase activity is regulated by the phosphorylation of the enzyme itself. Alternatively, it is possible that some other protein regulates the activity of tyrosine hydroxylase, and that it is this regulatory protein that is the substrate for the phosphorylation reaction. Also, although it is known that presynaptic impulse flow and cyclic AMP-dependent protein phosphorylation can each increase tyrosine hydroxylase activity, there is not yet any evidence to indicate that impulse flow affects presynaptic cyclic AMP levels, nor is there any data concerning the molecular mechanisms by which this process might be accomplished.

Calcium-Dependent Protein Phosphorylation in Synaptosomes

Recently, certain of the factors capable of regulating protein phosphorylation in intact synaptosomes have been investigated (Krueger, Forn, and Greengard, 1977). A crude mitochondrial preparation (P_2) that contained intact synaptosomes was preincubated with ^{32}P-labeled inorganic phosphate for 30 min, so that the synaptosomes could take up the labeled phosphate and synthesize their own endogenous labeled ATP. These synaptosomes were then treated with several agents known to increase the transport of calcium across membranes, including veratridine and high potassium. After 30 sec of

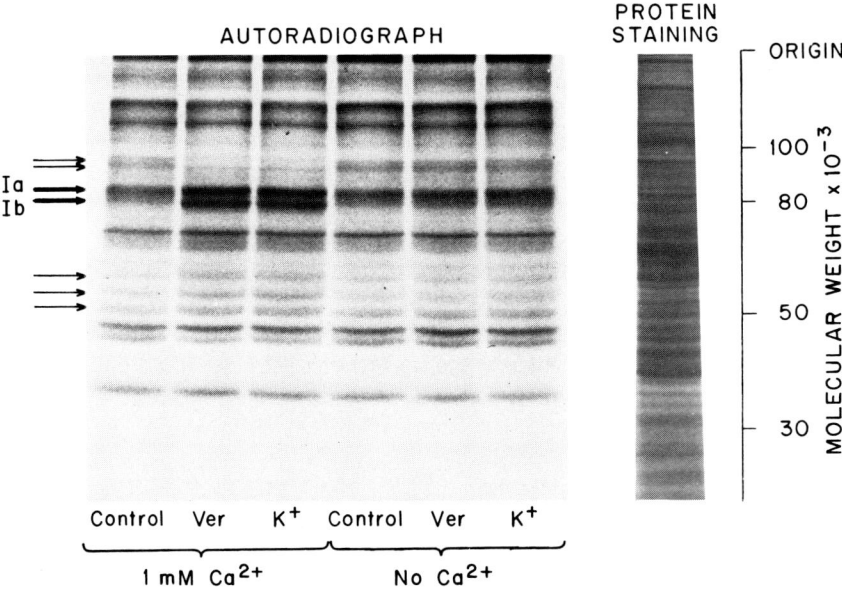

FIGURE 10. Effect of veratridine and of high K^+, in the absence and presence of Ca^{2+}, on the phosphorylation of endogenous proteins in a crude synaptosomal preparation from rat cerebral cortex. The synaptosomal fraction was preincubated with $^{32}P_i$ for 30 min in the absence of Ca^{2+}. Aliquots of this suspension were then incubated for 30 sec in the absence (control) or presence of 100 μM veratridine (Ver) or 60 mM K^+; 1 mM Ca^{2+} was present where indicated. The incubation was terminated by the addition of sodium dodecyl sulfate and the samples were subjected to sodium dodecyl sulfate polyacrylamide gel electrophoresis. Left, autoradiograph. The positions of Proteins 1a and 1b are indicated by bold arrows. Other arrows indicate the positions of other protein bands whose phosphorylation was affected by veratridine or high K^+. Right, protein staining. Taken from Krueger et al. (1977).

such treatment, aliquots of the synaptosome preparations were boiled in sodium dodecyl sulfate and subjected to sodium dodecyl sulfate polyacrylamide gel electrophoresis and autoradiography. As shown in Figure 10, when calcium was present in the incubation medium, both veratridine and high potassium had marked effects on the phosphorylation of a number of proteins, stimulating the incorporation of phosphate into certain proteins, and inhibiting the incorporation of phosphate into certain other proteins. When calcium was omitted from the external incubation medium, neither veratridine nor high potassium had any effect on protein phosphorylation. These and other results suggested that the observed changes in protein phosphorylation were due to the entry of calcium into an intact organelle. It is interesting that two of the proteins whose phosphorylation was stimulated by calcium entry have electrophoretic mobilities similar to those of Proteins Ia and Ib.

Further studies indicated that the intact organelles that exhibited the calcium-dependent changes in protein phosphorylation were, in fact, synaptosomes. In the experiment of Figure 11, the P_2 fraction was layered on a Ficoll gradient and centrifuged, to yield subfractions enriched in myelin, synaptosomes, and mitochondria. Veratridine produced stimulatory and inhibitory effects on protein phosphorylation, similar to those seen in the P_2 fraction, in that subfraction enriched in synaptosomes. Veratridine did not significantly influence protein phosphorylation in those subfractions enriched in myelin or mitochondria. In other experiments, it was found that the time course of the veratridine-induced protein phosphorylation in intact synaptosomes was similar to the time course of $^{45}Ca^{2+}$ uptake by the synaptosomes. These results raise the intriguing possibility that phosphoproteins may be involved in the regulation of certain presynaptic, calcium-dependent nerve terminal functions, such as neurotransmitter synthesis and release.

Multiple Roles for Cyclic Nucleotides and Phosphorylated Proteins in Neuronal Function

Evidence summarized in this article suggests that, at certain synapses, neurotransmitters may exert their postsynaptic electrophysiological actions through a mechanism involving cyclic nucleotides. Furthermore, it has been proposed that these effects are mediated by protein kinases, whose activation by cyclic nucleotides results in the phosphorylation of specific proteins in the postsynaptic membrane. It should be emphasized, however, that cyclic nucleotides

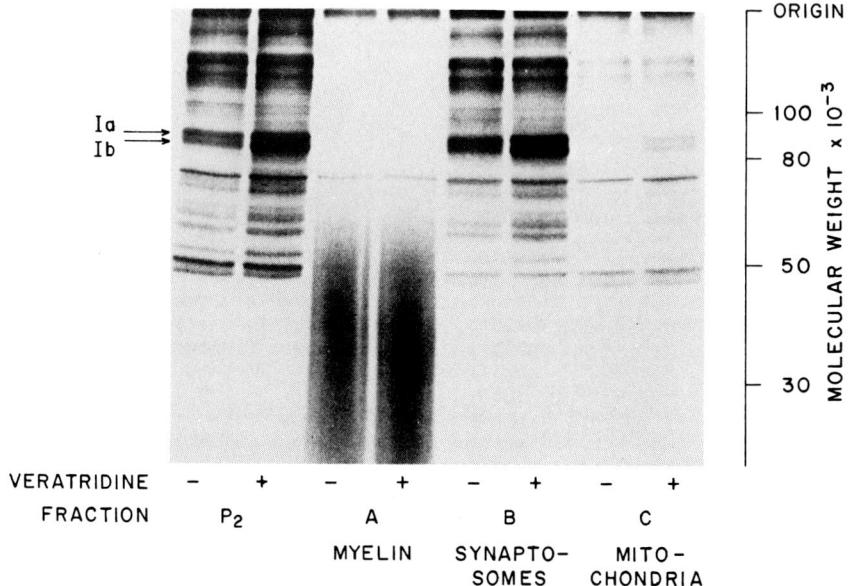

FIGURE 11. Protein phosphorylation in subfractions of a crude synaptomal preparation. The crude synaptosomal fraction (P_2) was subfractionated by centrifugation in a discontinuous Ficoll-sucrose flotation gradient. Protein phosphorylation, in the absence (−) and presence (+) of 100 μM veratridine, was then measured in the crude synaptosomal fraction (P_2) and in each of the subfractions of the gradient. The positions of Proteins 1a and 1b are indicated by the arrows. Krueger, Forn, and Greengard (unpublished data).

and phosphorylated proteins may have many other roles in the nervous system. Two such roles, the regulation of microtubular function and of neurotransmitter biosynthesis, have been discussed above. The increase in cyclic AMP during increased impulse flow may also serve to mobilize carbohydrate (Edwards, Nahorski, and Rogers, 1974) and lipid reserves and thus help to meet the additional energy requirements associated with elevated functional activity in nervous tissue. Furthermore, in certain invertebrate nerve networks, an increase in cyclic AMP mediated by serotonin has been shown to be responsible for the increased neurotransmitter release that accompanies behavioral sensitization (Brunelli, Castellucci, and Kandel, 1976). It is also of interest that in various model systems, cyclic AMP may act at a transcriptional level to regulate the de novo synthesis of a number of proteins with specific functional roles, such as tyrosine hydroxylase in neuroblastoma

(Waymire, Weiner, and Prasad, 1972; Richelson, 1973) and adrenal medulla (Costa, Guidotti, and Hanbauer, 1974), and N-acetyl transferase in the pineal gland (Klein and Berg, 1970; Romero, Zatz, and Axelrod, 1975). By analogy, one might anticipate that, in the CNS, elevation of the cyclic AMP content of postsynaptic cells in response to increased presynaptic impulse flow may also result in altered synthesis of certain proteins having specific functional roles in synaptic physiology. This might constitute one component of the mechanism by which long-term information storage (i.e., learning) and retrieval (i.e., memory) can occur.

It seems likely that continued investigations into the multiple roles for cyclic nucleotides and phosphorylated proteins in neuronal physiology, and into the manner through which these very diverse roles are coordinated in an orderly fashion, will help to elucidate many of the fundamental problems in neurobiology.

ACKNOWLEDGMENTS

This study was supported by Public Health Service grants MH-17387 and NS-08440 from the National Institutes of Health and a grant from Hoffmann-La Roche.

REFERENCES

Barbin, G., M. Garbarg, J.-C. Schwartz, and J. Storm-Mathisen (1976). Histamine synthesizing afferents to the hippocampal region, *J. Neurochem.* **26**:259–263.

Beam, K. G. and P. Greengard (1976). Cyclic nucleotides, protein phosphorylation, and synaptic function, *Cold Spring Harbor Symp. Quant. Biol.* **40**:157–168.

Black, J. W., G. J. Durant, J. C. Emmett, and C. R. Gannelin (1974). Sulfur-methylene isosterism in the development of metiamide, a new histamine H_2-receptor antagonist, *Nature (London)* **248**:65–67.

Bloom, F. E. (1975). The role of cyclic nucleotides in central synaptic function, *Rev. Physiol. Biochem. Pharmacol.* **74**:1–103.

Borisy, G. G. and J. B. Olmstead (1972). Nucleated assembly of microtubules in porcine brain extracts, *Science* **177**:1196–1197.

Brunelli, M., V. Castellucci, and E. R. Kandel (1976). Synaptic facilitation and behavioral sensitization in *Aplysia*: possible role of serotonin and cyclic AMP, *Science* **194**:1178–1181.

Clement-Cormier, Y. C., J. W. Kebabian, G. L. Petzold, and P. Greengard (1974). Dopamine-sensitive adenylate cyclase in mammalian brain: a possible site of action of antipsychotic drugs, *Proc. Natl. Acad. Sci. U.S.A.* **71**:1113–1117.

Clement-Cormier, Y. C., R. G. Parrish, G. L. Petzold, J. W. Kebabian, and P. Greengard (1975). Characterization of a dopamine-sensitive adenylate cyclase in the rat caudate nucleus, *J. Neurochem.* **25**:143–149.

Costa, E., A. Guidotti, and I. Hanbauer (1974). Do cyclic nucleotides promote the trans-synaptic induction of tyrosine hydroxylase? *Life Sci.* **14**:1169–1188.

Daly, J. (1975). Role of cyclic nucleotides in the nervous system, pp. 47–130 in *Handbook of Psychopharmacology*, Vol. 5, Iversen, L. L., S. D. Iversen, and S. H. Snyder, eds. Plenum Press, New York.

DeRobertis, E., R. DeLores Arnaiz, and M. Alberici (1967). Subcellular distribution of adenyl cyclase and cyclic phosphodiesterase in rat brain cortex, *J. Biol. Chem.* **242**:3487–3493.

Drummond, G. I. and Y. Ma (1973). Metabolism and function of cyclic AMP in nerve, pp. 119–176 in *Progress in Neurobiology*, Vol. 2, Kerkut, G. A. and J. W. Phillis, eds. Pergamon Press, New York.

Eccles, R. M. and B. Libet (1961). Origin and blockade of the synaptic responses of curarized sympathetic ganglia, *J. Physiol. (London)* **157**:484–503.

Edwards, C., S. R. Nahorski, and K. J. Rogers (1974). In vivo changes of cerebral cyclic adenosine 3′,5′-monophosphate induced by biogenic amines: association with phosphorylase activation, *J. Neurochem.* **22**:565–572.

Erlichman, J., R. Rosenfeld, and O. M. Rosen (1974). Phosphorylation of a cyclic adenosine 3′,5′-monophosphate-dependent protein kinase from bovine cardiac muscle, *J. Biol. Chem.* **249**:5000–5003.

Garbarg, M., G. Barbin, J. Feger, and J.-C. Schwartz (1974). Histaminergic pathway in rat brain evidenced by lesions of the medial forebrain bundle, *Science* **186**:833–835.

Goldstein, M., B. Anagnoste, and C. Shirron (1973). The effect of trivastal, haloperidol, and dibutyryl cyclic AMP on [^{14}C]dopamine synthesis in rat striatum, *J. Pharm. Pharmacol.* **25**:348–351.

Goodman, D. B. P., H. Rasmussen, F. DiBella, and C. E. Guthrow, Jr. (1970). Cyclic adenosine 3′:5′-monophosphate-stimulated phosphorylation of isolated neurotubule subunits, *Proc. Natl. Acad. Sci. U.S.A.* **67**:652–659.

Greengard, P. (1976). Possible role for cyclic nucleotides and phosphorylated membrane proteins in postsynaptic actions of neurotransmitters, *Nature (London)* **260**:101–108.

Greengard, P. and J. W. Kebabian (1974). Role of cyclic AMP in synaptic transmission in the mammalian peripheral nervous system, *Fed. Proc.* **33**:1059–1067.

Greengard, P. and D. A. McAfee (1972). Adenosine 3′:5′-cyclic monophosphate as a mediator in the action of neurohumoral agents, *Biochem. Soc. Symp.* **36**:87–102.

Haas, H. L. (1974). Histamine: action on single hypothalamic neurons, *Brain Res.* **76**:363–366.

Haas, H. L. and U. M. Bucher (1975). Histamine H_2-receptors on single central neurons, *Nature (London)* **255**:634–635.

Haas, H. L., P. Wolf, and J.-C. Nussbaumer (1975). Histamine: action on supraoptic and other hypothalamic neurons of the cat, *Brain Res.* **88**:166–170.

Harris, J. E., V. H. Morgenroth, III, R. H. Roth, and R. J. Baldessarini (1974). Regulation of catecholamine synthesis in the rat brain in vitro by cyclic AMP, *Nature (London)* **252**:156–158.

Hegstrand, L. R., P. D. Kanof, and P. Greengard (1976). Histamine-sensitive adenylate cyclase in mammalian brain, *Nature (London)* **260**:163–165.

Hoffer, B. J., G. R. Siggins, A. P. Oliver, and F. E. Bloom (1973). Activation of the pathway from locus coeruleus to rat cerebellar Purkinje neurons: pharmacological evidence of noradrenergic central inhibition, *J. Pharmacol. Exp. Ther.* **184:**553–569.

Johnson, E. M., T. Ueda, H. Maeno, and P. Greengard (1972). Adenosine 3′,5′-monophosphate-dependent phosphorylation of a specific protein in synaptic membrane fractions from rat cerebrum, *J. Biol. Chem.* **247:**5650–5652.

Kalix, P., D. A. McAfee, M. Schorderet, and P. Greengard (1974). Pharmacological analysis of synaptically mediated increase in cyclic adenosine monophosphate in rabbit superior cervical ganglion, *J. Pharmacol. Exp. Ther.* **188:**676–687.

Kanof, P. D., L. R. Hegstrand, and P. Greengard (1977). Biochemical characterization of histamine-sensitive adenylate cyclase in mammalian brain, *Arch. Biochem. Biophys.*, in press.

Kebabian, J. W., F. E. Bloom, A. L. Steiner, and P. Greengard (1975a). Neurotransmitters increase cyclic nucleotides in postganglionic neurons: immunocytochemical demonstration, *Science* **190:**157–159.

Kebabian, J. W. and P. Greengard (1971). Dopamine-sensitive adenyl cyclase: possible role in synaptic transmission, *Science* **174:**1346–1349.

Kebabian, J. W., G. L. Petzold, and P. Greengard (1972). Dopamine-sensitive adenylate cyclase in caudate nucleus of rat brain, and its similarity to the "dopamine receptor," *Proc. Natl. Acad. Sci. U.S.A.* **69:**2145–2149.

Kebabian, J. W., A. L. Steiner, and P. Greengard (1975b). Muscarinic cholinergic regulation of cyclic guanosine 3′,5′-monophosphate in autonomic ganglia: possible role in synaptic transmission, *J. Pharmacol. Exp. Ther.* **193:**474–488.

Klainer, L. M., Y.-M. Chi, S. L. Freidberg, T. W. Rall, and E. W. Sutherland (1962). Adenyl cyclase. IV. The effect of neurohormones on the formation of adenosine 3′,5′-phosphate by preparations from brain and other tissues, *J. Biol. Chem.* **237:**1239–1243.

Klein, D. C. and G. R. Berg (1970). Pineal gland: stimulation of melatonin production by norepinephrine involves cyclic AMP-mediated stimulation of N-acetyltransferase, pp. 241–263 in *Role of Cyclic AMP in Cell Function, Advances in Biochemical Psychopharmacology*, Vol. 3, Greengard, P. and E. Costa, eds. Raven Press, New York.

Krueger, B. K., J. Forn, and P. Greengard (1975). Dopamine-sensitive adenylate cyclase and protein phosphorylation in the rat caudate nucleus, pp. 123–147 in *Pre- and Postsynaptic Receptors*, Usdin, E. and W. E. Bunney, Jr., eds. Marcel Dekker, New York.

Krueger, B. K., J. Forn, and P. Greengard (1977). Depolarization-induced phosphorylation of specific proteins, mediated by calcium ion flux, in rat brain synaptosomes, *J. Biol. Chem.*, in press.

Kuo, J. F. and P. Greengard (1969). Cyclic nucleotide-dependent protein kinases. IV. Widespread occurrence of adenosine 3′,5′-monophosphate-dependent protein kinase in various tissues and phyla of the animal kingdom, *Proc. Natl. Acad. Sci. U.S.A.* **64:**1349–1355.

Libet, B. (1970). Generation of slow inhibitory and excitatory postsynaptic potentials, *Fed. Proc.* **29**:1945–1956.

Maeno, H. and P. Greengard (1972). Phosphoprotein phosphatases from rat cerebral cortex, *J. Biol. Chem.* **247**:3269–3277.

Maeno, H., P. L. Reyes, T. Ueda, S. A. Rudolph, and P. Greengard (1974). Autophosphorylation of adenosine 3′,5′-monophosphate-dependent protein kinase from bovine brain, *Arch. Biochem. Biophys.* **164**:551–559.

Makman, M. H., R. K. Mishra, and J. M. Brown (1975). Drug interactions with dopamine-stimulated adenylate cyclases of caudate nucleus and retina: direct agonist effect of a piribedil metabolite, pp. 213–222 in *Advances in Neurology*, Vol. 9, Calne, D. B., T. N. Chase, and A. Barbeau, eds. Raven Press, New York.

McAfee, D. A. and P. Greengard (1972). Adenosine 3′,5′-monophosphate: evidence for a role in synaptic transmission, *Science* **178**:310–312.

McAfee, D. A., M. Schorderet, and P. Greengard (1971). Adenosine 3′,5′-monophosphate in nervous tissue: increase associated with synaptic transmission, *Science* **171**:1156–1158.

Miller, R. J., A. S. Horn, and L. L. Iversen (1974). The action of neuroleptic drugs on dopamine-stimulated adenosine 3′,5′-monophosphate production in rat neostriatum and limbic forebrain, *Mol. Pharmacol.* **10**:759–766.

Miyamoto, E., J. F. Kuo, and P. Greengard (1969). Cyclic nucleotide-dependent protein kinases. III. Purification and properties of adenosine 3′,5′-monophosphate-dependent protein kinase from bovine brain, *J. Biol. Chem.* **244**:6395–6402.

Miyamoto, E., G. L. Petzold, J. F. Kuo, and P. Greengard (1973). Dissociation and activation of adenosine 3′,5′-monophosphate-dependent and guanosine 3′,5′-monophosphate-dependent protein kinases by cyclic nucleotides and by substrate proteins, *J. Biol. Chem.* **248**:179–189.

Morgenroth, V. H., III, L. R. Hegstrand, R. H. Roth, and P. Greengard (1975). Evidence for involvement of protein kinase in the activation by adenosine 3′:5′-monophosphate of brain tyrosine 3-monooxygenase, *J. Biol. Chem.* **250**:1946–1948.

Nathanson, J. A. (1977). Cyclic nucleotides and synaptic transmission, *Physiol. Rev.*, in press.

Nathanson, J. A. and P. Greengard (1973). Octopamine-sensitive adenylate cyclase: evidence for a biological role of octopamine in nervous tissue, *Science* **180**:308–310.

Nathanson, J. A. and P. Greengard (1974). Serotonin-sensitive adenylate cyclase in neural tissue and its similarity to the serotonin receptor: a possible site of action of lysergic acid diethylamide, *Proc. Natl. Acad. Sci. U.S.A.* **71**:797–801.

Perkins, J. P. (1973). Adenyl cyclase, *Adv. Cyclic Nucleotide Res.* **3**:1–64.

Pomerantz, A. H., S. A. Rudolph, B. E. Haley, and P. Greengard (1975). Photoaffinity labeling of a protein kinase from bovine brain with 8-azido-adenosine 3′,5′-monophosphate, *Biochemistry* **14**:3858–3862.

Rall, T. W. and A. G. Gilman (1970). The role of cyclic AMP in the nervous system, *Neurosci. Res. Program Bull.* **8**:221–323.

Richelson, E. (1973). Stimulation of tyrosine hydroxylase activity in an adrenergic clone of mouse neuroblastoma by dibutyryl cyclic AMP, *Nature (London) New Biol.* **242**:175–177.

Robison, G. A., R. W. Butcher, and E. W. Sutherland (1971). *Cyclic AMP.* Academic Press, New York.

Romero, J. A., M. Zatz, and J. Axelrod (1975). Beta-adrenergic stimulation of pineal N-acetyltransferase: adenosine 3',5'-cyclic monophosphate stimulates both RNA and protein synthesis, *Proc. Natl. Acad. Sci. U.S.A.* **72**:2107–2111.

Roth, R. H., P. M. Salzman, and V. H. Morgenroth, III (1974). Noradrenergic neurons: allosteric activation of hippocampal tyrosine hydroxylase by stimulation of the locus coeruleus, *Biochem. Pharmacol.* **23**:2779–2784.

Siggins, G. R., E. F. Battenberg, B. J. Hoffer, F. E. Bloom, and A. L. Steiner (1973). Noradrenergic stimulation of cyclic adenosine monophosphate in rat Purkinje neurons: an immunocytochemical study, *Science* **179**:585–588.

Siggins, G. R., B. J. Hoffer, and F. E. Bloom (1971*a*). Studies on norepinephrine-containing afferents to Purkinje cells of rat cerebellum. III. Evidence for mediation of norepinephrine effects by cyclic 3',5'-adenosine monophosphate, *Brain Res.* **25**:535–553.

Siggins, G. R., A. P. Oliver, B. J. Hoffer, and F. E. Bloom (1971*b*). Cyclic adenosine monophosphate and norepinephrine: effects on transmembrane properties of cerebellar Purkinje cells, *Science* **171**:192–194.

Sloboda, R. D., S. A. Rudolph, J. L. Rosenbaum, and P. Greengard (1975). Cyclic AMP-dependent endogenous phosphorylation of a microtubule-associated protein, *Proc. Natl. Acad. Sci. U.S.A.* **72**:177–181.

Ueda, T. and P. Greengard (1977). Adenosine 3':5'-monophosphate-regulated phosphoprotein system of neuronal membranes. I. Solubilization, purification and some properties of an endogenous phosphoprotein, *J. Biol. Chem.*, in press.

Ueda, T., H. Maeno, and P. Greengard (1973). Regulation of endogenous phosphorylation of specific proteins in synaptic membrane fractions from rat brain by adenosine 3':5'-monophosphate, *J. Biol. Chem.* **248**:8295–8305.

Uno, I., T. Ueda, and P. Greengard (1977*a*). Adenosine 3':5'-monophosphate-regulated phosphoprotein system of neuronal membranes. II. Solubilization, purification and some properties of an endogenous cyclic AMP-dependent protein kinase, *J. Biol. Chem.*, in press.

Uno, I., T. Ueda, and P. Greengard (1977*b*). Adenosine 3':5'-monophosphate-regulated phosphoprotein system of neuronal membranes. III. Study of enzyme systems involved in phosphorylation and dephosphorylation of two endogenous phosphoproteins, *Arch. Biochem. Biophys.*, submitted for publication.

Volle, R. L. (1966). *Muscarinic and Nicotinic Stimulant Actions at Autonomic Ganglia.* Pergamon Press, New York.

Von Hungen, K. and S. Roberts (1973). Adenylate cyclase receptors for adrenergic neurotransmitters in rat cerebral cortex, *Eur. J. Biochem.* **36**:391–401.

Von Hungen, K. and S. Roberts (1974). Neurotransmitter-sensitive adenylate cyclase systems in the brain, pp. 231–281 in *Reviews of Neuroscience*, Vol. 1, Ehrenpreis, S. and I. J. Kopin, eds. Raven Press, New York.

Walsh, D. A., C. D. Ashby, C. Gonzalez, D. Calkins, E. H. Fischer, and E. G. Krebs (1971). Purification and characterization of a protein inhibitor of adenosine 3′,5′-monophosphate-dependent protein kinases, *J. Biol. Chem.* **246:**1977–1985.

Walsh, D. A., J. P. Perkins, and E. G. Krebs (1968). An adenosine 3′,5′-monophosphate dependent protein kinase from rabbit skeletal muscle, *J. Biol. Chem.* **243:**3763–3765.

Waymire, J. C., N. Weiner, and K. N. Prasad (1972). Regulation of tyrosine hydroxylase activity in cultured mouse neuroblastoma cells: elevation induced by analogs of adenosine 3′:5′-cyclic monophosphate, *Proc. Natl. Acad. Sci. U.S.A.* **69:**2241–2245.

Weight, F. F., G. Petzold, and P. Greengard (1974). Guanosine 3′,5′-monophosphate in sympathetic ganglia: increase associated with synaptic transmission, *Science* **186:**942–944.

Weisenberg, R. D. (1972). Microtubule formation in vitro in solutions containing low calcium concentrations, *Science* **177:**1104–1105.

Wuerker, R. B. and J. B. Kirkpatrick (1972). Neuronal microtubules, neurofilaments and microfilaments, *Int. Rev. Cytol.* **33:**45–75.

Membrane Fluidity Implicated in the Regulation of Decay of Post-Tetanic Potentiation

S. H. Barondes, W. T. Schlapfer, and P. B. J. Woodson

University of California, San Diego; and Veterans Administration Hospital, San Diego, California

The efficacy of chemical synaptic transmission, measured as the amplitude of the postsynaptic conductance change produced by a presynaptic spike, is subject to various modulations. One synaptic modulation that is relatively long-lived (minutes to hours), and that is seen at many, but not all, synapses, is post-tetanic potentiation (PTP). PTP is a transient increase in the efficacy of synaptic transmission, after a period of repetitive stimulation (for example, see Figure 1). Wherever PTP has been studied in detail, it has been found to be a presynaptic process, i.e., a change in the amount of transmitter released per presynaptic spike (Liley and North, 1953; Gage and Hubbard, 1966; McLachlan, 1975; Zucker, 1974; Magleby and Zengel, 1975a,b; Schlapfer, Tremblay, Woodson, and Barondes, 1976). Furthermore, at frog (Magleby and Zengel, 1975a) and rat neuromuscular junctions (Bennett, Florin, and Hall, 1975), sympathetic ganglia (McLachlan, 1975), and *Aplysia* central synapses (Schlapfer et al., 1976; Woodson, Schlapfer, and Barondes, 1976a), there is evidence that the change in transmitter release per spike underlying PTP is due to a change in the fraction of available transmitter released (also called the probability of release), and not due to a change in the amount of transmitter in the pool available for release.

Relatively little is presently known about the molecular basis of PTP. A first approximation, the "calcium accumulation hypothesis," has been proposed and supported by work at a number of neuromuscular junctions (Katz and Miledi, 1968; Rahamimoff, 1968; Weinreich, 1971;

Wilson and Skirboll, 1974; Bennett and Florin, 1975; Bennett et al., 1975). The purpose of this paper is to consider recent work that allows further development of an analysis of the mechanism of PTP. Three types of experimental findings direct this elaboration. (1) The rate of decay of PTP is modifiable independent of the amplitude of PTP, a finding at both mammalian (Liley and North, 1953) and amphibian (Magleby and Zengel, 1975a) neuromuscular junctions, as well as at two central synapses (called RC1-R15 and L10-L5) in the marine mollusc *Aplysia californica* (Schlapfer et al., 1976; Woodson et al., 1976a). (2) Treatments that influence membrane fluidity, such as temperature changes or additions of alcohols, have specific effects on PTP decay rate. (3) Physiological treatments like heterosynaptic stimulation, as well as putative neurotransmitters, also have specific effects on PTP decay rate (Woodson, Tremblay, Schlapfer, and Barondes, 1976b; Tremblay, Woodson, Schlapfer, and Barondes, 1976).

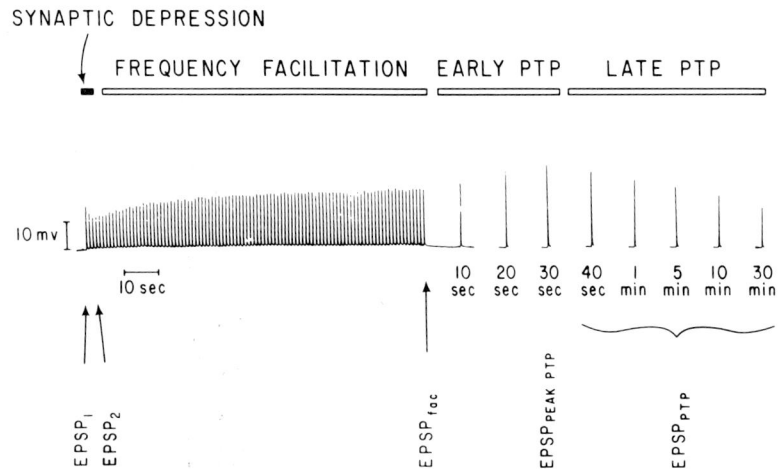

FIGURE 1. PTP recorded in cell R15 of the abdominal ganglion of *A. californica* after repetitive stimulation (100 pulses at 1/sec) of the right visceropleural connective with suction electrodes. The EPSPs (unitary and monosynaptic) were recorded intracellularly with one barrel of double barrel 3 M KCl filled microelectrodes; the second barrel was used to hyperpolarize R15 to −100 mV. The synaptic junction studied is called RC1-R15. Early PTP refers to the increase in EPSP amplitude after the train up to its peak value; late PTP decays thereafter. In addition to PTP, other modifications of synaptic transmission at this synapse are also shown. These are referred to as synaptic depression and frequency facilitation and are considered in detail in Schlapfer, Woodson, Tremblay, and Barondes (1974) and Schlapfer et al. (1976).

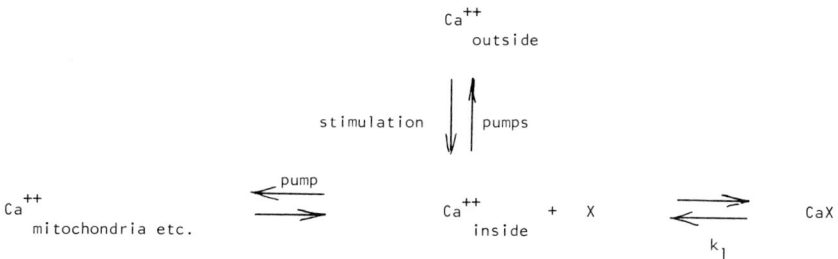

Efficiency of transmitter release = α [CaX]^n; n = 2 to 4

FIGURE 2. Calcium pools presumed to underlie the calcium accumulation hypothesis of post-tetanic potentiation. The amplitude of PTP is a function of the amount of CaX, whereas the rate of decay of PTP is a function of the rate constant of dissociation (K_1) of CaX.

The Calcium Accumulation Hypothesis

The sine qua non of transmitter release is the flow of calcium down a very steep concentration gradient into the presynaptic terminal upon the arrival of a spike (Llinás, 1977; Baker, 1972). The entry of calcium produces a tremendous acceleration and synchronization of the spontaneous exocytotic process. This is believed to be due to increased vesicle fusion with the presynaptic plasma membrane. The effect of calcium on exocytosis is thought to be mediated by its combination with a hypothetical molecular species, X (Figure 2), presumably located in the presynaptic terminal membrane (Parsegian, 1977). The exocytotic rate is controlled by the concentration of the complex CaX. In many systems, including neuromuscular junctions and the *Aplysia* CNS synapses cited above, the relationship between external Ca^{2+} and the amount of transmitter released per spike is a very steep accelerating function, often best described by power laws of $2 \leq n \leq 4$ (Rahamimoff, 1974). This would suggest that the amount of transmitter released per spike is proportional to a power of the concentration of the complex CaX (Figure 2). Such a relationship indicates that n CaX complexes must cooperate to produce the formation of an active release site at which one synaptic vesicle can fuse with the terminal membrane (Rahamimoff, 1974).

Given this analysis of the role of CaX in transmitter release, the central idea of the calcium accumulation hypothesis (or "residual calcium hypothesis") of PTP is that the rate of dissociation of CaX, k_1, is much slower than the rate of disappearance of active release sites, i.e., sites with n cooperating CaX complexes. The rapid rate of disappearance of active release sites, terminating spike-dependent transmitter release, may be a consequence of the following: (1) The intracellular calcium concentration is rapidly reduced after the spike by the active transmembrane calcium pumps and the sequestering of Ca^{2+} by mitochondria. This causes a shift in the equilibrium of the reaction $Ca^{2+} + X \rightleftarrows CaX$ toward dissociation of CaX. Because of the steep relationship between the exocytosis rate and the concentration of CaX, the rate of vesicle fusion events falls rapidly. (2) In addition, it is plausible to assume that a release site which was activiated by n CaX complexes is either destroyed by the vesicle fusion process or may have to wait a long time for the arrival of another synaptic vesicle.

Although exocytosis is rapidly terminated after a spike, the calcium accumulation hypothesis requires that k_1, the rate of dissociation of CaX (Figure 2), is much smaller than the rate at which exocytosis is terminated after a spike. There is, therefore, a residuum of CaX for some time after a spike, and calcium entering in response to a second spike will produce some CaX which will sum with the CaX remaining from the first spike. Therefore, the efficiency of the transmitter release process is increased for the second of two pulses. During repetitive stimulation there is a progressive accumulation of CaX and, therefore, a progressive increase in the efficiency of the transmitter release process.

According to the calcium accumulation hypothesis, the amplitude of PTP, i.e., the magnitude of the change in the efficiency of transmitter release upon repetitive stimulation, is the ratio of the nth power of the total (accumulated plus spike entered) amount of CaX evoking release after the train of stimulation to the nth power of the total (equilibrium CaX plus spike entered) amount of CaX evoking release after an isolated spike. The rate of decay of PTP is a function of k_1, the rate of dissociation of CaX. Because Ca_i is small, the rate of formation of CaX can be assumed to be small in the absence of stimulation.

The calcium accumulation hypothesis of PTP is supported at the rat diaphragm-phrenic nerve neuromuscular junction (Wilson and Skirboll, 1974), the frog sartorius neuromuscular junction (Rosenthal, 1969), the *Aplysia* synapse L10-L5 (Woodson et al., 1976a) and RC1-R15 (unpublished observations) by the observation that the magnitude of PTP is inversely correlated with the external calcium ion concentration.

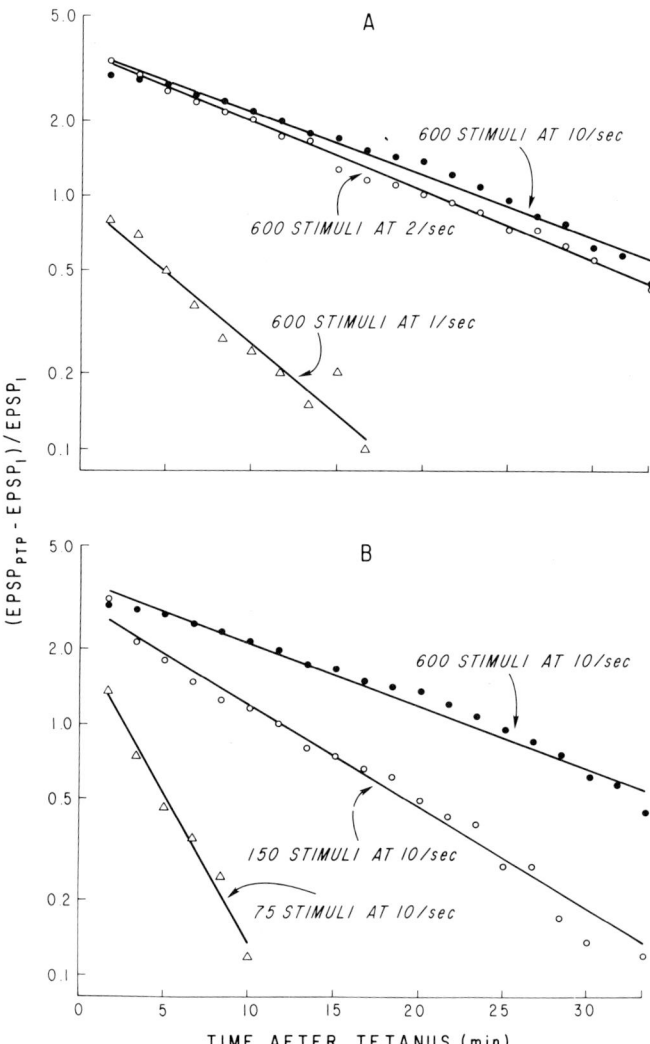

FIGURE 3. Decay of the PTP amplitude for different stimulus frequencies (A) and different numbers of stimuli at a constant frequency (B) at RC1-R15 in *Aplysia*. Test pulses were given every 100 sec after trains of the indicated duration and frequency. All data are from a single animal. A rest period of 20 min was allowed after the test EPSP had returned to control level before the next run was started. Return to the same stimulus paradigm (600 pulses at 10/sec) after 14 h of intracellular recording gave nearly identical results. The lines were obtained by linear regression analysis of the data points. From Schlapfer et al. (1976).

This relationship has been predicted for the calcium accumulation hypothesis by kinetic analyses (Rahamimoff, 1968).

The calcium accumulation hypothesis predicts that the magnitude of PTP should increase with longer trains of stimulation up to an asymptote, but the rate constant of decay of PTP should be invariant. The first prediction is indeed borne out (Liley and North, 1953; Schlapfer et al., 1976; Magleby and Zengel, 1975a,b; Woodson et al., 1976a). However, the rate constant of decay of PTP changes as a function of degree of stimulation. This latter observation occasions a modification of the calcium accumulation hypothesis.

The Rate Constant of PTP Decay Is Modified by Stimulation

At the frog sartorius neuromuscular junction (Magleby and Zengel, 1975a,b), the rat phrenic nerve-diaphragm neuromuscular junction (Liley and North, 1953), and at the central neuron-neuron synapses RC1-R15 and L10-L5 of *A. californica* (Schlapfer et al., 1976; Woodson et al., 1976a), PTP decays with a single exponential time course (Figure 3); i.e., the potentiated test postsynaptic potential (PSP) returns to the amplitude of the isolated control PSP (PSP_1) as a single exponential function of the time after a period of repetitive stimulation. On a plot of $\ln(EPSP_{PTP}\text{-}EPSP_1)/EPSP_1$ versus time (Figure 3), the zero time

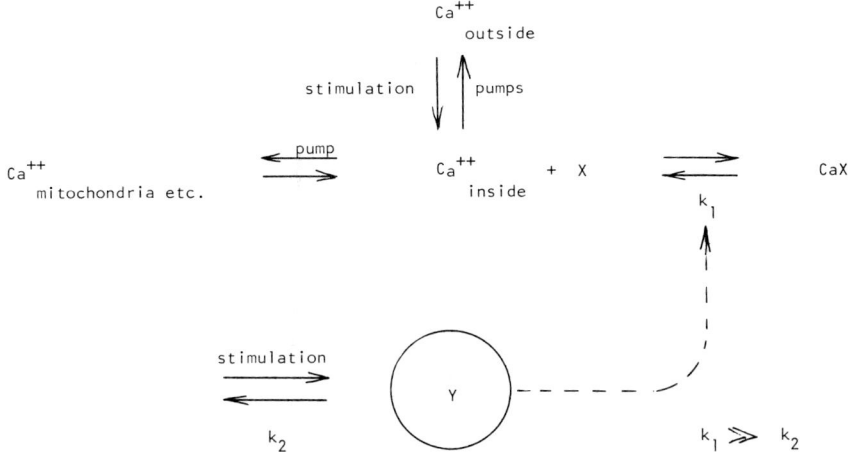

FIGURE 4. Elaboration of the calcium accumulation hypothesis to account for the modulation of the rate constant of PTP decay by a parameter, Y, dependent on stimulation. See text for discussion.

intercept is a measure of the PTP amplitude, i.e., the change in transmitter release per spike, and the slope represents the rate constant of decay of PTP. What is critical for the present discussion is that the rate constant of decay of PTP changes as a function of stimulus number or stimulus frequency (Figure 3). This observation is made not only at central synapses in *Aplysia* (Schlapfer et al., 1976; Woodson et al., 1976a), but also at neuromuscular junctions (Liley and North, 1953; Magleby and Zengel, 1975a).

These findings have led Magleby and Zengel (1975a) to propose that there must be a stimulus-sensitive parameter (Y of Figure 4) that controls the rate constant of PTP decay and that is distinct from the concentration of CaX. The possibility that k_1 is a function of the concentration of CaX is ruled out because CaX and, hence, PTP would then not decay with a single exponential time course. The value of the parameter Y is thought to be elevated by stimulation and to return to its resting value with a time course that is much slower than the time course of decay of PTP. In this way, the single exponential decay of PTP is preserved.

The Fluidity of the Particular Membrane Lipids Associated with CaX Could Determine Its Dissociation Constant

Insight into the possible nature of parameter Y has been provided by our experimental findings (described below) that agents that influence membrane fluidity influence the rate constant of decay of PTP. Prompted by three experimental results, we wish to examine the plausibility of the hypothesis that the freedom of movement in the membrane of the complex CaX is an important factor in determining the magnitude of k_1; and, furthermore, that the regulation of the freedom of movement of CaX by Y is the mechanism whereby the decay rate of PTP is physiologically regulated. We prefer to continue with the theoretical treatment before describing the experiments that prompted this analysis, to avoid interruption of the theoretical line of argument. To be considered, first, are general observations that support the idea that the freedom of movement of CaX can have a significant effect on the dissociation rate constant of CaX.

The Ca^{2+} to X bond will break when the vibratory energy along the bond axis equals the bond energy. Because X is confined to the presynaptic terminal membrane, the molecule X must vibrate within the medium of the lipids surrounding it. This medium is viscous and will offer opposition to the movement of X. The damping effect on the vibration of the CaX bond will slow down the rate of dissociation of CaX; and the effect will be even greater if X is either a polyvalent chelator of Ca^{2+}, making a number of separate bonds, or a group of molecules gathered together by the Ca^{2+}, which they complex. The possibility of multiple bonding to the Ca^{2+} is likely (Williams, 1975), and serves to amplify the vibration damping effect on k_1 by providing more routes for the dissipation of the vibratory energy of the CaX bond. Thus it is expected that the rate constant of dissociation should be very susceptible to the "fluidity" of the particular lipids (Miller and Pang, 1976) associated with CaX. The fluidity of a given patch of lipids is a way of speaking about the extent to which the lipids deviate from a solid crystalline structure and tend toward a looser, liquid crystal state.

Like any solvent, the lipids of a patch will exhibit a slowing down of molecular movement (decrease in fluidity) as the temperature is lowered, and, at some point, the lipid solvent will "freeze" and the fluidity will exhibit a sharp drop. The binding of Ca^{2+} to an artifical membrane of methyl phosphatidic acid has been studied as a function of the fluidity of the membrane (Träuble and Eibl, 1975). It was found that upon going through the freezing point, called the phase-transition temperature, the amount of Ca^{2+} bound to the membrane changed dramatically, such that more Ca^{2+} was bound to the membrane in the less fluid state. This observation supports the inference that the fluidity of the environment of a membrane Ca^{2+} complex can affect the rate of dissociation of the complex.

It may perhaps be objected that any but enormous changes in k_1 will be of little significance to the net rate of disappearance of CaX because of the high mass action drive to dissociate in the presence of low Ca_i. However, it should be noted that k_1 is very low according to the basic premise of the calcium accumulation hypothesis, and is indeed the rate-limiting factor in the decay of CaX. Otherwise, there can be no residual calcium for subsequent spikes to add to. Any change in the rate constant k_1 will then have a strong effect on the amount of CaX remaining at a given time after a train of stimuli.

We now turn our attention to a general consideration of the factors controlling the fluidity of membrane components, so as to be able to interpret the experiments that bear on our hypothesis. The fluidity of a patch of lipids is the result of a balance between forces that promote independent molecular movement and those that tend to correlate the movements of molecules (Träuble and Eibl, 1975). Among these factors (reviewed by Träuble and Eibl, 1975) are thermal vibrations, electrostatic interactions due to dipole moments and ionization in the phospholipid head groups, and structural irregularities in the fatty acid side chains (e.g., double bonds, especially in the *trans* configuration). Thus, changes in the biochemical composition of a membrane, such as alterations of the degree of unsaturation of the fatty acids or changes in the nature of the lipid head groups, will act to regulate the fluidity. We have already mentioned the effects of heating up the membrane; indeed, temperature appears to be a very common regulator of membrane fluidity. Changes in pH and ionic strength of the aqueous medium adjoining a membrane will change the degree of ionization of the head groups, and will also alter the screening of the charges and dipoles. Depending on the particular lipids, changes in pH or ionic strength can therefore either increase or decrease the membrane fluidity.

Another way to regulate the fluidity of a phase of lipids is by varying the concentration of small "solute" molecules in the phase. By the colligative properties of solutions (Andrews, 1976), such molecules will depress the freezing point of the phase, i.e., lower its transition temperature. If the molecule also has specific interactions with lipids, the forces between lipid molecules may be further modified. Such molecules can either fluidize or rigidify a given phase of lipids (Miller and Pang, 1976). Candidates for this sort of molecule are cholesterol, free fatty acids, and amphiphilic pharmacological agents, such as alcohols and general anesthetics (Seeman, 1972).

We should now also point out that Ca^{2+} itself, in appropriate concentrations, can influence membrane fluidity. It is not likely that this is an important regulator of PTP decay rate, since the amount of Ca^{2+} that enters per spike is probably not sufficient. Effects of Ca^{2+} on lipid fluidity in relatively homogenous systems require that the ratio Ca^{2+} per lipid be in the range of 1 (Träuble and Eibl, 1975). Considering the small number of Ca^{2+} molecules that enter per spike (Llinás, 1977), and the large number of lipid molecules in a nerve terminal membrane, the stoichiometry does not suggest this possibility. However, heterogeneities or special properties of nerve ending membrane lipids might make such a possibility operative. It may also be argued that the Ca^{2+} within CaX may locally regulate fluidity. Whereas this is possible, it should be emphasized that the *entity* CaX cannot control its own decay rate and yet decay with single exponential kinetics.

Experimental Evidence That the Fluidity of Critical Presynaptic Membrane Components Limits Decay Rate of PTP

Two types of experiments have led us to infer that the fluidity of a critical presynaptic membrane component, presumably contained

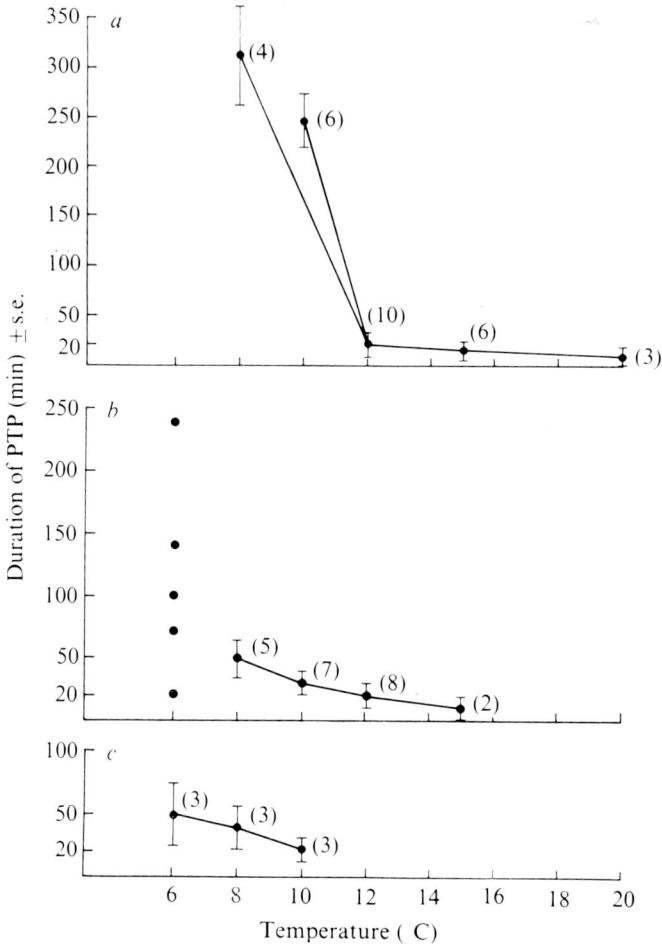

FIGURE 5. Dependence of the duration of PTP on temperature at RC1-R15 in *Aplysia*, and its adaptation. Trains of 100 pulses at 2/sec were given with the preparation kept at the temperature indicated. The duration of the PTP was estimated by administering test pulses at 10-min intervals at this same temperature until the size of the EPSP returned to the size of the first EPSP of the train. The number of experiments at each point is shown in parentheses. (a) Pooled data from 10 preparations. Every preparation was tested at 12°C. In six preparations, the temperature was then lowered from 12 to 10°C, whereas, in four other preparations, the temperature was taken from 12°C directly to 8°C. (b) Pooled data from four animals that were maintained at 11°C rather than the usual 20°C for 2 days before the experiment. The duration of the PTP was only slightly prolonged when the temperature was lowered from 12 to 10 or 8°C, but at 6°C, some preparations showed an abrupt prolongation of the PTP. None of the preparations treated in this fashion showed a temperature transition between 12 and 10°C. (c) Three isolated ganglia were maintained at 10°C for 4 h before stimulation. In these conditions, the duration of the PTP measured at 10°C was short compared with control animals (a), and no abrupt prolongation occurred when the temperature was lowered to 6°C. From Schlapfer et al. (1975).

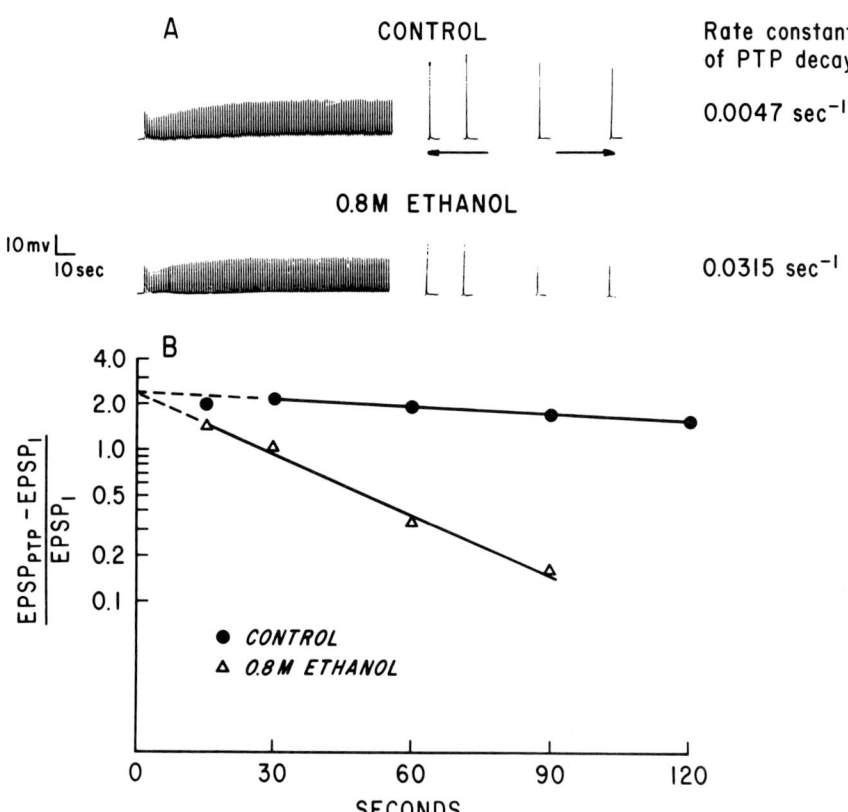

FIGURE 6. Bath application of 0.8 M ethanol increases the rate constant of the decay of PTP. (A) Intracellular record of the EPSPs recorded in cell R15 of the abdominal ganglion of *Aplysia* on stimulation of the right visceropleural connective during a train of 100 pulses at 1/sec was followed by test pulses at 15-sec intervals and then every 30 sec. Thirty minutes after a control train, ethanol perfusion was begun, and a train was given 30 min later in the presence of ethanol. Ethanol had no effect on the amplitude of the EPSPs during the train, but selectively shortened the duration of PTP. (B) During PTP, the amplitude of the test EPSP ($EPSP_{PTP}$) returned toward the size of the first EPSP of a train ($EPSP_1$) with a single exponential time course. The rate constant of the decay of PTP (the slope of the straight line fitted to the data points after the peak by linear regression analyses) was increased by the application of ethanol. The zero time intercept (a measure of the PTP amplitude) was not affected significantly by ethanol. Data are from a single preparation. Symbols: ●, control; △, 0.8 M ethanol. From Woodson et al. (1976a).

within the nerve terminal membrane, regulates parameter Y, and, hence, the rate constant of decay of PTP. To conduct these experiments we have used two of the classical treatments known to influence membrane fluidity in other systems—changes in temperature of the system and effects of addition of alcohols. These experiments have been published (Schlapfer, Woodson, Smith, Tremblay, and Barondes, 1975; Woodson, Traynor, Schlapfer, and Barondes, 1976c), and will be presented only briefly here.

Effects of temperature were studied by administering trains of stimulation at a number of temperatures between 20 and 7.5°C, and observing the duration of PTP. We found that at RC1-R15, the duration of PTP was a decreasing function of temperature. As the temperature was lowered from 20 to 12°C, the duration of PTP became slightly longer. The most striking finding, however, was that upon lowering the temperature from 12 to 10°C there was a striking 10-fold increase in the duration of PTP (Figure 5) (Schlapfer et al., 1975). This phenomenon resembles the temperature transition of lipid phases discussed above. The kinetics of decay of PTP at the transition temperature or below were actually more complex than observed at normal temperature (15°C). Our impression, subject to further experimental analysis, is that PTP first decayed to a higher "equilibrium" level of excitatory postsynaptic potential (EPSP) amplitude, rather than decaying to the amplitude of initial isolated EPSP. Whereas the details of decay at the transition temperature have not been completely analyzed as yet, what is clear is that there is a striking effect of temperature reduction on PTP decay reminiscent of temperature transitions of lipids. This is consistent with the possibility that fluidity of a presynaptic membrane component regulates PTP decay rate.

We have also studied the effect of ethanol and other aliphatic alcohols on PTP decay rate. These are small amphiphilic molecules that can interpolate into the membrane (Träuble and Eibl, 1975). We found that these agents strikingly accelerate the rate of decay of PTP (Figure 6). Furthermore, potency of the aliphatic alcohols correlates with their lipid solubility (Figure 7). Therefore, these experiments provide further support for the concept that fluidity of a critical presynaptic membrane component regulates the rate constant of decay of PTP. We also tested the possibility that addition of ethanol can affect the transition temperature. As expected, in the presence of alcohol the normal transition temperature behavior is not found consistent with the possibility that ethanol and temperature are influencing the same type of process.

An interesting and unexpected finding in these studies is that both the temperature effect (Figure 5) (Schlapfer et al., 1975) and the ethanol effect (Figure 8) (Traynor, Woodson, Schlapfer, and Barondes, 1976) show tolerance. Details of these experiments have been published elsewhere. What we mean by tolerance is that previous exposure to low

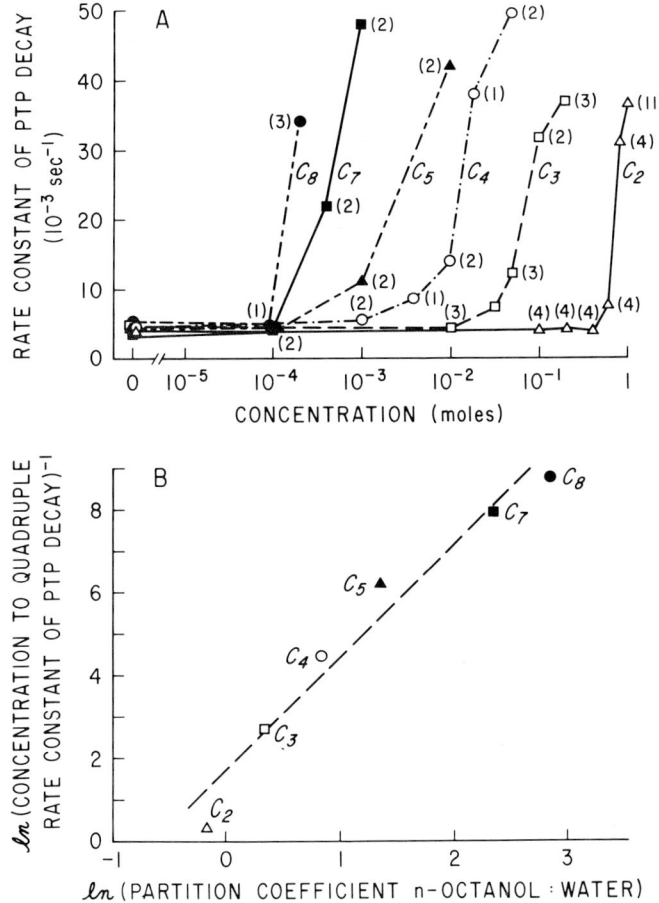

FIGURE 7. (A) Potency of aliphatic alcohols in increasing the rate constant of PTP decay at RC1-R15 in *Aplysia*. Symbols: ●, C_8; ■, C_7; ▲, C_5; ○, C_4; □, C_3; △, C_2. The size of the carbon chain is indicated by the number (C_2 is ethanol; C_8 is *n*-octanol). An aliphatic alcohol (in fortified artificial seawater) was perfused for 30 min, beginning 30 min after a control train; and then a train was given in the presence of the alcohol. In contrast with ethanol, the higher alcohols reduced the amplitudes of all EPSPs. PTP still decayed, however, with a single exponential time course with a rate constant that was readily determined. Each data point represents the average value obtained from three different preparations, except for ethanol, where the number of preparations at each data point is indicated. Note that the effect of each alcohol increases markedly over a narrow range of concentration. (B) The potency of the effect of the different alcohols (measured as the concentration, C, needed to increase the rate of decay of PTP fourfold) correlates with the lipophilicity of the alcohol (as measured by the *n*-octanol: water partition coefficient, P). The data points were obtained from (A) by interpolating the concentration of each alcohol that would give a rate constant of PTP decay of 20×10^{-3} sec^{-1}. A plot of $\ln(1/C)$ against $\ln P$ gives a straight line with the equation $\ln(1/C) = 2.71 \ln P - 1.66$. Other biological systems susceptible to alcohols similarly give straight lines in these coordinates. Symbols as in (A). From Woodson et al. (1976a).

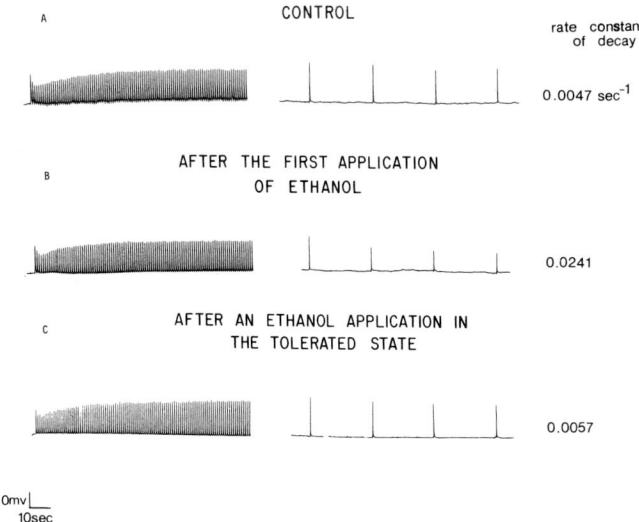

FIGURE 8. Tolerance of the specific effect of ethanol in accelerating PTP decay. Intracellular records of the EPSPs in cell R15 of the abdominal ganglion of *Aplysia* during stimulation of the right visceropleural connective by a train of 100 pulses at 1 pulse/sec were followed by two test pulses at 15-sec intervals and then test pulses every 30 sec. (A) Control preparation. (B) The stimulus pattern was given 30 min after starting the first application of artificial seawater containing 0.8 M ethanol. The response during the train of stimuli is similar to that of the control preparation; however, the PTP observed after the train decays with a much faster time course. Beginning 10 min after this train, the preparation was washed for 120 min before the second application of ethanol. (C) The stimulus pattern was given 30 min after starting the fifth application of 0.8 M ethanol. The rate of decay of PTP here is similar to that in the control preparation. The calculated rate constant of PTP decay (k) is shown for each case. From Traynor et al. (1976).

temperature or repetitive exposure to ethanol using a specific experimental paradigm (for details see Schlapfer et al., 1975; Traynor et al., 1976) blocks the effects of treatments on PTP decay rate. Such adaptation is reminiscent of adaptive processes in bacteria to alterations in membrane fluidity (Ingram, 1976; Sinensky, 1971). The fact that adaptive responses are seen both in bacterial reaction and PTP reaction to these types of treatments provides further evidence of similar regulatory processes operative in both systems.

This series of studies, therefore, provides some experimental support for the contention that the parameter Y that regulates the rate constant of decay of PTP is, or is influenced by, the state of fluidity of some critical component in the presynaptic membrane. This critical component is presumably associated with (contained within and/or around) and regulating the dissociation of CaX.

Effects of Biogenic Amines and Heterosynaptic Input on PTP Decay at RC1-R15

Although they have no direct bearing on the general line of theoretical development that we have presented, several other observations about the modifiability of the rate constant of decay of PTP at RC1-R15 should be noted. We have found that both heterosynaptic input and biogenic amines, including dopamine and serotonin, affect the rate constant of decay of PTP at this synapse. For example, upon administration of a burst of stimulation to the branchial nerve of the *Aplysia* abdominal ganglion at 4/sec for 5 sec during a train of stimuli to RC1-R15, the ensuing PTP observed when the train is terminated decays at a more rapid rate (Figure 9). This effect persists even though the transient depression of the EPSP recorded at RC1-R15 immediately after the

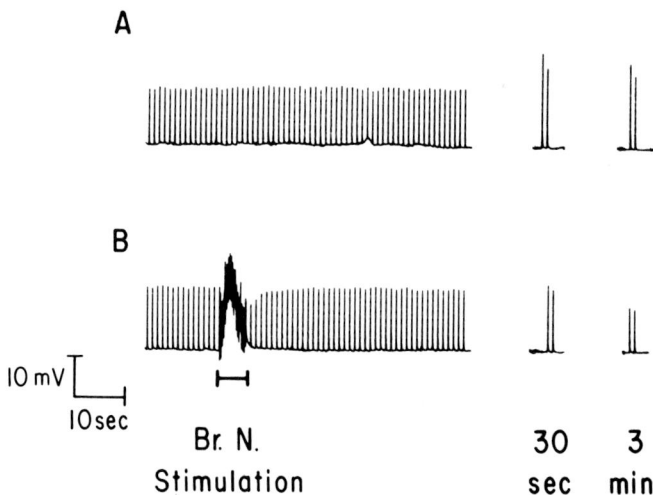

FIGURE 9. Effect of stimulation (4/sec for 5 sec) of the branchial nerve (BrN) on the EPSP amplitude in cell R15 of *Aplysia* during and after a train of EPSPs was obtained by stimulation of the right visceropleural connective. Only the end of each train of stimuli to the right connective is shown. Whereas the amplitude of the EPSP during the train returns very quickly to the control size after BrN stimulation, homosynaptic test EPSPs after the train (PTP) are decreased in amplitude for longer periods. From Woodson et al. (1976c).

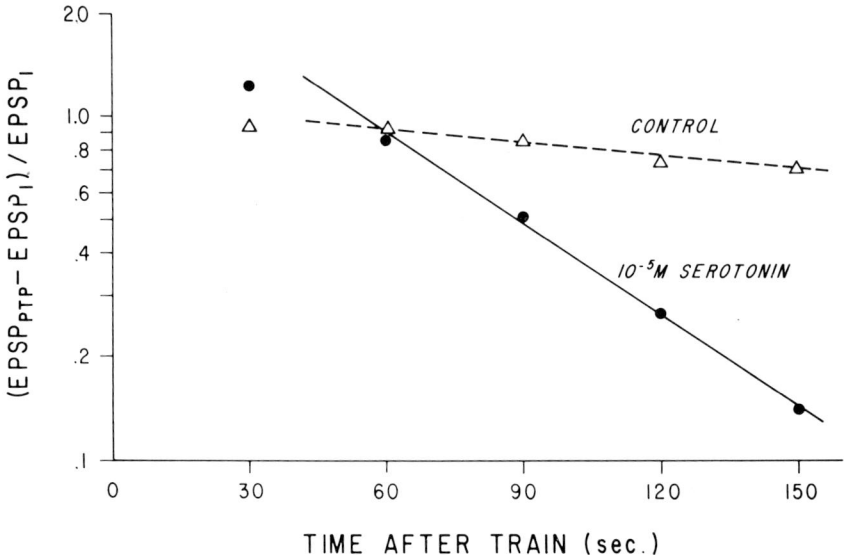

FIGURE 10. Decay of the PTP amplitude at RC1-R15 in *Aplysia* is accelerated by bath application of serotonin. Perfusion with 10^{-5} M serotonin was begun 30 min before a train of 100 pulses at 1/sec. The finding that peak PTP amplitude in serotonin is higher than control reflects the fact that $EPSP_1$ is lower in serotonin than in the control situation. From Tremblay et al. (1976).

branchial nerve stimulation is rapidly reversed by continuing homosynaptic stimulation (for details, see Woodson et al., 1976*b*). Therefore, there seems to be a special effect of the heterosynaptic input in controlling the rate constant of decay of PTP. Similar effects are observed when biogenic amines, including dopamine and serotonin, are added to the perfusion medium (Tremblay et al., 1976). For example, perfusion with serotonin leads to striking acceleration of PTP decay rate (Figure 10). Serotonin is more potent than dopamine; of the two, only the latter is antagonized by haloperidol and propanolol (Tremblay et al., 1976). The effects of heterosynaptic stimulation on PTP decay are also antagonized by haloperidol (Woodson et al., 1976*b*), raising the possibility that it may be mediated by a direct or indirect dopaminergic input onto the presynaptic nerve terminal at RC1-R15.

These experimental results are of interest in several regards. First, they show that treatments, including physiological treatment like heterosynaptic stimulation, can express their effects on synaptic transmission by modifying the rate constant of decay of a specific form of modifiable synaptic transmission, PTP. In addition, however, these results can be interpreted in the context of the membrane fluidity hypothesis mentioned above. There is indeed precedent for the inference that biogenic amines can affect membrane fluidity. For example, norepinephrine has been shown to significantly alter the fluidity of erythrocyte membranes, possibly through the accumulation of cyclic AMP (McConnel, 1975). Therefore our general analysis of a mechanism regulating PTP decay rate provides clues about a specific physiological regulatory mechanism (heterosynaptic stimulation) that acts on PTP decay rate.

CONCLUSION

This paper has been concerned with elaboration and expansion of a molecular analysis of PTP. We have reviewed the calcium accumulation

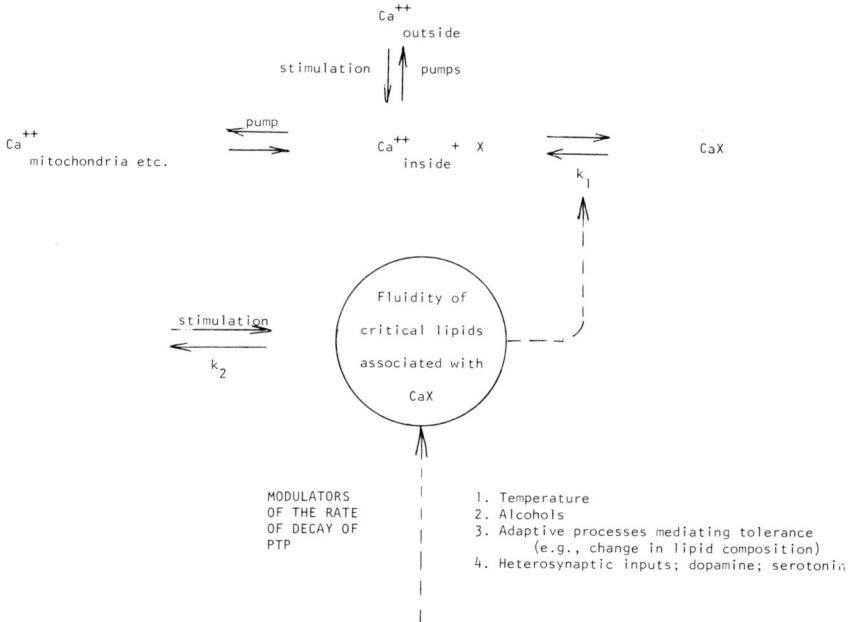

FIGURE 11. Further elaboration of the calcium accumulation hypothesis. We propose that the fluidity of the lipids associated with (either surrounding or part of) CaX molecules within the membrane is regulated and thereby controls the rate constant of dissociation (k_1) of CaX that in turn regulates the PTP decay rate. The fluidity of critical lipids is presumed to be influenced both by stimulation and by the treatments listed as modulators of the rate constant of decay of PTP.

hypothesis and shown why an additional parameter, called "Y," is necessary to explain the modifiable rate constant of decay of PTP. Furthermore, we have shown that experimental treatments, such as changes in temperature or addition of aliphatic alcohols, can change the rate constant of PTP decay. This suggests that the parameter Y is related to fluidity of critical membrane components associated with residual calcium complexes traditionally referred to as CaX. Finally, we have called attention to the fact that other treatments, such as heterosynaptic stimulation or biogenic amines, can also influence the rate constant of decay of PTP, and that these effects can be interpreted in the light of previous considerations. Figure 11, then, presents our current elaboration of the calcium accumulation hypothesis summarizing these various considerations.

ACKNOWLEDGMENTS

This research has been supported by the Veterans Administration Hospital, San Diego, and a grant from the National Institute on Alcohol Abuse and Alcoholism.

REFERENCES

Andrews, F. C. (1976). Colligative properties of simple solutions, *Science* **194**:567–571.

Baker, P. F. (1972). Transport and metabolism of calcium ions in nerve, *Progr. Biophys. Mol. Biol.* **24**:177–223.

Bennett, M. R. and T. Florin (1975). An electrophysiological analysis of the effect of Ca ions on neuromuscular transmission in the mouse vas deferens, *Br. J. Pharmacol.* **55**:97–104.

Bennett, M. R., T. Florin, and R. Hall (1975). The effect of calcium ions on the binomial statistic parameters which control acetylcholine release at synapses in striated muscle, *J. Physiol. (London)* **247**:429–446.

Gage, P. W. and J. I. Hubbard (1966). An investigation of the post-tetanic potentiation of end-plate potentials at a mammalian neuromuscular junction, *J. Physiol. (London)* **184**:353–375.

Ingram, L. O. (1976). Adaptation of membrane lipids to alcohols, *J. Bacteriol.* **125**:670–678.

Katz, B. and R. Miledi (1968). The role of calcium in neuromuscular facilitation, *J. Physiol. (London)* **195**:481–492.

Liley, A. W. and K. A. K. North (1953). An electrical investigation of effects of repetitive stimulation on mammalian neuromuscular junction, *J. Neurophysiol.* **16**:509–527.

Llinás, R. (1977). Electrophysiological measurements of presynaptic calcium currents and their relationship to transmitter release, pp. 139–160 in *Society for Neuroscience Symposia*, Vol. 2, Cowan, W. M. and J. A. Ferrendelli, eds. Society for Neuroscience, Bethesda, Md.

Magleby, K. L. and J. E. Zengel (1975a). A dual effect of repetitive stimulation on post-tetanic potentiation of transmitter release at the frog neuromuscular junction, *J. Physiol. (London)* **245**:163–182.

Magleby, K. L. and J. E. Zengel (1975b). A quantitative description of tetanic and post-tetanic potentiation of transmitter release at the frog neuromuscular junction, *J. Physiol. (London)* **245**:183–208.

McConnell, H. M. (1975). Changes in lipid bilayers, pp. 123–131 in *Functional Linkage in Biomolecular Systems*, Schmitt, F. O., D. M. Schneider, and D. M. Crothers, eds. Raven Press, New York.

McLachlan, E. M. (1975). An analysis of the release of acetylcholine from preganglionic nerve terminals, *J. Physiol. (London)* **245**:447–466.

Miller, K. W. and K. Y. Pang (1976). General anesthetics can selectively perturb lipid bilayer membranes, *Nature (London)* **263**:253–255.

Parsegian, V. A. (1977). Diffusion of calcium and its influence on vesicle-membrane interactions, pp. 161–171 in *Society for Neuroscience Symposia*, Vol. 2, Cowan, W. M. and J. A. Ferrendelli, eds. Society for Neuroscience, Bethesda, Md.

Rahamimoff, R. (1968). A dual effect of calcium ions on neuromuscular facilitation, *J. Physiol. (London)* **195**:471–489.

Rahamimoff, R. (1974). Modulation of transmitter release at the neuromuscular junction, pp. 943–952 in *The Neurosciences. Third Study Program*, Schmitt, F. O. and F. G. Worden, eds. MIT Press, Cambridge.

Rosenthal, J. (1969). Post-tetanic potentiation at the neuromuscular junction of the frog, *J. Physiol. (London)* **203**:121–133.

Schlapfer, W. T., J. P. Tremblay, P. B. J. Woodson, and S. H. Barondes (1976). Frequency facilitation and post-tetanic potentiation of a unitary synaptic potential in *Aplysia californica* are limited by different processes, *Brain Res.* **109**:1–20.

Schlapfer, W. T., P. B. J. Woodson, G. A. Smith, J. P. Tremblay, and S. H. Barondes (1975). Marked prolongation of post-tetanic potentiation at a transition temperature and its adaptation, *Nature (London)* **258**:623–625.

Schlapfer, W. T., P. B. J. Woodson, J. P. Tremblay, and S. H. Barondes (1974). Depression and frequency facilitation at a synapse in *Aplysia californica*: evidence for regulation by availability of transmitter, *Brain Res.* **76**:267–280.

Seeman, P. (1972). The membrane actions of anesthetics and tranquilizers, *Pharmacol. Rev.* **24**:583–655.

Sinensky, M. (1971). Temperature control of phospholipid biosynthesis in *Escherichia coli*, *J. Bacteriol.* **106**:449–455.

Träuble, H. and H. Eibl (1975). Molecular interactions in lipid bilayers, pp. 59–90 in *Functional Linkage in Biomolecular Systems*, Schmitt, F. O., D. M. Schneider, and D. M. Crothers, eds. Raven Press, New York.

Traynor, M. E., P. B. J. Woodson, W. T. Schlapfer, and S. H. Barondes (1976). Sustained tolerance to a specific effect of ethanol on post-tetanic potentiation in *Aplysia*, *Science* **193**:510–511.

Tremblay, J. P., P. B. J. Woodson, W. T. Schlapfer, and S. H. Barondes (1976). Dopamine, serotonin and related compounds: pre-synaptic effects on synaptic depression, frequency facilitation and post-tetanic potentiation at an identified synapse in *Aplysia californica*, *Brain Res.* **109**:61–81.

Weinreich, D. (1971). Ionic mechanism of post-tetanic potentiation at the neuromuscular junction of the frog, *J. Physiol. (London)* **212**:431–446.

Williams, R. J. P. (1975). The binding of metal ions to membranes and its consequences, pp. 106–121 in *Biological Membranes*, Parson, D. S., ed. Clarendon Press, Oxford.

Wilson, D. F. and L. R. Skirboll (1974). Basis for post-tetanic potentiation at the mammalian neuromuscular junction, *Am. J. Physiol.* **227**:92–95.

Woodson, P. B. J., W. T. Schlapfer, and S. H. Barondes (1976a). Amplitude and decay rate of post-tetanic potentiation controlled by separate stimulus-history sensitive systems, *Abstr. Annu. Meet. Soc. Neurosci.*, 6th, Toronto, p. 999.

Woodson, P. B. J., J. P. Tremblay, W. T. Schlapfer, and S. H. Barondes (1976b). Heterosynaptic inhibition modifies pre-synaptic plasticities of the transmission process at a synapse in *Aplysia californica, Brain Res.* **109**:83–95.

Woodson, P. B. J., M. E. Traynor, W. T. Schlapfer, and S. H. Barondes (1976c). Increased membrane fluidity implicated in acceleration of decay of post-tetanic potentiation by alcohols, *Nature (London)* **260**:797–799.

Zucker, R. S. (1974). Characteristics of crayfish neuromuscular facilitation and their calcium dependence, *J. Physiol. (London)* **241**:91–110.

KEY WORD INDEX

Acetylcholine, 85, 176, 217, 249, 269, 294, 322, 343, 403
N-Acetyltransferase, 378, 429
ACTH, 310
Action potentials, 356
"Active zones" in nerve terminals, 221
Adenylate cyclase, 384, 407
   diurnal variation of activity in pineal gland, 388
   neurotransmitter-sensitive adenylate cyclase, 410
   norepinephrine-sensitive adenylate cyclase, 414
   octopamine-sensitive adenylate cyclase, 414
   pineal gland β-adrenergic receptor, 384
Adrenal medulla, 294
β-Adrenergic receptor, 378
   pineal gland, 376
β-Adrenergic stimulation, 382
Adrenocortical cells, 196
Aequorin, 143
Alcohols, 446
Allophenics, 47
N-Allylnorcyclazocine, 294
γ-Aminobutyric acid (see GABA)
3-Aminopyridine, 144
4-Aminopyridine, 215
Amphid, 7
Angiotensin, 340
Angiotensin II, 250
   blockade by P 113, 326
   blood-brain barrier, 324
   direct neuronal effects, 322
   endogenous levels in brain, 331
   local ischemia hypothesis, 327
   metabolic pathway in brain, 308
   peripheral versus CNS effects, 311
   receptors in anterior ventral third ventricle, 324
   receptors in area postrema, 315
   receptors in subfornical organ, 320
   receptors in subnucleus medialis, 319
   sites of CNS receptors, 315
   surface receptor hypothesis, 330
   thirst hormone, 311

Angiotensinogenase, 309
Anterior commissure, 314
Antipsychotic drugs, 412
Aplysia californica, 341, 435
Area postrema, 315
Ariolimax californicus, 197
Aromatic amino acid decarboxylase, 377
Aspartate, 257
Atropine, 89, 294, 405
Autapses, 88
Axoplasmic transport, 121

Baclofen, 252
Bag cells, 344
Behavioral mutants, 1
Benzomorphans, 299
Biogenic amines, 449
Blood-brain barrier, 324
Bombesin, 243
Bradykinin, 243, 322
Brown widow spider venom, 224
Bursting pacemaker potential, 343

Caenorhabditis elegans, 1
   anatomical defects in sensory mutants, 13
   chemoreceptor structure, 7
   chemotactic behavior, 3
   chemotactic receptor location, 5
   classification of sensory mutants, 12
   isolation of sensory mutants, 8
   nervous system, 2
   reproductive physiology, 18
   sperm-defective mutants, 16
   sperm structure, 17
Calcium, 139, 218
   accumulation hypothesis, 435
   action potentials in pedal glands, 202
   Ca^{2+} gates, 149
   channels, 221
   charge neutralization of vesicles, 165
   conductance, 173
   diffusion in presynaptic terminal, 164
   extrusion, 178
   intraterminal storage, 184

mathematical model of Ca^{2+} gates, 149
mucous secretion from pedal gland, 209
neurotransmitter release, 356
presynaptic I_{Ca}, 144
regulation of neurosecretory peptides, 360
regulation of pacemaker conductance, 351
regulation of peptide effects on neurons, 362
squid giant synapse, 140
stimulus-secretion coupling, 195
studies in synaptosomes, 172
transmitter release, 139
two uptake mechanisms in nerve terminals, 187
vesicle-membrane interaction, 161
Calcium-dependent protein phosphorylation, 426
Carbachol, 328
Catecholamine, 86
Caudate nucleus, 411
Cell culture
  sympathetic neurons, 83
Cell-substratum adhesion, 67
  developmental implications, 78
  direction of neuronal growth, 72
  effect on neuronal growth, 70
  growth cone function, 77
  types of substrata, 69
Cerebellum, 409
  development, 60
  Purkinje cell degeneration, 54
  reeler mutant, 55
  staggerer mutant, 57
Cerebral cortex
  development, 27
Chemotactic behavior, 3
Chemotaxis, 3
Chimeras, 47
  β-glucuronidase, 52
  muscular dystrophy (dy) gene, 59
  photoreceptor degeneration, 48
  production, 48
  Purkinje cell, 52
  Purkinje cell degeneration, 60
  Purkinje cell degeneration (pcd) gene, 54
  reeler (rl) gene, 55

retinal degeneration (rd) gene, 48
retinal dystrophy (rdy) gene, 50
staggerer (sg) gene, 57
β-Chlorophenyl-GABA, 252
Cholera toxin, 379
Cholinergic receptor, 399
Cholinergic synapses, 85
Cilia, 7
Coated vesicles, 230
Cobalt, 203
Colchicine, 121
Compound exocytosis, 198
Compound eye, 92
Contact guidance, 104
Corpus callosum, 30
Corpus striatum, 412
Cyclic AMP, 3, 378, 401, 451
Cyclic AMP-dependent protein kinase, 380
Cyclic GMP, 3, 403
Cyclic nucleotides, 376, 399
  cerebellar Purkinje cell, 409
  diurnal variation in β-adrenergic response in pineal gland, 382
  effect of norepinephrine on cyclic GMP in pineal gland, 394
  effect on N-acetyltransferase activity in pineal gland, 378
  influence on activity of CNS tyrosine hydroxylase, 424
  neurotransmitter-sensitive adenylate cyclases, 410
  phosphorylation of microtubular protein, 422
  phosphorylation of synaptic membrane proteins, 416
  possible role in modulation of membrane potential, 415
  regulation of protein synthesis, 428
  role in protein phosphorylation, 414
  sensitivity to β-adrenergic stimulation in pineal gland, 383
  superior cervical ganglion, 404

Daphnia, 106
Delayed rectifying conductance, 354
Denervation supersensitivity, 389
Desensitization, 344

KEY WORD INDEX

Desmethylimipramine, 85
Development, 1, 68, 82, 92
  cerebellum, 60
  cerebral cortex, 27
Differentiation, 83, 105
[^{3}H]Dihydroalprenolol, 384
Dinitrophenol, 185
Dopamine, 83, 282, 294, 401, 449
  receptor, 411
Dopamine-sensitive adenylate cyclase, 404
Drosophila, 107

Electrically coupled cells, 196
Eledoisin, 243, 322
Endocrine, 195
Endocytosis, 215
Endoplasmic reticulum, 191
α-Endorphin, 292
β-Endorphin, 292, 369
γ-Endorphin, 292
Endorphins, 369
  antinociceptive agents, 301
  binding assays for opiate receptors, 296
  bioassay for opiate activity, 298
  inactivation, 303
  role in sexual function, 303
  structure-activity relationships, 291
Enkephalins, 258, 369
  antinociceptive agents, 301
  binding assays for opiate receptors, 296
  bioassay for opiate activity, 298
  putative neuromodulators, 293
  structure-activity relationship, 291
Epinephrine, 294, 368, 386
Erythrocyte, 451
Ethanol, 446
Ethylketocyclazocine, 299
Exocrine, 195
Exocytosis, 176, 215, 437

Facilitation, 185, 344
Fast green, 202
Fertilization, 15
Fertilization-defective mutants, 15
Filaments, 20
Filopodia, 114
Fixation of peripheral nervous tissue, 217
Fluphenazine, 412

Foramen of Monroe, 314
Freeze fracture, 219
Freeze substitution, 219

GABA, 176, 282, 409
Gap junctions, 315
Gastrin, 308
Glucagon, 308
β-Glucuronidase, 52
Glutamate, 247, 269
Gramicidin-D, 173
Granule cells, 30, 57
Growth cones, 68, 105

Haloperidol, 329, 450
Helisoma, 196
Heterosynaptic stimulation, 436
Hexamethonium, 88, 294
Hippocampus, 412
Histamine, 401
Histamine-sensitive adenylate cyclase, 412
Horseradish peroxidase, 176, 324
6-Hydroxydopamine, 329
Hydroxyindole-*O*-methyltransferase, 377
Hypertension, 333
Hypothalamic peptide hormones, 241, 265, 308, 341
Hypothalamus, 333

Immunofluorescent techniques, 405
Infundibular recess, 315
Insect visual systems, 92
  anatomy, 93
  axon trajectories, 98
  development of fiber pathways, 100
  differentiation of interneurons, 105
  growth cones, 109
  ommatidial development, 106
  synaptogenesis, 115
Insulin, 250, 308
Ionophore, 399
  A-23187, 189
Islet cells, 196
Isolated pedal gland cells, 212
Isoproterenol, 380

Ketocyclazocine, 294
Kinin, 243

Lanthanum, 232
Lateral geniculate nucleus, 33
Lateral olfactory tract, 33
Leptazol, 244
Leucine-enkephalin, 291
LHRH, 265
  analogues, 275
  direct action on neuronal activity, 274
  distribution in CNS, 271
  effect on sexual behavior, 274
  origin of LHRH-containing fibers, 273
  regulation by sex hormones, 272
  subcellular distribution, 273
Lineage of a cell, 108
Lioresal, 252
Lipids, 442
β-Lipotropin, 291, 369
Locus coeruleus, 409
Luteinizing hormone, 303
Luteinizing hormone-releasing hormone (see LHRH)

Magnesium, 235
Manganese, 203
MAP_1, 424
MAP_2, 424
Mechanosensory receptors, 120
Meclofenamate, 328
Median eminence, 279, 315
β-Melanocyte-stimulating hormone, 369
Melatonin, 377
Membrane
  fluidity, 236, 435
  fusion, 218
  interactions, 166
Mepyramine, 412
Merkel cells, 127
Metiamide, 412
Methionine-enkephalin, 291
5-Methoxy-N-acetyltryptamine, 377
Microculture, 87
Microspikes, 68
Microtubule-associated proteins 1 and 2 (see MAP_1, MAP_2)
Microtubules, 422
Mitochondria, 185
Mitral cells, 55
Molluscs, 196

Monoamines, 269
Morphine, 258, 294, 369
Morphogenesis, 67, 92
Morphology, 1
Mosaic patterns, 60
Muscular dystrophy chimeras, 59
Mucus, 197
  secretion, 207
Mutant genes: CNS, 47
Myocytes, 87

Nalorphine, 294
Naloxone, 257, 293, 369
Nematode, 2
  behavioral mutants, 1
Neocortex, 412
Nerve growth factor (NGF), 82
Nerve sprouting, 120
  regulation, 121
Neural crest cells, 90
Neurite, 105
Neurogenesis, 92
Neurohormonal communication, 365
Neuromuscular junctions, 140, 215, 435
Neuronal specificity, 67
Neuropil, 94
Neurosecretion, 215
Neurostenin, 169
Neurotransmitter
  biosynthesis, 424
  receptors
    models for induced changes in ion permeability, 399
  release, 357
Neurotransmitter-sensitive adenylate cyclase, 410
Norepinephrine, 83, 176, 282, 294, 377, 401, 451
Norepinephrine-sensitive adenylate cyclase, 414
Normorphine, 299
Nucleus accumbens, 411
Nucleus mesencephalicus profundus, 319

Octopamine, 401
Octopamine-sensitive adenylate cyclase, 414
Olfactory bulb, 33

Olfactory tubercle, 411
Oligomycin, 187
Ommatidium, 93
Opiate receptors, 258
  antinociceptive action, 301
  binding assays, 295
  bioassay, 298
  comparison with adrenergic system, 303
  different types, 294
  interaction with substance P, 258
Organum vasculosum, 315
Otala, 341
Oxytocin, 241, 341

P 113, 326
Pacemaker conductances, 349
Pacemaker potential, 343
Pancreatic islet cells, 196, 207
Papaverine, 328
Pedal gland, 197
Peptidergic neural elements, 265
Peptidergic neuron, 241
Peptides
  effects on behavior, 310
  functional role(s) in nervous system, 340
Phase-transition temperature, 442
Phentolamine, 405
Phosphodiesterase, 416
  activity, 390
  pineal gland, 390
Phospholipase, 169
Phospholipid bilayers, 166
Phosphoprotein phosphatase, 416
Phosphoproteins, 416
Phosphorylated proteins, 399
Photoreceptor
  cells, 55
  degeneration, 48
Physalaemin, 243, 322
Picrotoxin, 244
Pigment epithelial cells, 49
Pineal gland, 376
  action of β-adrenergic agonists on melatonin synthesis, 378
  anatomy, 377
  biosynthesis of melatonin, 377
  cyclic GMP and norepinephrine, 394

  diurnal variation in N-acetyltransferase activity, 382
  diurnal variation in adenylyl cyclase activity, 389
  diurnal variation in β-adrenergic binding sites, 387
  diurnal variation in cyclic nucleotide response to β-adrenergic stimulation, 382
  effect of denervation, 389
  influence of external light, 381
  physiological response to adrenergic stimulation, 381
  properties of adenylyl cyclase, 384
  properties of phosphodiesterase, 390
  properties of protein kinase, 391
Pituitary-endocrine axis, 265
Pituitary gland, 303
Polylysine, 70
Polymorphic cells, 28
Polyornithine, 70
Post-tetanic potentiation (see PTP)
Potassium conductance, 205, 351
Primary afferent fibers, 257
Prolactin, 265
Propranolol, 89, 380, 450
Prostaglandin E, 328
Protein
  I, 416
  II, 416
  kinase, 380, 414
    properties in pineal gland, 391
  phosphatases, 422
  phosphorylation, 415
PTP, 185, 435
  calcium accumulation hypothesis, 438
  effect of aliphatic alcohols on decay, 446
  effect of biogenic amines on decay, 449
  effect of heterosynaptic input on decay, 449
  effect of membrane fluidity on decay, 441
  effect of temperature on decay, 446
  rate constant of decay, 440
Purkinje cells, 52, 409
  degeneration, 54
Pyramidal cells, 28
Pyramidal neurons, 30

Receptors, 5, 367
Reeler mutant mouse, 27, 55
 cortical development, 38
 developmental implications, 42
 distribution of axon terminals from corpus callosum, 30
 distribution of lateral olfactory tract connections, 33
 distribution of thalamo-cortical connections, 30
 intrinsic organization within neocortex, 35
 neocortical efferent systems, 33
 organization of cell types within cortex, 28
 synaptology of lateral olfactory tract, 38
Renin, 308
Renin-angiotensin, 368
Reserpine, 83, 384
Residual calcium hypothesis, 438
Retinal degeneration, 48
Retinal dystrophy, 50
Rhabdome, 93
Rhabdomere, 93
Ruthenium red, 185

Salivary gland, 196
 cells, 196
Sarcoplasmic reticulum, 191
Scorpion venon, 175
Second messenger, 399
Secretagogues, 196
Secretory mechanisms, 195
 ionic requirements, 207
Sensory mutants, 2
Sensory neurons, 8
 cell culture, 68
Serotonin, 330, 343, 377, 401, 449
 N-acetyltransferase, 377
Serotonin-sensitive adenylate cyclase, 414
SIF cells, 404
Skin
 effect of sensory denervation, 131
 mechanosensory innervation, 124
 regeneration, 132
 touch receptors, 127
Slug, 197
Snail, 196

Sodium, 209, 334
 channels, 155, 175
 conductance, 202, 351
Sodium-calcium exchange, 178
Somatostatin, 265, 308
 direct action on neurons, 277
 distribution, 275
 effect on Ca^{2+} flux, 277
 "somatostatinergic" neural pathways, 276
 subcellular distribution, 276
Sperm, 2, 55
Sperm-defective mutants, 15
Spinal cord, 245
Spinal ganglia, 245
Squid giant synapse, 140, 195
Staggerer, 57
Stellate cells, 35
Stimulus-secretion coupling, 195
Strontium, 235, 362
Subcommissural organ, 315
Subfornical organ, 314
Subnucleus medialis, 319
Substance P, 308
 antagonism by Lioresal, 252
 direct action on neurons, 245
 discovery, 241
 distribution in nervous system, 244
 effects of analogues, 251
 evidence for transmitter function, 255
 excitatory neurotransmitter? 249
 purification and synthesis, 242
 role in nociceptive pathways, 257
 transport by axoplasmic flow, 245
Superior cervical ganglion, 82, 377, 404
Superior colliculus, 33
Suppression potential, 141
Sympathetic ganglia, 435
Sympathetic nervous system, 376
Sympathetic neurons, 82
 cell culture, 83
 dual-function single neurons, 89
 influence of myocytes, 87
 influence of non-neuronal ganglionic cells, 85
Synaptic modulation, 435
Synaptic potentials, 344
Synaptic transmission, 139, 365, 435

Synaptic vesicles, 157, 176, 191
  charge neutralization by Ca^{2+} and/or Mg^{2+}, 165
  dehydration in membrane fusion, 168
  directed movement, 163
  effects of divalent cations, 235
  endocytosis, 230
  exocytosis, 215
  influence of Ca^{2+}, 161
  membrane fluidity, 236
  model for fusion with membrane, 169
  number of exocytoses, 224
  presynaptic membrane "compression," 226
  random movement, 162
  recycling, 215
  secretion at "active zones," 224
  "specific" membrane retrieval, 232
  use of 4-aminopyridine, 221
  vesicle collapse, 226
  vesicular "particles" in presynaptic membranes, 230
Synaptogenesis, 115
Synaptosomes, 172, 426
  calcium conductance, 173
  critical evaluation, 177
  functional integrity, 172
  transmitter release, 176

Tectum, 35
Temperature transition of lipid, 446
Testosterone, 303
Tetraethylammonium, 141
Tetraethylammonium chloride (TEA), 204
Tetraparentals, 47
Tetrodotoxin (see TTX)
Thalamo-cortical connections, 30
Thalamus, 35
Theophylline, 407
Thyrotropin-releasing hormone (see TRH)
Thyrotropin-secreting hormone (see TSH)
Tolerance, 446
Transmitter release, 139, 176, 185, 438
TRH, 265
  direct action on neuronal activity, 269
  distribution in CNS, 266
  phylogenetic distribution, 268
  sites of synthesis, 266
  subcellular distribution, 268
  synthetic analogues, 269
Tryptophan, 377
  hydroxylase, 377
TSH, 265
TTX, 141, 175, 203
TTX-insensitive sodium current, 204
Tuberoinfundibular neurons
  electrophysiological studies, 278
  electrophysiology, 281
  localization, 279
  neuropharmacology, 282
  site of hypothalamic peptides, 279
Tubocurarine, 294
  D-tubocurarine, 88
Tubulin, 422
Tyrosine hydroxylase, 82, 424

Vacuoles, 232
Vas deferens, 298
Vasoactive intestinal peptide, 308
Vasopressin, 241, 320
  comparison with ACh, 343
  excitatory effects on invertebrate neurons, 341
  facilitated release of transmitter, 358
  inhibitory effects on invertebrate neurons, 361
  regulation of pacemaker conductances, 349
  voltage-clamp studies, 346
Ventricular system, 311
  anatomy, 314
Ventrobasal nucleus, 30
Veratridine, 84, 173, 426
Vision, 92
Visual cortex, 35
Voltage clamp, 143, 206, 346
Voltage-dependent conductances, 347
Voltage-independent conductances, 344